Family
NURSING

Research, Theory, & Practice

fourth edition

Family NURSING

Research, Theory, & Practice

fourth edition

Marilyn M. Friedman, RN, MS, MA, PhD
Professor and Chair, Graduate Studies Programs in Nursing
California State University, Los Angeles
Los Angeles, California

Appleton & Lange
Stamford, Connecticut

Prentice Hall International (UK) Limited, *London*
Prentice Hall of Australia Pty. Limited, *Sydney*
Prentice Hall Canada, Inc., *Toronto*
Prentice Hall Hispanoamericana, S.A., *Mexico*
Prentice Hall of India Private Limited, *New Delhi*
Prentice Hall of Japan, Inc., *Tokyo*
Simon & Schuster Asia Pte. Ltd., *Singapore*
Editora Prentice Hall do Brasil Ltda., *Rio de Janeiro*
Prentice Hall, *Upper Saddle River, New Jersey*

Friedman, Marilyn M.
      Family nursing : theory, research, and practice / Marilyn M.
   Friedman. — 4th ed.
         p.   cm.
      Includes bibliographical references and index.
      ISBN 0-8385-2525-3 (pbk. : alk. paper)
      1. Family nursing.   I. Title.
      [DNLM: 1. Nursing Process—programmed instruction.   2. Family—
   nurses' instruction.   3. Family Health—nurses' instruction.   WY
   18.2 F911f 1997]
   RT120.F34F75   1997
   610.73—dc21
   DNLM/DLC
   for Library of Congress   97-2151
                                                              CIP

Acquisitions Editor: Lauren Keller
Production Editor: Lisa M. Guidone
Designer: Libby Schmitz

ISBN 0-8385-2525-3

90000

9 780838 525258

Contents

Contributors

Cynthia D. Connelly, RN, PhD
Postdoctoral Research Fellow
Psychosocial and Community Health Nursing
School of Nursing
University of Washington
Seattle, Washington
Revisor of Chapter 6, Family Developmental Theory

Shirley May Harmon Hanson, RN, PMHNP, PhD, FAAN, CFLE, LMFT
Professor
School of Nursing
Oregon Health Sciences University
Portland, Oregon
Author of Chapter 4, Theoretical Approaches to Family Nursing

Susan A. Heady, RN, PhD, CS
Associate Professor
Department of Nursing
Webster University
St. Louis, Missouri
Revisor of Chapter 12, Family Role Structure

George K. Hong, PhD
Professor
Division of Administration and Counseling
California State University, Los Angeles
Los Angeles, California
Author of Chapter 21, The Asian-American Family

Joanna Rowe Kaakinen, RN, PhD
Associate Professor
School of Nursing
University of Portland
Portland, Oregon
Co-author of Chapter 4, Theoretical Approaches to Family Nursing

Anne Marie C. Levac, RN, MN
Director
Nursing Professional Development and Research
Children's Hospital of Eastern Ontario
Ottawa, Ontario, Canada
Revisor of Chapter 3, The Family Nursing Process

Darlene E. McCown, RN, PhD, FNPCS, PNP
Associate Professor
Department of Nursing
St. John Fisher College
Rochester, New York
Revisor of Chapter 14, The Family Affective Function

Marilyn McCubbin, RN, PhD, FAAN
Associate Professor
School of Nursing
University of Wisconsin, Madison
Madison, Wisconsin
Co-revisor of Chapter 17, Family Stress and Coping Processes: Family Adaptation

Kim Miller, RN, PhD
Professor
Department of Nursing
California State University, Los Angeles
Los Angeles, California
Co-revisor of Chapter 6, Family Developmental Theory

Irene S. Morgan, RNC, FNP, MS
Doctoral Candidate, University of Colorado
Associate Professor
Division of Nursing
California State University, Chico
Chico, California
Co-author of Chapter 16, The Family Health Care Function

Erla Kolbrun Svavarsdottir, MSC
Doctoral Candidate, School of Nursing
University of Wisconsin, Madison
Madison, Wisconsin
*Revisor of Chapter 17, Family Stress and Coping
Processes: Family Adaptation*

Rhea P. Williams, RN, PhD
Professor
Department of Nursing
California State University, Los Angeles
Los Angeles, California
Co-revisor of Chapter 6, Family Developmental Theory

Preface

This text is intended for undergraduate and graduate family nursing students and practitioners who are not practicing advanced family therapy or family systems nursing. Advanced family nursing practice requires the completion of a specialized program at the Masters level. Hence, I included family nursing interventions that are basic and straightforward; these suggested interventions, although certainly necessary within family nursing practice, are insufficient for working with the very complex family where more sophisticated, indirect interviewing and advanced counseling skills are required.

Based on the need to more adequately address the full practice of family nursing, rather than primarily its theoretical and research foundations and assessment, the text's focus in the third and fourth edition has been broadened to include family nursing diagnoses and interventions. Chapter 3, "The Family Nursing Process," and Chapter 18, "Family Nursing Interventions," have been expanded to cover the new literature appearing in the counseling, education, case management, and family nursing process areas. Since there are still few published books and articles on family nursing diagnoses and interventions, my discussion of these areas reflects the embryonic state of knowledge about family nursing interventions. Some of the interventions described in Chapter 18 are adapted from individually oriented nursing and mental health literature, due to the paucity of writing in the family nursing area.

In this edition, as in the first through third editions, the same basic comprehensive family assessment tool is presented, with some modification. The family assessment model is based primarily on three theoretical perspectives: a systems perspective, a structural–functional perspective, and a family developmental perspective. A multicultural perspective is also integrated throughout. Each chapter has been updated and contains a research, theoretical, and applied component that is related to each of the practice areas.

This textbook began and continues to represent the product of my teaching of family nursing at both the undergraduate and graduate level. I first started out with a very rudimentary family assessment tool (back in the mid-1970s). Gradually, as the result of insights gained from usage, student and faculty feedback, and knowledge acquired through the family literature, the family assessment tool grew into a series of self-learning modules which have been incorporated in much of the content within this book. The learning objectives and study questions were retained from the original modules to assist students with their own learning. The study questions (evaluation) at the end of the chapter test the reader's understanding of the chapter.

The assessment content and process presented in the following chapters has proved to be a valuable teaching–learning tool in both undergraduate and graduate courses. One obvious limitation to its usage in its pure form is that it is quite detailed and elaborate, precluding use in everyday practice. I believe, however, that a detailed approach is initially necessary to learn family nursing meaningfully. Once the content and skills are grasped, a more practical, attenuated assessment process may be initiated.

One way of using the comprehensive assessment tool with more clinical efficiency is to use the broad categories of assessment as *guides* to screen the family as to its basic strengths and problems. In comprehensively screening families, one or two presenting problem areas are usually identified. An in-depth assessment of these specific problem areas can then be accomplished, saving the practitioner considerable time and effort. Using interviewing skills to gain the family members' perceptions of experiences/events and observations of family interactions are important data collection methodologies to utilize in family nursing practice.

This book is subdivided into five broad areas. Part I includes three introductory chapters that discuss the family's importance and family definitions (Chap. 1), family nursing's evolution, focus, and goals (Chap. 2), and the family nursing process (Chap. 3). In Chapter 1, the sections outlining demographic trends impacting the family and the varied family forms have been updated and enlarged.

The chapter on family nursing (Chap. 2) covers the gamut of emerging goals and roles of the family nurse—from health promotion through rehabilitation. The rising costs of medical care, the implementation of diagnostic related groups (DRGs), managed care, the rising proportion of older, chronically ill individuals, and the recognition that many chronic illnesses can be prevented or ameliorated with lifestyle changes are prominent trends that have greatly expanded the role of the family nurse in both health promotion and acute and long-term care.

Chapter 3, "The Family Nursing Process," has been updated and revised with the assistance of Anne Marie Levac. Because of Anne Marie Levac's participation in the Family Nursing Unit at the University of Calgary with Drs. Wright, Watson, and Bell, she has an excellent understanding of their model of family nursing practice and has strengthened the nursing process components by integrating some of their key ideas and processes within this chapter.

Part II addresses the basic theoretical approaches used in family nursing practice (Chaps. 4 through 7). Chapter 4, "Theoretical Approaches to Family Nursing," is a new chapter written by Shirley Hanson, Joanna Kaakinen, and me. The chapter reviews the various theories used in family nursing practice, with much better coverage of nursing theories and family therapy theories than in the previous edition. Integrated family nursing theories are also described and advocated.

Chapter 6, "Family Developmental Theory," has been revised and updated with the assistance of Cynthia Connelly, Kim Miller, and Rhea Williams. In this chapter, family developmental theory is applied to single-parent and stepparent families, in addition to the two-parent nuclear family. Greater depth of

content is presented on the older family. Chapter 7, "Systems Theory," contains greater coverage of holism, cybernetics, and communication theory as more focused, mid-range theories subsumed under general systems theory.

Part III introduces the reader to the actual family assessment model or tool, family nursing diagnoses, and family nursing interventions. In each of these chapters, pertinent research and theory have been incorporated. The specific topical areas where theory, research, assessment, nursing diagnoses, and intervention are addressed are found in chapters focused on identifying family and sociocultural data, family structure, family functions, and family stress and coping. Family structural dimensions are crucial to family nursing practice, since they cover family dynamics as seen in family communication patterns and processes (Chap. 10), the family power structure (Chap. 11), the family role structure (Chap. 12), and family values (Chap. 13). The affective function (Chap. 14), family socialization function (Chap. 15), and the health care function (Chap. 16) are the three most relevant family functions to assess in family nursing. Family stress and coping processes and family adaptation (Chap. 17) are also essential components within family nursing assessment and intervention.

Chapter 8, "Family Identifying Data: Sociocultural Assessment and Intervention," is significantly expanded, covering the latest conceptual and research developments in this area. Social support research and theory, as well as family nursing interventions tailored to ethnic families, are elaborated on in this fourth edition.

Chapter 10, "Family Communication Patterns and Processes," contains recent research and theoretical discussions of gender differences in communication and how these impact on family communication. Family communication patterns across cultures are also described.

Chapter 12, "Family Role Structure," has been revised with the assistance of Susan Heady. Research on family role changes during illness, the family caregiver role, and the role of the father in families today significantly strengthens this chapter.

Chapter 14 was revised with the assistance of Darlene McCown and covers the process of family bereavement more thoroughly than in the previous editions. In Chapter 15, "The Family Socialization

Function," findings are incorporated from the latest socialization research. There is also broadened coverage of multicultural aspects of parenting, socialization in single-parent and stepparent families, and family nursing interventions.

Chapter 16 was again revised with the aid of Irene Morgan. The critical thrust of family health promotion is clearly evident in this chapter, with Pender's revised Health Promotion Model providing the theoretical foundation for identifying the multiple factors influencing family health promotion. Recent research findings on health care practices among families (such as lifestyle practices and patterns) has also been incorporated.

Erla Svavarsdottir, Marilyn McCubbin, and I completed a major revision of Chapter 17, now titled "Family Stress and Coping Processes: Family Adaptation." The Resiliency Model of Family Stress, Adjustment, and Adaptation is fully described, and other research and theoretical developments in the area of family stress and coping have been updated.

Part IV (Chap. 18) addresses general family nursing interventions. New intervention areas are highlighted under a discussion of nursing case management.

In Part V, cultural differences among families from the three largest minority groups in the United States, Hispanic-American, African-American, and Asian-American, are addressed in Chapters 19, 20, and 21. Current literature about each of these families, coupled with an expanded description of family nursing interventions that are culturally sensitive and appropriate, make these chapters quite useful for working with culturally diverse clients. Chapter 21, "The Asian-American Family," is a new chapter in this fourth edition, written with the assistance of George Hong, an expert counselor of Asian-American families (and professor of counseling). Because Asian-Americans are proportionally the fastest-growing minority group in the United States and their Eastern legacy is so disparate from our Western tradition, this chapter is an important addition to the fourth edition.

The Appendices contain the Friedman Family Assessment Model (long form and short form), a family case description, and a case example of the use of the family nursing process. The family nursing example is included to give students a concrete model of family nursing practice and also an oppor-

tunity to retest themselves on the use of the Friedman Family Assessment Model and application of the family nursing process. Chapters in Part III describe the knowledge base needed to complete the family assessment and to develop family nursing diagnoses and intervention guidelines.

The other contributors and I have attempted to retain the important references and writings from the earlier editions (making it somewhat "historical"), while describing and inserting the recent theory, research, and practice-oriented literature and references. We have drawn from a wide range of literature. In addition to nursing and family nursing in particular, the literature in family mental health, family social sciences, and psychology, as well as the multicultural literature has been surveyed and described.

I tell my friends who ask why I am so busy that I am working on a book I started in 1978. Who would ever imagine that one project could take so long and I could be so slow? So as to not be totally misleading, I should clarify that this was the year I authored the first manuscript of this text's first edition. At that time it was much easier to write the text—because there was so little to cull from the literature as compared to today. (Of course, I was a lot younger then too—an even more significant factor.) At that time there were only three family-centered texts published. None of these texts, however, discussed family theory, assessment, or intervention in any depth. Now in 1997, there is a proliferation of texts in family nursing that contain in-depth discussions of theories, research, and practice. The growth of publications about family nursing; the inception of the *Journal of Family Nursing* in 1995; the growing incorporation of family nursing into ANA Standards of Nursing Practice, NANDA nursing diagnoses, and the Nursing Intervention Classification (NIC); the holding of national and international family nursing conferences; the continuing activity of the family and health section of the National Council for Family Relations; and the increase in family nursing courses in both undergraduate and graduate nursing programs present strong evidence of the development of family nursing as both an integral part of generalist practice and as a specialty area in advanced practice nursing.

Moreover, there is a growing recognition that family nursing is conceptually and empirically distinct from nursing of family members (Hanson & Boyd, 1996; Whall & Fawcett, 1991a). Due to the profound influence of family therapy and the application of systems theory, family nurses are increasingly "thinking interactionally" in their writings and conversations about families and family nursing practice.

In spite of the remarkable progress and advancements made in family nursing, I continue to be awed by the contrast between what is promulgated and what is practiced. A family-centered approach remains a stated ideal rather than a prevailing practice—not only in the inpatient but also in the community and clinic setting (Bruce, 1994). Nevertheless, among nurses who incorporate family nursing interventions, positive outcomes are evident. For example, Kirschling and associates (1994), in a survey of 201 nurses who were asked to describe family nursing interventions, identified successful outcomes. These included that families were able to identify problems and effectively seek care, make positive behavioral changes, feel more satisfied with their own competency in solving problems, and have greater knowledge about and understanding of family members' beliefs and perceptions.

My ardent belief is that health professionals, regardless of the setting, must broaden their commitment so that they serve families as units, as well as family subsystems (e.g., parental subsystems) and individual family members. One of the primary obstacles to providing family health care is the gap between the substantive family nursing science knowledge and family nursing practice. Vast amounts of literature are available on the family—in the fields of sociology (family sociology), social psychology, anthropology (cross-cultural family studies), family therapy, social work, and nursing. Nurse educators are increasingly including this foundational knowledge base in the courses they teach—both in family nursing courses and integrated courses (Hanson & Boyd, 1996). In many advanced practice nursing programs, however, there continues to be an enormous concentration on the individual client or patient with minimal focus on the family system. No one would negate the importance of studying the individual client comprehensively, but individual, family, and community clients must be the enlarged focus of professional nursing.

The New Edition: A Reflection of Expanded Vistas in Family Nursing

Leaders in family nursing have recently acknowledged that systematic family assessment is emphasized in nursing curricula and publications, but that there is a lack of published writing about and emphasis on family nursing interventions (Bell, 1995; Gilliss & Davis, 1993; Robinson, 1994; Wright & Leahey, 1988). I certainly agree with them.

Family nursing continues to be a very exciting and rewarding dimension of professional nursing, as well as an emerging, vital, advanced practice nursing area. I hope this text is able to convey some of my excitement about family nursing to you. Happy reading!

Marilyn M. Friedman

Acknowledgments

I would like to thank the twelve contributors to this fourth edition. Without their significant work and great cooperation, this edition would still be "in the making." A very special thanks goes to the authors of the two new chapters, Chapter 4, "Theoretical Approaches to Family Nursing," and Chapter 21, "The Asian-American Family." Drs. Shirley Hanson, Joanna Kaakinen, and George Hong were wonderful co-authors, and I very much enjoyed and learned from our joint authoring experience. I would also like to acknowledge the assistance and support received from my editors at Appleton & Lange. Their leadership, "prodding," and continual encouragement brought the new edition to fruition. Mary Strycharske, our California State University, Los Angeles, nurse practitioner program secretary, also made this edition possible by so ably handling the many tasks at school when I was furiously working at home to meet my latest deadline. And lastly, my husband, Amnon, and my dogs, Tasha and Muffin, should be recognized. They spent countless hours tolerating the noise from the computer and a year having our bedroom filled with boxes of books and articles and a camp table set up for my writing desk. (Of course, I don't think the dogs noticed the mess.)

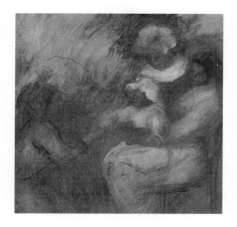

one

INTRODUCTORY CONCEPTS AND PROCESSES

Part I includes foundational knowledge for family nursing practice. Chapter 1 presents basic information about the family, its importance, and family definitions. Chapter 2 covers family nursing's evolution, prime goals, and the roles of the family nurse. In Chapter 3, the process of providing family nursing care is described. The steps within the nursing process are used as a framework for this discussion.

Introduction to the Family

Marilyn M. Friedman

▶ learning objectives

▶ learning objectives

1. Describe the basic purposes the family serves for society and the individual family members.
2. Explain why it is important for nurses to work with families.
3. Describe how family and society mutually affect each other.
4. Give examples of how the family influences the health status of its members, and of how the family is influenced by an illness of one or more of its members.
5. Define family, nuclear (conjugal) family, extended family, and family of orientation or origin.
6. Explain the difference between the meaning of health and family health.
7. Identify several demographic trends that have had major impact on the American family.
8. Discuss some of the factors associated with the growth of childless families, single-parent families, cohabiting families, and unmarried teenage mothers.
9. Define variant family forms and give examples of several diverse family forms.
10. Identify several stressors commonly found in single-parent and in stepparent families.

One of the most important aspects of nursing is the emphasis placed on the family unit. The family—along with the individual, group, and community—is nursing's client or recipient of care.

Empirically we realize that the health of family members and the quality of family life are closely related. Until the last decade, however, remarkably little attention has been paid to the family as an object of systematic study in nursing. Apart from simple evaluative labeling of families with terms such as "good," "problem," "multiproblem," or "dysfunctional," nurses in the past were generally unable to describe objectively the families they were caring for. This situation is changing. Today the study of families in both undergraduate and graduate programs has grown significantly.

This chapter will set the stage for a systematic study of family theories and research (sometimes referred to as family science and family nursing science) and for family nursing practice by describing basic purposes of the family, the rationale for nurses working with families, how the society and family mutually influence each other, and most importantly, the salient interrelationship between the health status of family and the health status of its individual members. The chapter also discusses the state of the American family and its future, basic family definitions, the family's various forms, and characteristics of healthy families.

▶ TWO BASIC PURPOSES OF THE FAMILY

Because the family forms the basic unit of our society, it is the social institution that has the most marked effect on its members. This basic unit so strongly influences the development of an individual that it may determine the success or failure of that person's life.

The family unit occupies a position between the individual and society (Bronfenbrenner, 1979). Its basic purposes are twofold: (1) to meet the needs of the society of which it is a part, and (2) to meet the needs of the individuals in it. These functions, which are fundamental to human adaptation, cannot be fulfilled separately. They must be joined in the family.

For society, the family, through its procreation and socialization of new members, functions to fill a vital need. It forms a grouping of individuals that society treats as an entity; it creates a network of kinship systems that help stabilize a society, even in its industrialized state; it generates new members in order to assure the survival of the community; and it provides new "recruits" for society, preparing children to assume productive roles in society (Williams & Leaman, 1973).

The family serves as the critical intervening variable (or as some authors term it, "buffer" or "bargaining agent") between society and the individual. In other words, a basic purpose of the family is *mediation*—taking the basic societal expectations and obligations and molding and modifying them to fit the needs and interests of its individual family members.

The family also functions to meet the *needs of its members*. For the spouse or adult members it serves to stabilize their lives—meeting their affective, socioeconomic, and sexual needs. For the children, the family provides physical and emotional care, and concomitantly directs their personality development. The family system is the main learning context for an individual's behavior, thoughts, and feelings.

Parents are the primary "teachers," because parents interpret the world and society to children. The environment—outside forces—is important, particularly as it affects parents when children are young, because parents are the ones who translate to their children the major meanings these outside forces have.*

The family has long been seen as the most vital context for healthy growth and development. It has a crucial influence on the formation of an individual's identity and feelings of self-esteem. Minuchin (1974), a noted family therapist, so beautifully summarizes the dual role that the family plays:

> The family, then, is the matrix of its members' sense of identity—of belonging and of being different. Its chief task is to foster their psychosocial growth and well-being throughout their life in common. . . . The family also forms the smallest social unit which transmits a society's demands and values, and thus, preserves them. The family must adapt to society's needs while it fosters its members' growth, all the while maintaining enough continuity to fulfill its function as the individual's reference group. (p. 3)

An individual is the repository of group (especially primary group or family) experience. His or her identity is both individual (intrapersonal experiences) and social (interpersonal experiences). A person's intrapsychic experiences are largely developed from his or her interpersonal experiences, as through the parent–child relationship (Mead, 1934). A meaningful conception of an individual's mental health status can be achieved only when we relate the functioning of the individual to the human relation patterns of that person's primary group or family.

▶ WHY WORK WITH THE FAMILY?

Why has there been a renewed interest and commitment to working with families? Tinkham and

---

* The interpretation parents give of the world and society is naturally based on their experiences and their "reality." If they have been discriminated against or lived in a crime-ridden community, they may see the world as being dangerous, hostile, a place to avoid, and thereby impart these perceptions to their children. If, on the other hand, the world has provided stability and security for them, this perspective will be transmitted to their children.

Voorhies (1984) believe that the family provides the critical resource for delivering efficacious health services to people. They refer to the family as being the community health nurse's "patient," with the major focus being family health needs and their resolution.

The following summary highlights the most cogent reasons why the family unit must be a central focus of our care.

1. The family is a critical resource for delivering health care. For instance, significant inroads can be made to curtail risks that lifestyle and environmental hazards create. A primary health promotion goal is to raise the level of wellness of the whole family, which should then significantly raise the wellness level of each of its members.

2. In a family unit, any dysfunction (illness, injury, separation) that affects one or more family members may, and frequently will, in some way affect other members as well as the unit as a whole. The family is a closely knit, interdependent network whose members mutually influence each other. The problems of one family member "seep in" and affect the other family members and the whole system (this is called the "ripple effect"). If a nurse assesses only the individual and not the family, he or she may be missing the gestalt needed to gain a holistic assessment of the situation. One of the important tenets of family therapy is that the symptoms of the identified patient (the family member with the overt behavioral problems or psychosomatic illness) are indices of the family's level of adaptation, or in this case, maladaptation.

3. There is such a strong interrelationship between family and health status of its members that the role of the family is crucial during every facet of health care of its individual family members—from preventive strategies through the rehabilitative phase. Assessing and rendering family health care is critical for assisting each family member to achieve an optimum level of wellness.

4. Case finding is another good reason for providing family health care. The presence of health problems in one member which provides an entrée into the family, may lead to discovery of disease or risk factors in other family members; this is often the case when visiting families with chronic health problems or communicable disease at home. The family-centered nurse often works through one family member to reach its other members.

5. One can achieve a clearer understanding of the individuals and their functioning when they are viewed within their family context.

6. Inasmuch as the family is a vital support system for individuals, this resource needs to be assessed and incorporated into treatment plans for individual clients.

▶ THE FAMILY–SOCIETY INTERFACE

As the basic unit in society, the family shapes and is shaped by the external forces (community and larger social systems) surrounding it. Most sociologists would agree that the influence of society on the family is greater than that of the family on society, although the family also exerts an effect on the society. The family should not, however, be considered a passive, reactionary agent in the process of social change. Throughout history the family has demonstrated tremendous resiliency and adaptiveness, just as political, educational, and other societal institutions have shown their ability to change as need dictates. Moreover, the forces operating in society and in the family are continually intervening, interacting, and changing.

Society, with its beliefs, values, and customs, pervades every facet of family life, such as the age at which children may go to work and the age at which they are legally given adult status. Society also sanctions illness definitions, sick-role behaviors, and the appropriateness of treatments. The adulation of youth by society, the participation of women in the labor force, and health care entitlement programs such as Medicare have altered the functions of the family relative to its role in assisting parents and grandparents. Liberal divorce laws and loosening of social mores have led to a growth in various family forms.

On the other hand, the family influences society, which in turn may alter social norms. For instance, the egalitarian roles that women have assumed in family life have made drastic changes in the way society now views women and their roles and capacities. The ongoing controversies over family planning services and abortion laws further exemplify the way in which the family exerts political pressure on society to change. With rising expectations for accessibility to comprehensive health services, families also continue to push for health reform legislation.

▶ INTERACTION OF HEALTH/ ILLNESS AND THE FAMILY

Family members' health/illness status and the family mutually influence each other. An illness within the family affects the whole family and its interactions, while the family in turn affects the course of an illness and members' health status. Hence, the impact of the health/illness status on the family and the family's impact on the health/illness status are reciprocal or highly interdependent (Gilliss et al., 1989; Wright & Leahey, 1994). Families tend to be both a reactor to family members' health problems and an actor in determining their health problems.

Turning to the interaction between the family and its members' health status, the family is the primary source for health and illness notions and health behavior. In one way or another, the family tends to be involved in the decision-making and therapeutic process at every stage of a family member's health and illness, from the state of being well (when promotion of health and preventive strategies are taught) to diagnosis, treatment, and recuperation (Doherty, 1992). The process of becoming a "patient" and receiving health services encompasses a series of decisions and events involving the interaction of a number of persons, including family, friends, and professional providers of care. Moreover, the role the family plays in this process varies over time depending on an individual's health, the type of health problem (e.g., whether it is acute, chronic, severe), and the degree of familial concern and involvement.

Six stages of health/illness and family interaction will be presented (Table 1–1) to further illustrate the interdependency of the family and its members' health

▶ TABLE 1–1

SIX STAGES OF HEALTH/ILLNESS AND FAMILY INTERACTIONS

Stage 1	Family Efforts at Health Promotion
Stage 2	Family Appraisal of Symptoms
Stage 3	Care-seeking
Stage 4	Referral and Obtaining Care
Stage 5	Acute Response to Illness by Client and Family
Stage 6	Adaptation to Illness and Recovery

Partially adapted from Doherty (1992), Suchman (1965).

status.* These stages also present a temporal sequencing of a family's experience with illness/disability.

Stage 1: Family Efforts at Health Promotion

The family can play a vital role in all forms of health promotion and risk reduction (Doherty, 1992). It is also true that the family may expose its members to health hazards. Many forms of health promotion, prevention, and risk reduction involve lifestyle issues such as the cessation of smoking and engaging in regular exercise. Whether a child gets a particular immunization, a father is encouraged to get more exercise and eat a more nutritious diet, or a mother receives proper prenatal care, all involve, to a great degree, family decisions and participation. Health promotion begins in the family. Wellness strategies, to be successful, usually require improvements in the lifestyle of an entire family. Moreover, within a family, members learn about their own health status and body image—such as whether they are frail and sickly or healthy and resilient.

Families unfortunately may also be the *genesis* of illness among family members. Family social disorganization often has negative health consequences for family members. A variety of specific health problems have been found more frequently in troubled or dysfunctional families, among them tuberculosis (Holmes, 1956), mental disorders (Bemak, Chung,

---

*The following six stages represent an adaptation of Suchman's (1965) five stages of illness and medical care and Doherty and Campbell's (1988) five stages of the family health and illness cycle.

& Bornemann, 1996), hypertension (Harburg et al., 1973), coronary heart disease (Syme et al., 1964), and stroke fatalities (Neser, 1975). Many studies, as illustrated in a decade literature review (Ross, Mirowsky, & Goldstein, 1990), demonstrate the pervasive influence of family on health. These reviewers found that four family factors provided explanations for a causal relationship between family and illness: marital relationship, parenthood, and the family's social support system. A couple's type of marital relationship can also affect family health status according to a well-documented study, the California Health Project (Fisher & Ransom, 1995). These researchers found that husbands and wives from "balanced" and "traditional" families reported higher health scores than marital partners from "disconnected" and "emotionally strained" families.

Stage 2: Family Appraisal of Symptoms

This stage begins when an individuals' symptoms are (1) recognized; (2) interpreted as to their seriousness, possible cause, and importance or meaning; and (3) met with varying degrees of concern by the symptomatic individual and his or her family. The stage consists of the family's beliefs about the symptoms or illness of a family member and how to deal with the illness (Doherty & Campbell, 1988).

Because the family serves as the basic point of reference for assessing health behavior and provides basic definitions of health and illness, it influences the individual's perceptions. In the American family, the mother is usually the major interpreter of the meaning of particular symptoms, the decision maker on what action should be taken, and the informal health caregiver (McGoldrick, 1989). The central family member (usually the mother) who influences health appraisal is called in some of the literature the "family health expert" (Doherty & Baird, 1987).

Families influence recognition and interpretation of symptoms of illness. Poor families are often slower to respond to initial symptoms or may not recognize symptoms as signs of disease (Koos, 1954).

Stage 3: Care-seeking

The care-seeking stage begins when the family decides that the ailing member is really sick and needs help. The ill person and family start to seek alleviation, information, advice, and professional validation from extended family, friends, neighbors, and other nonprofessionals (the lay referral structure). The decisions as to whether a member's illness should be treated at home or in a medical clinic or hospital tends to be negotiated within the family (Doherty, 1992). For example, Richardson (1970), in a study of low-income, urban households, found that about one-half of those with illnesses reported consulting another family member concerning what they should do about the situation. Knapp and associates (1966) also found that the family was the most frequently mentioned source of information concerning home remedies and self-medication.

Not only does the family provide the basic definitions of health, but family members may press a family member into this stage if they believe he or she is failing to react favorably. This process may be extremely difficult for the family, particularly when a psychiatric disorder is the major problem (Pederson, Draguns, Lonner, & Trimble, 1996). This may be because the family has to label the person as mentally ill and make the problem public and/or acknowledge their own feelings of guilt and shame. The problem is compounded when the affected person denies the disorder or blames the family (Vincent, 1970).

Stage 4: Referral and Obtaining Care

This stage commences when contact is made with a health agency or professional and/or with an indigenous or folk practitioner. Studies have clearly shown that the family is again instrumental in deciding where the treatment should be given and by whom (Pratt, 1976). The family health expert will refer a family member to whatever types of service or practitioner is deemed appropriate. The family serves as primary health referral agent (Williams & Leaman, 1973). Of course, decisions about what services to use are also determined by the availability and accessibility of health care to the family.

Most health care utilization data show that while the more affluent families use primary care physicians and medical specialists for their care, the most common resource for initial medical care for poor families is the emergency room. Among working- and middle-class families with health insurance, there has also been a growth in the use of prepaid group practice (health maintenance organization) and other managed care systems.

The type of health care sought varies tremendously. The folk or Eastern practitioner, the unorthodox "healer," the holistic health practitioner (using sometimes alternative modalities such as acupressure and acupuncture), the superspecialist (such as a neurosurgeon), the nurse practitioner, the primary care physician, and the family or individual therapist, should all be considered as possible sources of health care (thus broadening antiquated definitions of medical care providers).

How do families decide what clinic or health provider to contact? Although such variables as acceptability, appropriateness, perceived adequacy of service, and seriousness of condition are important, the accessibility and proximity to a primary care facility seems to also be a prime determinant of whom families contact (Abernathy & Schrems, 1971).

Stage 5: Acute Response to Illness by Client and Family

As the client accepts care of health practitioners, he or she surrenders certain prerogatives and decisions, and is expected to assume the patient role, characterized by a dependence on the health professional's advice, the willingness to comply with medical advice, and a striving to recover. Parsons (1951) coined this social state, "the sick role." How this role is further defined and enacted at home will be influenced by the family's sociocultural and idiosyncratic background. Some families exclude the sick member from all responsibilities and "serve and assist" to the fullest extent. Other families expect little change in the ill member's behavior, hoping that he or she can carry on as usual; this approach is seen frequently when it is the mother who is sick. Litman (1974) explains the difficulty mothers often have when sick:

> In view of both her rather pervasive and pivotal role as an agent of cure and care within the family setting, the mother may find it not only extremely difficult to fulfill her obligations to all the members of the household when one or more is ill, but she may experience considerable difficulty in maintaining her normal role and responsibility when she herself is the one who is ill. (p. 505)

Hence, mothers generally have a great deal of reluctance in accepting a patient role.

Thus the family unit plays a pivotal role in determining the sick member's patient role behaviors. The family is also instrumental in deciding where the treatment should be given—hospital, clinic, or home (Doherty, 1992). Efforts by health professionals to treat illness and promote good health may often conflict with family values and attitudinal patterns, making medical compliance problematic.

During the acute response stage, the family must make an adjustment to the family member's illness, diagnosis, and treatment. For serious or life-threatening illness, a family crisis may ensue, wherein the family undergoes a period of disorganization in response to the powerful health stressor event (Hill, 1949).

Stage 6: Adaptation to Illness and Recovery

The process of a family member's adaptation to illness as well as the family's adaptation and coping as a unit has been studied extensively by family scientists and family nurse researchers. The adaptation stage is a period when family nurses are called upon to assist families to cope with health stressors.

The presence of a serious, chronic illness in one family member usually has a profound impact on the family system, especially on its role structure and the carrying out of family functions. The disruptive effect may, in turn, negatively affect the outcome of rehabilitation efforts. Can the patient resume his or her prior (pre-illness) role responsibilities or is he or she able to establish a new, "workable" role in the family? The way in which this issue is resolved usually has to do with two factors: (1) the seriousness of the disability and (2) the "centrality" of the patient within the family unit (Sussman & Slater, 1963). When either the nature of the person's condition is serious (greatly disabling or progressively deteriorating) or the family member is a pivotal, crucial person to the family's functioning, the impact on family is much more pronounced.

Families play an important supportive role during the course of a client's convalescence or rehabilitation. In the absence of this support, the success of convalescence/rehabilitation decreases significantly.

▶ FAMILY DEFINITIONS

The family has been defined in various ways. Definitions of the family differ depending on the theoretical orientation of the "definer"—that is, by the kind of explanation the writer seeks to make concerning the family. For instance, writers who follow the interactionist theoretical orientation of the family see the family as an arena of interacting personalities, thus emphasizing the family's dynamic transactional characteristics. Writers who espouse a general systems perspective define the family as a small open social system composed of a set of highly interdependent parts and affected by both its internal structure and external environment. Therefore, there are multiple definitions, with theories shaping these definitions and our expectations of family life (Smith, 1995).

The U.S. Bureau of Census uses a traditionally oriented definition of the family which is as follows: The family is composed of persons joined together by bonds of marriage, blood, or adoption and residing in the same household. This traditional definition of the family is limiting today, both in terms of its applicability and inclusiveness. Any definition of the family must cover the wide array of family forms present today, which traditional definitions do not. Some family scholars have argued that we have defined the family according to a middle-class, white, nuclear family model and have tended to view families that do not conform to this model as "deviant" (Smith, 1995).

Whall (1986b), in her concept analysis of the family as the unit of care in nursing, defines family as "a self-identified group of two or more individuals whose association is characterized by special terms, who may or may not be related by blood lines or law, but who function in such a way that they consider themselves to be family" (p. 241). Taking into account who individuals identify as family members is a crucial component of this definition. Bozett (1987) incorporates the individual's definition by referring to family as "who the patient says it is" (p. 4). Family Service America (1984) also defines family in a comprehensive manner—as "two or more people joined together by bonds of sharing and intimacy" (p. 7).

Incorporating the central notions from the above nontraditional definitions, **family** in this text refers to *two or more persons who are joined together by bonds of sharing and emotional closeness and who identify themselves as being part of the family.* Because this definition is purposefully broad, it then encompasses the variety of relationships that are outside the legal perspective, including families not related by blood, marriage, or adoption. This includes extended family living in two or more households, cohabiting couples, childless families, gay and lesbian families, and single-parent families, as well as the two-parent nuclear family.

The following additional family definitions are presented to facilitate an understanding of family literature.

- **Nuclear (conjugal) family**—The family of marriage, parenthood, or procreation; it is composed of a husband, wife, and their immediate children—natural, adopted, or both.
- **Family of orientation (family of origin)**—The family unit into which a person is born.
- **Extended family**—The nuclear family and other related (by blood) persons, who are most commonly members of the family of orientation of one of the nuclear family mates. These are "kin" and may include grandparents, aunts, uncles, nephews, nieces, and cousins.

▶ FAMILY HEALTH

Given that family nursing is ultimately concerned with the health of the family, the concept of family health—or as Dunn (1961) calls it, family wellness—needs to be clarified. In reviewing the literature in this area, it is clear that this concept is probably even less consistently and clearly defined than the concept of health. In both cases the concepts are defined so broadly and abstractly that to fully operationalize them becomes a most difficult task.

Using systems theory as a starting point, we first need to assume that family health is more than just a sum of its parts (the health status of each of the family members). It is greater than and different from its parts. Yet, in the literature we see that the term "family health" or "familial health" is used ambiguously (Johnson, 1984), sometimes referring to the health of the individual family members and sometimes to the health of the family unit itself. Medical diseases are sometimes listed under "family health." Because only individuals can have medical diseases, it is obvious that the former usage of the term is flawed.

In family research, family health is most often conceptualized as family functioning or family adaptation (McCubbin & Patterson, 1983a), although variations within this broad definition exist. The World Health Organization (1974) proposes a similar definition to this latter definition. They state that familial health "connotes the relative functioning of the family as the primary social agent in the promotion of health and well-being" (p. 17).

The meaning of family health also differs depending on the discipline of the author or the theoretical perspective he or she adopts. For instance, in family mental health where an interactional perspective is taken, family health is referred to as the state of the family's internal processes or dynamics such as their interpersonal relationships. The focus is on relationships between the family and its subsystems, such as the parental or parent–child subsystem, or between the family and its members.

If a systems perspective is adopted, the outcome of internal interactions and exchange between the family and its environment are emphasized. One of the outcomes is a balance between growth or change and stability or equilibrium in the family (Wright & Leahey, 1994). Both tendencies are needed in the proper balance for a family to be functional or healthy.

Public health and community welfare authors use biostatistical indicators of family health. These address the relationships of family to the community and its stability as a unit. They include poverty and divorce rates among families, presence of criminal and juvenile problems, and high school dropout and unemployment rates as indicators of family health.

Family nursing authors tend to use a family mental health or systems perspective in defining family health. There is also growing interest in using nursing theories in family nursing. One example of the application of a nursing theory to working with families comes from Tadych (1985). Applying Orem's self-care theory, family health refers to the extent to which the family assists its members to meet their self-care requisites, as well as the extent to which it fulfills its family functions and accomplishes the tasks appropriate to the family's developmental level (p. 52).

▶ CHARACTERISTICS OF HEALTHY FAMILIES

The characteristics of healthy families are described in various ways by several widely cited authors. Even the terms these authors use to describe healthy families varies. For example, Pratt (1976) called healthy families "energized families." Beavers (1977) and Beavers and Hampson (1993) describe healthy families as "competent" or "optimally functioning" families, while McCubbin and McCubbin (1993) call families who are functioning well, "resilient families."

The Beavers Systems Model is perhaps best known for including an observational rating scale of families in terms of their level of competence in six areas: (1) family structure—power, parental coalition, and closeness; (2) mythology; (3) goal-directed negotiations; (4) autonomy; (5) family affect; and (6) a global appraisal of health pathology, which ranges from optimal/adaptive to severely dysfunctional. The model incorporates clinical observations of families in treatment and research settings over a 30-year period and emphasizes family competence, i.e., "how well the family performs the necessary and nurturing tasks of organizing and managing itself" (Beavers & Hampson, 1993, p. 74).

The following is a summary of Beavers's (1977) and Beavers and Hampson's (1993) description of optimally functioning families. They are characterized as:

- Consistently demonstrating high degrees of capable negotiation skills in dealing with their problems.

- Being clear, open, and spontaneous in their expression of a wide range of feelings, beliefs, and differences.

- Being respectful of members' feelings.

- Encouraging autonomy of their members.

- Expecting members to take personal responsibility for their actions.

- Demonstrating affiliative attitudes (closeness and warmth) towards each other. The parents in these families are clearly the leaders and care for each other. Family leadership is egalitarian and flows from the marital/parental dyad. The parents form a strong parental coalition and provide models of respect and affection/closeness for the children. The family is optimistic and enjoys each other (Beavers & Hampson, 1993).

Some limitations to Beavers's portrayal of optimally healthy families have been noted. The most cogent of these criticisms is that the families about which observational ratings have been made are largely white, middle-class, two-parent families (Gershwin & Nilsen, 1989). Thus, we must consider that families from diverse socioeconomic and cultural backgrounds, as well as families with differing structures, may not "fit" well into Beavers's attributes of a competent family.

Pratt (1976) and McCubbin and McCubbin (1993) stress how important the family's interaction with the community is in facilitating high-level family health. According to McCubbin and McCubbin (1993), family functioning is being redefined to include the degree to which families are able to adapt to the social context in which they live. That is, when families fit well into the community in which they live, they are generally considered to be well-functioning. Pratt (1976) concurs when she says that energized families have varied and active contacts with a wide range of other groups and organizations, so as to enhance, support, and fulfill the interests and needs of family members.

The pace of social change in recent decades has accelerated, with the family especially feeling its impact. In this process the family has demonstrated remarkable resiliency and ability to adapt to environmental flux. As the family interfaces with multiple institutions in society, it is in a perpetual state of evolution (Berardo, 1988). It mediates, translates, and incorporates social change within its structure (Goode, 1964).

With the family evidencing increasing complexities in household and family patterns, family members now have more options to pursue lifestyles that reflect their differences and preferences. Nevertheless, many family social scientists and family health professionals are concerned about the state of the American family and see many of the rapid family changes as having detrimental effects on the family (Tiesel & Olson, 1992). Their concerns often focus on the effects these various family changes have on the children.

▶ SOCIETAL CHANGES AFFECTING FAMILIES

Recent and ongoing societal changes have influenced family life. Evidence of the profound changes and enormous diversity within American families comes from demographic data primarily compiled by the U.S. Bureau of the Census. Naisbitt in *Megatrends* (1984) colorfully describes the changes in the 1980s as a "decade of unprecedented diversity"; and this trend has continued. There is no longer such a thing as the typical family.

Economic trends and changes are believed to have exerted the greatest impact on the family, but in addition to this factor, technological advances, demographic trends, sociocultural trends, and political trends are important factors that have influenced the family (Clark, 1984; Toffler, 1990).

The most obvious economic trend today is the rising costs in all areas of family life. This is particularly true in terms of the cost of health care (Nelson & Roark, 1985), particularly burdensome for poor families, older families (who are living on preinflationary dollars), and beginning families. Under the rubric of technological advances is included the knowledge explosion (Toffler, 1970); the increased ability to prolong life (Clark, 1984); environmental pollution (air, water, food, and noise); the use of nuclear energy and automation (Clark, 1984); and birth control advances. Automation has made a great difference in the home. The majority of women are now working and have had to reallocate their time; automation has allowed working wives to spend less time working in the home. Birth control advances are the last major technological advance to be mentioned here. Having better control over reproduction has literally transformed the family, in particular the life cycles of families. Women are no longer having as many children and, equally important, are having their children in a shorter period of time, making the child-rearing period of the family's life shorter. Couples now have more time alone—before the advent of children and after they have been launched (Duvall, 1977).

Demographic Trends

Major demographic and prevailing characteristics of the population influence the type of family services required and to whom these services should be targeted. The following trends are highlighted in Table 1–2.

Continuing Population Growth.

The population of the United States has steadily grown—by 56 million persons in 25 years (1965–1990). Current population rate of growth is modest, less than 1 percent per year (Rosenblatt, 1996). It is predicted that U.S. population growth will decline, but that is not expected until well into the 21st century. The size of the post-war (1945–1964) baby boomer generation and large inflows of immigrants are primary causes for the present rate of growth (Marshall, 1991).

Aging of the Population.   Probably the most important trend in demography is the increased general life expectancy and the fact that the majority of the population now survives into old age. Because of this, the United States is in the midst of a demographic revolution, the inexorable aging of our population (Fig. 1–1). The aging of America will be

> ▶ TABLE 1–2

U.S. DEMOGRAPHIC TRENDS

- ■ CONTINUING POPULATION GROWTH
  - Aging of the population
  - Changing racial and ethnic composition of the population
- ■ CHANGES IN THE FAMILY
  - Economic status changes: Growing disparity between rich and poor families
  - Decline in household size
  - Delayed marriage and high rates of marriage, divorce, and remarriage
  - Increase in first births to older mothers
  - Increase in the proportion of single parent and stepparent families
  - Changing gender norms
  - Growth in women's employment
  - Increase in family heterogeneity

particularly pronounced after 2000, when the baby boomers reach age 55 (Marshall, 1991). There is a concomitant decrease in the number of younger children in the home. Senior citizen growth is particularly rapid in the group over 75 years of age (Fig. 1–2).

The aging population will have an enormous impact on the family and on health care. For instance, because women live 7 to 8 years longer than men, on average, most older persons, especially over 75, are women who live alone and are poor. In terms of health care, with over 13 percent of the U.S. population in 1995 being over 65 years of age (and the proportion expected to rise steadily to 24 percent in 2050), the nation's health care will be critically strained. The rapid growth of the very old, who are the biggest users of health care services as well as caregiver assistance, will have a profound effect on family life (Pifer & Bronte, 1986).

Changing Racial and Ethnic Composition of the Population.   Dramatic changes are also occurring in the racial/ethnic portrait of the United States. Latinos and Asians will constitute more than half of the growth in the U.S. population for the next half century and beyond, the U.S. Bureau of the Census predicts (Rosenblatt, 1996). The population of non-Latino whites, now at 74 percent, will shrink to 53 percent by the year 2050. Latinos will increase from 10 percent to 25 percent, African-Americans from 12 to 14 percent, Asians from 3 to 8 percent, and Native Americans from 0.7 to 0.9 percent according to census projections. Latino growth is due to both immigration and higher fertility rates (two-thirds higher than non-Latino whites). A modest growth in African-Americans is due to a somewhat higher fertility rate, while the growth in Asians is due to immigration (Pew Health Professions Commission, 1991).

Changes in the Family

Economic Status Changes: Growing Disparity Between Rich and Poor Families.   At the family level, the U.S. economy is producing a greater disparity between affluent and poor families. In 1978, there were 11.7 percent of families below the federal poverty line, by 1989 the percentage had increased to 12.8 percent. During that same period, income stratification dramatically widened. The poorest 20 percent of the population became 8 per-

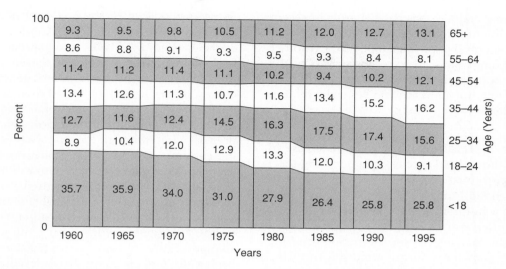

Figure 1–1. The U.S. population is getting older (age distribution of the U.S. population). *(Source: U.S. Bureau of the Census, 1982, 1992.)*

cent poorer, while the richest 20 percent became 13 percent richer (Pew Health Professions Commission, 1991). Decline in the economic resources of families in the lower levels will inevitably impact negatively on their health status.

Who are these poor families? Over 38 percent of them are in female-headed households, with 61.5 percent of poor African-Americans, 39 percent of poor whites, and 39 percent of poor Latinos living in female-headed households in 1988 (Marshall, 1991).

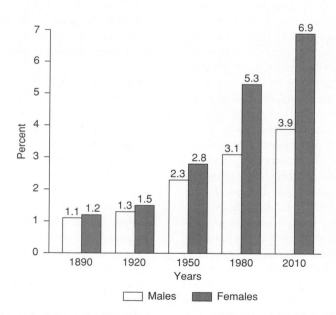

Figure 1–2. Increase in the very old population (percent of population 75 years and older, by sex). *(Source: U.S. Bureau of the Census, 1978, 1992.)*

Poverty among children has risen sharply in recent years. One-fifth of all children are poor; they constitute 40 percent of all poor (Marshall, 1991). Another alarming finding comes from recent surveys of the homeless population. The largest proportion of those becoming homeless are families with children (Schraneveldt & Young, 1992).

Decline in Household Size.   The decrease in family and household size is a major long-term demographic trend. According to the U.S. Bureau of the Census (1988), the size of the American household was at a historic low of 2.66 persons in 1987. Concomitantly, women also have experienced a shortened childbearing period, this period referring to the years they have raising children, from the youngest to the oldest child. These recent decreases in family size reflect the cumulative impact of a recent decline in fertility (down to 1.8 children per mother), and the increases in age of first marriage and rates of out-of-wedlock births (Santi, 1987).

Delayed Marriage and High Rates of Marriage, Divorce, and Remarriage.   Since the mid-1950s, marriages have been increasingly delayed (about 3 to 4 years on the average), as more young adults are attending school longer, more women are working, and more young couples are living together before marriage (Glick, 1994; Marshall, 1991). Despite these trends, the United States still has one of the highest marriage rates among developed countries. This is partly due to having one of the highest divorce and subsequent remarriage rates (Glick, 1994). The divorce rate in the United States is high but has leveled off since the mid-1980s. Weed (1990) estimates that 50 percent of recent marriages will end in divorce. Although remarriage rates are still high, reflecting an overall preference for marriage over single life, they have fallen sharply during the last 20 years (Glick, 1994). Inasmuch as men remarry more than women, many divorced women live in a state of poverty or near poverty because of their disadvantaged economic position. The prominence of no-fault divorce has enhanced the disadvantageous economic position of the divorced woman by effectively removing legal support for the husband's long-term commitment to support the mother of his children (White, 1988).

Increase in First Births to Older Mothers.   In a report from the National Center for Health Statistics (Ventura, 1989), national data from 1988 were summarized that indicated there has been a significant increase in the numbers of first births to older mothers, ages 30 to 34 and particularly ages 35 to 39 (Ventura, 1989). These women tend to be better educated and during their pregnancy to receive prenatal care. Although the typical ages of childbearing continue to be 15 to 29 years, women in their early 30s accounted for 12 percent of all first births in 1986 compared with just 3 percent in 1970.

The dramatic rise in first births among older women is the result of several other demographic trends. First, marriage has been postponed by a sizable proportion of young people; second, there has been a sharp decline and then a leveling off of first births for women in their 20s, leaving large numbers of women still childless at age 30 and older. In addition, there was a substantial growth in the number of women age 25 to 39 from 1970 to 1986. These are the children born during the baby boom years following World War II. And lastly, national surveys show that most women intend to have at least one child, with only about 10 percent of women in their early 30s expecting to remain childless (Ventura, 1989).

Increase in the Proportion of Single Parent and Stepparent Families.   Both of these family forms have significantly increased in number recently. Discussion of these trends is found in the next section.

Changing Gender Norms.   Since the 1980s, numerous studies and extensive feminist writing have addressed the issue of femininity and masculinity and their impact on family power and role relationships (Ellman & Taggart, 1993). Because of traditional notions of "women's work," women's roles, and what was considered feminine, women have had diminished power in the family. Gender relationships are based on power, and power differences still greatly favor men. As women become educated, work outside of the home, and share in the provider role, however, their power in the family increases and norms about women's and men's roles in the family change. Women are also much freer to chose their own lifestyles and the type of family they wish or need to live in.

Among middle-class and upper-middle-class educated families and immigrant families in which wives work, changing gender norms have made major differences in the family. No longer does the man automatically wear "the pants in the family." We are in an era of transition with respect to gender. Even though many women and men do not feel comfortable with the past, gender habits die hard (Ellman & Taggart, 1993). Further discussion of changing gender roles is found in Chapters 11 and 12.

Growth in Women's Employment. In the aftermath of World War II, the labor force participation of women, particularly married women, rose steadily. Women now constitute almost half of the U.S. workforce and continue to enter the labor market in increasing numbers. Women working has had mixed effects on the family (Schraneveldt & Young, 1992). On the one hand, it provides the family with a higher standard of living (many families cannot survive unless both parents work). On the other hand, there is less shared time with family members. There is a greater need for marital sharing of family responsibilities, which often happens only partially (see Chap. 12).

Increase in Family Heterogeneity. Never in recorded history has a society been composed of a greater multiplicity of attitudes, values, behaviors, and lifestyles. These social, behavioral, and cultural differences are reflected in a variety of family forms. Hence, families using health services come from all walks of life and represent all types of lifestyles. Many, if not most, of our clients are not part of the idealized traditional nuclear family. It is imperative for health care professionals to understand and appreciate the wide varieties of family forms, as well as some of the reasons for their existence.

The *postmodern family*, the term sociological literature uses to refer to today's families, reflects the "ascendence of diversity over uniformity—persons throughout their life course creating living arrangements in response to ever-shifting situations, some of their own choosing, others imposed on them" (Scanzoni & Marsiglio, 1993, p. 125). Each family form has its own particular strengths and vulnerabilities. Nonetheless, it is probably true that certain family arrangements are probably more suitable for fulfilling certain basic functions than other forms. In studies that compare different family forms with each other, it has been very difficult to sort out the effect of the family form from the many other variables that

also influence the outcomes being studied, such as socioeconomic factors, family developmental stage, and child care arrangements (Macklin, 1988).

Controversy exists between the effects on children of one family form versus another. Gottfried and Gottfried (1994) conclude from their review of numerous studies that the different family forms in themselves are not detrimental to children's development. However, Bronstein et al. (1993), Bianchi (1995), and Popenoe (1995), in summarizing numerous studies, assert that children from two-biological-parent families show better psychological, social, and educational adjustment than children from other family forms.

▶ VARIED FAMILY FORMS

In family sociology, the various family forms are classified as traditional and nontraditional, and as **variant family forms**. Variant family forms refer to those family structures that are a variation from the norm. They include those family forms that are different from the traditional nuclear family, which is characterized by households of husband, wife, and children living apart from both sets of parents. In this text, I have used the terms "variant" and "different" interchangeably in referring to family forms in an attempt to avoid negative connotations toward any existing type of family and to recognize the diversity of options available to people and families. Table 1–3 presents a series of nine questions the reader can use to evaluate his or her definitions of and beliefs about families.

As can be seen in Table 1–4, a multitude of different family forms exist. Because of their significance for family nursing, the major types of family forms will be described.

The Nuclear Family

The "vanishing" nuclear family constitutes one of the most significant demographic and social transformations in recent history. With the acceleration of the divorce rate, out-of-wedlock births, and cohabitation from 1965 to the present, family forms other than the nuclear family have rapidly proliferated. According to the 1990 U.S. Census the nuclear family, consisting of a husband provider, a wife homemaker, and children

► TABLE 1–3

WHAT ARE YOUR ATTITUDES ABOUT FAMILIES?

1. Do you consider a two parent nuclear family the *ideal and best* type of family?

☐ Yes   ☐ Usually   ☐ It depends . . .   ☐ No

2. Do you consider your own family traditional?

☐ Yes   ☐ No, because   ☐ Don't know
                   ―――――――

3. Do you believe fathers can raise children on their own?

☐ Yes   ☐ No, because ____   ☐ Usually   ☐ No
         ――――――――――――   not

4. Who determines whether a unit is a "family"?

☐ Society's   ☐ Religious   ☐ The family   ☐ Other
  legal   doctrine   itself
  definition

5. Do you think that the definition of the family is changing today?

☐ Yes   ☐ To some extent   ☐ No   ☐ Don't know

6. Could a person living alone be a familiy?

☐ Yes   ☐ Maybe   ☐ No   ☐ Don't know

7. Do you think a childless couple is a family?

☐ Yes   ☐ No   ☐ Don't know

8. Should gay and lesbian couples be allowed to marry?

☐ Yes   ☐ No   ☐ Perhaps   ☐ Don't know

9. Do you believe that the American family is in serious trouble today?

☐ Yes   ☐ Probably   ☐ No   ☐ Difficult to say

---

that was once the norm, accounts for 26 percent of all households (U.S. Bureau of the Census, 1991a). Only 50.8 percent of American children live in a traditional nuclear family today. The percentage of children living in nuclear families varies significantly by race and ethnicity. Fifty-six percent of white children lived in "traditional nuclear families," while 26 percent of African-American and 38 percent of Latino children did in 1990 (U.S. Bureau of the Census, 1991a).

Although it is recognized that the traditional nuclear family is no longer modal, family scientists have asked "to what extent is the traditional family the norm?" This type of family still appears to be the "ideal" norm, but not the "real" norm. Surveys suggest the majority of Americans still wish for traditional family life but have a greater tolerance for nontraditional living arrangements than in the past. Although at any one point in time the majority of adults are not living in traditional nuclear households, over the course of their lives, most will do so.

Yet increasing numbers, as previously described, are living in nontraditional family forms.

Two growing variations within nuclear families are the dual-earner/dual-career and the childless family. Adoptive families are another type of nuclear family noted in the literature as having special circumstances and needs.

The Dual-earner Family.

With the striking increase in employment among married women, almost two-thirds of two-parent families are now dual-earners (Piotrkowski & Hughes, 1993). From 1974 to 1994, there was a 46 percent increase in dual-earner households, and in 1995, a national survey conducted by Louis Harris showed that 55 percent of working women contribute half or more of their family income (Walters, 1995). In most dual-earner families, where both spouses are employed either part- or full-time, the majority of women have jobs that are undertaken because of economic necessity. Yet, despite wives' need to work, Harris's survey found

▶ TABLE 1–4

DIFFERENT FAMILY FORMS IN THE UNITED STATES

Traditional Variant Family Forms	Nontraditional Variant Family Forms

The most common traditional variant family forms now existing are:
1. Nuclear family—one parent working, living in same household
  a. First marriage families
  b. Stepparent families
2. Nuclear family—dual-earner/dual-career, husband, wife, and children living in same household.
  a. First marriage families
  b. Blended or stepparent families
3. Nuclear dyad—husband and wife alone; childless, or no children living at home.
  a. Single career
  b. Dual career
4. Single-parent family—one head (female- or male-headed) as a consequence of divorce, abandonment, or separation.
  a. Working/career
  b. Unemployed
5. Single adult living alone.
6. Three-generation extended family—may characterize any of above family forms (1 to 4 above) living in a common household.
7. Middle-aged or elderly couple—husband as provider, wife at home (children have been launched into college, career, and/or marriage).
8. Extended kin network. Two or more nuclear households of primary kin or unmarried members living in close geographical proximity and operating within a reciprocal system of exchange of goods and services.
	The most common nontraditional variant family forms are:
	1. Unmarried parent and child family—usually mother and child.
	2. Unmarried couple and child family—usually a common law–type of marriage.
	3. Cohabiting couple—unmarried couple living together.
	4. Gay/lesbian family—persons of the same sex living together as "marital partners."
	5. Augmented family—household composed of nuclear or single-parent family with one or more unrelated persons.
	6. Commune family—household of more than one monogamous couple with children, sharing common facilities, resources, and experiences; socialization of the child is a group activity.

Adapted partially from Sussman (1974), Macklin (1988).

that many women (48 percent) want to work part- or full-time regardless of whether they need to or not (Walters, 1995).

In dual-earner families, the major challenges focus on: (1) managing housework and child care; (2) having two paid jobs; and (3) family relationships (Piotrkowski & Hughes, 1993). "Family work" represents the household chores and child care tasks, the first-noted challenge above. Despite women's changing roles outside the family, within the family traditional sex-role attitudes often shape family life. Women, according to numerous studies, still do the "lion's share" of family work. In turn, this workload imbalance frequently leads to role overload and sometimes marital conflict (Piotrkowski & Hughes, 1993). When children are young, the greatest challenge to dual-earner families is in arranging and coordinating the care of children while parents are at work. Child care arrangements are difficult to find and are often transient.

The challenge of managing two jobs is influenced by the types of jobs the couple have and the stress these jobs produce. Excessive job demands coupled with a lack of control over job demands generally produces high stress levels. Occupational stress is not just a personal problem but also a family problem.

For example, job stress may have an adverse effect on parent–child relationships.

The third challenge, managing family relationships, is influenced by the previous two challenges. If "family work" and/or managing two jobs is stressful, then family relationships are negatively impacted.

A crucial concern in the dual-earner family literature revolves around possible effects on the couple's children of having two parents who work. There is no evidence to date, however, to suggest that the dual-earner lifestyle, in and of itself, is stressful for children.

In a growing minority of dual-earner families, both husband and wife pursue careers while maintaining a family. Career-oriented people tend to view their positions as a primary source of personal satisfaction and identity. Both Skinner (1984) Goldenberg and Goldenberg (1990) note that a significant feature of the dual-career lifestyle is that it is associated with considerable stress and strain, with more stress and strain reported by the wife than her husband. The basis of this stress is primarily the competing demands of the occupational structure and those associated with the family—child care, homemaking, and marital responsibilities. Two-career couples tend to do more sharing of traditionally female tasks than do one-career or dual-worker families, particularly in the area of child care (Barnett & Baruch, 1987; Macklin, 1988). But it appears that in many families, the wife still assumes the major responsibility for domestic tasks (Piotrkowski & Hughes, 1993).

There is also growing research interest in family dynamics about the dual-career families—particularly commuter families, in which spouses voluntarily live in separate residences for at least a majority of each week because of geographically separated jobs. Although usually a temporary pattern, research findings point to the difficulties that this lifestyle impose (Macklin, 1988).

The Childless Family. One type of traditional variant nuclear family is the family without children. About 5 percent or more of all ever-married women in the United States are voluntarily childless. The rate is expected to go up to 10 percent in the near future not only because of delayed marriage and childbearing patterns but because of the many career and educational options now available to women (Houseknecht, 1987; Macklin, 1988).

The Extended Family

The traditional extended family is one in which the couple shares household arrangements and expenses with parents, siblings, or other close relatives. The children are then reared by several generations and have a choice of models after which to pattern their behavior. This type of family is more frequent in working-class and recent immigrant families. As people live longer, and divorces, teenage pregnancies, and out-of-wedlock births increase, houses also have become home to several generations, usually on a temporary basis. Demographers also have found that because of increased longevity, four- and five-generation families are becoming commonplace among poor and working-class families (Otten, 1989).

There is also another form of extended family—the extended kin network family. Here two or more nuclear households of primary kin or unmarried kin live in close proximity and operate within a reciprocal system of social support, including the exchange of goods and services. This type of family form is modal in the Latino community (see Chap. 19 for greater detail).

Although the great majority of Americans do not live in the two types of extended families mentioned, greater extended family ties are possible and widespread today due to advances in transportation and communication. The nuclear American family is not as isolated as it superficially appears. The many ways in which families rely on one another create an extended family context that has been verified in several important studies.

The frequently repeated myth that the nuclear family is isolated from family supports is not borne out by this research, the evidence showing that a modified extended family usually exists within a rich network of generational interaction (Hill, 1970; Kingson et al., 1986). Primary kin—parents and siblings of spouses—form the most important network of extended kinship relations. The common modified extended family of today differs from the isolated nuclear family in that it provides significant support and continuing assistance to other nuclear families within the extended-family network (Shanas et al., 1968). This type of extended family is typically set up on an egalitarian basis and is composed of a series of nuclear families that equally value these extended-family bonds (Litwak, 1972).

The Single-parent Family

The single-parent family is one in which there is one head of household, mother (80 percent of families) or father (20 percent of families) (Bianchi, 1995). The traditional variant single-parent family is one in which the head is widowed, divorced, abandoned, or separated. The nontraditional variant single-parent family is one in which the head—practically always the mother—has never been married (see Table 1–4).

Demographic Trends.

One of the most dramatic demographic changes taking place in the United States is the radical shift in the modal household from one headed by a marital pair rearing their dependent-age children to a household headed by a single adult (Bianchi, 1995; Rossi, 1986). Since 1940, the number of single-parent families has increased in the United States, from 8 percent in 1950 to 29 percent in 1990 (Fig. 1–3). Breaking these statistics down by race and ethnicity, significant differences are apparent (Fig. 1–4). According to U.S. census data (U.S. Bureau of the Census, 1993b) in 1990, about 50 percent of all African-American families were single-parent families, while 15 percent of all white non-Latino families were single-parent families. The

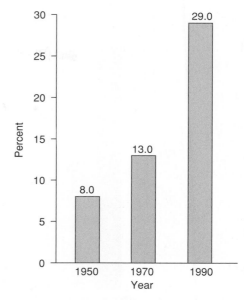

Figure 1–3. Percentage of American families consisting of single-parent households with children under age 18. *(Source: U.S. Bureau of the Census, 1992.)*

growth of mother-child families, however, slowed during the 1980s, while growth of father-child families increased, accounting for more than one-third of the overall growth in the number of one-parent fami-

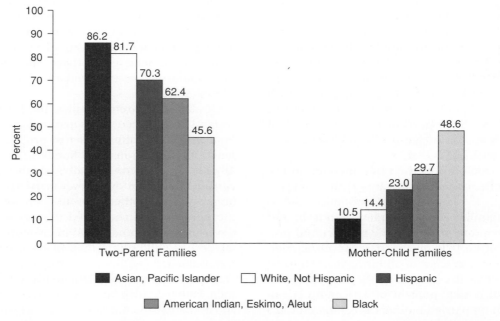

Figure 1–4. Percentage of two-parent or mother-child families with children under age 18, broken down by race/ethnicity. Note: Persons of Hispanic ethnicity may be of any race. *(Source: U.S. Bureau of the Census, 1993b.)*

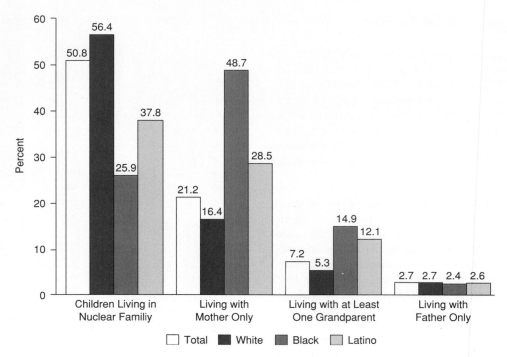

Figure 1–5. Percentage of children in various household structures broken down by race/ethnicity. One out of two children live in a nuclear family, which is defined as composed solely of both biological parents and full brothers and sisters. *(Source: Census Bureau's Survey of Income and Program Participation, based on national-level estimates of children under age 18, for the period June through September, 1991b.)*

lies (Bianchi, 1995). Eighty percent of this growth is among white father-child families.

The proportion of children nationally who are under the age of 18 and are cared for by a single parent, however, has skyrocketed, from 9 percent of all children in 1960 to 24 percent of all children in 1991. Among black children the proportion is much greater, from 22 percent in 1960 to 51 percent in 1991 (Fig. 1–5). Sixty percent of all children will spend about a year or longer in a single-parent home before they reach the age of 18.

Factors associated with the rapid increase in the numbers of one-parent families are (1) the high rate of divorce, (2) the large amount of financial aid to one-parent families with dependent children, and (3) the tremendous growth in the number and proportion of births that occurred to never-married mothers—from 5 percent of all births in 1960 to 34 percent of all births in 1992 (U.S. Bureau of the Census, 1993b). Sixty percent of African-American births were to unmarried mothers as compared to 20 percent of white births.

Among never-married mothers, the significant increase is within the teenage mother group. From 1970 to 1987 there was a 22 percent increase in births among unmarried women ages 15 to 17. Ninety percent of these teenage mothers had not completed high school and were on welfare (U.S. Bureau of the Census, 1985).

Of all single-parent families, the largest group is headed by divorced and separated mothers. These families have a different set of problems and challenges than never-married families. They are generally better off economically, which gives them a considerable edge over never-married families with largely young mothers. Seventy percent of divorced mothers work as compared to only 38 percent of never-married mothers, and many more proportionally receive child support payments in comparison to never-married families (Bianchi, 1995).

About 20 percent of all single parents in 1992 were men. Father-headed families have more than doubled since 1970 (U.S. Bureau of the Census, 1992). Although courts still favor mothers as custodial parents, men are making more vigorous claims to custody rights. Single fathers experience the same role change and role overload problems as single mothers. They are on average, however, much better off financially.

Goldenberg and Goldenberg (1990) and Mendes (1988), in reviewing the research on single-parent families, emphasize the fact that single-parent families are not homogeneous. They are, in fact, very diverse in terms of their resources, opportunities, and limitations. Mendes (1988) identifies five common lifestyles of the single parent:

1. Sole executive lifestyle. Here the single parent is the only parent actually involved in the lives and care of the children. In some cases, he or she attempts to fulfill both father and mother roles and is very much prone to stress, fatigue, and role overload. In other families, the sole executive handles what he or she can do without undue stress, and then coordinates the allocation of some of the other functions by assigning them to competent persons within or outside the family.

2. Auxiliary parent. In this lifestyle the custodial parent shares one or more of the parental responsibilities with an auxiliary parent, usually the father of one or more of the children.

3. Unrelated substitute. In this lifestyle the custodial parent shares one or more parental functions with a person who is not related to the family, such as a live-in housekeeper who is "like a mother" to the children.

4. Related substitute. Here the related substitute is a blood or legal relative who assumes a parental role. These persons are often grandmothers, but could also be aunts, uncles, cousins, or siblings of the children. There has been a large increase in the number of grandmothers, particularly in African-American families, who care for their teenage children's children.

5. Titular parent. The titular parent lives with the children, but has, for all intents and purposes, abdicated the parental role. Teenage mothers or mothers who are alcoholics, drug addicts, or mentally disturbed are sometimes parents in name only. In these cases there may be a parental child acting as parent, or a parent of the titular parent who assumes the child care and domestic responsibilities.

Each of these types of single-parent families has its own set of problems and strengths. Crucial to the successful functioning of any of these types of families, however, is the family's integration into a viable psychosocial support system.

Generic Features of Single-parent Families.   As a group, single-parent families are disadvantaged when compared to other forms of families. They are characterized as having a high rate of poverty, are disproportionately from disadvantaged minority backgrounds, are more mobile, and the single parents are relatively undereducated. This is more often the case in female-headed than in male-headed families.

Of the generic features of single-parent families, poverty is the most serious. Furthermore, the gap between single-parent and two-parent families is increasing (Hogan, 1990). Families headed by women (over 10 million in 1985) had a poverty rate of 34.5 percent and accounted for nearly half of all poor families (Bowen, Desimone, & McKay, 1995). *Newsweek* (Gelman et al., 1985) calls these women a "new class of poor." Single parenthood appears to be a major factor in "the feminization of poverty." Several variables are cited as causative factors: the minimal to nonexistent child support from fathers; the inequities of the workplace for women; cutbacks in social welfare programs since 1980; and the lack of education and work skills of young, never-married mothers.

Role changes, role overload, and role conflicts are other generic features of single parents. Role problems revolve around playing both mother and father roles; and the role overload of working, raising a family, domestic responsibilities, and of attempting to have a personal life. And lastly, since most single divorced parents will remarry, there is the necessity of making another major role change—relinquishing the other parent role and forming new marital and parental roles on remarriage (Goldenberg & Goldenberg, 1990; Hogan et al., 1984; LeMasters, 1974; Macklin, 1988).

Accumulated evidence from studies of single-parent families consistently demonstrates that children in single-parent families are worse off than children in two-parent families. Children in single-parent families are two to three times more likely to have emotional and behavioral problems than children in two-parent families, when family income is equal. They are twice as likely to drop out of high school and 2.5 times as likely to become teenage mothers (Popenoe, 1995).

The Unmarried Teenage Mother.

As mentioned earlier, a very large increase of pregnancies is occurring within the unmarried teenage group, particularly among adolescent African-American girls. Births to unmarried teenagers are also high, and would be even higher if not for abortion. It is estimated that about half of teenage pregnancies are resolved by abortions (Chilman, 1988). The causes for the increase in unmarried teenage families are multiple. The major factors cited in the literature are early sexual activity, no use or ineffective use of contraceptives, poverty, failing to marry before the child's birth, and relatively greater acceptance of unwed adolescent motherhood among lower-class African-Americans (Chilman, 1988; Prater, 1995). The fact that over 50 percent of urban male African-American youths are unemployed is one reason for the low marriage rate in the African-American teenage group. The shortage of young African-American men as compared to young women also explains why so many young African-American teenage mothers do not marry.

Services to adolescent single parents to date are sorely inadequate. A continuum of services is needed. They range from primary preventive services in sex education and birth control to outreach programs, support networks, counseling, and school-based clinics and parenting classes, as well as services to the extended families of unmarried teenage mothers.

Single parents as a whole also have special needs. In addition to providing parenting classes and peer support networks, social policy changes are required so that adequate child care facilities and institutional supports such as flexible working hours can be established.

The Single Adult Living Alone

The number of people living alone has also grown. In 1986, 24 percent of all households were made up of people living alone. A preponderance of elderly women live alone, but the large increase in lone living is among those adults in their 20s and 30s (Glick, 1988a).

Many home health clients, especially older chronically ill or disabled individuals, are single people living alone. Although these solitary people do not appear to fit into the text's definition of family, they probably have extended family members, siblings or children being the most common, whom they identify as their family. Most solitary people are part of some loosely formed family network. If this network is not made up of relatives, then it may be composed of friends such as those residing in the same retirement home, nursing home, or neighborhood. Pets can also be important family members.

Then there are those individuals who are truly "loners." They have a greater need for health and psychosocial services, because they have no support system and sometimes are not interested in developing one. Long-term and home care nurses can help these types of clients by developing a supportive relationship with them, thereby reducing the client's social isolation.

The Stepparent Family

Although divorce has been increasingly common, this trend has been accompanied by high rates of remarriage. Seventy-two percent of recently divorced women eventually remarry (Glick, 1994). Hence, this situation has produced a dramatic growth in stepparent or blended families. These families are also known as "remarried families," in which there may or may not be children, and "reconstituted families." It was estimated that in 1990 in two-parent families about one child in seven was living with a stepparent (Glick, 1994). Usually these types of families are composed of a mother, her biological children, and a stepfather.

This family form typically is one that initially is a complex and stressful merger. Many adjustments need to be made, and different individuals and subgroups of the newly created family often move toward adaptation at different rates (Visher & Visher, 1993). Although all family members must adjust to the new family situation, children often have greater problems coping because of their age and concomitant developmental tasks, as well as their "dual citizenship" (membership in two households and cultures) (Visher & Visher, 1993).

Coleman, Ganong, and Goodwin (1994) reviewed 26 marriage and family textbooks and summarized both the strengths and stressors identified in stepparent families within these texts. They first mention that stressors and a deficit-comparison model are prevalently used in texts when discussing stepparent families—evidence perhaps of society's negative stereotyping. Three strengths are identified, as follows:

1. Remarriage is another opportunity for marital success, as the remarried adults may be wiser and more mature "the second time around."

2. For stepchildren, stepparents can serve as additional positive role models, providing them with care, knowledge, and interests that the biological parent may not have been able to supply.

3. Improved finances may also be a significant benefit of forming a stepparent family, particularly for divorced women and their children.

Several sources of stress are mentioned by Coleman and associates (1994) and Visher and Visher (1993):

1. The relationship between stepparents and stepchildren is a primary source of many family difficulties. Discipline problems and the stepchildren's difficulty in accepting a stepparent as parent because of "divided loyalties" typically strain relationships in remarried families. Marital power issues may also be evident. Divorced women who during their divorced period become the primary decision-maker and authority figure often have no interest in having anything but an egalitarian relationship with their new spouse. The new spouse may, however, have different expectations. In stepfamilies, children may also vie for power with the "conquer and divide" strategy—pitting their two biological parents against each other.

2. The increased complexity of stepparent families is a significant feature that impedes adjustment. Complex and multiple roles and relationships can be a major source of difficulties for both parents and children, as they attempt to maintain previous and existing kin relationships and to cope with new kin relationships. Children, especially, feel divided loyalties as mentioned previously.

3. Role ambiguity is often a major stepparent family stressor (Visher & Visher, 1993). Stepparents often have little idea how to act as a stepparent; their marital partners may have high, unrealistic expectations for them in this role, and the stepchildren may not accept the new member in the stepparent role. Additionally, there are few societal guidelines to help stepparents learn their new roles.

4. Financial pressures may be present. Stepparents may have to provide financial support to two sets of children, placing a financial strain on both families.

5. Former spouse relationships may be strained and a source of tension and conflict, particularly when tied to child support, visitation issues, and how children should be raised.

6. Negative stereotyping of stepfamilies in society may cause stepfamily members to hide their status from outsiders to avoid shame. Communities are often unsupportive of this family form. For instance, there is no legal status between stepparent and stepchild.

7. Unrealistic expectations about what family life should be like create another primary source of dissatisfaction and disagreements in stepparent families, especially in the early months of the new family.

Stepparent development as a family system differs from the traditional two-parent nuclear family development. In Chapter 6, Carter and McGoldrick's (1989) Model of Stepparent Development is outlined as consisting of three phases or steps along with concomitant developmental issues to be addressed.

Only a few authors have discussed factors that help stepparent families adjust positively. The most helpful discussion of characteristics of successful stepparent families comes from Visher and Visher (1993). They list five characteristics found in large part in healthy stepparent families, as follows:

1. Expectations for the stepparent family are realistic. The adults realize that initially things will

be rocky, that it takes time to adapt, and that adaptation cannot be forced. Losses have to be mourned. Stepfamilies are "born of loss" (p. 246), being formed following either divorce or death. Adults support and assist their children in coping with the losses accompanying the creation of a new family.

2. Satisfactory step-relationships have been formed. This not only includes the marital relationship, but the relationship between marital partners.

3. A strong, unified couple relationship exists.

4. The separate households have learned to cooperate—to make satisfactory arrangements involving the children.

5. Satisfying rituals are established. The stepfamily members are able to decide what rituals and ways of doing things they would like to adopt.

The Binuclear Family

The binuclear family refers to the postdivorced family in which the child is a member of a family system composed of two nuclear households, maternal and paternal, with varying degrees of cooperation between and time spent in each household (Ahrons & Perlmutter, 1982). With the movement toward sex-role equity, increased participation by some fathers in parenting, and the growing awareness of the loss of being a noncustodial parent and the negative consequences to children when there is no father contact, various ways of active coparenting have emerged. The most widely discussed form of active coparenting is joint custody, where both parents have equal legal rights and responsibilities to the minor child irrespective of residential arrangements.

There has been increased attention given to coparenting and joint custody. Nevertheless, these family arrangements are only seen among a small fraction of divorced families. A case in point: in a nationally representative sample of children in single-parent and stepparent families, almost half of the children had not seen their nonresidential parent in the past year. The residential parent assumed a disproportionately large amount of the child care (Furstenberg & Nord, 1985).

The Nonmarital Heterosexual Cohabiting Family

There is a substantial growth in the number of U.S. couples living together unmarried (U.S. Bureau of the Census, 1985; Koeninn, 1997). This wave of cohabitation appeared in the 1960s and has continued, with over a 100 percent increase nationally in the number of cohabiting household units from 1970 to 1995 (from nearly 523,000 to 3.7 million households). This trend has continued. In an earlier era, cohabitation was limited to the very rich, those in the theater, and the very poor. But today, cohabitation has become a much more acceptable nontraditional family form for young adults before and in between marriages (Koeninn, 1997; Weiss, 1988).

It is estimated that perhaps as many as half of all couples live together before marriage. In fact, increasingly cohabitation has come to be looked upon as a normative process leading to marriage. It is not only young people who are living together without being married; older persons and widowed or divorced persons also have begun to live together, often for companionship and to share limited financial resources (Goldenberg & Goldenberg, 1990).

Gay and Lesbian Families

There is no consensus as to what constitutes a gay and lesbian family. Allen and Demo's (1995) definition is presented here as it is broad and inclusionary of the rich diversity of gay and lesbian families. They suggest that gay and lesbian families refer to "the presence of two or more people who share a same-sex orientation (e.g., a couple), or by the presence of at least one lesbian or gay adult rearing a child" (p. 13). Although there are no official estimates of the number of gay and lesbian families, this family form represents a significant minority of U.S. households (Allen & Demo, 1995; Eliason, 1996). Very little research has been presented or published about gay and lesbian families according to Allen and Demo (1995), who conducted an extensive literature review in this area. Allen and Demo (1995) and Laird (1993) concluded that very little is known of family relationships and what is presented or published is based on small samples of predominantly white, urban, middle-class, highly educated respondents.

Gay and lesbian families are richly diverse in their form and composition. First of all, they are families formed from lovers, friends, biological and adopted children, blood relatives, stepchildren, and even ex-lovers. In addition, families do not necessarily reside in the same household (Laird, 1993). Therefore, there is no normative or uniform family form among gay and lesbian families. Usually gay and lesbian families are same-sex couples, but they could also be headed by singly gay or lesbian parents or multiple parenting figures.

According to Goldbenberg and Goldenberg (1990), who counsel gay and lesbian families, cohabiting homosexual couples have much in common with heterosexual cohabiting couples. There are, however, notable differences. One strikingly apparent difference is the greater stigmatization that gay and lesbian families face or potentially face if they disclose their homosexuality and nontraditional living arrangements (Laird, 1993). Efforts at concealment, self-condemnation because of their gayness, the negative self-labeling that occurs as a result of society's negative labeling, and for gay men, fear of disenfranchisement as a result of the AIDS crisis are also stresses particular to gay and lesbian families (Goldenberg & Goldenberg, 1990).

In marked contrast to heterosexual marriages, there is no legal sanction for homosexual marriages. Homosexual unions are not "institutionalized," meaning that rules, standards, practices, and social sanctions for continuance are not present. Thus, lack of legal basis is a problem today in terms of inheritance and parental rights. For instance, the "lesbian baby boom" has brought to light some perplexing problems for lesbian couples who separate. In these cases, the lesbian partner who is not the biological parent, has no legal relationship with her child. In other cases, children have been legally removed from a lesbian family home because the lesbian parent has been deemed an "unfit mother" due to her sexual orientation alone (Eliason, 1996). Although the vast majority of studies have found no differences in childrearing and child's adjustment by lesbian/gay parents versus heterosexual parents, legal barriers still exist in adoption and child custody matters.

▶ LOOKING AT THE FUTURE OF THE AMERICAN FAMILY

In reviewing the many articles and chapters that discuss the state of families and their future, I agree with Hunter (1994), who comments that the family appears as the most conspicuous field of conflict in society—or as an institution under siege. A case in point was the heated political debate over "family values" in 1992. Hunter (1994) and Rodman and Sidden (1992) identify the following battleground family issues that so prominently fill our newspapers today: the concerns over "latchkey" child; the status and role of women, particularly those who have children (i.e., the debate about whether mothers who work "hurt" their children); the moral legitimacy of abortion; the appropriate pace of children's development; the legal and social status of homosexuals; the increase in family violence; the rise of illegitimacy, especially among African-American teenagers and young adults; and the growing demand for adequate day care.

The controversy over these family issues and the future of the family as an institution has been interpreted by some as one between optimists and pessimists. Although both sides acknowledge that the family is undergoing profound changes, they disagree sharply over the extent, meaning, and consequences of those changes (Hunter, 1994). The pessimists have deep-seated anxiety over the decline of the American family. They see the previously mentioned issues (and more) as cause for their gloomy outlook (Rodman & Sidden, 1992). The optimists, on the other hand, view change as positive and mention such changes as rising egalitarianism and shared gender roles, the ability for women to work and have a family; and the technological advances that give the family more leisure time together. They point to the age-old adage that the family, being resilient and adaptive to new social conditions, is "here to stay" (Hunter, 1994).

A major problem with most pessimists is that they have a rather narrow time frame within which they analyze the family. History teaches us a lesson here. Attacks on the family and its status and future are *not* new. Coontz (1996), a family historian, impressively argues that "American families have been under siege more often than not during the past 300 years" (p. 38) and somehow have been able to adapt to social and economic changes. Coontz (1996) also remarks that "we can take comfort from the fact that American families have always been in flux and that a wide variety of family forms and values have worked well for different groups at different times. Our challenge is to grapple with sweeping transformations we are currently undergoing" (p. 43).

▶ FAMILY NURSING IMPLICATIONS

The preceding description of family forms illustrates the broad array of structures prevalent in families today. There is no "right," "wrong," "proper," or "improper" form of family. Families must be understood within their own context. Labels and types serve only as a reference to the family's living arrangements and primary group network. Every effort must be made to understand the uniqueness of each particular family. Society places complex and often conflicting demands on people; hence, the need for a range of family forms to coexist. Health professionals serving families must be tolerant and sensitive to the diversity of family lifestyles and should abandon the traditional model of the "ideal family."

We need, as a society and through our public policy and health care programs, to promote and strengthen the family and seek ways to make communities more supportive (especially in the area of child care) to children and parents who live in diverse family forms. In short, in our roles as family nurse and informed citizen, we need to make our programs and community "family friendly."

We also must recognize that many families are in trouble. It is only by recognizing the stressed state of these families that social action, broadened family-focused health services, and urgently needed domestic policy changes will occur.

▶ study questions

Choose all correct answers to the following questions.

1. Which of these characteristics belong in a broadened, inclusionary definition of "family"?
    a. Composed of one or more persons.
    b. Geographic dispersion.
    c. Emotional involvement and commitment.
    d. Sense of identity as a family.

2. Which is correct?
    a. The family of parenthood/procreation is the family into which you were born.
    b. The family of orientation/origin is the family of marriage.
    c. The extended family includes the family's close family and friends.
    d. None of the above.

3. The family functions to meet the *needs of society* by (select best answer):
    a. Mediating between society's expectations and the needs of the individual.
    b. Providing recruits for society's job market.
    c. Rearing of children.

4. The family functions to meet the *needs of its members* by (select best answer):
   a. Providing recruits for society.
   b. Serving as a "buffer" between society and the individual.
   c. Facilitating the personality development of the individual.

5. Which of these is (are) the main reason(s) for nurses to work with the family?
   a. The entire family is affected by the health problem of a family member.
   b. Promotion of healthy functioning of the whole family will positively affect each family member and his or her health status.
   c. By working with the whole family, the nurse may be able to discover health problems that other family members are having.

6. Which of these is (are) example(s) of how the ill family member can adversely affect the family?
   a. Birth of handicapped child disrupts the marital relationship.
   b. Emotional disturbance of the husband disrupts the economic and emotional stability of the family.
   c. Family is brought together in a common effort to help the ill member get well.

How does the family affect the health of its family members in each of the following six stages of health/illness?

7. Stage 1: Family efforts at health promotion.

8. Stage 2: Family appraisal of symptoms.

9. Stage 3: Care-seeking.

10. Stage 4: Referral and obtaining care.

11. Stage 5: Acute response by client and family to illness.

12. Stage 6: Adaptation to illness and recovery.

13. Some ways in which society has been able to influence/change family values, attitudes, or sanctions are:
    a. Judicial rulings on constitutional rights of people.
    b. Postponement of marriage and childbearing.
    c. Health legislation.
    d. Advances in technology.

14. How does the meaning of family health differ from the meaning of health?

Fill in the correct answers to the following questions.

15. What does the phrase "variant family forms" refer to?

16. Give three examples of traditional variant family forms.

17. Give three examples of nontraditional variant family forms.

18. Name three stressors that commonly affect single-parent families.

19. List two major recent general demographic trends and two family demographic trends in the United States today.

Choose the correct answer(s) to the following questions.

20. What are the usual ties between nuclear and extended family? (circle all accurate descriptions)
    a. A modified extended family exists within a network of generational interaction.
    b. Parents and siblings of spouses form the most important network of extended kinship relations.
    c. The extended family network provides significant support and continuing assistance to nuclear families.

21. Relative to the nuclear childless family, the cohabiting family, and the family with an unmarried teenage mother, which factor is associated with *all three of these family forms?*
    a. Need for birth control information
    b. Poverty
    c. High divorce rates
    d. Unavailability of males
    e. Postponement of marriage
    f. Early premarital coitus

22. Gay and lesbian families have much in common with cohabiting heterosexual couples, but also have major differences. These differences are:
    a. Among gay and lesbian families there is no uniform or normative family structure.
    b. Greater stigmatization of family among gay and lesbian families.
    c. The family developmental stages differ considerably between these two types of families.

23. The Beavers Systems Model identifies indicators of family competence including:
    a. An emphasis on traditional roles and decision making.
    b. Family members are optimistic and enjoy being with each other.
    c. Autonomy of family members is encouraged.
    d. Family members display capable negotiation skills in dealing with their problems.

▶ chapter 1 study answers

1. c, d.

2. d.

3. a.

4. c.

5. a, b, and c.

6. a and b.

7. *Stage 1: Family efforts at health promotion.* Family reinforces health promotion and preventive measures, or may expose family members to health hazards.

8. *Stage 2: Family appraisal of symptoms.* Family recognizes and defines meaning of symptoms/illness.

9. *Stage 3: Care-seeking.* Family persuades individual to seek care.

10. *Stage 4: Referral and obtaining care.* Family is the primary health referral agent (to whom, and when). Contact is made with health practitioner.

11. *Stage 5: Acute response by client and family to illness.* Family defines appropriate roles for client during this stage; the illness also impacts on family and in serious, life-threatening situations can produce crisis.

12. *Stage 6: Adaptation to illness and recovery.* Family either supports or hinders client's recovery pattern. Nature of health problem also affects the family's adaptation.

13. a, c, and d.

14. Whereas health refers to the individual's state of functioning (i.e., the extent to which an individual functions as an integrated whole person, maximizing his or her potential within his or her environment), family health refers to the adequacy of functioning of the family as a unit or system. Beyond this difference, many finer distinctions exist, such as the use of different indicators to measure family health and health.

15. Variant family forms refer to all family arrangements that are different from the traditional nuclear family of husband/father, the wife/mother, and children residing together.

16. Examples of traditional variant family forms are nuclear dyads (childless couples), single-parent (divorced) families, single adults living alone, and extended three-generation families.

17. Examples of nontraditional variant family forms are commune families, never-married parent and child families, unmarried couple and child families, cohabiting heterosexual couples, and gay/lesbian families.

18. Role conflicts/role overload, role changes, and poverty.

19. General demographic trends: continual growth; increasing racial and ethnic diversity; aging population. Family demographic trends: more working women/mothers; high marriage, divorce, and remarriage rates; decrease in household/family size (fertility control, postponement of marriage, and childbearing are factors creating the decreased size of household/family); increase in births to older mothers; growth in variant family forms; growing disparity between rich and poor families.

20. a, b, and c.

21. a.

22. a, b, and c.

23. b, c, and d.

2

Family Nursing: Focus, Evolution, and Goals

Marilyn M. Friedman

► learning objectives

1. Explain the differences in how the family is conceptualized in the four levels of family nursing practice.
2. Compare how the family is incorporated into the American Nurses Association's standards of practice in community health nursing and maternal–child nursing versus psychiatric–mental health nursing.
3. Differentiate between how goals and priorities are set by the family nurse versus how goals are set and prioritized by the family-centered community health nurse.
4. Identify the four specialty areas in nursing that historically have been most ardently involved in family health care.
5. Briefly describe the three levels of prevention.

6. Explain why health promotion is a primary thrust within family nursing.
7. Discuss the primary factors leading to increased interest in health promotion and health maintenance today.
8. Identify factors that have impeded the growth of health promotion, self-care, and family nursing.
9. Identify the five key dimensions of wellness, as described by Ardell.
10. Explain the purpose of risk appraisal as a tool in disease prevention.
11. Describe the family nurse's role in primary, secondary, and tertiary prevention.

This text is about family nursing and the basic knowledge base—consisting of theory, factual information, research, and clinical implications—needed to practice basic family nursing. The chapter begins the discussion of family nursing by addressing what family nursing encompasses, its evolution, and the incorporation of family into professional standards of care. Finally, the primary goal of family nursing, promotion and maintenance of family health, is analyzed by using Leavell and associates' (1965) levels-of-prevention framework as a vehicle for discussing the family nurse's role within the three levels of prevention. Particular emphasis is given to primary prevention, especially health promotion, because this focus is seen as the main thrust of family nursing. Discussions of family health, the wellness lifestyle, and risk appraisal and reduction are also elaborated upon as part of primary prevention. The family nurse's role in secondary and tertiary prevention completes the discussion of the family nurse's role in health and illness.

▶ FAMILY NURSING: DEFINING THE SPECIALTY

Family nursing is a specialty area that cuts across the various other specialty areas of nursing. Although as a distinct specialty it is still relatively young, there is strong evidence that family nursing is a growing, dynamic specialty area of focus in practice, education, and research. Significant progress is being made in broadening nursing's practice paradigm to include the family as client. Yet, a gap between conceptualization and practice still exists (Friedemann, 1989). Interestingly enough, there are several names of this specialty: family health care nursing (Bomar, 1996; Hanson & Boyd, 1996); nursing of families or family systems nursing, depending on focus and the level of practice (Wright & Leahey, 1994); and system-focused or systemic family nursing (Friedemann, 1995).

When the first edition of this text was written in 1979 to 1980, there were no definitions of family nursing. Several texts discussed family nursing (Ford, 1979; Sobol & Robischon, 1975); family-centered community nursing (Reinhardt & Quinn, 1973); family-focused nursing (Janosik & Miller, 1980); and family health care (Hymovich & Barnard, 1979); but notions about a specialty called family nursing were absent. Today, texts, articles, and professional presentations in the area of family nursing are extensive. The specialty even has its own journal, *The Journal of Family Nursing*, begun in 1995.

There is, however, disagreement over what family nursing actually encompasses (Hanson & Boyd, 1996; Wright & Leahey, 1994), and how it differs from community health nursing (Friedman, 1986) and family therapy (Gillis et al., 1989; Wright & Leahey, 1994). A review of the family nursing literature reveals that within the definition of family nursing four levels of family nursing practice or foci are evident. The level of family nursing that is practiced depends on how the family nurse conceptualizes the family and works with it. The degree of family-centeredness also is dependent on the phi-

losophy of the system within which the nurse works. The work environment (what leadership rewards and negatively reinforces) is also a major determinant of behavior. Each of these four levels or foci of family nursing are components of family nursing.

Level I: Family As Context

In level I, family nursing is conceptualized as a field where the family is viewed as context to the client or family member (Bozett, 1987; Robinson, 1995) (Fig. 2–1). Nursing care is individually focused. The family, as typically the client's most important primary group, is visualized as a stressor of or resource to the client. The family is the background or secondary focus and the individual, the foreground or primary focus relative to assessment and intervention.

The nurse may involve the family to varying degrees. In some cases the nurse may assess the family as part of the client's social support system, but with little incorporation of the family into the client's plan of care. In other cases, the nurse may show extensive involvement of the family in the client's care. The family's potential or actual as well as tangible and socioemotional impact on the client, is assessed and integrated into the treatment plan.

Most nursing theories conceptualize the family's role in this light. Most specialty areas also view the family as a crucial social environment of the client and hence a primary social support resource. A case in point is the definition of family-centered care promulgated by the interdisciplinary Association for the Care of Children's Health (1989). They state that family-centered care is a philosophy of pediatric health care that considers and treats the child in the context of the family and recognizes the family as the primary and continuing provider of care for the child. Where the family is incorporated into the assessment and plan of care of the patient, some authors call this family-centered or family-focused care (Bozett, 1987).

Level II: Family As Sum of Its Members

In the second type of family nursing practice, the family is seen as an accumulation or sum of the indi-

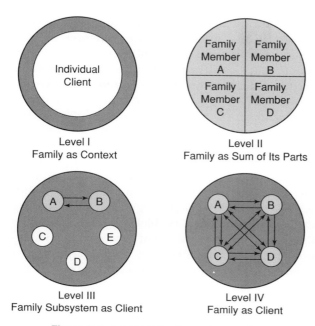

Figure 2–1. Levels of family nursing practice.

tions, caregiving issues, and bonding-attachment concerns are examples of the nursing foci here.

Level IV: Family As Client

In the fourth type of family nursing practice conceptualization, the entire family is viewed as client or as the primary focus of assessment and care. The family is now in the foreground, with the individual family members in the background or context. The family is viewed as an interactional system. The focus is on internal family dynamics and relationships, the family's structure and functions, as well as the relationships of family subsystems with the whole and of the family with its outer environment. It is in this latter type of conceptualization and care that the unique contributions of family nursing are evident.

When systems theory and cybernetics, especially the notions of interaction, circularity, and reciprocity, become the prevailing way the family is viewed and analyzed, Wright and Leahey (1990) call this family systems nursing. Here the connections between illness, family members, and the family are assessed within this interactional perspective and incorporated into the treatment plan. This type of practice involves using a different paradigm or epistemological framework for assessment and care, one characterized by holism and circular causation. Family systems nursing utilizes advanced clinical assessment and intervention skills based on an integration of nursing, family therapy, and systems theory (Wright & Leahey, 1988). It represents advanced nursing practice, as its concentration is simultaneously on not only the whole family as the unit of care, but on multiple systems, such as the individual, the family, and larger systems (Bell, 1996).

Family nursing is seen in this text as consisting of the third level of conceptualization or practice. This is not to say that visualizing and working with the family as context is not important; in fact, working with families in this way is critical to providing comprehensive nursing care to individual clients. Focusing on family nursing as the third level of practice also does not preclude nurses from practicing at two or three levels simultaneously or over time. In order to define the knowledge base needed and the nursing processes involved, however, clarity as to the level of care is imperative. Therefore, the focus of

vidual family members. When care is made available to or provided for all the family members, family health care is seen as being provided. This is a model that is implicit to much of practice within family primary care and community health nursing. No explicit model of this conceptualization of family nursing practice exists.

Fortunately, there is a growing effort in family primary care to see the family as a whole as the focus of care (Doherty & Campbell, 1988) rather than as a sum of its parts, but with cost-containment efforts and lack of reimbursement for family care, these efforts are not widespread. In this level, the foreground is each of the clients, seen as separate rather than interacting units.

Level III: Family Subsystem As Client

In the third type of family nursing practice, family subsystems are the focus and recipient of assessment and intervention. Friedemann (1993b) and Robinson (1995) refer to this model as being the basis for interpersonal family nursing. Family dyads, triads, and other family subsystems are the unit of analysis and care. Parent–child relationships, marital interac-

family nursing in this text refers to nursing practice where the family is seen and treated as the client or recipient of care.

There is a fifth conceptualization of family and family nursing described by Hanson and Boyd (1996b). That is, the *family as a component of society.* Here, the family is visualized as one subsystem within a larger system—the community, society. This view of the family will be discussed in Chapter 5. Because this model is not, however, a primary model through which care is delivered to families, it is only cursorily mentioned here.

Defining Family Nursing

Family nursing encompasses all the five models described above, even though the fourth model is uniquely family nursing. Family nursing practice is defined in this text as the provision of care involving the nursing process, to families and family members in health and illness situations. Hence, families and family members may be healthy and/or may be experiencing health problems. Family nursing may be rendered in any health setting and many other settings where families are being served, e.g., educational and multipurpose service centers, and to all forms of families.

It is practice that is informed by nursing, family, social science, and family therapy theories. (Refer to Chapter 4 for more in-depth discussion of theoretical foundations.) The emphasis of family nursing practice should be health-oriented, incorporating holistic, systemic, and interactional perspectives and drawing on and forth family strengths (Bell, 1996; Friedemann, 1995; Wright & Leahey, 1994).

Distinguishing Family Nursing from Other Practice Areas

Because family nursing historically has been aligned primarily with community health nursing (Whall, 1986a), some confusion exists between what is community health or public health nursing and family nursing. Whereas family nursing focuses on the family as its target or recipient of care, community health nursing's target of service is the community (Williams, 1996). The health of the community rather than the health of the family is the ultimate goal of commu-

nity health nursing. It is through families that community health nurses improve and preserve the health of communities. The difference here is a matter of ultimate goals and priorities. The implications of this difference are that in rendering personal health services to a family—for example, a single-parent family of mother and young children—the "noncommunity-oriented" family nurse would be concerned with the family's unique problems first, and second with the community health problems common to young families (the first commitment being a client and family). In a community health setting, the nurse would be cognizant of the pressing maternal–child health problems in the community that were relevant to the client family, such as immunizations and family planning, and prioritize these needs along with the unique health needs of the family.

Another point of confusion is the difference between family nursing and family therapy (Gilliss et al., 1989). In Wright and Leahey's text, *Nurses and Families* (1994), they distinguish nursing of families from family therapy and family systems nursing. Wright and Leahey (1994) believe that advanced preparation is needed to practice as a family systems nurse clinician. However, nursing of families, consisting of basic family nursing assessment and intervention, should be part of baccalaureate nursing education. The nurse here is able to complete family assessments of healthy/functional and dysfunctional families. The family nurse or interviewer intervenes using educative–supportive strategies that are direct and straightforward. In family systems nursing or family therapy, the nursing interventions include more complex and indirect psychosocial interventions (Wright & Leahey, 1988, 1994) and the clinician works with multiple systems simultaneously (Bell, 1996).

Family nurse researchers working as a special interest group under the auspices of the Family Nursing Continuing Education Project, Oregon Health Sciences University (Kirschling et al., 1989), were also interested in clarifying what family nurses actually do. To address this question they conducted a national survey of 263 nurses who identified themselves as being family nurses, asking them about their practice and interaction with their clients. From this data, the researchers identified unique characteristics of family nursing practice. The following four major themes emerged when participants were queried as to what they did differently when they cared for families rather than individuals:

- Recognition and integration of family concepts.
- Application of a broader perspective as identified in the nurses' approach to nursing care, primarily by assessing the family.
- A focus on family interaction and family dynamics.
- Involvement of family members in care, particularly in areas of decision making and caregiving.

▶ THE INCORPORATION OF FAMILY INTO ANA'S STANDARDS OF CARE

Ideally, in all clinical areas of nursing practice, family nursing should be a reality. In some settings and specialty areas, however, incorporating the family as client is more difficult to achieve than in others. For instance, in episodic settings—especially in intensive care units and emergency departments, where immediate lifesaving measures are needed—a predominant patient focus is understandable.

Evidence of what specialty areas believe to be the appropriate standards and scope of their practice are found in publications from the American Nurses Association (ANA), which is responsible for defining and establishing the scope of nursing practice and standards in both the general field and in areas of specialization.

We reviewed the ANA's *Social Policy Statements* (1980; 1995a) and *Standards of Clinical Nursing Practice* (general standards) (ANA, 1991), and standards/scope of practice statements in seven specialty areas to see the extent to which the family was incorporated into standards of care documents. Standards from psychiatric–mental health nursing (ANA, 1994), gerontological nursing (ANA, 1995), community health nursing (ANA, Council of Community Health Nurses, 1986), home health care nursing (ANA, 1986); maternal and child health nursing (1983); rehabilitation nursing (1988); and primary health care nursing practitioner (1987) were reviewed. This survey revealed that there was a recognition of the family as context, i.e., as an important

resource to the individual client in all standards documents. All the standards—except rehabilitation nursing and primary care—also stated that the client may be an individual, family, group, or community. However, when specific descriptions of standards and scope of practice were delineated, the family was clearly not considered as client in some of the specialties. The standards documents, again with the exception of rehabilitation nursing, following the general *Standards of Clinical Nursing Practice* lead, used the nursing process framework to describe their standards of practice. Hence, the same basic framework, the nursing process, was used in all standards of care, but the description of practice varied widely with respect to family inclusion.

In the ANA's important social policy statements of 1980 and 1995, the association describes the family, along with the individual client and community, as nursing's recipient of care. The family is also identified as a necessary unit of nursing services. The generic standards of clinical practice also state that the family is a client along with individuals, groups, and communities.

In the psychiatric–mental health nursing standards (ANA, 1994), family psychotherapy is discussed as an intervention appropriate for a psychiatric–mental health nurse functioning at an advanced practice level (Masters prepared advanced practice nurse).

In the *Standards of Community Health Nursing Practice* (ANA, 1986) and *Standards of Home Health Nursing Practice* (ANA, 1986), the nursing process is utilized to assess, plan, diagnose, intervene, and evaluate *families*. Collaboration with families is stressed. Family nursing care is promulgated as a vital component of practice.

In the *Standards of Maternal and Child Health Nursing Practice* (ANA, 1983), family is heavily identified and integrated throughout the standards. For instance, the standards state that nurses assist families to achieve health promotion and to cope with health problems and role transitions.

In the gerontology nursing practice standards (ANA, 1995) and rehabilitation nursing standards (ANA, 1988), the family in the specific standards is clearly seen as a resource to the individual client. And lastly, in the standards of practice for primary care nurse practitioners (ANA, 1987), there is no mention of family. The ANA 1985 scope of practice document did mention family in the introductory section, stating primary care's orientation "to the family and/or broader systems of which the individual is a part" (p. 3), but nowhere else in the document is the family identified. Perhaps because the primary care statements are older, they do not represent standards of clinical practice today.

▶ FAMILY NURSING'S HISTORICAL LEGACY

"The concept of family nursing has always been with us in nursing" (Ford, 1979, p. 4). It has, however, seen decline and regrowth.

In the preindustrialized, colonial era, when family members worked at home in cottage industries or farming, family care predominated. Then came industrialization, with family members moving into factories to work. Health care gradually moved from the home to the hospital.

In England, Florence Nightingale was aware of the importance of the family and home environment in the care of the sick. She mentions the needs of family members in military camps and the need "to keep whole families out of pauperism by nursing the breadwinner back to health" (Beard, 1915, as cited in Whall, 1986a, pp. 242–243).

During the 1800s and early 1900s in the United States, public health nurses and their equivalents in England served families in the home (initially the poor, but later also those with communicable diseases). With bureaucratization in society, specialization in medicine grew (obstetrics, pediatrics, surgery, and so forth). Nursing also became specialized, and family medicine and nursing practice fell into disuse. Insurance coverage limitations, private and public reimbursement policies and referrals, and lack of preventive funding also were policies that later mitigated against family-focused care (Ford, 1979).

Public health nursing, maternal–child health, and midwifery managed to bridge the gap in some instances and stand as examples of both family-centered and fractionalized care. For instance, obstetrics often ignores the baby and family, and communicable disease public health nursing services typically only include the family with regard to case finding. An example of where family nursing contin-

ued was in the Frontier Nursing Service. Here, the Frontier Nursing Service provided both midwifery and public health nursing services to families.

The four specialty groups in nursing that have been the most ardent in focusing on the family have been community health nursing, which sees the family as client; parent–child nursing, which sees the family as context and client; psychiatric–mental health nursing, which sees extensive family involvement within the family therapy specialization; and the family primary care or nurse practitioner specialty, which sometimes sees the family as a sum of its members and as context. Each of these specialty groups has been informed by both specific developments in its own area of specialization and by more general developments within nursing, social science, and society. For instance, in community health nursing, the legacy was to consider the family as a focus of service. But not until the 1970s was there much substantive content within nursing programs that addressed family theory, assessment, and intervention. In the 1970s we saw texts focusing on family theory and its application to family-centered community health nursing. In community health nursing, sociological and cultural theories of family behavior (such as family socialization, poverty, roles, values, dynamics, and cultural diversity) were important in influencing the field.

Psychiatric–mental health nursing, in contrast, was more heavily influenced by the theories and clinical writings within the family therapy movement. Since these nurses work with troubled families, this knowledge base was more important to assist them in assessing and intervening with dysfunctional families. Family therapy theories and practice models, however, are only one psychotherapeutic modality in mental health. Hence, family nursing assessment and intervention are not widespread throughout the whole specialty area.

Maternal or parent–child nursing has a long history of family involvement—beginning with the early days of midwifery and visiting of mothers and children in the home. It has long been recognized that when caring for mothers and children, the family is crucial. Family-centered texts in pediatrics and maternity are the norm. Most texts primarily see the family as context. Parent–child family-focused nursing has been particularly influenced by growth and development, mother–child bonding, role, and socialization theories.

Family and pediatric nurse practitioners are the fourth specialty area identified as being family focused. In the 1960s it was recognized among health care planners and legislators that specialization in medicine was not meeting the primary health care needs of the whole population in the United States. Federal monies were granted to medical schools to open up family practice programs. The nurse-practitioner movement grew on the coattails of this larger movement concerned with cost-effective, accessible care to all sectors of society. Nurse-practitioner programs have also been heavily federally funded. Family nurse practitioners care for the whole family, but their predominant focus is to see the family as a sum of its members. Both pediatric and family nurse practitioners view the family as context to the individual client. This is changing, however, as some nurse-practitioner programs are incorporating advanced family nursing content into their curricula to attempt to broaden services and to help students "think family" (Wright & Leahey, 1984) or to "think interactionally" (Wright & Leahey, 1994).

In addition to the more specific influences each of these specialty areas experienced, certain more general factors enhanced the growth of family nursing. These include:

1. The increased recognition in nursing and society of the need for health promotion and a health focus, rather than the practically exclusive disease orientation.
2. Our aging population and the growth of chronic illness, which have brought self-care and the needs of family caregivers into prominence.
3. The widespread awareness concerning the pervasiveness of troubled families in our communities.
4. The promulgation and general acceptance of certain interpersonal and family-based theories, such as attachment and bonding theory, general systems theory, and family stress and coping theories.
5. The marriage and family therapy movements and the growth in child guidance, marriage, and family clinics and services.
6. The growth of family research and the significance of its findings. Two cases in point are:

(a) the extensive and influential family communication research in the 1950s and 1960s which showed that troubled parents, particularly mothers and their communication patterns, were associated with troubled children; and
(b) the growing number of family nursing research studies that demonstrate the impact of health stressors and coping on family health outcomes.

▶ LEVELS OF PREVENTION

Leavell and associates (1965) developed a framework, referred to as levels of prevention, which is used here to explain the goals of family nursing. The levels of prevention cover the entire spectrum of health and illness, as well as the goals appropriate for each of the levels. The three levels are:

1. Primary prevention, which involves health promotion and specific preventive or health protective measures designed to keep people free of disease and injury. Specific preventive measures or health protective behaviors are also called health maintenance.
2. Secondary prevention, consisting of early detection, diagnosis, and treatment.
3. Tertiary prevention, which covers the stage of recovery and rehabilitation, is designed to minimize the client's disability and maximize his or her level of functioning (Fig. 2–2).

The three levels of prevention constitute the major goals of family nursing. They consist of the health promotion and maintenance (primary prevention), detection and treatment, and restoration of health. Health promotion is a major thrust of family nursing. Certainly, however, early detection, diagnosis, and treatment are also important goals. In addition, tertiary prevention or rehabilitation and restoration of health are especially important goals in family nursing today, given the growth in home health care and the prevalence of chronic disease and disability among our rapidly increasing older population.

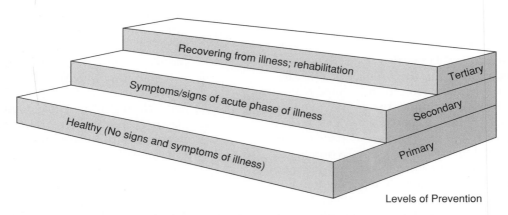

Figure 2–2. Relationship of levels of prevention to health–illness stages.

▶ PRIMARY PREVENTION: FAMILY HEALTH PROMOTION AND MAINTENANCE

Factors Leading to Renewed Interest in Primary Prevention

Six important factors that have led to the renewed interest in primary prevention are briefly discussed below (Table 2–1).

Need for a Change in Focus. In today's health care system, most health resources go toward curative, acute care. Our present health care system spends most of its resources on crisis-oriented and high-tech curative health care, with the treatment given in many cases being too little, too late. In the case of chronic illness—our prevailing cause of morbidity and mortality—we are not treating and eradicating disease, but only minimizing its impact, repairing the damage as much as possible, and treating its complications. We are spending most of our money treating the end result of self-destructive lifestyles rather than focusing on the causative factors of ill health, such as lifestyle and environmental hazards (Ardell & Newman, 1977; Pender, 1987). Only 3 percent of all health care expenditures are for preventive services (Smith & Wesley, 1993).

There is widespread concern among lay persons, legislators, and health care professionals that the present system of health care is both costly and relatively

---

▶ TABLE 2–1

FACTORS LEADING TO RENEWED INTEREST IN PRIMARY PREVENTION

1. Need for a change in focus
   - Most health resources are spent on acute care
   - Rising costs have produced minimal evidence of improvement
   - National efforts to encourage health promotion and disease prevention are on the rise
   - There is greater recognition of the inseparability of mind and body and role of stress in illness and recovery
2. Consumerism and popular demand for increased self-control
3. The wellness movement
4. Growing acceptability of alternative health modalities by health professionals and the public
5. Lack of access to health services
6. Growing emphasis on health in advanced nursing practice

ineffective. Only minimal cost containment or conservation of health resources is in sight. Managed care is the most significant way in which costs are being contained. Yet, in spite of managed care and integrated health systems, enormous amounts of money are being spent for hospital and medical care with little improvement to show for it. Longevity, a major measure of our health system effectiveness, has not significantly improved in recent years. Compliance studies show that there is a widespread lack of medical compliance by patients, which naturally raises costs even more. Ardell (1977) reminds us that Americans spend vast amounts of money on the treatment of diseases and last-minute miracles; however, many of these problems could have been prevented for free (Castro, 1991).

In spite of the major emphasis and allocation of resources to acute care, a national shift towards health promotion and health protection is evident in the United States and Canada throughout the last decade (Loveland-Cherry, 1996). The Surgeon General's landmark report, *Healthy People* (U.S. Public Health Service, 1979) and its companion report, *Promoting Health/Preventing Disease: Objectives for the Nation* (U.S. Public Health Service, 1980) emphasized the fact that lifestyle modifications were the most significant changes needed to achieve health gains in our nation. Six lifestyle changes were identified: cessation of smoking; reduction of alcohol misuse; dietary changes to reduce excess calories, fat, salt, and sugar; exercise; periodic screening procedures for major disorders such as high blood pressure and diabetes; and use of seatbelts and following speed limits on highways. More recent publications such as *Healthy People 2000* (U.S. Public Health Service, 1991) continue to influence health care in the direction of providing more and better health promotion and maintenance activities.

There is a growing realization that mind and body are inseparable—each mutually influencing the other—and that an integration of body and mind are needed for recovery and wellness to occur. This recognition has resulted in the incorporation of a holistic approach in both nursing and the mental health professions whereby the whole person is considered in assessment and care (ANA, 1995a).

Along with the awareness of mind–body interaction, the role that stress plays in illness is increasingly acknowledged. It is estimated that 80 percent of all illnesses are stress induced, with stress being responsible for aggravating all illnesses and illnesses aggravating existing stress. Multiple studies have shown the negative role stress plays on an individual's or family's health status (Pelletier, 1979). Because of this, treatment of the medical problem alone is not adequate.

Consumerism and Popular Demand for Increased Self-Control.

Consumers today are more assertive than in the past (Bomar & McNeely, 1996) and expect to be informed about their medical services and to be given more self-control over their lives. This usually translates into being given sufficient information to be reasonably informed about available options so that they can make their own choices and evaluate services. The need for greater self-control is related to present societal values, anti-authority sentiments, and the growing professional value being given to client empowerment, i.e., the shifting of decision-making power from the health provider to the client (Labonte, 1989).

Individuals and families should have control over their own actions. The responsibility for one's health lies not with the health care professional, but with the individual and/or his or her family (Leonard, 1976). Wellness training, holistic health care, and self-care, all part of health promotion, share in the fundamental belief that taking responsibility for and being in control of one's own health are necessities.

There have been unprecedented public disclosures of the inadequacies and inequities of the health care system, which have only intensified consumer demand to be in control over one's own health care. The women's movement is an example of successful pressures being applied for self-control. The women's movement has focused national attention on the inferior or inappropriate health care received by women in a male-dominated system and has encouraged women to retain control over their health. With the trend toward more primary health care being provided by nurse practitioners, who emphasize teaching and supportive counseling, primary care has been demystified and more control has been transferred from providers to individual and family clients.

The Wellness Movement.

Since the mid 1970s, there has been increasing interest in and incorporation of healthy lifestyles into the lives of many middle-class and affluent Americans. The wellness movement of the 1970s evolved outside the traditional health system. It was a lay-initiated movement (Armentrout, 1993). Today, a greater value is being placed on health, personal fulfillment, and quality of life (Harris & Gurin, 1985). Although the general level of health knowledge in our society is still relatively low, more educated persons, through reading of health-oriented articles and books and exposure to mass media, have become well informed about general health promotional strategies and environmental hazards and risks.

A wellness lifestyle, according to Ardell (1977), consists of five dimensions: self-responsibility, self-care, nutritional awareness, stress management, exercise and physical fitness, and environmental awareness (see Chap. 16 for greater detail on a health promotion wellness lifestyle).

Growing Acceptability of Alternative Health Modalities by Health Professionals and the Public.

Various alternative health promotion modalities have become respectable in most health care professional circles; even the most esoteric modalities for stress reduction and pain control are being looked on as helpful by many health care practitioners. There is much more openness and acceptance of alternative modalities, including yoga, meditation, herbal medicine, massage, relaxation techniques, acupressure, acupuncture, guided imagery, visualization, and body therapies. Many of these approaches to health emphasize health promotion, holism, and client empowerment (Rodwell, 1996).

Many consumers—who are increasingly from cultures where alternative medicine is the convention—are turning to herbal medicine, Eastern medical modalities, and other holistic health approaches which promote and restore health (Picker, 1996). The *New England Journal of Medicine*, for example, reported that one third of Americans visited at least one alternative practitioner in 1990 (McCall, 1996).

Lack of Access to Health Services.

There is some evidence that as health services have become more inaccessible because of lack of insurance and high cost, consumers are turning more to health promotion and disease prevention self-care strategies. Thus an impetus to self-care may arise from situations where professional health services are not readily available or accessible (Levin et al., 1976). In 1987, a shocking 37 million Americans had no health insurance and 19 million were underinsured (Smith & Wesley, 1993; U.S. Department of Health and Human Services, 1989b), and estimates are even higher today. It is unclear, however, how many of these uninsured individuals use self-care for health promotion and maintenance in addition to using self-care to treat common primary health care problems.

Growing Emphasis on Health in Advanced Nursing Practice.

Health professionals, particularly advanced practice nurses, are being socialized to incorporate health promotion and disease prevention as integral and necessary parts of their nursing care. In fact, one study by Brown and Waybrant (1988), who surveyed nurse practitioners, demonstrated that nurse practitioners actively engage in a wide array of health promotion and maintenance activities. More nurses are assuming positions in community-based, primary care settings where health promotion and disease prevention can be addressed effectively in practice (Rodgers, 1993).

Family Health Promotion

A primary goal of family nursing is health promotion of the family as a whole and each of its members (Bomar, 1996; Hartrick, Lindsey, & Hills, 1994). Health behaviors, values, and attitudes are learned in the family (Crooks et al., 1987; Pender, 1987). One of the basic functions of the family is the health care function, the purpose of which is to meet family members' health needs. Because teaching of healthy behaviors in the family context is typically more effective than teaching individuals, it is perhaps the most important health promotion strategy.

Health promotion is one of the two components of primary prevention (Leavell et al., 1965). A clear distinction needs to be made between health promotion and disease prevention or health-protective behaviors (Tripp & Stachowiak, 1992). Health promotion is not disease or health problem specific. It is designed to contribute to the growth, enlargement, or excellence of health. It is a positive, dynamic process that focuses on improving the quality of life and well-being, not merely avoiding disease (Pender, 1987). Health promotion involves "approach" behaviors consisting of a number of actions and activities whose end is high-level wellness (Dunn, 1961).

In contrast, health maintenance or prevention (of illness) is disease or health problem specific and involves "avoidance" of risk behaviors as well as specific preventive or protective measures like immunizations. Both health promotion and health protection/health maintenance are important goals, and are complementary to each other (Duncan & Gold, 1986; Pender, 1987).

Family health promotion involves both promoting family members' health and promoting family system health (Loveland-Cherry, 1988, 1996). In the former case the emphasis is on the individual family members in the context of the family, while in the latter case the focus is health promotion of the family system both internally and in interaction with its external interacting systems, such as the social welfare or educational systems. Here the goals are the promotion of the health of the family unit.

Practically all the health-promotion literature deals with the individual rather than the family unit. Nevertheless, health promotion can be easily applied to the family as a whole. Because the family is a small interactional system, it means, however, that different areas need to be assessed (such as family functioning, family dynamics, communication patterns, parent–child relationships, and the family's interaction with the community) and different strategies applied. Refer to Chapter 1 for a review of the characteristics of healthy families. These characteristics are the behaviors and attitudes that we need to encourage families to acquire or maintain—given, of course, that they are mutually valued by and appropriate for the family in question. In the family assessment and intervention chapters that follow, health promotion of the family system is incorporated.

Health promotion and primary prevention of acute and chronic health problems pose the greatest health challenge to our society. Perhaps our most important goal should be to assist people (individuals and families) to learn how to be healthy in a natural, enjoyable way, rather than just focusing on assisting clients about how not to get sick, or worse yet, assisting clients only when they are sick.

Impediments to Primary Prevention

Although there has been a substantial growth in professional and public commitment to primary prevention, certain factors have created major impediments or obstacles to the incorporation of primary prevention, particularly family-focused health promotion and health protection efforts in all sectors of society. A major impediment is money or, more accurately, how we chose collectively to spend our money. Lack of third-party reimbursement for family assessments and interventions and for health promotion and preventive activities creates a situation whereby only the more affluent or the very needy can afford to obtain professional help or access to the needed education.

A second obstacle is the attitudes and socialization of physicians and nurses in the United States. We are still very illness-oriented and often only pay lip service to the importance of disease prevention and health promotion. The medical model is still the dominant model for practice, policy-making, and funding. The adherence of health professionals to the medical model—in which health and illness are looked on as discrete, separate entities and the client is seen as a set of physiological systems—has led us and society (the consumers) to view health care primarily in terms of curative medical care. Individuals, when ill, "turn themselves over" to health providers. There has been little encouragement or reward from society or health care professionals for assuming self-responsibility for staying well or striving to improve one's total functioning (Bruhn & Cordova, 1978).

A third obstacle is the fact that many health care professionals act as poor role models for their clients. These professionals often are sedentary, overweight, and under apparent stress; thus they are not in a position to speak effectively about improving anyone's lifestyle. They do not ask about the family, do not view their client as the family, and do not recognize the reciprocal impact of family and health/illness. Thus, the psychosocial and family factors involved in health care are given insufficient attention (Doherty & Campbell, 1988).

Other obstacles to primary prevention are our materialistic value system; the presence of social problems such as inadequate health care, employ-ment, and educational opportunities for stigmatized members of society (e.g., the poor, minorities, senior citizens, and women); and widespread environmen-tal hazards (e.g., air and water pollution and expo-sure to toxic substances) extant in our communities.

Family Health Promotion/Health Maintenance: Preventive Measures and Risk Appraisal

Primary prevention, in addition to health promo-tion, involves maintaining and improving the level of individual and family resistance to particular dis-eases. Risk appraisal and risk reduction methods are ways to decrease the possibility that a client will acquire specific illnesses or diseases.

Specific Preventive Measures. Increasing resistance to social, emotional, and biological forces that precipitate disease is a goal of primary prevention. As mentioned previously, a wellness lifestyle should enhance this resistance. (This is cov-ered in more depth in Chap. 16.) Nevertheless, dis-ease prevention is also needed. Prevention involves "a defensive set of actions that ward off specific ill-ness conditions or their sequelae that threaten the quality of life or longevity" (Pender, 1986, p. 38). Specific preventive measures are part of disease pre-vention. Examples of specific preventive measures are immunizations and fluoride treatment.

The Risk Approach to Health Care and Prevention. Because most people are concerned more with the threat of illness than with their health, the concept of risk has become part of our thinking about disease prevention. "Risk" implies that the probability of adverse consequences is increased by the presence of one or more charac-teristics or factors (Backett, Davies, & Petros-Barvazian, 1984). Risk, then, is a probability or statistical measure—the probability of a future occurrence. When the probability of the occurrence of an injury, disease, or death can be reduced or nullified if an anticipatory action is taken, then this action uses the risk approach at an individual or family level (Backett, Davies, & Petros-Barvazian, 1984). The risks that individuals and families pos-

sess are, in fact, a type of shorthand expression of their probable future need for preventive and/or curative care. Collective community risks also exist, e.g., the presence of gang violence, poverty, or poor health care services. The degree of risk in these cases is also an expression of need and should be the basis for determining priorities in the allocation of scarce resources. Often it leads to calls for greater emphasis on primary prevention and primary care services.

In terms of disease prevention, one of the most common ways in which primary prevention is prac-ticed is by determining long-term risks to which a client is exposed and then by prescribing measures that will reduce the individual's risk factors. In many cases, a health hazard appraisal method or tool is used. In this approach, the total personal risks to a client are estimated by identifying the average risk for the major causes of death in the client's own age, sex, and racial group. From this, one can develop a prognosis for the well client. Using this appraisal method, the health care practitioner can estimate those causes most likely to bring about disease and death in the client, and recommend lifestyle changes, specific protective measures, and health treatments to reduce risk. Table 2–2 is an example of a health hazard appraisal tool for an individual client.

Families, as well as individuals, can be appraised as to the extent of risks a family may be exposed to. An example of a risk appraisal tool for a family is found in Table 2–3.

The Family's Role in Primary Pre-vention. Families have been found to be the most important source of help for American adults who have changed their lifestyles to a more well-ness-oriented one. A Gallop national survey in 1985 confirmed that when it comes to health matters, most people get more help from their family than any other source, even their doctor (Gurin, 1985). Moreover, the family plays a significant role as to the extent to which family members are exposed to risks (Duffy, 1988). The family discourages or encourages risk behaviors such as smoking, alcohol use, seatbelt use, good or poor nutrition and exer-cise, and so forth.

In summary, primary prevention—health promo-tion and disease prevention—is a primary thrust of

► TABLE 2-2

HEALTH HAZARD APPRAISAL TOOL: INDIVIDUAL CLIENT

Name: John Doe
Age: 43
Race and Gender: White male
Occupation: Small businessman

Rank—Disease/Injury	Prognostic Criteria	Client Findings	Recommendations
1. Arteriosclerotic heart disease	Blood pressure	120/70	
	Cholesterol level	280	Reduce saturated fats, calories, and red meats; prescribe lovastatin 10 mg daily.
	Diabetes	No	
	Exercise	Sedentary—none	Initiate regular exercise program.
	Family history	None	
	Smoking	2 packs a day for 20 years	Referred to stop-smoking clinic.
	Weight	200 lb (5 ft 10 in)	Weight reduction diet. Reduce to 165 lb.
2. Auto accidents	Alcohol	Drinks occasionally (socially); no automobile accidents	
	Drugs	None	
	Mileage	30,000/year	
	Seatbelts	Occasional use	Recommended to always use seatbelts in car.
3. Suicide	Depression	None observed, client denies	
	Family history	Negative	
4. Cirrhosis of liver	Alcohol use	Social occasions only	

Adapted in part from Edelman and Mandle (1986). Robbins and Hall (1970).

family nursing. Family nurses should help families take responsibility for their own health and incorporate wellness lifestyle changes into both their family's lifestyle and their members' personal lives. The family continues to play a crucial role in helping its members learn new ways to live more healthy lives. By believing in families' abilities to provide their own self-health care and to act in their own best interests, we will provide positive support and more effectively become resource persons and facilitators to families. Thus, primary prevention is a most exciting and vital role for family nurses. Primary care is an important instrument for achieving a stronger emphasis on primary prevention (Donaldson, Yordy, & Vanselow, 1994). Primary care providers (nurse practitioners and community-based nurses) are particularly well placed to provide family health promotion and health protection in their practice (Broering, 1993). Fortunately, the emphasis on this role is becoming more pronounced in practice (Venegoni, 1995), education, and research (Duffy, 1988).

Primary prevention emphasis is particularly crucial in working with school-aged children and young families. Nurses in school settings have great occasion to teach primary prevention to their student clients and their families. Intervening with this population gives nurses the opportunity not only to help prevent the onset of health-damaging risk behaviors but to discourage health-compromising behaviors that may be less firmly established as part of a lifestyle. Early intervention provides an opportunity to introduce, reinforce, and help further establish healthy lifelong patterns.

► SECONDARY PREVENTION

Case finding and detection are keys to secondary prevention so that early diagnosis and prompt treatment can be instituted. If the nature of the disease precludes cure, then the goal is to control the progression of the disease and prevent disability.

> ► TABLE 2-3

HEALTH HAZARD APPRAISAL TOOL: FAMILY CLIENT

Family Name:	Sawyer
Developmental Stage:	Family with preschool children
Race/Ethnicity:	African-American
Family Form:	Two-parent nuclear family
Family Composition:	Husband, 27; wife, 25; son, 3; daughter, 13 months
Parents' Occupation:	Both full-time high school teachers

Common Health Problems	Prognostic Criteria	Family Findings	Recommendations
1. Marital relationship strains	Poverty Wife battering History of family instability Social isolation	Mother reports husband and she co-parent children and have active church and social network.	
2. Sibling rivalry	Sibling fighting Acting out by older sibling(s)	Older son occasionally resentful of parents' attention to baby sister.	Spend time alone with older son everyday. Encourage him to help care for his little sister.
3. Developmental lag(s)—Lack of growth and developmental information	Slowed development Parental expectations are incongruent with child's developmental age Poverty	Parents are well informed. Children's development is within normal limits.	

The nurse's role here would be to refer all family members for screening, health histories, and physical examinations (or complete the screening and checkups himself or herself). Additionally, depending on the setting, initiation and follow-through of referrals for diagnosis and treatment may be indicated. Health teaching, along with careful referral and follow-up, are concomitant functions at this time.

Using Guidelines for Periodic Health Assessments and Laboratory Testing

Health assessment (physical examinations and histories) and laboratory testing should be individualized rather than carried out as a routine "standard annual physical." In fact, annual physicals are no longer recommended for healthy adults. Several important health and medical associations (the American Medical Association, American Heart Association, Canadian Task Force on the Periodic Health Examination, and American College of Physicians) have promulgated recommendations for health main-

tenance checkups (Oppenheim, 1984; Parachini, 1987), according to age and gender, for when physicals should be completed on healthy persons and what exams and tests should be performed. For instance, the AMA now advises healthy adults until age 40 to have a checkup every 5 years, then every 1 to 3 years thereafter. Four diseases can be effectively and easily screened for in the physical examination: cervical cancer (Pap smear), hypertension (blood pressure readings), bowel cancer (stool blood test), and breast cancer (breast exam and mammogram). Blood cholesterol testing for atherosclerosis is also simple and effective (Oppenheim, 1984). These guidelines inform primary care providers about what their priorities should be with a client. The timing of regular health examinations, health promotion education, and specific preventive recommendations are based on these guidelines (Ryan, 1996). These guidelines incorporate much of the same content as the risk approach/risk appraisal tool discussed previously.

When clients come in for physicals, primary care practitioners are encouraged to go beyond their interest in secondary prevention, to ask more comprehensive questions about clients' health behaviors, and using a family-centered approach to follow up more concertedly on needed lifestyle modifications and other primary prevention strategies.

▶ TERTIARY PREVENTION

Rehabilitation is the primary focus of tertiary prevention. Recovery and maintenance care for chronically ill people are also included under this rubric. Rehabilitation involves restoring individuals disabled by disease or injury to a level of functioning optimal for them—or to their greatest usefulness—physically, socially, emotionally, and vocationally. In learning to live with a permanent disability, the client and family need tremendous support and extensive teaching of self and dependent care. The nurse plays central roles in tertiary prevention, particularly in view of the growth of home health care. In addition to direct caregiving, the family nurse's most significant roles are that of coordinator or case manager, client/family advocate, teacher, counselor, and environmental modifier.

This chapter has described the several levels of family nursing. The text will primarily address the third level of practice in which the family is considered the client. The historical legacy and growth of family nursing was presented as well as the extent to which some specialty areas have incorporated family into their respective standards of practice. The goals of family nursing are described by using the levels of prevention as an organizing framework. Because of the pervasive health problems among American family members, family health promotion is an especially critical goal for family nurses in various settings today.

▶ study questions

1. One major difference between the three levels of family nursing practice is:
    a. The setting in which family nursing is practiced.
    b. The conceptualization of the family.
    c. The specialty area of the nurse.
    d. None of the above.

2. What are the differences between nursing of families and family systems nursing, as defined by Wright, Leahey, and Bell? (Select all correct answers.)
    a. Family systems nursing deals simultaneously with two or more systems.
    b. Family systems nursing is more concerned with cause-and-effect relationships.
    c. Family systems nursing represents advanced nursing practice in the family nursing specialty area.
    d. Family systems nursing is theoretically based in developmental theory and social learning theory.

3. What is the different mission of the family-centered community health nurse versus the family-centered nurse working in other settings?

4. Which of the following statements is/are true about the levels of prevention? The levels:
    a. Specifically identify the nurse's role in prevention of disease.
    b. Cover the entire spectrum of health and disease.
    c. Identify goals for each of the three levels of prevention.
    d. Are generally synonymous with preventive, curative, and rehabilitative phases of health care.

Match the correct level of prevention from the right-hand column (items 5–13) with the description in the left-hand column.

5. Case finding.
6. Health promotion.
7. Specific preventive measures.
8. Early detection and treatment.
9. Convalescence.
10. Minimizing the complications of the disease.
11. Rehabilitation.
12. Health maintenance.
13. Risk avoidance and reduction.

a. Primary prevention.
b. Secondary prevention.
c. Tertiary prevention.

14. The family as client is an integral part of the ANA standards of practice in *two* specialty areas in nursing. Which are these?
    a. Rehabilitation nursing.
    b. Medical–surgical nursing.
    c. Psychiatric–mental health nursing.
    d. Community health nursing.
    e. Maternal–child nursing.
    f. Family nurse practitioners.

15. Identify four factors that have led to increased interest and involvement in primary prevention.

16. Identify five key dimensions making up a wellness lifestyle.

17. The health hazard appraisal tool contains and asks for what kinds of information?

18. Why is the risk approach used in health care today?

19. How does the meaning of family health differ from the meaning of health? What factors would a family nurse assess related to health promotion?

20. Why is health promotion considered a primary thrust of family nursing?

21. Which of the following impeding factors with respect to family health promotion is said to be the most significant?
    a. Health care professionals' socialization and attitudes.
    b. Allocation of fiscal resources.
    c. The American value system.
    d. Presence of societal social problems.

► chapter 2 study answers

1. b.

2. a and c.

3. The ordering of priorities is different. The community health nurse is committed to providing services to families to help resolve major *community health* problems in addition to services designed to meet unique health needs of family. The family nurse in other settings/specialties prioritizes the family's particular health needs.

4. b, c, and d.

5. b.

6. a.

7. a.

8. b.

9. c.

10. b.

11. c.

12. a.

13. a.

14. d and e.

15. Any four of the following:
    1. Recognition of need for a change in focus from crisis-oriented acute care (often the end result of self-destructive life patterns and environmental hazards) to causative factors of major chronic illnesses (lifestyle and environmental improvements).
    2. The wellness movement.
    3. Consumerism and popular demand for increased self-control.
    4. Problems with accessibility and availability of primary care health services.
    5. Growing acceptability of alternative health modalities.
    6. Growing emphasis on health in advanced nursing practice.

16. 1. Self-responsibility and self-care.
    2. Nutritional awareness.

3. Stress management.
4. Physical fitness.
5. Environmental sensitivity.

17. The health hazard appraisal tool lists basic identifying data on an individual or family and the rank and nature of the major health problems (causing death) for persons or families of that age and sex (individual) or developmental stage (family). Prognostic criteria for each of these major health problems are also identified adjacent to problem. The tool then asks for information about the client relative to each of these criteria and has space next to the client data for recommendations to reduce risks.

18. Identifying risks assists professionals in determining their priorities for assessment and intervention. It uses probability data to look at future, long-term risks or possible health needs.

19. Whereas health refers to the individual's state of functioning, family health refers to the adequacy of functioning of the family as a unit or system. Family dynamics (internal family functioning) and family's relationship with its external environment would be two broad components that would need to be assessed relative to family health promotion.

20. If family nurses can help families incorporate family health-promotion strategies or incorporate a wellness lifestyle, most health problems can be alleviated or forestalled. Health promotion is much more cost-effective than illness care.

21. b.

The Family Nursing Process

Marilyn M. Friedman with Anne Marie C. Levac

▶ learning objectives

1. Explain the difference between using the nursing process in family nursing and using the nursing process in working with individuals.

2. Describe each of the five basic steps within the nursing process relative to its purpose and meaning.

3. Discuss the preparation needed to adequately conduct a family interview or home visit.

4. Identify several sources of family assessment data.

5. Explain the advantages of using the problem, etiology or contributing factors, and defining characteristics when making a family nursing diagnosis.

6. Explain why family strengths are helpful to include as part of the family assessment.

7. Describe several variables that the family nurse would consider when determining priorities for nursing care.

8. Identify within what phases of the nursing process the identification of resources is included.

9. Apply the premise that "families have the right and responsibility to make their own health decisions" at each step of the nursing process.

10. Name the classification system of client problems used in community health nursing.

11. Identify strengths and limitations of the North American Nursing Diagnoses Association (NANDA) in terms of making family nursing diagnoses.

12. Describe several factors that influence the particular family nursing intervention selected.

13. Identify the three domains of family functioning in the Calgary Family Intervention Model and describe one intervention directed at each domain.

14. Select two concepts of change that are important to assist families in changing their behavior.

15. List two family problems that confront family nurses and interpret the meaning of these problematic behaviors.

Comprehensive family nursing is a complex process, making it necessary to have a logical, systematic approach for working with families and individual family members. This approach is the nursing process. According to Yura and Walsh (1988), "The nursing process is the core and essence of nursing; it is central to all nursing actions, applicable in any setting and within any theoretical–conceptual frame of reference" (p. 1). "Process" refers to a deliberate and conscious act of moving from one point to another (in this case through a series of circular, dynamic steps or phases) toward goal fulfillment. It is basically a systematic problem-solving process that is utilized when working with individuals, families, groups, or communities. The American Nurses Association (ANA) descriptions of the nursing process within their social policy statements (1980, 1995a) are particularly informative because they link process to nursing standards of care (Fig. 3–1).

▶ THE FAMILY NURSING PROCESS

The family nursing process will differ relative to who is the focus of care. This focus difference depends on the nurse's conceptualization of the family in his or her practice. If he or she sees the family as the background or context of the individual patient, then the individual family members become the focus and the nursing process is individually oriented, as is the tra-

ditional way of proceeding. If, however, the nurse conceptualizes the family as the unit of care, then, even though the process itself does not vary, the family as a unit or system is the focus.

Most family nurses in practice work simultaneously with both individual family members and with the family and its subsystems. This means the family nurse will utilize the nursing process on two levels—on the individual and on the family and family subsystem level. In this case, assessment, diagnosis, planning, intervention, and evaluation will be more extensive and complex.

If feasible, it is important to assess and focus on both levels of analysis. Our nursing services are typically very specialized if we only assess and work with the family as a system. And conversely, an adequate understanding of each family member cannot be gained without viewing that member within the context of the primary group—the family.

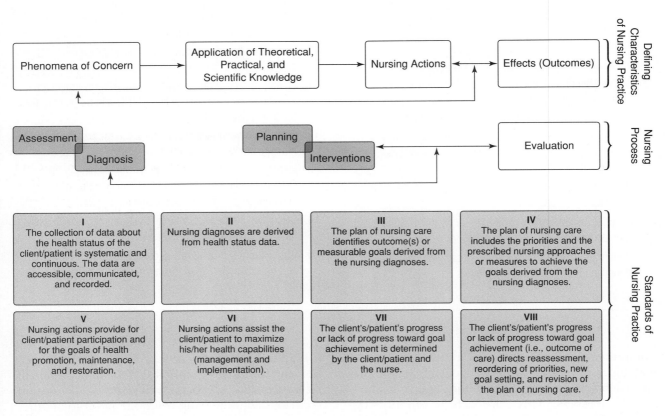

Figure 3–1. Relationship of the nursing process to the standards of nursing practice. "Client/patient" refers to individuals, families, and communities. *(Adapted from American Nurses Association, 1980, 1991, 1995a.)*

This two-level approach to assessing and carrying out family nursing care is illustrated in Figure 3–2. In reality, the steps in the diagram are interdependent and not strictly sequential or linear in organization. In practice, one or more steps or phases may overlap or take place simultaneously, with movement back and forth among the various steps.

▶ FAMILY ASSESSMENT

Family Assessment: An Interactional Level of Analysis

Although in the above section we have stated that family nursing care often involves assessment and intervention at both the individual and family level,

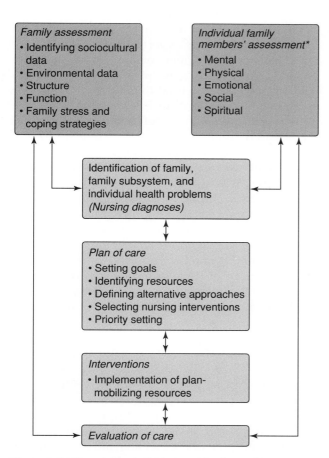

Figure 3–2. Steps in the individual and family nursing process. *Individual client nursing process is not covered in this text.

for purposes of this text and in this chapter, only family assessment, planning, and intervention is discussed. Many texts cover the nursing process used with individual clients.

In order to work effectively with family clients, conducting assessments and providing care, the family nurse must "think interactionally" (Wright & Leahey, 1984, 1994). Wright and Leahey (1994) explain that perhaps the most significant variable that promotes or impedes family nursing is how the nurse conceptualizes problems. Knowledge of family theory and research as well as a systematic framework for assessing and working with families greatly helps the nurse to make the transition from an individualistic to a familistic perspective. To this end, this text presents foundational family science knowledge, as well as a comprehensive family assessment tool.

The Assessment Process

The process of nursing assessment is highlighted by continuous information gathering and professional judgments that attach meaning to the information being gathered. In other words, data are collected in a systematic fashion (using a family assessment tool), classified, and analyzed as to their meaning. Often cursory data are collected on each of the major areas. When the assessor then finds significant probable or potential problems, he or she then probes those areas more deeply. Additionally, family strengths should be explored in the assessment process. The amount and type of information is also dependent on the client, who may wish to convey more information in one area than another. Data collection is the *sine qua non* of problem and strength identification. Although assessment is the first step of the nursing process, data continues, however, to be gathered throughout the provision of services, showing the dynamic, interactive, and flexible nature of this process.

Sources of Assessment Data. Family data collection comes from many sources: client interviews relative to past and present events, objective findings (e.g., observations of home and its facilities), subjective appraisals (e.g., reported experiences of family members), written and oral information from referrals, various agencies working with family, and other health team members.

The interview is a face-to-face meeting with one or more family members. It is desirable when possible to interview the whole family during the initial assessment phase. This gives everyone a chance to share their perceptions, and gives the nurse an opportunity to see the interactions of family members (Holman, 1983). The interview should be focused, but, according to the purpose of the interview, varies in its degree of structure.

There may be times when the nurse conducts an interview with only one family member. In these cases, it is essential to "think family" by asking questions that include other family members. For instance, a question such as "What would your husband say if he were here?" could shift an individually focused interview toward one that draws forth family data.

One of the important roles of the family health nurse is that of an active participant observer in the family. While the nurse is working with families, he or she must also have the ability to "stand back" and observe the conditions and situations existing in the home.

Several family system tools are used to gather information during a family interview. The genogram, ecomap, and family sculpture are commonly used for this purpose. They are discussed in later chapters. The Friedman family assessment tool used in this text can be used to structure interview questions and foci.

More structured checklists, inventories, and questionnaires can be used in data collection (Holman, 1983). They may be especially useful when a great deal of information is needed to be gleaned or recorded. When a nurse is seeing a family over an extended period of time, or there is more than one nurse working with the family, checklists and other structured, easily completed tools may be useful.

One of the most frequent uses of structured family assessment tools is in the area of family research. There are numerous good family assessment instruments. Most of these can be found in three family assessment instrument texts listed in the References: Grotevant and Carlson (1989), Jacob and Tennenbaum (1988), and McCubbin & Thompson (1991).

Building a Trusting Relationship.

The establishment of a trusting relationship in which there is mutual respect and open, honest communication goes hand in hand with the assessment process and orientation phase of working with a family. Reciprocal trust (Thorne & Robinson, 1989; Robinson, 1996) in the nurse–family relationship sets the stage for and is the cornerstone of effective family nursing care. By promoting trust, the nurse is also creating a context for the family to be open to implementing future family nursing interventions.

Trust is developed when the nurse conveys an acceptance of the family and acknowledges the family's abilities, rights, and beliefs irrespective of the nurse's goals, values, or expectations. Wright and Leahey (1994) maintain that families should be encouraged to state their expectations for health care explicitly at the outset. This clarification between nurse and family promotes trust in the nurse–family relationship and may prevent family disappointment with services later on. Embedded in this conversation is a message of caring and an acknowledgment that the nurse respects the family's perspective and their expertise in managing their lives. This acknowledgment of family strengths serves to increase the family's own problem-solving abilities and to decrease potential dependency. A positive nurse–family relationship is enhanced when the nurse assumes an active, confident approach; builds upon family strengths; cultivates a context of racial and ethnic sensitivity; maintains a nonjudgmental stance; and takes an equal interest in all family members (Levac, Wright, & Leahey, in press).

The orientation phase in working with families is seen as the time for assisting the family to begin to express its present concerns so that the nurse may more fully understand the family and the meaning of its experience; the family members may deepen their understanding of their own concerns during this phase; the family may begin to problem solve; and family members may feel some sense of relief from sharing their concerns.

Preparation for Family Interviews and Home Visits.

Before interviewing the family, the nurse must be prepared both conceptually and practically to conduct a family assessment. In terms of conceptual preparation, Wright and Leahey (1994) propose that the nurse needs to be clear about the purpose of the meeting and ascertain with the family where the meeting will be held. Before interviewing the family, the nurse can read available records, discuss the family with health care team members who know the family well, and anticipate the family needs (both common developmental and unique situational needs). The nurse should then formulate some beginning ideas about the family system and develop purposeful assessment questions to ask family members. When interviewing the family in the home, anticipation of family needs is even more critical because home visits are quite costly in terms of both time and money.

In order to be practically prepared for a home visit, the nurse should gather information, assessment, and intervention tools (e.g., tongue blades, developmental screening kit, dressings) that are needed before leaving the agency. Flexibility, of course, is essential, because unanticipated or priority needs often become apparent, and part of the preparation may not be needed—or at least not on the particular visit. When the family has a telephone, calling to introduce oneself, stating the reason for the visit and making arrangements, is preferable (Leahy et al., 1977).

After having collected data on a systematic family assessment tool, the next step is analyzing the data. The data need to be summarized and collated, grouping similar data together and arranging them in orderly form so that accurate conclusions and problems can be identified. It is also at this time that gaps in information become obvious, indicating where further probing and detailing of information are needed.

Family Strengths.

In analyzing the data, several family health care professionals recommend that family strengths be identified (Clemen-Stone et al., 1987; Power & Dell Orto, 1988; Wright & Leahey, 1994). The strengths can be used as resources to draw upon when planning nursing interventions. Several authors have identified family strengths, most notably Otto (1973), Pratt (1976), Curran (1983), and most recently Beavers and Hampson (1990) and Power and co-workers (1988). They deal with the family atmosphere, flexibility and adaptibility, the extent of autonomy of members, as well as cohesiveness, the relationship of the family to the community, and communication skills. Table 3–1 gives the family strengths identified by Power and Dell Orto (1988). Characteristics of healthy families discussed in Chapter 1 are also family strengths.

► FAMILY NURSING DIAGNOSES

The family assessment culminates in an identification of family problems. Many family health problems are within the nurse's scope of practice, and are called **family nursing diagnoses**. Other family problems, however, fall under the scope of practice of other professions and fields, such as medicine, law, education, recreation, or social welfare. In these cases, the family's problems still need to be identified and discussed with the family, which serves to verify that the need or problem is mutually perceived. Often the nursing role here is to refer the family to appropriate resources and to provide the necessary coordination, teaching, and support related to the problem and referral. Other family problems are the concern of several health care professionals, with each having a different way of assessing and working with the family. In these instances, collaboration and coordination with the other team members is imper-

► TABLE 3–1

FAMILY STRENGTHS

Communication Skills
- The ability to listen.
- The ability of the family members to discuss their concerns (family expressiveness).

A Shared Family Paradigm
- Shared common perceptions of reality within the family.
- Family's willingness to have hope and appreciate that change is possible.

Intra-family Support
- The ability to provide reinforcements to each other.
- The ability of family members to provide an atmosphere of belonging.

Self-Care Abilities
- The ability of family members to take responsibility for health problems.
- Family members' willingness to take good care of themselves.

Problem-solving Skills
- The ability of family members to use negotiation in family problem-solving.
- The ability to focus on the present, rather than on past events or disappointments.
- Family members have the capacity to use everyday experiences as resources.

Adapted from Power & Dell Orto (1988).

ative to avoid unnecessary client confusion and lack of efficient, effective services. These problems are called **collaborative problems** (Carpenito, 1987).

Family nursing diagnoses are an extension of nursing diagnoses to the family system and its subsystems and are the outcome of the nursing assessment. Family nursing diagnoses include actual or potential health problems that nurses, by virtue of their education and experience, are capable and licensed to treat (Gordon, 1978, 1982). They are used "as a basis for projecting outcomes, planning intervention, and evaluating outcome attainment" (Gordon, 1985, p. viii).

At the family level, the nursing diagnosis can be derived from using one of the family or nursing theories or from using North American Nursing Diagnosis Association (NANDA) diagnoses. For instance, if a structural-functional or interactional framework is utilized, family nursing diagnoses might include role conflicts or transitions, child-rearing problems, value conflicts, or communication problems. If a systems framework is utilized, then the family's closed boundaries relative to interactions with the community, lack of an intact parental subsystem, or excessive separateness of family members from each other are possible nursing diagnoses. In the discussions of each of the assessment and intervention areas that follow (Chaps. 8 to 17), the reader will be able to gain insight into the types of family nursing diagnoses and other family problems that may result from deficiencies in the family system, its structure or functions.

Nursing Diagnoses: The NANDA Classification

The nursing diagnosis movement represents a very significant effort on behalf of nurse leaders to systematize nursing practice and promote the use of a standardized list of diagnoses in practice. At the Ninth National Conference of the North American Nursing Diagnosis Association (NANDA), the following definition of nursing diagnosis was adopted (1988):

> A nursing diagnosis is a clinical judgment about individual, family, or community responses to actual or potential health problems/life processes. Nursing diagnoses provide the bases for selection of nursing interventions to achieve outcomes for which the nurse is accountable.

Although family is included in NANDA's definition of nursing diagnosis, the list of accepted diagnoses remains primarily individually oriented. In examining a recent list of the 98 accepted NANDA nursing diagnoses, there are some diagnoses that can or do address family system and subsystem health problems. Table 3–2 lists these selected nursing diagnoses.

In addition to the NANDA nursing diagnoses being individually oriented, four other features which may be limitations are apparent in the use of NANDA diagnoses in family nursing practice.

1. They are atheoretical, which can be both a strength and a weakness, depending on one's viewpoint. This limitation is generally noted in the literature.

▶ TABLE 3–2

NANDA NURSING DIAGNOSES RELEVANT TO FAMILY NURSING

Altered Family Processes
Altered Health Maintenance
Altered Nutrition: Less than Body Requirements
Altered Nutrition: More than Body Requirements
Altered Nutrition: Potential for More or Potential for Less than Body Requirements
Altered Parenting
Altered Patterns of Elimination: Inadequate Sanitary Disposal Conditions
Altered Role Performance
Altered Sexuality Patterns
Anticipatory Grieving
Decisional Conflict (specify)
Dysfunctional Grieving
Family Coping: Potential for Growth
Health Seeking Behavior
Ineffective Family Coping: Compromised
Ineffective Family Coping: Disabling
Impaired Adjustment
Impaired Home Maintenance Management
Impaired Social Interaction
Knowledge Deficit (specify)
Noncompliance (specify)
Parental Role Conflict
Risk for Altered Parenting
Risk for Trauma (injury)
High Risk for Violence
Powerlessness
Social Isolation

Source: NANDA diagnoses are described in McFarland & McFarlane (1993).

2. For the most part, the family-oriented nursing diagnoses are very broad and may not be sufficiently specific to guide nursing interventions. However, specifying the signs and symptoms of the problem and etiological or contributing factors can handle this limitation.

3. They are essentially illness oriented (Donnelly, 1990).

4. The present list is incomplete and does not cover the array of family nursing actual or potential problems/diagnoses that clinicians see.

Donnelly (1990) describes one large gap in the NANDA accepted list. She notes with concern the essential absence of standardized diagnostic categories that address family health promotion. She identifies only one NANDA diagnosis that "hints" at family health promotion concepts: "Family coping: Potential for growth." Although health-seeking behavior has been added since Donnelly's 1990 article, efforts are still needed to broaden the accepted list of diagnoses to adequately cover family-as-client throughout the broad spectrum of health–illness concerns.

Gordon's (1985) and the NANDA format for stating nursing diagnoses consists of the statement of the diagnosis, signs and symptoms (defining characteristics) and etiologic or contributing factors. This formatting provides a rich and broadened resource for goal setting and formulating treatment plans. An example of a common family health problem is "Impaired verbal communication (NANDA diagnosis) between mother and daughter characterized by mutual hostility; related to (contributing factors) values, control, and limit-setting conflicts and mother's low self-esteem." In this case the diagnosis from NANDA was used but the signs and symptoms and contributing factors were not identified by NANDA and thus were generated by the author. Another common family nursing diagnosis from NANDA is an alteration in parenting. Here there is an array of defining characteristics that may help the clinician in identifying the signs and symptoms. This diagnosis appears to be more broadly described. For example, the alteration in parenting could be characterized by inadequate child care provision and multiple parental surrogates with etiological factors being economic, knowledge deficit (mother), and social isolation (family). The nursing care plan shown in

Table 3–3 illustrates how this aspect is schematically handled in a nursing care plan tool.

Ross (1990) noted that "progress in the development of nursing diagnosis specific to types of clients is apparent, especially in the 1994 additions to the NANDA classifications" (p. 135). Based on the work of NANDA, Thomas, Barnard, and Sumner (1993) developed a framework for family assessment based on five family diagnoses categories: family processes, family coping, parenting, health maintenance and management, and home maintenance and management. Along with other clinical assessment measures (such as interviews, observation, and questionnaires), the authors provide clinicians with an extensive list of clinical family assessment tools to assess each family diagnostic category. Thus, the use of family diagnoses provides a basis for identifying many common family nursing problems.

It should be noted that some family nursing clinicians challenge the relevance of the NANDA classification system. Wright and Levac (1993) have voiced their concern over the use of NANDA diagnoses, particularly in regard to the "existence of" noncompliance. Based on a meta-theory of cognition (Maturana & Varela, 1992) they argue that diagnostic statements are based on the biologically impossible assumption that individuals (such as nurses) have access to an objective reality—that our observations/assessment of a family member's behavior are "*true.*" Since nursing assessments are based on observer perspectives and not ultimate truths, we cannot claim that a family is "noncompliant" or that a "parent is ineffective." Wright and Levac (1993) propose collaborative interactions with families that eliminate pathologizing language such as "noncompliant," "dysfunctional," and "inability" as descriptors of families or family behavior.

Rather than a nursing diagnosis, Wright and Leahey (1994) propose the formulation of a list of both problems and strengths such that a balanced view of the family is identified. The notion of "hypothesizing" about family problems and strengths (Watson, 1992; Wright & Leahey, 1994) allows the nurse to offer speculations about family structure, development, and functioning in a "spirit of wondering" rather than in a hierarchical stance of certainty. Hypothesizing may both guide the continuous assessment process and form the basis for nursing interventions.

► TABLE 3-3

STUDENT TOOL USED TO ASSESS, PLAN, AND IMPLEMENT FAMILY NURSING CARE

I. Assessment
  A. Assessment of individual family members
  B. Assessment of family[a]
      1. Identifying and sociocultural data
      2. Environmental data
      3. Family structure
      4. Family functions
      5. Family stress coping strategies
II. Nursing care plan (family)

Family Nursing Diagnosis Including Etiological or Contributing Factors	Signs and Symptoms of Problem (Defining Characteristics)	Goals	Intervention	Evaluation
Family overprotection of son, Bobby, due to parental: 1. Guilt about unwanted pregnancy. 2. Anxiety about child's health condition: asthma.	Mother dresses Bobby even though at age 4, he is able to do this himself. Mother won't let Bobby play outside for fear of his hurting himself. Child is clinging to mother when strangers present. Parents view Bobby as a special, "fragile" child.	Mother will let Bobby dress himself, with help only in realistically difficult tasks. Mother will let Bobby play with brother and friends outside in the afternoon.	***Modifying Behavior*** Explored parents' feelings and behavior toward child. Discussed with parents their child's developmental needs. Discussed with sibling activities he and Bobby might enjoy playing together. ***Manipulation of Contributing Factors*** Advised mother to discuss with her doctor child's health condition and prognosis.	Mother is letting Bobby dress himself when there is time. Bobby enjoys doing so. Under mother's supervision, Bobby is playing in the outside garden of house. Father is beginning to play ball at the park with both of the boys.

[a] To be discussed in later chapters.

Nursing Diagnosis: The Omaha System

Another classification system of client problems that has received favorable evaluation from home health agencies who have used the system is the Omaha system, developed by the Visiting Nurse Association of Omaha (VNA of Omaha, 1986). As part of a larger operationalization of the nursing process, an orderly, comprehensive list of client problems has been generated and tested.

Martin and Scheet (1992) described three components of the Omaha system: problem classification scheme, intervention scheme, and problem rating scale for outcomes. The problem classification scheme consists of 40 problems that fall into one of the four domains (environmental, psychosocial, physiological, and health-related behaviors). Modifiers appear at the third level of the problem classification scheme. One set of modifiers includes "family" and "individual," enabling the nurse "to clarify ownership and acknowledge involvement of one or more significant others (Martin & Scheet, 1992, p. 67). An implementation manual is available (VNA of Omaha, 1986) as well as a comprehensive textbook (Martin & Scheet, 1992) describing its application to community health nursing.

Specifying the Level of the Problem

In terms of family problem identification, the nurse needs to indicate at what family system level the problem lies—at the family unit level or at the level of one of the family subsystems or sets of relationships such as the marital dyad, the parent–child subsystem, or the sibling subsystem.

Importance of Family Participation

Active family participation through the nursing process should be of central concern. In terms of identifying problems and strengths, the family nurse and the family are jointly responsible for this part of the process. This process of mutually determining problems and strengths will also enhance the nurse–family relationship.

Diagnosis involves the process of putting information together with the family to formulate the problem(s) and to explore a possible course of action. A case in point: It is not enough for the nurse working with a family to observe that the family is under stress and is not following its plan for bringing in family or friends to help. Together with the family, the nurse needs to generate a diagnosis as to what is happening and why the family is not able to follow through with its intended action. If the nurse has collected adequate information and verified it with the family, the diagnosis will be reasonably accurate. His or her diagnosis should then lead to goals and interventions aimed at assisting the family to cope more effectively.

Interrelationship of Data and Problems

One of the problems in determining health needs or problems of families is that all the information gathered is interrelated, and there are almost insurmountable difficulties involved in sorting out the cause-and-effect relationships. This is because, according to systems theory, there is circular causality. Feedback loops exist (which will be discussed in Chap. 6) wherein one person's behavior (A) sets off another person's behavior (B) causing A to act in response to his or her (A's) previous behavior plus B's response. Also, there is an overlapping of family problems such as role and power conflicts, and cer-

tain problems are not of the same type or level of generality or specificity as others.

Potential Problems. The problems identified in family nursing often focus on the family's ability to cope with a health or environmental problem. In many situations there will be no present medical illness or disability. In these cases the most frequent diagnoses are preventive or health promotional, such as reduction of risks (nutritional modification—salt, caloric, sugar, and fat reduction; lowering stress levels) and lifestyle improvements (regular exercise, more rest and relaxation, better communication).

By definition, a nursing diagnosis may involve potential health problems that originate from existing or anticipated conditions. Freeman (1970, p. 58) calls these "foreseeable crisis or stress points." Because of anticipated periods of unusual demand on the family and its members, anticipatory guidance or health teaching, health counseling, and the initiation of referrals to community resources are often indicated. Examples of foreseeable stressors are pregnancy, movement into a new community, retirement, adolescence, a wife beginning full-time employment, and the progressive deterioration of an aging parent.

Determining Priority Needs. One word of caution is necessary concerning the problems identified by a referring agency. The presenting problem, or reason for referral to the agency, is rarely the only problem. In fact, it may be the least serious problem the family faces. Archer and Fleshman (1975) recommend that family-centered community health nurses use a sorting or triage process when working with families, because there is always too much to do and a scarcity of resources. They recommend that priorities be established based on a hierarchy of needs.

Of low priority and hierarchy relative to providing services are those needs that are impossible to do anything about, because of either client or agency constraints. Other needs or problems will resolve themselves or can be handled by the family's support system or someone less costly and more available, such as a homemaker-home health aide.

There are also needs and problems that are beyond the control of the client or the control and/or level of expertise of the nurse. These limitations must be recognized. If a problem is not within our area of expertise, it needs to be referred.

The needs for which family health nurses can affect change or on which we can make a discernible, positive health impact in an efficient manner are the problems we should be assisting families to alleviate or ameliorate.

Once family and individual health problems have been identified, they should be listed in order of priority, according to their importance to the family. There is often a disjuncture between how the professional views client needs and how the client (or members within the family) view their own problems. In these cases, it is essential that the nurse explore and listen to each family member's perspective in a nonjudgmental way. Then nurse and family may codetermine the direction for nursing care. This process enhances collaboration, and it demonstrates respect for the family's abilities to be active decision makers in their health care.

Only by ranking needs and priorities from the client's perspective can plans for intervention have any chance of success. Some nurses assign low-, medium-, and high-priority ratings, with high-priority needs being those that must be addressed immediately or very soon. In addition to client safety or life-threatening situations, two important factors to consider in assigning priorities are (1) the client's sense of urgency (this is important in building rapport), and (2) actions that will, or might have, therapeutic effects on future client and family health behaviors. These problems will then form the basis for setting goals and planning interventions.

▶ PLANNING

Mutual Goal Setting

Planning first involves joint formulation of client-centered measurable goals. The mutual setting of goals involves identifying outcomes (ANA, 1991). Delineating alternative approaches to meeting goals, selecting specific nursing interventions, identifying and mobilizing resources (including the family's own strengths and self-care capacities), and operationalizing the plan (setting of priorities and spelling out how the plan will be phased in) follows the goal-setting process. The nursing care plan serves as a blueprint for action.

Mutual goal setting with families is the cornerstone of effective planning. One of the basic premises of family nursing is that clients have the ultimate responsibility for managing their own lives (the principle of self-determination) and that we respect others' beliefs (Carey, 1989). Tinkham and Voorhies (1977) help families determine their own health goals by providing them with relevant information about themselves and/or their concerns. This allows them to make sounder decisions about what goals and services they wish to plan. Thus, the main determinant of what goals are set is the family, not the nurse (Otto, 1973).

Mutual goal setting with family members is consistently superior to unilateral goal setting for several reasons: (1) the process of mutual goal setting has a positive effect on interactions with families; (2) people tend to resist being told what to do, but are likely to work toward goals that they themselves choose and support; and (3) people who make decisions tend to feel accountable for them (Carey, 1989).

Goal setting has been increasingly recognized as a highly important component in planning. The development of clear-cut, specific, and acceptable goals is crucial. If family goals are not clear, it does not make much difference what activities are carried out because the end point is not known. To the extent that the stated objectives are defined and accepted as valid by the family, the desired action is likely to follow. In addition to the acceptability, clarity, and specificity of goals, goals also need to be stated in behavioral terms so that they can be measured (evaluated).

There are several levels of goals. The first level includes the specific, immediate, and measurable short-term goals; in the middle of the continuum are intermediate-level goals; and at the other end of the continuum are the long-term, more general, ultimate goals that indicate the broad purposes the nurse and family hope to achieve. Short-term goals are necessary to motivate and give confidence to the family and individuals that progress is being made, as well as to guide the family toward the larger, more comprehensive goal.

In goal setting it is desirable to work with the family in differentiating those problems that need to be resolved by nursing intervention, those problems the family as the self-care agent can handle by itself, and those problems that need to be referred to other members of the health care team or handled on a collaborative basis. A case in point is an elderly couple that needs (1) assistance in obtaining Medicaid, (2) diet counseling, and (3) basic nursing care for the nonambulatory husband. The nurse may decide to handle diet counseling herself, refer the couple to a social worker for Medicaid assistance, and suggest a home health aide to provide the routine nursing care needed for the husband. As a member of the health care team serving families, the family-centered nurse must also be continually alert to situations where team conferences (formal or informal) might be beneficial to the clients. Collaborative planning and goal setting with other team members helps foster a better understanding of client's needs, in addition to mapping out who will do what.

Generating Alternative Approaches and Identifying Resources

After setting goals, the health care professional and family need to generate alternative ways for reaching the stated goals. As these are delineated, possible resources for handling needs are identified. Such resources include use of family inner strengths, including their self-care resources, the family's support system, and physical and community sources of assistance.

Family strengths, as discussed previously, are most useful in assisting nurse and family in resolving family health problems. There is an increased movement, particularly in the family therapy field, toward models that focus on resources, strengths, and solutions (deShazer, 1991; Minuchin & Fishman, 1981). Often family strengths and abilities go unnoticed. Thus, it is important for health care professionals to draw forth individual and family strengths and to share these often unspoken observations with the family. To solicit strengths, the nurse might ask "What are the strengths in your family?" or "What family qualities would you *not* want to change?" (Wright & Levac, 1993). Otto (1973) also reports that he has successfully used a family-strength method in counseling of families. He explains that family strengths are first identified and then progressively shared with family members so as to increase their

awareness of their resources and to take inventory of further potentials or strengths they have. Members are encouraged to discover latent strengths and unfulfilled potentials as part of their problem-solving efforts.

Specific actions or approaches facilitated by the nurse are selected by family members from the available alternatives and resources. These are approaches that both family and nurse feel are appropriate and, hopefully, have a high probability of success. Some of the strategies may involve some or all family members, other health care team members, or extended family and friends, as well as the nurse.

In thinking through the planning of nursing approaches, the nurse needs to ask the following questions:

- Is this plan being developed in collaboration with the family?
- Will the proposed approaches enhance family strengths and increase family member independence?
- Is this action within the information and skill level of the family members or their own resources?
- On a scale of 1 to 10 (with 10 being highest), how committed and motivated are family members in regards to adhering to the plan?
- Are there adequate resources available to carry out the plan?
- How would family members respond to these questions?

Families have the right and responsibility to make their own health decisions. Because of this premise of family nursing, there will be certain actions that fully informed families choose that we may personally and professionally disagree with. So important is the issue of client information and understanding of possible consequences of action (so that families can make a reasonable decision), that we now have informed consent laws in most states. Archer and Fleshman (1975) cite the example of a client who was exposed to rubella during the first trimester of pregnancy, with tests showing no immunity to the rubella virus. The nurse's responsibility in such an instance would be to discuss with the parents the risk of having an infant who is deformed and to inform them of possible alternatives (obtain abortion, continue pregnancy, seek further consultation). The parents need time and an opportunity to discuss their feelings and thoughts, as well as assistance with problem solving. However, we cannot make decisions for them. We may draw on professional judgment and knowledge to recommend a particular course of action after hearing their concerns, but we should in no way reject or withdraw our support if the client makes a decision counter to our advice.

Some of the approaches we plan with families may be less than ideal, but are intended to improve the client's (family's) present situation. Seeking obtainable ways to reach goals is both realistic and pragmatic.

Priority Setting

The operationalization of the nursing care plan follows the mutual selection of approaches designed to reach each of the stated goals. Priority setting of interventions and a phasing in and coordinating of the plan leads to its implementation.

Factors that apply to setting priorities with regard to family needs (as previously discussed) also apply to setting priorities with respect to interventions. Additionally, reality factors such as agency policies, time and money constraints, and availability of personnel and other resources may also influence priorities.

▶ FAMILY NURSING INTERVENTION

There are several different definitions for nursing interventions in the literature. The ANA *Social Policy Statement* (1995) defines them as, "the actions nurses take on behalf of patients, families or communities" with an aim "to assist patients, families and communities to improve, correct or adjust to physical, emotional, psychosocial, spiritual, cultural and environmental conditions for which they seek help" (p. 9). Bulechek and McCloskey (1994) define nursing interventions as: "any direct-care treatment that a nurse performs on behalf of a client. Nursing interventions include nurse-initiated treatments and physician-initiated treatments. Nursing intervention labels are at the conceptual level and require a series of actions or activities to carry them out" (p. 130). As defined by

Wright and Bell (1994), nursing interventions are: "action(s) or response(s) of the nurse, which include the nurse's overt therapeutic actions, that occur in the context of a nurse–client relationship to affect individual, family or community functioning for which nurses are accountable" (p. 3).

The intervention phase begins with the completion of the nursing care plan. In collaboration and/or consultation with the nurse, implementation may be carried out by a number of people: the client (individual or family), health care team members, the extended family, and other persons in the family's social network.

During the time that nursing interventions are being offered, new data will continue to evolve and surface. As this information (client's responses, changes in situation, and so on) is collected, the nurse needs to be sufficiently flexible and adaptable to reassess the situation with the family and extemporaneously make modifications to the plan.

Indications for Family Nursing Intervention

Subsequent to the family assessment and a joint discussion of family concerns and problems, the family nurse and family need to decide whether family intervention is indicated. Criteria for making this decision includes the family's interest and motivation in receiving help and working on its problems, the family's level of functioning, the nurse's own skill level, and the resources available (Wright & Leahey, 1994). In addition to routine health promotional and preventive care, Wright and Leahey (1994) suggest that family nursing intervention may be indicated when:

1. A family presents with a problem(s) in which the relationships between family members are affected.
2. A family member presents with an illness that is having an obvious detrimental impact upon the other family members.
3. The family members are contributing to the symptoms or problems of an individual.
4. One family member's improvement leads to symptoms or deterioration in another family member.

5. A family member is first diagnosed with an illness.

6. A child or adolescent develops an emotional, behavioral, or physical problem in the context of a family member's illness.

7. A chronically ill family member moves from an institution back to the community.

8. An ill family member dies (p. 8).

Levels of Family Nursing Intervention

There are different levels of family nursing interventions with respect to the complexity of the interventions themselves. Wright and Leahey (1994) define two levels of expertise in the nursing of families—generalists and specialists. According to Wright and Leahey, generalists conceptualize family as the context for working with an individual patient. They are prepared at a baccalaureate level. Specialists conceptualize family as the unit of care with competency in clinical interviewing skills and knowledge of family systems theory, family research, and models of family assessment and intervention; they are prepared at the masters or doctoral level. In contrast to Wright and Leahey's belief that baccalaureate graduates function as generalists (according to their definition), Friedman (1992) believes that baccalaureate graduates, in completing family system coursework, are usually effective in working with families as units. More complex families would, nevertheless, need to be referred to specialists with advanced preparation.

Guidelines for Family Nursing Intervention

Recently, several useful principles to keep in mind while intervening with families have been developed. A foundational concept is that interventions can only be offered to families and that the best work that the nurse can do is create a context for the family to discover solutions (Wright & Leahey, 1994). In other words, the nurse applies experience and knowledge to devise interventions in collaboration with the family but cannot force or direct change (Maturana & Varela, 1992; Wright & Levac, 1993). It is important

that the nurse not blame himself or herself or the family should the family choose not to implement a particular intervention or idea. Thus, rather than reacting negatively towards oneself or the family, the nurse could become more curious about the family's functioning and collaboratively develop new or re-adjust prior interventions with the family to meet the goals. Vosburgh and Simpson (1993) maintain that "a focus for intervention becomes searching for strengths, welcoming differences in families and being respectfully curious about their uniqueness" (p. 232). Interventions need to be devised with sensitivity to the family's language and ethnic and religious preferences. Robinson (1996) found that interventions that made a difference to families were those that promoted and enhanced relationships between the family and the nurse. Robinson (1996) stressed that "these relationships are not central to care, they *are* care" (p. 153). Thus, the nature of the nurse–family relationship is not a prerequisite to effective interventions, but rather may be considered an intervention in and of itself.

As the definitions outlined above imply, the primary aim of intervening with families is to invite change such that suffering may be alleviated and/or high-level family wellness may be achieved. For the nurse working with a family over a period of time, change may seem slow or even nonexistent. It must be remembered that change in families comes about "over time through a sequence of interventive moves, each one growing out of information gained, in part, through observing the outcomes of the previous interventions" (Hartman & Laird, 1983, p. 306). Thus, the astute nurse pays particular attention to differences over time, even though they are subtle, and punctuates progress regularly. Wright and Leahey (1994) have highlighted some important concepts of change that they have found critical in assisting families with health problems:

- Change is dependent on the perception of the problem.
- Change is dependent on context.
- Change is dependent on co-evolving goals for treatment.
- Understanding alone does not lead to change.
- Change does not necessarily occur equally in all family members.

- Facilitating change is the nurse's responsibility.
- Change can be due to a myriad of causes (p. 25).

Nursing Intervention Classifications

Freeman (1970), in her classic community health nursing text, generally classifies nursing intervention as being:

1. Supplemental. Here the nurse acts as a direct provider of nursing services by intervening in areas where the family is unable to do so.
2. Facilitative. In this case the family nurse removes barriers to needed services, such as medical, social welfare, transportation, or home health care services.
3. Developmental. Nursing goals are aimed at facilitating the capacity of the family to act on their own behalf (e.g., promoting family group self-care and self-responsibility). Assisting families to utilize their own self-health care resources, such as their internal and external social support systems, is one such intervention (Milardo, 1988). Chapter 8 discusses social support in more detail.

The classification and description of more specific nursing interventions remains in an early stage of development. This is a necessary accomplishment if nurses are to provide evidence for the effectiveness of their interventions on the health of families. To date, commendable progress has been made by Bulechek and McCloskey and associates (1994) to develop a standardized language for nursing interventions. This nursing research team from the University of Iowa has worked diligently to construct and validate a taxonomy of interventions. In 1992, the Nursing Interventions Classification (NIC) was published containing 336 direct-care nursing interventions (McCloskey & Bulechek, 1992). A major strength of the NIC is that it provides a broad range of interventions for both generalists and specialists. It also includes interventions for high-acuity patients (Moorhead, McCloskey, & Bulechek, 1993).

Additionally, Craft and Willadsen (1992) from the University of Iowa surveyed 130 nurse experts (of whom 54 responded) in order to develop and validate nursing interventions related to family. In a movement toward a standardized language for family interventions these researchers concluded with the specification of nine family intervention labels and their defining activities (Table 3–4). The reader is encouraged to read the original source, which

► TABLE 3–4

FAMILY INTERVENTION LABELS AND DEFINING ACTIVITIES

Label	Defining Activity
Family Support	Promotion of family interests and goals[a]
Family Process Maintenance	Minimization of family process disruption effects[a]
Family Integrity Promotion	Promotion of family cohesion and unity[a]
Family Involvement	Family participation in the emotional and physical care of the patient[b]
Family Mobilization	Utilization of family strengths to influence the patient's health in positive direction[b]
Caregiver Support	Provision of the necessary information, advocacy, and support to facilitate primary patient care by people other than health care professionals[c]
Family Therapy	Interaction with the family as a change agent to move the family toward a more productive way of living[a]
Sibling Support	Promotion of interests of siblings when a brother or sister experiences an illness[c]
Parent Education: Adolescent	Provision of assistance to parents to understand and help their adolescent children[c]

[a] Interventions directed toward family as a unit.
[b] Interventions directed toward both family as unit and family as context.
[c] Interventions directed toward family as context.
From Craft and Willadsen (1992), p. 529.

describes the study in detail and lists sources used to identify each label.

Calgary Family Intervention Model

Another milestone in developing and languaging nursing interventions was the birth of the Calgary Family Intervention Model (CFIM) by Wright and Leahey (1994). CFIM is "an organizing framework for conceptualizing the intersection between a particular domain of family functioning and the specific intervention offered by the nurse" (p. 99). Specifically *CFIM focuses on promoting, improving, and/or sustaining effective family functioning in three domains: cognitive (thoughts), affective (emotions), and behavioral (actions)* (Table 3–5). CFIM assists the nurse "to conceptualize a fit between domains of family functioning and interventions offered by the nurse" (p. 101).

Using this model, the nurse needs to determine which domain of family functioning needs to change and then determine the most appropriate intervention(s) that would target that domain. In a collaborative manner, the nurse seeks input from the family about which interventions may be most useful. For example, if a problem were identified as a lack of information, the nurse may determine that the domain of family functioning that needs to be changed is the cognitive domain. By offering an intervention (such as providing information), the nurse may assist the family to learn better ways of managing a problem. If the problem is that of inadequate exercise, the nurse may determine that the behavioral domain of family functioning needs to change and may offer an intervention that will change the family's exercise (behavioral) patterns. However, there will be situations when more than one domain needs changing or when one intervention could effect change in more than one domain of family functioning. This is not surprising since a change in one part (of family functioning) will likely effect change in another.

In order to determine the fit between the domain that needs changing and the intervention of choice, the nurse may need to experiment with different interventions. Continuous evaluation of the effectiveness of the interventions is necessary. Table 3–5 defines the three above-mentioned domains and provides examples of interventions that may be used for each domain. Table 3–6 illustrates application of CFIM to the problem: An elderly parent is requesting more visits from his adult children; the adult children do not enjoy visiting their parent, who is always complaining. Note specific skills the nurse can use to operationalize the intervention of "caregiver support."

▶ TABLE 3–5

CALGARY FAMILY INTERVENTION MODEL: THREE DOMAINS OF FAMILY FUNCTIONING

1. **Cognitive**—Interventions directed at the cognitive domain of family functioning provide new ideas, opinions, information, or education on a particular health problem or risk.
   Some examples are: offering information/opinions, reframing, offering education, and externalizing the problem. Additionally, interventive questions may be formulated to trigger change within the cognitive domain of family functioning.

2. **Affective**—Nursing actions directed at the affective domain of family functioning are intended to assist families with intense emotional responses that may be blocking their problem-solving efforts.
   Some examples are: validating/normalizing emotional responses, storying the illness experience, and drawing forth family support. Interventive questions may be developed to effect change within the affective domain of family functioning.

3. **Behavioral**—Nursing strategies directed at assisting family members to interact/behave differently with each other and with those outside of the family are included here.
   Some examples are: encouraging family members as caregivers, encouraging respite, and devising rituals. Interventive questions may be devised to invite change within the behavioral domain of family functioning.

Adapted from Wright and Leahey (1994).

Specific Family Nursing Interventions

As indicated in the previous discussion, a myriad of family nursing interventions exist that may be used in working with families. Which interventions are selected are often influenced by the level of nurse competency, the theoretical model the family nurse utilizes in the care of a particular family, as well as the family nursing diagnosis made and the goals formulated. For example, anticipatory guidance (a type of teaching strategy) is emphasized in the developmental model, while crisis intervention strategies are used frequently when a family stress and coping model is applied in practice.

APPLICATION OF CFIM*: CAREGIVER SUPPORT

Parent–Child System Problem: Aging parent requests more visits from his adult children; adult children do not enjoy visiting their father because he frequently complains about their lack of visits.

Domains of Family Functioning	Interventions (Encouraging family members to be caregivers and caregiver support)
1. Cognitive	Teach adult children that their aging parent is having difficulty remembering their visits (short-term memory deficits), which is a common phenomenon of aging. Therefore, it is not useful to remind their aging parent of when they visited last.
2. Affective	Empathize with the aging parent; say that you understand that it must be lonely at times being a resident in a geriatric care center. The adult children would appreciate knowing that their parent is lonely so that they can respond appropriately. Therefore, advise the elderly parent to avoid complaining to the children that they do not visit enough and instead, to tell them when they come that "sometimes, I feel lonely here. I'm really glad you came to visit me."
3. Behavioral	Advise the adult children to stop giving excuses and explanations as to why they cannot come more often. Instead, obtain a guest book or calendar and write down each visit. Write down *who* visited and on *what* day, and perhaps any interesting news, so that the aging parent may read this between visits.

From Wright and Leahey (1994).
* Calgary Family Intervention Model.

Moreover, the specific intervention strategies health care professionals utilize with families may depend on the level of functioning of the family. Leavitt (1982) classifies families into highly functional, moderately dysfunctional, highly dysfunctional, acute and highly dysfunctional, and chronic. Depending on the nurse's perspective about the family's degree of functionality, nursing interventions

vary. For instance, with a highly functional family, the family nursing actions are largely preventive and health promotive (teaching, providing information). In contrast, with the highly dysfunctional, acute family, short-term and long-term therapeutic, supportive, and preventive actions are advised (Leavitt, 1982).

The particular interventions implemented also depend on the families, as they are active participants in goal setting and selection of interventions. In any case, educative (teaching) and supportive strategies are core intervention strategies regardless of all the other factors involved.

In each of the assessment and intervention chapters, specific interventions stressed in that particular area are identified. Further discussion of the specific family nursing interventions outlined in Table 3–7 is found in Chapter 18.

Barriers to Implementing Interventions

Family-related Barriers: Apathy and Indecision. Barriers to implementing interventions may be either family behaviors and/or nurse behaviors. Dyer (1973) in his work with culturally diverse and poor families in the community identified problematic family behaviors that confront nurses. The first of these behaviors is apathy. It is

FAMILY NURSING INTERVENTIONS

Behavior modification
Contracting
Case management, including coordination and advocacy
Collaboration
Consultation
Counseling, including support, cognitive reappraisal (reframing), crisis intervention, and group work
Empowerment strategies
Environmental modification
Family advocacy
Lifestyle modification, including stress management
Networking, including use of self-help groups and social support
Referring
Role modeling
Role supplementation
Teaching strategies
Values clarification

manifested when the family responds to nursing actions with an apparent "so what" attitude and gives no sign of action or concern. Does the family really not care? Usually they do care. Often, however, there are differences in values or beliefs that influence the family's responses, particularly if the family is of a different socioeconomic or ethnic background than the nurse. Behaviors that may be related to apathy include hopelessness (the belief that "whatever the family does, it won't matter anyway") and fatalism (the feeling that "what will be, will be"). Fatalism is a central theme among poor and powerless families. Apathetic behavior also may be related to a sense of futility about the effectiveness or availability of services. Without a perception that effective and accessible treatment exists, clients are not going to seek health services (Becker, 1972).

Dyer (1973) also describes family indecision as a problem. In this instance, family members have difficulty making decisions or tend to use a "de facto style" when making decisions (letting things just happen). Such families often need the nurse to explore with them their feelings and the pros and cons about various options. Rather than assuming responsibility for making the family's decisions and inadvertently encouraging dependency, it is recommended that the nurse assume the role of a supportive resource person to the family.

In any of these situations, it is important for the nurse to probe into what is happening within the family and to be curious about the root of the problem so that it can be identified and subsequently addressed.

Nurse-related Barriers.
Often we think of barriers to implementing interventions as behaviors separate and apart from ourselves. However, some barriers to effective implementation of interventions may be related to the nurse's ideas or behaviors. As professional nurses, we must routinely reflect on our own beliefs and behaviors as we work with families to ensure that we are not inadvertently closing down options for them. Some common barriers are listed below with an example of a self-reflective question that the nurse may routinely ask himself or herself to avoid such barriers:

Barrier 1: Imposing Ideas.   The nurse assumes, and thus engages, in a noncollaborative relationship (a "one up" stance) with the family. Here the nurse may fall into the trap of imposing her or his ideas on the family without fully considering their expertise and ideas. The nurse assumes full responsibility for the nursing plan and its implementation (as opposed to an equal, nonhierarchical approach in which both nurse input and family input are respected and encouraged).

Self-reflective Question: "How frequently are decisions about the patient's health care made mutually by the patient, family, and myself?" (Leahey & Harper-Jaques, 1996, p. 139).

Barrier 2: Negative Labeling.   The nurse may negatively label the family (or himself or herself) when interventions appear unsuccessful. For example, if a family returns for a clinic visit and has not implemented the nurse's ideas, the nurse may refer to this family as "resistant" or view his or her actions as "ineffective."

Self-reflective Question: When interventions are not successful, what might I do differently? What might the family do differently?

Barrier 3: Overlooking Strengths.   The nurse highlights weaknesses and problems in the family and pays little or less attention to the strengths and resources that exist.

Self-reflective Question: "What interventions can I use to further enhance this family's strengths?" (Leahey & Harper-Jaques, 1996, p. 145).

Barrier 4: Neglecting Cultural or Gender Implications.   The nurse does not sufficiently take into account ethnic or cultural diversity or gender issues when planning interventions with the family.

Self-reflective Question: In what ways does my plan of care reflect the cultural needs of this family? What, if any, are my own cultural or gender biases that may be constraining my work with this family?

▶ EVALUATION

The fifth component of the nursing process is evaluation. The evaluation is based on how effective the interventions were that the family, nurse, and others instituted. Effectiveness is determined by looking at *family member outcomes* (how the family responded), rather than the interventions implemented. The evaluation, again, is a joint endeavor between the nurse and the family.

Although a client-centered approach to evaluation is most relevant, it is often frustrating because of the difficulties in establishing objective criteria for desired outcomes and because of factors other than planned interventions that intervene and affect family/client outcomes. Because of such factors, one never gets a clear-cut, "pure" look at the efficacy of nursing intervention.

The nursing care plan contains the framework for evaluation. If clear, specific behavioral goals have been delineated, these can then serve as the criteria for evaluating the degree of effectiveness achieved. In some instances there may be a need to develop even more specific criteria for evaluation of goals. For example, the goal, "The family will seek medical services for their sick baby," may need more specific criteria to judge whether the goal has been attained. Criteria for evaluation might include the fact that the family has been seen by a pediatrician and has received treatment for the baby's illness. In many cases, however, the goal is written in more specific terms to avoid further criteria development, such as, "The child will obtain diagnostic and treatment services from pediatrician within 1 to 3 days."

Evaluation is an ongoing process that occurs each time a nurse updates the nursing care plan. Before care plans are expanded or modified, certain nursing actions will need to be looked at jointly by the nurse and family to see if they are really helpful. Unless family responses to nursing intervention are jointly evaluated, ineffective nursing action may persist.

The following questions should be contemplated when evaluating:

1. Is there a consensus between the family and other health care team members on the evaluation?

2. What additional data need to be collected to evaluate progress?

3. Were there any unforeseen outcomes that need to be considered?

4. If the family's behavior and perceptions indicate that the problem has not been satisfactorily resolved, what are the reasons?

5. Were the nursing diagnoses, goals, and approaches realistic and accurate?

Various methods of evaluation are used in nursing. Martin (1994) discussed some methods for measuring the quality of nursing practice. To this end, she recommended the use of: case conferences; shared evaluation visits and observations, record audits, peer reviews, and utilization reviews; client satisfaction surveys; and external audits. The most important factor is that the method needs to be tailored to the goals and interventions being evaluated.

▶ MODIFICATION

Modification follows the evaluation plan and begins the cyclical process of returning to the assessment and reassessing—feeding in the new information obtained from previous encounters, and then continuing to revise each phase in the cycle as needed.

Modification is often difficult to do, as it can be frustrating and ego deflating to admit our plan and implementation were ineffective. So often in working with families on a long-term basis we see only very slow results or perhaps no movement of a family at all—at least not when we are working with them. At this point we need to make sure that if we continue our search for a more accurate diagnosis or a more effective plan, our efforts have some chance of success and the resources to be expended will be commensurate with the gain achieved. It is most important, however, to keep foremost in our minds the principle of self-determination—that families have a right to decide what is best for them and to make their own health decisions.

Table 3–3 presents a family nursing care plan example, using the process outlined in this chapter.

▶ TERMINATION

There is a dearth of literature about effectively terminating work with families. It is difficult to know when the time is right to put closure on the nurse–family relationship. Wright and Leahey (1994) state that the most important indicator of termination "is the family's ability to master or live with problems, not to eliminate them" (p. 211). Discussion about termination should occur early on, so that both nurse and family are clear about expectations. Regular review of goals and progress helps to prevent problems with termination. Final termination may be initiated by the nurse, the family, or by another professional or agency (Wright & Leahey, 1994). It is ideal when termination is mutually agreed upon by family and nurse and when time is set aside, to have a final conversation about the work completed. Nurses need to be cautious about continuing to work with families when they are showing an ability to live with their problems, otherwise continu-

ing to work with the family may encourage unnecessary family dependency. Wright and Leahey (1994) provide a list of nursing actions that can be used in the therapeutic termination of the nurse–family relationship: review contracts, decrease the frequency of sessions, give credit to the family for changes it has made, evaluate family interviews, and offer follow-up services or referrals. These actions help to place a closure on the relationship and are intended to assist the family to sustain positive gains.

▶ study questions

Choose the correct answer(s) to the following question.

1. The primary difference between the nursing process when working with families versus working solely with individual clients is (select the best answer):
   a. The community setting must be assessed.
   b. The level of assessment, diagnosis, planning, implementation, and evaluation is broadened to include the family, its subsystems, and its members.
   c. The level of assessment, diagnosis, planning, implementation, and evaluation is the family system.
   d. Prevention and health promotion are the aim versus cure and rehabilitation when working with individuals.

2. Match the correct process characteristics in the left-hand column with the nursing phase/component on the right.

Process Characteristics

   a. Continuous data collection
   b. Approaches based on identified goals
   c. Client outcome appraisal
   d. Anticipated behaviorally stated client responses
   e. Setting of priorities
   f. Nursing action, therapy, or approaches
   g. Execution of the nursing care plan
   h. Existing or potential family and individual health problem
   i. Mobilizing community resources
   j. Identification of resources
   k. Refinement and revision efforts
   l. Defining alternative approaches

Phase/Components of Nursing Process

   1. Assessment
   2. Diagnosis
   3. Goal setting
   4. Plan of care
   5. Intervention
   6. Evaluation
   7. Modification

3. The nursing assessment is (choose the best answer):
   a. Based on initial gathering of data.
   b. Done by all persons involved in providing client care.
   c. A sensitive and continuing process conducted by all involved health providers.

4. One objective in terms of completing a family assessment process is the setting up of priorities for intervention.
   a. True.
   b. False.
   c. Uncertain.

Match the nurse's statements with the appropriate step in the nursing process.

   a. Establishing a relationship.
   b. Obtaining information.
   c. Clarification of focal problem.
   d. Assessment of strengths and resources.
   e. Formulation of a therapeutic plan and mobilization of client's and others' resources.

5. "How have things been with your family?"

6. "I'm concerned about your problem and would like to know more."

7. "Can you tell me about the fight with your wife?"

8. "How can I be most helpful to you and your family at this time?"

9. "When you discuss your worries with your sister, what is her response?"

10. List three activities the family health nurse could carry out in preparation for a home visit.

Fill in the space in the following question.

11. NANDA recommends that a nursing diagnosis contain the statement of the problem, its etiology or contributing factors, and defining characteristics. Explain one advantage to using this method for diagnosing client problems.

   _____

   _____

Choose the correct answer(s) to the following question.

12. In planning nursing intervention, priorities need to be established. These variables are significant when establishing priorities:
    a. Family/individual interests and perceptions.
    b. Degree of urgency or acuteness of problem.
    c. Availability of resources.
    d. Agency policies.
    e. Actions that are prerequisite to other actions.

Fill in the space in the following question.

13. Active family involvement in the nursing process should occur during

    _____

    _____

    _____ phase(s) of the nursing process.

After reading the vignette, answer the following questions.

14. Mr. and Mrs. Wong's daughter, age 5, has been observed several times by kindergarten teachers in grand mal seizures. The school nurse, while visiting the family, discusses the convulsions and need for medical follow-up at a special clinic in a nearby community. She notes that the parents change the subject, brushing off observed seizures as temper tantrums. They state that the family does not have time to take her to a doctor and that "professionals don't ever listen to us."
    a. What type of family-related barrier does the school nurse have in working with this family?
    b. What may be the basis for this family-related barrier?
    c. What might be a possible nurse-related barrier that might be contributing to the problem?

15. List two situations when family nursing intervention may be indicated according to Wright and Leahey (1994).

Select one answer to the following questions.

16. A widely used (in community health nursing) classification scheme for client problems is the:
    a. NANDA system of nursing diagnosis.
    b. Freeman classification.
    c. Omaha system.
    d. None of the above.

17. In the list below select two *major* concepts of change that are important to consider when assisting families to make changes.
    a. Change depends on the nature of the stressors families face.
    b. Change only occurs if both parents are in agreement.
    c. Gaining the right information leads to change.
    d. Change is situationally determined.
    e. The client's perception of the problem is critical in considering change.

Provide the short answers indicated.

18. What are three sources of data for family assessment? _____
    _____

19. Which classification of interventions contains "supplemental," "facilita-
    tive," and "developmental" categories? _____

20. List the three domains of family functioning discussed in the Calgary
    Family Intervention Model and one possible intervention that could be
    directed at each domain.

21. State two family intervention labels developed by Craft and Willadsen.

22. Relative to family nursing practice, indicate whether the following about
    NANDA nursing diagnoses classification is a strength, a limitation, or
    neither in the list below (s = strength, l = limitation, and n = neither).
    ____a. Diagnoses are individually oriented.
    ____b. Diagnoses are predominantly problem- or illness-oriented.
    ____c. Diagnoses cut across all nursing settings.
    ____d. Diagnoses are each generated by a group of experts, submitted to
            NANDA, and carefully considered.
    ____e. Diagnoses are in state of expansion and refinement.
    ____ f. Statements of family problems are broad.

23. According to Wright and Leahey (1994), the most important indicator of
    therapeutic termination with a family is _____.

► chapter 3 study answers

1. b.

2. a. 1.   g. 5
   b. 5.   h. 2.
   c. 6.   i. 5.
   d. 3.   j. 4.
   e. 2 and/or 4.   k. 7.
   f. 5.   l. 4.

3. c.

4. b.

5. a and b.

6. a, b, and c.

7. b or c.

8. e.

9. d and e.

10. Any three:
    a. Review written records.
    b. Discuss the family with other health care team members who know the family well.
    c. Gather whatever information, teaching supplies, and assessment and intervention equipment are needed or anticipated.
    d. Call family on phone to set up visit if possible.

11. One advantage to using this method of diagnosing is that the symptoms and etiologic factors lead to more comprehensive setting of goals and approaches.

12. All choices (a–e) are correct.

13. All phases, since the family and its members are the crucial, central focus of our services and must be involved in all phases in order for each phase to be accomplished.

14. a. Apathy.
    b. Any of the following: difference in value system, difference in perception of problem due to ignorance or fear, and sense of futility about available resources.
    c. Possible nurse-related barriers to consider are: imposing ideas, overlooking strengths, neglecting cultural or gender implications.

15. Any of these: a family presents with a problem(s) in which the relationships between family members are affected; a family member presents with an illness that is having an obvious detrimental impact on the other family members; family members contribute to the symptoms or problems of an individual; one family member's improvement leads to symptoms or deterioration in another family member; a family member is first diagnosed with an illness; a child or adolescent develops an emotional, behavioral, or physical problem in the context of a family member's illness; a chronically ill family member moves from an institution back to the community; an ill family member dies.

16. c.

17. d and e.

18. Interview data, observational data, responses from questionnaires, checklists, and agency written records.

19. Freeman's classification.

20. Three domains of family functioning and their respective intervention(s) are:

Domain	Possible Interventions
1. Cognitive	Offering information/opinions, reframing, offering education, externalizing the problem, and interventive questions directed at the cognitive domain.
2. Affective	Validating/normalizing responses, storying the illness experience, drawing forth family support, and interventive questions directed at the affective domain.
3. Behavioral	Encouraging family members as caregivers, encouraging respite, devising rituals, and interventive questions directed at the behavioral domain.

21. Any of the family intervention labels are correct: family support, family process maintenance, family integrity promotion, family involvement, family mobilization, caregiver support, family therapy, sibling support, and parent education: adolescent.

22. a. l.
     b. l.
     c. s.
     d. s.
     e. s.
     f. n.

23. The family's ability to master or live with problems, not necessarily to eliminate them.

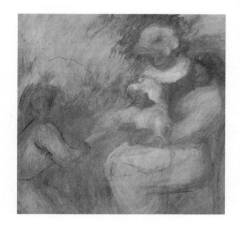

two

THEORETICAL FOUNDATIONS

The theoretical foundations for family nursing practice are described in Part II. Theoretical perspectives used in family nursing are reviewed in Chapter 4. Although family social science and family therapy theories still form the basis for most of family nursing practice to date, notable progress is being made to reformulate family theories to fit a nursing perspective and to use nursing theories in family nursing practice. Chapters 5 through 7 present the three theories that are the primary basis for the Friedman Family Assessment Model (see Appendices A and B for the complete model). These three theoretical perspectives are structural–functional theory (Chap. 5), family developmental theory (Chap. 6), and systems theory (Chap. 7).

4

Theoretical Approaches to Family Nursing

Shirley May Harmon Hanson, Joanna Rowe Kaakinen, and Marilyn M. Friedman

► learning objectives

1. Explain the advantages inherent in deriving family nursing practice from a theoretical framework model.
2. Discuss the three sources of family nursing theory and their contribution to the specialty.
3. Explain how family nursing theory contributes to family nursing practice.
4. Describe the basic assumptions of each nursing model, family social science theory, and family therapy theory presented in this chapter.

5. Discuss the current state of the art in regard to theory development in family nursing.
6. Identify the theoretical legacy of the three integrated family systems nursing models: Calgary Family Assessment and Intervention Models, the Family Stressor–Strengths Model/Inventory, and the Friedman Family Assessment Model.

Theoretical and conceptual frameworks are necessary to guide the practice and research of family nursing. This background is even more critical in respect to family nursing because thinking interactionally and systematically in family nursing requires a paradigm shift from the individual-as-client approach to that of family-as-client. The purpose of this chapter is to provide a basic grounding in the major theoretical/conceptual approaches used to practice family nursing and to conduct family nursing research.

► WHAT IS THEORY?

The function of theory is to characterize, explain, or predict phenomena evident within nursing. Thus, nursing theories ideally represent logical and intelligible patterns for observations within nursing practice (Fawcett & Downs, 1992). The relationship of theory to practice constitutes a dynamic feedback loop rather than a static linear progression. That is, family nursing theory informs practice, and family practice, in turn, facilitates the development of family nursing theory. Thus, the theory, practice, and research related to family nursing are mutually dependent on each other.

A conceptual model is defined as a set of abstract and general concepts and propositions that integrate concepts into a meaningful configuration (Fawcett, 1995). Conceptual models evolve from the empirical observations and intuitive insights of scholars and/or from deductions that creatively combine ideas from several fields of inquiry. Conceptual models provide a distinct frame of reference and a coherent internally unified way of thinking about nursing.

A conceptual model consists of concepts and propositions. Concepts are words that describe mental images of phenomena (Fawcett, 1995). The "family" is an example of a concept that should be in any conceptual model for family nursing. Propositions are statements that describe or link concepts. An example of a proposition would be the notion of "interaction" linking the concept of "family" to another concept such as "community," i.e., the family interacts with the community.

A *theory* is less abstract than its parent conceptual model. Theories are subject to rules of organization and are composed of concepts, relationship between concepts (propositions), relationships between propositions, and connections between propositions and the empirical world of observation (Klein & White, 1996). Theories purport to account for or organize some phenomena and are used to describe, explain, or predict specific and concrete phenomena (Fawcett, 1995). Theories vary tremendously in their level of abstraction or generality, as well as in their scope of applicability and the number of phenomena they address. Theories are generally classified as grand, middle range, or low level (also called single domain).

Within the various theories, theoretical perspectives, conceptual models, or "streams of influence," to be described in this chapter, much overlap of ideas can be seen. There has been a substantial amount of cross-fertilization between theorists, whereby concepts originating in one theory have been translated into similar concepts in another theory. Many of the notions within nursing theories incorporate concepts borrowed from earlier grand and middle-range theories of sociology, anthropology, and psychology. Concepts such as interaction,

stressors, environment, self-concept, or self-esteem are examples of nursing concepts borrowed from the behavioral and social sciences. Likewise the family social science theories have used the earlier grand theories and concepts of developmental theory, symbolic interactionism, structural–functional, social change, and general systems theory, and applied them to the family. Also family therapy theories have adapted concepts and propositions from the family social sciences, particularly general systems theory, as foundations for their theory development.

▶ WHY THEORY?

According to Klein and White (1996), the major function of theory is to provide knowledge to improve our services to families. There are seven ways in which theories directly contribute to the immediate goals of science and more indirectly to the improvement of family services:

1. Accumulation. Theories assist in the accumulation and organization of research findings.

2. Precision. Theories articulate ideas more clearly and specifically than is possible in everyday language.

3. Guidance. Theories direct researchers to develop and test hypotheses (i.e., empirical statements about what the data are expected to look like).

4. Connectedness. Theories demonstrate how ideas are connected to each other and to other theories. They are systematic sets of ideas.

5. Interpretation. Theories help to make sense about how the phenomena they address operate.

6. Prediction. Theories point to what may or could happen in the future.

7. Explanation. Theories provide answers to "why" and "how" questions.

For the purpose of this chapter, the terms conceptual frameworks and theories may be used interchangeably. Typically, we call the work from nursing, conceptual frameworks, and the work from family social science and family therapy, theories.

► CONCEPTUAL SOURCES FOR FAMILY NURSING THEORIES

Family nursing theories are an evolving synthesis of the scholarship from three traditions (Fig. 4–1) (Hanson & Boyd, 1996b). At the present time, there is no singular theory/conceptual framework from nursing, family social science, or family therapy that fully describes the relationships and dynamics for family life and family nursing. Thus, an *integrated* approach is necessary for the theory, practice, research, and education of family nursing. One theoretical perspective does not give nurses a sufficiently broad knowledge upon which to assess and intervene with families. Hence, nurses must draw upon multiple theories to work effectively with families. (See Table 4–1 for criteria for evaluating family theories useful to family nursing.)

Of the three genres of theory, the family social science theories are the most well developed and informative with respect to how families function, the environment–family interchange, interactions within the family, how the family changes over time, and the family's reaction to health and illness. One striking limitation in using the family social science theories as a basis for assessment and intervention in family nursing is that their clinical application is parsimonious, although recent work has made some strides in this direction (Berkey & Hanson, 1991; Hanson & Boyd, 1996b; Wright & Leahey, 1994).

Family therapy theories, although less developed than family social science theories, are more relevant to family nursing practice because they emanate from a professional/practice heritage rather than academic

► TABLE 4–1

CRITERIA FOR EVALUATING FAMILY THEORIES

1. *Internal consistency:* A theory does not contain logically contradictory assertions.
2. *Clarity or explicitness:* The ideas in a theory are expressed in such a way that they are unambiguous. They are defined and explicated where necessary.
3. *Explanatory power:* A theory explains well what it is intended to explain.
4. *Coherence:* The key ideas in a theory are integrated or interconnected, and loose ends are avoided.
5. *Understanding:* A theory provides a comprehensible sense of the whole phenomenon being examined.
6. *Empirical fit:* A large portion of the tests of a theory have been confirmatory or at least have not been interpreted as disconfirming.
7. *Testability:* It is possible for a theory to be empirically supported or refuted.
8. *Heuristic value:* A theory has generated or can generate considerable research and intellectual curiosity (including a large number of empirical studies, as well as much debate or controversy).
9. *Groundedness:* A theory has been built up from detailed information about events and processes observable in the world.
10. *Contextualization:* A theory gives serious consideration to the social and historical contexts affecting or affected by its key ideas.
11. *Interpretive sensitivity:* A theory reflects the experiences practiced and felt by the social units to which it is applied.
12. *Predictive power:* A theory can successfully predict phenomena that have occurred since it was formulated.
13. *Practical utility:* A theory can be readily applied to social problems, policies, and programs of action (i.e., it is useful for teaching, therapy, political action, or some combination of these).

Adapted from Klein, D.M. & White, J.M. (1996). Family theories: An introduction—understanding families. Thousand Oaks, Calif.: Sage Publications.

disciplines, such as family social science. Many of the family therapy theories stem from a foundation in family social science theories. Increasingly so, family nursing theory, practice, and research are drawing from family therapy theories as the profession grows more sophisticated within the specialty of family nursing. Family therapy models are also more applicable to advanced nursing practice. Whall (1986b) urged family nurse therapists to reformulate existing family therapy theories to fit the nursing perspective in accordance with nursing theory.

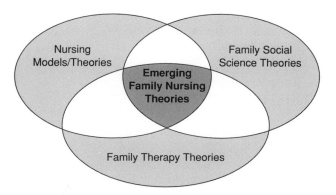

Figure 4–1. Conceptual source of family nursing theories.

Finally, of all three genres of theories, nursing models/theories are the least developed in regard to family nursing. During the 1960s and 1970s, one of nursing's emphases was on the development of nursing models. Of the major nursing models, some fit some nursing settings and functions more than others. The major drawback to nursing models is that they originated in an individual paradigm and only a few evolved to fit a family nursing focus (Berkey & Hanson, 1991). The nursing models, in large part, represent a deductive approach to the development of nursing science and embody an important part of our nursing heritage. However, in the 1990s, the nursing frameworks and their deductive approach (general to specific) are being viewed critically. More inductive approaches (specific to general) to nursing theory development are being advocated.

The remainder of this chapter presents each of the three genres of theories that are significant to evolving family nursing theories (see Tables 4–2 and 4–3). The major nursing conceptual frameworks that are most applicable to family nursing are presented. First, some nursing models/theories are summarized, then the dominant family social science theories that are central to family nursing are highlighted. Three significant family therapy theories are then presented that contribute significantly to family nursing. And finally, several integrated models are briefly discussed.

► NURSING MODELS AND THEORIES

Historically nursing drew from the knowledge base of many disciplines, but the development of nursing models and theories during the last three decades has profoundly influenced the discipline of nursing. In the evolving conceptual models of family nursing, the *first tradition* that influenced family nursing theory came from the legacy of nursing theorists such as Nightingale, King, Roy, Neuman, Orem, and Rogers.

The discipline of nursing is concerned with the concepts of person, environment, health, and nursing, which are melded together with the following three propositions:

1. Nursing is concerned with the principles and laws that govern the life process, well-being,

---

► TABLE 4-2

THEORETICAL APPROACHES USED IN FAMILY NURSING PRACTICE

Nursing Theories/Conceptual Models

Systems orientation
  • Neuman's systems conceptual model
Developmental orientation
  • Orem's self-care model
Systems and interactional orientations
  • Roy's adaptation model
  • King's interacting systems model
Systems and developmental orientations
Rogers's life process model
Others:
  • Nightingale
  • Friedemann

Family Social Science Theories

Developmental theory
Systems theory
Structural–functional theory
Interactional/Communications theory
Family Stress theory
Change theory
Others:
  • Conflict theory
  • Social exchange theory
  • Multicultural theory

Family Therapy Theories

Structural family therapy theory
Family systems therapy theory
Interactional/Communications family therapy theory
Others:
  • Psychodynamic therapy theory
  • Experiential therapy theory
  • Strategic therapy theory
  • Behavioral therapy theory
  • Solution-oriented therapy theory
  • Narrative therapy theory

---

and optimum function of human beings, sick or well.

2. Nursing is concerned with the patterning of human behavior in interaction with the environment in normal life events and critical life situations.

► TABLE 4–3

DIFFERENCES AMONG NURSING THEORIES, FAMILY SOCIAL SCIENCE THEORIES, AND FAMILY THERAPY THEORIES

Criteria	Nursing Theories	Family Social Science Theories	Family Therapy Theories
Purpose of theory	Descriptive and prescriptive (practice models); guide nursing assessment and intervention efforts.	Descriptive and explanatory (academic models); explain family functioning and dynamics.	Descriptive and prescriptive (practice models); explain fully dysfunction and guide therapeutic actions.
Discipline focus	Nursing focus.	Interdisciplinary (although primarily sociological).	Marriage and family therapy, and family mental health.
Target population	Primarily those families with health and illness problems.	Primarily "normal" families (normality-oriented).	Primarily "troubled" families (pathology-oriented).

Adapted from Jones and Dimond (1982).

3. Nursing is concerned with the processes by which positive changes in health status are effected (Whall & Fawcett, 1991b, p. 3).

Whall and Fawcett (1991b) augmented the above propositions of nursing to address family:

1. Family [nursing] is concerned with the principles and laws that govern family process, family well-being, and optimum function of families in various states of illness and wellness.

2. Family [nursing] is concerned with the patterning of family behavior in interaction with the environment, in normal life events and critical life situations.

3. Family [nursing] is concerned with the processes by which positive changes in family health status may be effected (Donaldson & Crowley, 1978; Gordner, 1980, cited by Whall, 1991b, pp. 3–4).

The person aspect of the discipline of nursing began with the focus on the individual. However, to stay current with the nursing educational system, the concept of client should be broadened to include individual, family, and/or community (ANA, 1995). We agree with Gilliss (1991) who argued that replacing the term "family" for "individual" within a nursing theory negates the complexity of the family system. Hence, to apply the major nursing theories to family, one must look to other nurse scholars who have delved into a variety of interdisciplinary theo-

ries and developed family theoretical approaches to nursing practice. Some nursing theorists have amplified their original theoretical works to include family in their conceptual frameworks and nursing models.

Whall and Fawcett (1991a) suggested that family is articulated differently in the metaparadigm of nursing from other disciplines addressing the family by the following three aspects:

• Considering environmental influences on family health and the effect of actions taken by nurses on behalf of or in conjunction with the family,

• Incorporating comprehensive biopsychosocial or holistic perspective of health, and

• Focusing on family well-being, rather than pathology (p. 4).

Whall and Fawcett (1991a) stated that there is little evidence of formal family theory in nursing. Yet, the concept of family-as-client has been accepted in the nursing discipline as is evidenced in the literature from 1950 through 1990 (Whall & Fawcett, 1991a) and in the recent ANA *Social Policy Statement* (1995) and the various ANA's *Standards of Clinical Nursing Practice* (see Chap. 2 for details). Family has become a specific unit of study, but "there remains virtually no evidence of formal middle-range family theory that is unique or distinctive to nursing" (Whall & Fawcett, 1991a, p. 15). This lack of interdisciplinary focus gives strong support for the interdisciplinary model presented in Figure 4–1.

Several nursing conceptual frameworks and nursing theories, however, are specifically suited to family nursing practice. Distinct aspects of these theories are presented in historical order. The reader is referred to the bibliography for more detailed resources and specifics of each framework.

Nightingale

Florence Nightingale did not actually present a theory of nursing or family nursing. Nevertheless, she acknowledged the family in many of her writings and in much of her nursing practice (Nightingale, 1859). In 1852, at the age of 32 years, Florence Nightingale wrote:

> The family? It is too narrow a field for the development of an immortal spirit, be that spirit male or female. The family uses people not for what they are, not for what they are intended to be, but for what it wants them for—for its own uses. . . . This system dooms some minds to incurable infancy, others to silent misery. (Nightingale, 1949, p. 37)

Obviously, Nightingale was chafing under the sexist restraints of her time and class. But in spite of her personal sense of family-induced constraints, she firmly believed that the family was one supportive institution that followed its members from cradle to grave. She supported helping women and children toward good health by promoting both nurse-midwifery and home-based health services. In 1876, in a document entitled "Training Nurses for the Sick Poor," she admonished nurses to engage in both sick nursing and health nursing in the home environment. She appeared to have given both home-health nurses and maternal–child nurses the charge to carry out nursing practice with the whole family as the unit-of-service (Nightingale, 1949).

King

Imogene King (1981, 1987) developed an interacting systems conceptual framework and a middle-range Theory of Goal Attainment. In her earliest works, King included a family-as-context approach. She broadly defined family as a small group of individuals who are bound together for the socialization of its members. The family was viewed as both an interpersonal and a social system. King's concept of individual client can be expanded to include family, which represents the interpersonal system. The social system aspect of family was presented as transmitting values and norms of behavior across the life span (King, 1983; Frey & Sieloff, 1995). "The Theory of Goal Attainment encompassed several concepts that are relevant to families, including perception, interaction, communication, transaction, space, time, growth and development, and stress" (Whall & Fawcett, 1991a, p. 17).

Roy

In 1976, Sister Callista Roy presented the Adaptation Model, which viewed the individual as an adaptive system that responds to environmental stimuli via four response modes: physiological, self concept, role function, and interdependence. In Roy's original work (1976) the family is seen as context to the individual. Later, Roy and Roberts (1981) altered this family-as-context conceptualization to the "family as an adaptive system that, like the individual, has inputs, internal control and feedback processes, and output" (Whall & Fawcett, 1991a, p. 23).

Describing her Adaptation Model and how the family is incorporated, Roy explained that the family, as well as the individual, group, social organization, and community, may be the unit of analysis and a focus of nursing practice. Roy's Theory of Adaptation seems to hold promise in terms of describing and explaining family nursing phenomena. McCubbin and Figley (1983) suggested that the concept of coping in Roy's model could easily be broadened to the family unit, where ineffective family coping patterns lead to family functioning problems. Moreover, Roy's theory stressed health promotion and the importance of assisting clients in manipulating their environment, which are significant elements in family nursing.

Neuman

The Neuman Health Care Systems Model (Neuman, 1982) addressed the family as a client from the beginning of the development of this framework. Betty Neuman (1983) defined the family as "a group of two or more persons who create and maintain a common culture; its most central goal is one of continuance" (p. 241). According to Neuman, the family may be viewed as a system composed of family member subsystems. The focus of Neuman's theory is primarily on relationships among individual family members. The family system is exposed to stressors that affect its stability and threaten its state of wellness. The family's goal is to maintain stability by preserving the integrity of its basic structure (Whall & Fawcett, 1991b).

Hanson and Mischke (1996) and Berkey and Hanson (1991) presented a Family Assessment Intervention Model that was adapted from Neuman's Health Care Systems Model. They modified Neuman's assumptions so that they incorporate a family focus. These assumptions are:

1. Good assessment requires knowledge of all factors that influence the family's perceptual field.

2. Most nursing care delivered to families occurs during transition periods.

3. The well family demonstrates a spectrum of abilities, insights, and strengths.

4. Family members of the dynamic unit are engaged in tasks aimed at personal development and continuation of the family system.

5. The family, as well as the caregiver, validates the meaning a stressor holds for the family.

6. Factors in the nurse's perceptual field that influence assessment of the family situation will become apparent (Hanson & Mischke, 1996, pp. 175–176).

Hanson and Mischke (1996) stated that families are consistently exposed to stressors on a daily basis that challenge the stability of the family unit. Families develop coping strategies to maintain equilibrium and conserve energy resources. The family unit is influenced when any member experiences a stressor or the whole family experiences a stressor that threatens the ability of the family system. Working together, family nurses and families strive for the goal of family stability. Each family responds to stress events based on (1) the perception of the situation, and (2) the family's ability to adjust and restore the impaired family function created by the stressor.

The Family Assessment Intervention Model (Hanson & Mischke, 1996; Berkey and Hanson, 1991)

focuses on (1) wellness/promotion and classification of the problems, (2) family reactions and the degree of instability, and (3) restoration of family stability and function. This model is an excellent example of an adaptation of the Neuman conceptual framework based on actual family nursing practice. The Family System Stressors Strengths Inventory (FS³I) is an instrument that evolved from this model and is used for family assessment as well as family measurement.

Tomlinson and Anderson (1995) further analyzed Neuman's model. They defined family health as "a holistic function of the family system and its health promotion capability" (p. 134). Anderson and Tomlinson (1992) presented a Family Health System paradigm that merged concepts of family health, nursing practice, and Neuman's Health Care Systems Model. Within five broad areas, these nursing scholars make specific statements that demonstrate ways in which Neuman's theory interfaces with the Family Health System paradigm (Tomlinson and Anderson, 1995). These address:

1. Complexity of the system. "The level of complexity would need to shift when using the family health systems perspective to consider not only the individual stressor response in relation to the family but also the family's response relative to lines of defense and resistance . . . The concept of health in families must include the collective family system's definition of health. . . Perception of health thus rests within the family's construction of the meaning of health and illness (p. 138–139)."

2. The core of the family. "The family health systems paradigm goes beyond looking at the family as composed of individual members and postulates that consideration for individual family members should be viewed from the perspective of the collective tension between the individual, dyadic, and family systems in meeting their unique goals in relation to the environment (p. 139)."

3. The goal of family health. "From a family health system perspective, it is most desirable to facilitate client system wellness using strengths to reduce stressor effects and enhance family growth toward positive transformation of its central structure as a result of a significant illness experience (p. 140)."

4. Nurse entry point in caring for families. "The nurse enters a partnership with the family which empowers the family "in making decisions about their own family health issues (p. 140)."

5. Nursing interaction. "In the Family Health Systems concept, family systems approach by the caregiver becomes 'shared caregiver role' to help conserve family system energy as it moves toward optimal stability or wellness (140)."

The Neuman conceptual nursing model may become even more important in the 21st century as the emphasis of health care continues to move toward community-based health care. (See Hanson and Mischke [1996] for further development of this model to families.)

Orem

Dorothea Orem's (1971) Model of Self-Care can be extended beyond its original parameters of individual to family self-care. In the original work, Orem (1971) did not address family in the self-care theory other than to indicate that nurses will need to work with family members to help the family member achieve self care. Orem (1983a, 1983b) described the family as a basic conditioning unit in which the individual learns culture, roles, and responsibilities. Later, Orem (1985) suggested that people receive health care as individuals and as members of a multiperson unit, i.e., a family. In Orem's theory, the family is viewed mostly as the context of the individual client and not as a recipient of care itself.

Gray (1996) presented the following paradigm for family nurses based on a set of assumptions for self-care:

1. Self-care can be evaluated by families in a variety of situations. Orem's theory permits the assessment of families in relation to their self-care potential as it relates to health promotion and health protection. Each individual family member is viewed as a self-care agent who makes a personal continuous contribution to his or her own health.

2. Self-care relates to the personal values and health beliefs of the family. This allows

the family's self-care behavior to evolve through a combination of social and cognitive experiences that have been learned through interpersonal relationships, communication, and culture that are unique to each family.

3. Self-care can be administered to families by self-care agents. Specifically, this allows the family members, either individually or collectively, to initiate and perform self-care requisites that includes attitudes about their health and their ability to perform self-care behaviors.

4. Self-care can be used to foster the promotion of health in families and to recognize and evaluate areas where diminished health may exist (p. 88).

Orem's Self-Care Nursing Model can be expanded to include families as a unit of care.

Rogers

Martha Rogers (1970, 1986, 1990) viewed the human being as a unitary multidimensional energy field that is engaged in a continuous mutual process with the environment. Her conceptual framework is known as the Science of Unitary Human Beings. Much of Rogers's model reflects the influence of general systems theory. Fawcett (1991), in expanding Rogers's model, posited that the family is a constant open system energy field that is ever-changing in response to its interaction with the environment. Casey (1996) described five assumptions of Rogers's theory that apply to family nursing:

1. The family unit is viewed in its wholeness; unity is composed of subsystems that are interdependent and that together form a unity that is different than the sum of the family subsystems.

2. Families are continuously influenced by information within the environment, and depending on the degree of permeability of the boundaries, they are constantly responding to this input.

3. The family system is subject to change, which takes place along a space–time axis. The family moves through stages of development in a sequential, unidirectional manner.

4. The family is an open system in constant inter-action with the environment through exchange of matter and energy that evolves toward a growing level of complexity.

5. The family has the capacity for feeling, for knowing, for comprehending, and for using these processes to determine patterns, make choices, and recognize its environment (pp. 56–57).

Rogers's conceptual framework has been used by nurse researchers as a base for grounding nursing theory and as a base for family nursing practice.

Friedemann

Marie-Louise Friedemann (1995) developed a Framework of Systemic Organization. In her work, family is viewed as a social system that has the expressed goal of transmitting culture to its members. She postulated the following assumptions about families:

1. The family embedded in the civil system transmits culture, the total of human system patterns and values.

2. With the civil system and the environment at large, the family shares the responsibility to provide physical necessities and safety, teach social skills to its members, provide for personal growth and development, allow emotional bonding of family members, and promote a purpose for life and meaning through spirituality.

3. The family satisfies its members' needs for control over their environment and guides them in finding their place in the network of systems through spirituality.

4. All family processes include collectively accepted and coordinated behaviors or strategies that aim at regulating the earthly conditions of space, time, energy and matter in pursuing the four system targets: family stability, growth, control, and spirituality.

5. Family strategies fall into the four process dimensions of system maintenance, system change, coherence, and individualization. The dimensions share collinearity (interdepen-

dence) but exist independently in that none is emphasized at the expense of another in healthy families (pp. 16–17).

Four specific elements that are central to Friedemann's theory are family stability, family growth, family control, and family spirituality. The family offers safety to its members as they learn the group values, norms, and acceptable behaviors. The family grows as its members grow and interact with other civil systems, i.e., schools, church, and work. Family growth is facilitated by communication among its members. By selectively opening or closing its boundaries, the family serves as a buffer from society for its members. Family control is maintained via the organizational structure of the family. Family spirituality connects the family members together emotionally and encourages self-growth of the members (Freidemann, 1995).

Other Nursing Models and Theories

Only a few major nursing frameworks with potential for family nursing were mentioned here. In the future, the major role of seminal nursing theory development will be to provide the foundation for nurses to explore specific phenomena regarding families that surface from their nursing practice. The integration of the nursing frameworks and perspectives with family social science theory and family therapy will be essential as the subspecialty of family nursing becomes more clearly delineated within the discipline of nursing.

▶ FAMILY SOCIAL SCIENCE THEORIES

The *second tradition* that contributes to our model of family nursing theory as depicted in Figure 4–1 comes from the family social sciences. These theories were developed from various family social science disciplines (largely sociology) and originally evolved with little conscious awareness of their potential use by clinicians (Jones & Dimond, 1982). These theories proliferated during the first half of the 20th century so that by the early 1950s there was an attempt to organize the accumulated conceptual knowledge about the family.

Reviewing the literature on social science theoretical frameworks used to study families, it is clear that there has been little consensus as to what theories constitute the major theoretical frameworks. Since the 1960s, it was generally recognized that three family conceptual approaches dominated the field of marriage and the family: (1) structural–functional, (2) interactional, and (3) developmental (Broderick, 1971; Nye & Berardo, 1981, pp. xxv–xxvi). Presently, there is an emergence of other frameworks for studying the family: conflict, exchange, psychoanalytic, social–psychological, developmental, economic, and legal.

More recently three new resources have tracked the state of family social science with more emphasis on their practice utility. In a source book of family theories and methods (Boss, Doherty, LaRossa, Schumm, & Steinmetz, 1993), recent scholars traced the development of family theory, from its origins in religion and philosophy, through the construction of theory and methodology in the mid-20th century, to emerging models emphasizing the interaction between theories and methods. Klein and White (1996) reviewed what they deemed are the major family social science frameworks of today: exchange, symbolic interaction, family development, conflict, systems, and ecological frameworks. Winton (1995) summarized the different frameworks for studying families. In essence, family social science theories are also evolving which have served to make the knowledge base more user friendly for practice disciplines such as family nursing.

The following is a summary of the major theories from the family social science area that have been useful to the understanding of families and family nursing.

Structural–Functional Theory

The structural–functional framework defines the family as a social system. Family analysis consists of examining the family in terms of its relationship with other major social structures (institutions) such as medicine, religion, education, government, and the economy. This perspective looks at the arrangement of members within the family, relationships between the members, and relationships of the members to the whole (Artinian, 1994; Friedman, 1992). The primary focus is to determine how family patterns are related to other institutions and to consider the family in the overall structure of society. Emphasis is placed on the basic functions of families (Hanson & Boyd, 1996b): economic, reproductive, protective,

culture, socialization, status conferring, relationships, and health functions. A central issue of the structural–functional theorist is how well the family structure allows the family to perform its functions. Family theorists who use this approach want to understand the social or family system and its relationship to the overall social system (Nye & Berardo, 1981). This approach characterizes the family as open to outside influences; yet at the same time, the family maintains its boundaries. The family is seen as a passively adapting institution rather than an agent of change. The framework has tended to emphasize a static view of the societal structure and to neglect change as a structural dynamic. Assumptions of this perspective include:

- A family is a social system with functional requirements.
- A family is a small group that has generic features common to all small groups.
- Social systems such as families accomplish functions that serve the individuals in addition to those that serve society.
- Individuals act in accordance with a set of internalized norms and values that are learned primarily in the family through socialization.

This perspective is a useful framework for assessing families and health. Illness of a family member results in alteration of the family structure and function. For example, if a single mother is ill, she cannot carry out her various roles, so grandparents or siblings may have to assume child-care responsibilities. The power structure and communication patterns of the family are affected with illness of parents. Assessment includes determining whether changes due to illness influence the family's ability to carry out its functions. Using this perspective, sample assessment questions could be: How did the death alter the family structure? What family roles were changed with the onset of the chronic illness? Intervention becomes necessary when changes in family structure alter the family's ability to function. Examples of intervention using this model are: assisting families to use existing support structures, and assisting families to modify their organization so that role responsibilities can be distributed.

The major strength of the structural–functional approach to family nursing practice is that it is comprehensive and views families within the broader community context. The major weakness of this approach is its static view, which tends to view families at one moment in time rather than as a system that changes over time. The structural–functional approach was one of this text's three organizing and theoretical frameworks and as such is elaborated in Chapter 5.

Systems Theory

Systems theory is one of the most influential and generative of all the family frameworks. This approach to understanding families was influenced by theory derived from physics and biology by von Bertalanffy (1950, 1968a as cited in Mercer, 1989). A system is composed of a set of interacting elements; each system is identifiable as distinct from the environment in which it exists. An open system exchanges energy and matter with the environment (negentropy) while a closed system is isolated from its environment (entropy). Systems depend on both positive and negative feedback, in order to maintain a steady state (homeostasis). Assumptions of the systems perspective applied to the family system include:

- Family systems are greater than and different from the sum of their parts.
- There are hierarchies within family systems and between subsystems (i.e., mother–child) and the family and community.
- There are boundaries in the family system and they can be open, closed, or random.
- Family systems increase in complexity over time, evolving to allow greater adaptability, tolerance to change, and growth by differentiation.
- Family systems change constantly in response to stresses and strains from within as well as from outside environments. Change in one part of family systems affects the total system.
- Causality is modified by feedback; therefore, causality never exists in the real world.
- Family systems patterns are circular rather than linear, therefore change must be directed toward the cycle.
- Family systems are an organized whole, with individuals in the family being interdependent and interactive.

- Family systems have homeostasis features to maintain stable patterns, which can be adaptive or maladaptive.

The family system perspective encourages nurses to see clients as participating members of a family. Nurses using this perspective assess the effects of illness or injury upon the entire family system and the reciprocal effects of the family on the illness or injury (Wright & Leahey, 1994). Emphasis is on the whole rather than on individuals. Relevant concepts in family systems theory include: subsystems, boundaries, open systems, feedback loops, family interactions, adaptation, and change. A sample of assessment questions includes: Who makes up the family system? How has a family member's critical illness affected the family and its members? Interventions need to address subsystem and whole family processes and functioning.

Four major strengths of the general systems framework are that it is: (1) a grand theory that covers a large array of phenomena, (2) a contextually based theory in that it views the family within the context of its suprasystems (the large community in which it is embedded) and subsystems, (3) an interactionally focused theory, and (4) a holistic theory. It looks at processes in the family rather than content, and at relationships between parts (the relationship between and within subsystems and the relationship between the family and its interacting and suprasystems). The family is viewed as a whole, not as merely a sum of its parts. Two limitations of using this theoretical orientation in family nursing practice are: (1) it is broad and very general, and more specific concepts and practice guidelines need to be developed outside the theory; and (2) this approach may not be as helpful as individually oriented theories for addressing individual client concerns.

General systems theory, because of its broad applicability and noted strengths, was selected in this text as one of the three theoretical perspectives foundational to the Friedman Family Assessment Model. Systems theory is discussed in detail in Chapter 7.

Family Developmental Theory

Individual developmental theory has always been at the core of nursing. Developmental stages were introduced by Freud and expanded by Erikson, Piaget, and others. Basic assumptions of the developmental model include:

- Developmentally-based tasks occur at a specific period.
- Successful achievement leads to happiness and success with later tasks.
- Failure to achieve tasks leads to unhappiness, disapproval, or difficulty in achieving later tasks.

Evelyn Duvall (1977) in her classic book, *Family Development*, took the principles of individual development and applied them to the family as a unit. Her stages of family development were based on the age of the eldest child. She identified overall family tasks that needed to be accomplished for each stage of family development. The stages started with the marriage of couples and ended with death. Developmental concepts include movement to a higher level of functioning implying unidirectional progression. Disequilibrium occurs during the transitional periods from one stage to the other. The intimate small group, called the family, has a predictable natural history designated by stages, beginning with the simple husband–wife pair. The group becomes more complex with the addition of each new position/member over time. The group again becomes simple and less complex as the younger generation leaves home to jobs or marriage. Finally the group comes full circle to the original husband–wife pair. At each family life cycle stage, there are family developmental needs and tasks that must be performed (Duvall & Miller, 1985).

Developmental theory was an attempt to transcend the structural–functional (large-scale analysis) and interactional (small-scale analysis) frameworks: it addressed the passage of time. Its goals were to integrate the small- and large-scale analyses of the other two approaches while viewing the family as an open system in relation to other configurations in society (Jones & Dimond, 1982, p. 13). Developmental theory explains how and what developmentally based changes occur to human organisms or groups over time. Achievement of family developmental tasks assists individual members to accomplish their tasks.

The framework assists family nurses in anticipating clinical problems in families as well as in identifying family strengths. The framework serves as a guide for assessing the family's developmental stage, the extent to which families are fulfilling the tasks associated with their respective stage, the family's developmental history, and the availability of resources essential for performing developmental tasks.

In conducting an assessment of families using the developmental model, several questions can be asked, including: Where does this family place on the continuum of family life cycle stages? What are the developmental tasks that are and are not being accomplished? Typical kinds of nursing intervention strategies using this perspective would be: helping families to understand individual and family growth and development stages, and helping families to deal with the normalcy of transition periods that fall between developmental periods (i.e., tasks of the school-aged family versus tasks of the adolescent family). Family nurses must recognize that in every family there are both individual and family developmental tasks that need to be accomplished for every stage of the individual/family life cycle.

Basic assumptions include:

- Families change and develop in different ways because of internal and environmental stimulation/demands.
- Developmental tasks are goals worked toward rather than specific jobs completed at once.
- Each family is unique in its composition and in the complexity of its age-role expectations and positions.
- Individuals and families are a function of their historical milieu as well as the current social context.
- Families have enough in common despite their uniqueness to chart family development over the family life span.
- Families may arrive at similar developmental levels, through quite different processes.

The major strength of the family developmental approach is that it provides a basis for forecasting what a family will be experiencing at any period in the family life cycle, e.g., role transitions and family constellation changes. The major weakness is the fact that the model was developed at a time in history when the traditional nuclear family was emphasized. The perfect linear progression of families, from marriage through death, is simply not a reality of our times. What happens to the stages of the individual/family life cycle when there is a divorce, death, adoption, and the other multiple forms that we now call family?

Developmental theory was selected in this text as one of the foundational theories guiding the Friedman Family Assessment Model, and will be discussed in detail in Chapter 6.

Family Interactional Theory

The family interactional approach stems from a grand theory in social psychology and sociology, symbolic interaction. Hill and Hansen (1960), Turner (1970), Rose (1962), and others applied the constructs and propositions of this theoretical perspective to the family. The interactional approach focuses on families as units of interacting personalities and examines internal family dynamics, including communication processes, roles, decision making and problem solving, and socialization patterns (Rose, 1962).

In understanding internal family dynamics, one major focus is on family roles. Within the family, each member occupies formal and informal positions. Family members define their role expectations through their perceptions of role demands. They judge their own behavior by obtaining feedback from others in the family. The responses of others serves to challenge or reinforce how family members enact their roles (Nye, 1976). Central to the family interactional approach is the process of role taking (Turner, 1970). In role taking, roles emerge as a consequence of the social interaction between two or more family members (Turner, 1970). Through the process of role taking, family members develop informal roles which may or may not be functional to the family in the long run.

This approach to understanding families' internal dynamics is most relevant to family nursing. Hence, a major strength of its approach is its focus on internal processes within families. Processes rather than outcomes of social interactions are the major focus. The major limitation in using this approach is that the family is examined in a vacuum, with no consideration of the family's context (environment, history, culture, socioeconomic status, etc.). Interactionalists consider families to be comparatively closed units, with the external world having little effect on what occurs within the family.

Assessment of families within an interactional framework emphasizes assessment of interaction/communication between and among family members, family role and power analysis, family coping, relationships between marital partners, siblings, parents, children, and family socialization patterns. Interventions are then generated, based on the family's needs for health promotion, health maintenance, or health restoration in the six above areas.

In this text, the family interactional approach is integrated into the family structural and functional focus. Six chapters address internal family dynamics, including assessment and intervention guidelines: Chapter 10, "Family Communication Processes and Patterns"; Chapter 11, "Family Power Structure"; Chapter 12, "Family Role Structure"; Chapter 14, "The Family Affective Function"; Chapter 15, "The Family Socialization Function"; and Chapter 17, "Family Stress and Coping Processes: Family Adaptation."

Family Stress Theory

The family stress model is especially germane to health care situations because of the pervasive illness-related stress the family experiences (Artinian, 1994). Reuben Hill (1949), who originally developed family stress theory, conducted research on war-induced separation and reunion within families to discover the factors that determine how families under stress adapted. Two important theoretical perspectives emerged from his research. First, he conceptualized that families facing stress sometimes experience a roller-coaster profile of adjustment, which may result in crisis. A decline in family functioning or family disorganization from crisis is followed by an upward recovery curve, and a new level of family organization. Second, he developed the "ABCX" model of family stress, which identified how key factors (stressor, definition/interpretation of stressor event, and resources) result in crisis or noncrisis (Hill, 1965).

In Hill's model, the A variable is the provoking event or stressors with its associated hardships. This event may be such magnitude as to cause change in the family system. The B variable refers to the family's strengths or resources available to assist it in dealing with stressor events. Family resources include religious faith, finances, social support, physical health, family flexibility, and/or family coping mechanisms. The C variable refers to the definition families make of the seriousness of stressor events or the subjective meaning the family attaches to the events. The family's definition of the events determines how it deals with them and how stressful the events will be for the family. This last point is critical, because sometimes nurses cannot understand from the reality of situations why families react in certain ways to events, when indeed they are reacting from their perceptions rather than the reality. All three of these variables influence the family's ability to prevent changes associated with stressor events. Changes created by stressful illness may lead to a crisis, the X variable. The X variable refers to the amount of disruption or incapacitation within the family system due to the stressful event. Susceptibility to crisis is a function of both a deficiency in family resources and the tendency to define hardships as crisis producing. Assumptions of the family stress model include (Artinian, 1994):

- Unexpected or unplanned events are usually perceived as stressful.
- Events within families, such as serious illness, and defined as stressful, are more disruptive than stressors that occur outside the family, such as war, flood, or depression.
- Lack of previous experience with stressor events leads to increased perceptions of stress.
- Ambiguous stressor events are more stressful than nonambiguous events.

Hill's theory was later expanded by McCubbin and Patterson (1983a) to cover the postcrisis period. Called the Double ABCX Model, each of Hill's variables was modified; the notion of coping was inserted as a central predictor of family adaptation. The latest family stress theory, the Resiliency Model (McCubbin & McCubbin, 1993) builds on the former two models and is discussed in depth in Chapter 17.

Assessment areas should cover the prominent variables within the theory itself (i.e., stressors, perception of the stressor event, family resources, family coping, and how much the crisis has disrupted the family functioning). Questions nurses could ask include: Did the family have time to prepare for the event or was it unexpected (i.e., sudden unexpected death versus death after long-term fatal illness)? Has the family experienced similar stressor events? Interventions include: helping families to enhance their resources and support systems, and helping families to modify their subjective perceptions of the events.

The major strengths of this framework are that it is fairly simple to understand, i.e., it makes sense, and it fits what nurses see and do in clinical settings. The model emphasizes that perception of stressor(s) is more important than objective reality and by identifying resources and strengths, family nursing approaches can be developed that empower families. The model is limited in its usefulness for addressing the needs of healthy families in terms of health promotion and disease prevention.

Change Theory

The process of change is important for family nursing theory and practice. The family nurse works with families in order to facilitate change and, therefore, needs to understand the application of change theory as it applies to families.

Nurses are confronted with the paradoxical relationship between persistence (stability) and change in families. Maturana (1978) noted that change is an alteration in the family's structure that occurs as compensation for perturbations and has the purpose of maintaining structure (i.e., stability). According to Wright and Watson (1988) "the most profound and sustaining change [within a family] will be that which occurs within the family's belief system (cognition)" (p. 425).

Watzlawick, Weakland, and Fisch (1974) referred to first- and second-order changes. In first-order change, the system itself remains unchanged while its parts undergo some type of change. For example, learning a new behavioral strategy to discipline a child; the family remains the same but a new approach is used. It is like treating the symptom instead of the cause. In second-order change, a change occurs in the system itself, hence, a "change of change." In second-order change, there are actual changes in the rules governing the system and, therefore, the system is transformed structurally and/or communicationally, sending the family to a different level of functioning. Second-order change is said to occur when parents begin to treat their teenager as a growing adult instead of as a young child.

Families do not change in smooth linear progression, but rather in discontinuous leaps, a form of transformation in which new patterns appear that did not exit before. Bateson (1979) suggested that we are unaware of changes and that we become accustomed to a new way of being before our senses advise us. To effect change within a family system, nurses need to be able to maintain a metaposition to the family, observing the connections between systems (e.g., between the family and community).

Wright and Leahey (1994) proffered a number of concepts relative to change theory that assist family nurses in their practice.

1. Change is dependent on the perception of the problem. Nurses must recognize that there are as many truths or realities as there are members of a given family. The nurse must accept all these perceptions and offer the family another view of their problems.

2. Change is dependent on context. Efforts to promote change in family systems must take into account the contextual constraints and resources. In the assessment of families, nurses must be cognizant of the family's relationship to larger or suprasystems.

3. Change is dependent on co-evolving goals for treatment. It is important that goals are mutually developed between nurses and families with a realistic time frame. Nurses often set one-sided, unrealistic goals for families. One of the primary goals in family nursing is to change or alter the family's view of the problem. Nurses can assist families to find alternative behavioral, cognitive, and affective responses to problems.

4. Understanding alone does not lead to change. Understanding problems does not bring about change but rather change occurs through alterations in belief and behavior. Nurses often search for the "why" answers with families rather than focusing energies into the "what" questions. Focusing on *what* is being done here and now to perpetuate the problem and *what* can be done to effect a change provides the family with alternative avenues for action.

5. Change does not occur equally in all family members. Change can lead to a variety of reactions, with some family members changing more dramatically and quickly than others.

6. Nurses are responsible for facilitating change. Nurses cannot make families change, as that responsibility belongs to the family. Nurses facilitate a context for change.

7. Change can be due to a myriad of causes. Change is influenced by many different factors; thus, it is difficult to know what specifically precipitated the changes.

Other Family Social Science Theories

Only the major frameworks that have historically been used in family social science and that are relevant for family nursing practice were presented. Other frameworks that support family nursing include: chaos theory, social exchange theory, conflict theory, ecological framework, anthropological/multicultural approach, and phenomenology theory (Nye & Berardo, 1981; Klein & White, 1996; Friedman, 1992). The multicultural approach to family nursing is presented in Chapter 8, while conflict theory is discussed in Chapter 10.

▶ FAMILY THERAPY THEORIES

Family therapy theories, in contrast to family social science theories, are practice theories. They have been developed to work with troubled families and, therefore, are pathology-oriented for the most part (see Table 4–2). Even so, these theories describe family system dynamics and patterns that exist in all families to some extent. Because this genre of theories are concerned with what can be done to facilitate change in "dysfunctional" families (Whall, 1983), they are both descriptive and prescriptive (suggesting treatment or intervention strategies).

Both family social science theory and family therapy have a short history, with family therapy theories being of even more recent vintage. Yet, over the last 35 years there has been extensive theory development in the field of family therapy.

Multiple family therapy theories exist; these all have been influenced by the multiple theories that are extant in the psychological and sociological disciplines. No single approach to family therapy can be put forth as the "right" or "wrong" approach; each is simply an alternative explanation of family phenomena and a specific approach to family assessment, diagnoses, and treatment. Over time, family therapy theories have been classified in various ways by a variety of theorists. One classification list is composed of the following theoretical perspectives: psychoanalytic, experiential, communication, strategic, behavioral, cognitive, structural, narrative, and solution-focused (brief therapy) (Gladding, 1995; Becvar & Becvar, 1996).

Three of the most prominent of the family therapy theories (Goldenberg & Goldenberg, 1996) are presented here: structural family therapy theory, family systems theory, and family interactional/communications theory. These three theories share a general systems theory orientation (Doherty & Baird, 1983), including an interactional focus and the notions of interdependency of the family subsystems, circular causality, nonsummativity (the family is greater and different than the sum of its parts), the ripple effect (a change in one part affects all other parts of the whole), and holism (the need to view the family as a whole).

Structural Family Therapy Theory

Minuchin and associates (Minuchin, 1974; Minuchin & Fishman, 1981; Minuchin, Rosman & Baker, 1978) developed this systems-oriented approach to family therapy in the early and mid-1970s. The theory's uniqueness results from its use of spatial and organizational metaphors, both in describing problems and in identifying solutions (Goldenberg & Goldenberg, 1996). Minuchin (1974) described the family "structure" as a covert set of functional demands that organize the ways in which family members interact. Moreover, in his intervention strategies, he set the prime goal of therapy to be "restructuring the family."

Minuchin (1974) conceptualized the family as an open sociocultural system that is continually faced with demands for change from within and outside the family. Individuals within the context of the family must learn to adapt to these demands and the resultant stress. The family's underlying organizational structure, i.e., its enduring transactional patterns and flexibility in responding to demands for change, helps determine the functionality or dysfunctionality of the family.

Four major concepts that are central to understanding structural family therapy are: (1) transactional patterns, (2) adaptation, (3) subsystems, and (4) boundaries. **Transactional patterns** refer to repeated patterns of transactions that become laws that govern the interactions and conduct of various family members. **Adaptation** refers to the availability of alternative transactional patterns, as well as the family's ability to mobilize these alternative transactional patterns to meet external and internal demands for change. Transactional patterns help the family to be stable or homeostatic. Family dysfunction is the product of dysfunctional transactional patterns and, hence, poor adaptation. **Subsystems** are the ways in which the family system differentiates and carries out its affective and socialization functions. These subsystems in families are usually individuals or relation/relational subsystems such as the marital, parent–child, and sibling subsystem in the two-parent nuclear family. **Boundaries** ensure differentiation of the family subsystems. The clarity of these boundaries provides a prime barometer of how well the family functions. As part of the notion of boundaries, Minuchin introduced the idea of two pathological extremes in boundaries: the disengaged, where boundaries are too rigid, to the point where there is little cohesiveness between family members; and enmeshed, where the boundaries are diffuse or porous to the point where subsystems do not function autonomously or independently at all. As Minuchin (1974) explained, in the enmeshed family, one person sneezes and everyone runs for the Kleenex.

The goal of family therapy is to facilitate a transformation in family structure. The clinician using this approach attempts to change family patterns through in-session manipulation of family interaction. Therapy is present-centered, action-oriented, and problem-focused. Clarifying boundaries and power hierarchies (who is in charge), i.e., creating second-order family change, alters the presenting problem.

Assessment of families occurs through asking questions, observing family transactions, and staging enactments (having family members interact with each other about a particular situation in the interview itself). Evaluating the whole system, its subsystems, boundaries, coalitions, as well as family transactional patterns and covert rules, is part of the assessment. Intervention includes joining with the family by respecting the current family structure, intervening directly to restructure the family, and working with family success through praise and support (Minuchin & Fishman, 1981). The role of the therapist is active, directive, and action-oriented.

The strengths of this approach are that the concepts are fairly clear, well integrated, developed, and tested. The limitation of the model is that the approach calls for a very directive and active role on the part of the therapist. Some practitioners and/or families may feel uncomfortable with such a direct, active, and sometimes confrontational approach.

Family Systems Therapy Theory

Family systems theory partially stems from general systems theory, which was identified earlier in the family social science tradition. (In actuality, all of the different models in family therapy are viewed to be systemic in nature.) Murray Bowen first developed family systems theory in the mid-1970s. He is recognized as being the leading family therapy theorist and one of the prominent pioneers in family therapy. His family systems theory is the best developed and integrated of the family therapy theoretical frameworks (Goldenberg & Goldenberg, 1996). After Bowen's death in 1990, his work has continued to evolve through the work of Michael Kerr (Kerr & Bowen, 1988) and David Freeman (1992).

The underlying assumption or premise in this theory is that chronic anxiety is an inevitable, omnipresent part of life (Goldenberg & Goldenberg, 1996). Chronic anxiety is the underlying basis for dysfunction. Its only "antidote is resolution through differentiation," the key concept within Bowen's theory (Goldenberg & Goldenberg, 1996, p. 169). In order to address chronic anxiety and emotional processes in families and society, Bowen emphasized eight interlocking concepts (Gladding, 1995) (see Table 4–4). According to Bowen, understanding these concepts provided a theory-based framework for working with families.

The key concept within his theory is **differentiation of self**. This notion refers to the ability of persons to distinguish themselves from their family of origin on an emotional and intellectual level. There are two counterbalancing life forces: togetherness and individuality. On one end of the continuum is autonomy, which signals an ability to think through a situation clearly and separate out feelings from rational thought. At the other end of the continuum is undifferentiated ego mass, which implies an emo-

▶ **TABLE 4–4**

BOWEN'S FAMILY SYSTEMS THEORY— EIGHT INTERLOCKING CONCEPTS

- Differentiation of self
- Nuclear family emotional system
- Multigenerational transmission process
- Family projection process
- Triangling
- Sibling position
- Emotional cutoff
- Societal regression

tional dependence on the family of origin even if living away from the family. An individual's level of differentiation or the use of logical reasoning over time indicates whether that person displays his or her solid or pseudo-self. People are ranked on a scale of differentiation of self. The greater the differentiation of self, the more individuals are able to adapt to change and stress from their surroundings and, therefore, the less apt they are to run into emotional difficulty.

There are seven remaining interlocking concepts in Bowen's family systems theory (these concepts are indicated in bold). The nuclear family is conceptualized as a **nuclear family emotional system**. Coping strategies and patterns in families tend to be passed on from generation to generation, a phenomenon known as the **multigenerational transmission process**. Families that present dysfunction have carried the problematic behavior(s) over several generations. People tend to marry partners at their own level of differentiation and couples tend to produce offspring at the same level of differentiation as themselves. The **family projection process** refers to the tendency of spouses who are anxious and have poor differentiation of self to transfer their anxiety and low level of differentiation to a susceptible child. **Triangles** are another major concept and are seen as a basic building block of any emotional system and the smallest stable relationship system. Triangles are a way of dealing with anxiety in which tension between two persons is projected onto another object/person in the family. In stressful situations, anxiety may spread from one central triangle within the family to triangles with a person(s) or object outside the family. **Sibling position** addresses the importance of birth order. People are seen as developing fixed personality characteristics based on their functional birth order in their family of origin (Toman, 1961). The more closely a marriage replicates one's sibling position in the family of origin, the better chance that couple has of having a successful marriage. **Emotional cutoff** refers to emotional withdrawal from parents and family due to unresolved attachments with them. In this circumstance, children who are emotionally fused to their parents and family of origin may live near or far from them. They try to keep emotionally distanced, but are fused regardless of their physical proximity. **Societal regression** is the analogue on a societal level for differentiation of self. It refers to a society that is under so much stress that it regresses because excessive toxic forces counter the tendency to achieve differentiation.

The major focus of Bowen's family systems therapy is on promoting differentiation of self from family and of intellect from emotion (Becvar & Becvar, 1996). By examining the processes mentioned above, family members gain insight and understanding into the past and are freed to choose how they will behave in the present. Assessment using the Bowen model consists of having individuals or couples discuss their family tree with the therapist. The roles of the therapist are coach and teacher. Intervention consists of asking questions about people's history while constructing a multigenerational genogram. People are given homework assignments to "go home again," such as asking questions of their own family members to gain a history of the past, to develop person-to-person relationships with family members, and to end emotional cutoffs. Bowenian therapists coach people on how to detriangulate, develop interpersonal relationships, and end cutoffs, and how to understand their intergenerational patterns, thus gaining insight into ways they currently interact.

One major strength of this therapeutic approach is its objective and neutral approach, which serves to take blame out of what people bring to the therapist. The logic of the approach appeals to many people who lead with their intellect rather than their feelings; thus it has been noted to appeal to male clients. A major weakness of this therapy is that it often requires long and expensive work. Many people are not inclined to stay in therapy long enough to see it to its completion. An emphasis on the past rather than on the present (i.e., the presenting problem) means that the presenting problem may not be addressed or resolved as soon as it is in other approaches.

Interactional/Communication Family Therapy Theory

The interactional/communication therapy approach was heavily influenced by ideas derived from general systems theory, cybernetics and information processing theory (see Chapter 7 for description of these latter two theories) (Goldenberg & Goldenberg, 1996). This theory embodies communication approaches to family therapy that have been seminal to the entire field of family therapy. The interactional/communication perspective has undergone major revisions over four decades, but the original theory development was done by the Mental Research Institute (MRI) in Palo Alto, California (Don Jackson, John Weakland, and Paul Watzlawick) and Virginia Satir (Becvar & Becvar, 1996).

Therapists using the interactional paradigm conceptualize the family as a system of interactive/interlocking behaviors or communication processing. Based on clinical research findings, interactional family therapists have rejected linear role theory and psychoanalytic constructs in the assessment and treatment of families (Jones and Dimond, 1982). Essential to this approach are the redundant patterns of family communication and the interaction within and between systems. Emphasis is on circular causation and the here-and-now rather than the past. The key question asked is "What?" That is, what is being processed, rather than "Why?", which is consistent with systems theory thinking. Causality is conceptualized as circular and recursive. Families are seen as error-activated and goal-directed systems (Jackson, 1965a).

The unit of analysis in this approach was derived from the dynamics of interchange between individuals, thus the term "interactional" analysis. Basic to this perspective is the assumption that psychiatric problems result from the way people interact with each other in the context of the family. "Individual symptoms reflect family system dysfunction and these symptoms persist only if they are maintained by that family system" (Goldenberg & Goldenberg, 1996, p. 211). Problem alleviation, therefore, results when the social context is successfully manipulated; in this sense, the locus of pathology is seen as outside the person. Different from structural family therapy theory, the interactional paradigm outlines the dynamic interaction of the patterns between family members with a focus on the communication process. A breakdown in family functioning occurs when dysfunctional family communication predominates and when the rules of family functioning become ambiguous.

The fundamental rules of communication theory developed by Watzlawick, Beavin, and Jackson, 1967, in *Pragmatics of Human Communication,* are as follows:

1. One cannot not behave, thus one cannot not communicate. All behavior is communication at some level.

2. All communication has a report (digital) level and a command (analog) level. The command level defines the nature of the relationship.

3. All behavior/communication must be examined in context. Without contextual awareness, complete understanding is not possible.

4. All systems are characterized by rules, which maintain homeostatic balance and preserve the system.

5. Relationships may be described as either symmetrical or complementary. Symmetrical implies equality and complementary implies oppositeness (a dominant–submissive relationship).

6. Each person punctuates his or her reality according to his or her own reality. Behavioral sequences are understood and meaning is experienced relative to the epistemology of the observer.

7. Problems are maintained within recursive feedback loops of recurrent patterns of communication.

8. The functional or normal family is able to maintain its basic integrity even during periods of stress. Changes are accommodated as needed and clear, congruent communication is present.

9. Dysfunctional families are said to be "stuck." Symptomatic behavior maintains the family's current equilibrium and needed change is avoided. A problem is a symptom of system dysfunction.

Satir (1982) built on the above communication ideas by adding four fundamental assumptions. First, the natural movement of all individuals is toward positive growth and development and that a symptom indicates an impasse in the growth process. Second, all individuals possess the resources necessary for growth and development. The goal of the therapist is to facilitate this process. Third, families possess mutual influence and shared responsibility. Therefore, no person in the family is to blame, only multiple stimuli and multiple effects. Fourth, therapy is a process involving interactions between both clients and therapists. Although the therapist may take the lead in facilitating growth, each person is in charge of his or her own growth. Therapy provides a supportive context for such development. A primary goal of family therapy is to understand the communication rules and processes that the troubled family uses and to teach the family functional communication rules and processes.

Key interventions, in addition to those of Satir, focus on establishing clear, congruent communication as well as clarifying and changing family rules (Jackson, 1965b; Satir, 1967). The strength of this approach is its focus on communication within the family environment. It addresses the interaction problems among family members. The weakness of this theory is that it looks primarily at internal family behavior and not at how the family is impacted by the larger culture and environment of which it is a part.

Other Family Therapy Theories

Due to limitations of space, only three of the family therapy frameworks were presented. Other frameworks and approaches from family therapy which contribute to family nursing theories include: psychodynamic (Ackerman, 1966), experiential/humanistic (Whitaker & Keith, 1981), strategic

(Madanes, 1991), behavior/cognitive (Falloon, 1991), and narrative (White and Epston, 1990).

▶ FAMILY NURSING THEORIES: INTEGRATED MODELS

Integrated approaches are needed to guide family nursing practice, as no singular theory provides a comprehensive framework for the diversity of families with whom we work. Presently there are three family nursing practice models that are cited widely and used extensively in family nursing (Hanson & Boyd, 1996a). These are the Family Systems Stressor–Strength Model and Inventory (Berkey & Hanson, 1991), the Friedman Family Assessment Model (the model used in this text), and the Calgary Family Assessment and Intervention Models (Wright & Leahey, 1994). Although there is much overlap in the content and processes involved in these three models, there are also substantial differences in approach.

Berkey and Hanson (1991), and Hanson and Mischke (1996), developed an integrated family nursing model by extending Neuman's Health Care System Model. Using family theory, Neuman's theoretical concepts were expanded to focus on the family as client. The Family Assessment Intervention Model and Family Systems Stressor Strength Inventory (FS³I) are more focused than the other two models, in that they involve the appraisal of family stressors and strengths, as well as the restoration of family stability and family functioning by the application of primary, secondary, and tertiary preventive approaches. The FS³I can be used for assessment and intervention as well as a measurement tool for both practice and research. The model and its assumptions are discussed earlier in this chapter under the Neuman Health Care Systems Model.

The Friedman Family Assessment Model constitutes an integrated approach by utilizing general systems theory, family developmental theory, structural–functional theory, and cross-cultural theory as primary theoretical foundations for a family assessment model and tool. Other mid-range theories are also incorporated into the various structural and functional dimensions assessed, such as communi-

cation theory, role theory, and family stress theory. Chapters 3 and 6, as well as the chapters in Part II of this text (Chaps. 8 through 17) elaborate on these family assessment content and process areas. Family nursing diagnoses and intervention strategies are also discussed relative to each of the identifying data, sociocultural, developmental, structural, functional and stress coping assessment areas.

The third integrated family systems nursing model is the Calgary Family Assessment Model (CFAM) and the Calgary Family Intervention Model (CFIM), developed by Wright and Leahey and associates (Wright & Leahey, 1994; Wright, Watson, & Bell, 1997). The Calgary family systems nursing model integrates theories from general systems theory, cybernetics, communication theory, and change theory. Increasingly, the Calgary family systems nursing model is informed by family therapy theories and approaches, more specifically Maturana's and Varela's theory of the biology of knowing, Gregory Bateson's theory of mind, and constructivist and narrative approaches (White & Eptston, 1990; Wright, Watson, & Bell, 1997).

These theories and ideas are incorporated into a nursing paradigm or perspective focusing on families experiencing health problems. The Calgary Family Assessment Model emphasizes identification of family strengths and resources. Intervention strategies are planned with the strong recognition that families should and must decide what is best for them. They are designed to assist families to empower themselves. The assessment and intervention models are grounded in solid clinical practice observations and qualitative clinical research.

Chapter 3 highlights the Calgary model. Chapter 18 summarizes particular intervention strategies that are cornerstones of the Calgary family systems nursing model, particularly strategies used to assist families to have facilitative beliefs and modify their constraining beliefs.

▶ SUMMARY AND CONCLUSIONS

At the present time, there is no single theory/conceptual framework from nursing, family social science, or family therapy that fully describes the relationships and dynamics for family life and family nursing theory. Thus, an *integrated* approach is necessary to guide practice, research, and education in family nursing. One theoretical perspective does not give nurses a sufficiently broad knowledge base from which to assess and intervene with families. Hence, nurses must draw on multiple theories to work effectively with families.

Of the three genres of theory, the family social science theories are the most well developed and informative with respect to how families function, the environment–family interchange, interactions within the family, how the family changes over time, and the family's reaction to health and illness. One striking limitation in using the family social science theories as a basis for assessment and intervention in family nursing is that their clinical application is parsimonious, although recent work has made some strides in remedying this situation (Berkey & Hanson, 1991; Wright & Leahey, 1994; Hanson & Boyd, 1996a).

Family therapy theories are the next most developed theories and emanate from a professional/practice heritage rather than the academic disciplines. Many of the family therapy theories stem from a foundation in family social science theories, but they are more practice-oriented. Family nursing theory, practice, and research are increasingly drawing from family therapy theories as the specialty of family nursing grows more sophisticated. Not all family therapy theories are applicable to nursing. For example, with nursing's focus on the entire health–illness continuum and on health promotion, family therapy theories may not be as germane for working with healthy families or families with some types of health problems. Also, family therapy models are more applicable to advanced nursing practice and, thus, may be beyond the level of expertise of baccalaureate-prepared nurses. Whall (1986b) urges family nurse therapists to reformulate existing family therapy theories to fit the nursing perspective in accordance with nursing theory.

Finally, of all three genres, nursing models are the least developed. During the 1960s and 1970s much effort was placed on the development of nursing models by nursing theorists. As concepts and propositions were explicated, different models fit some nursing settings and functions better than others. The major drawback to the nursing models is that they originated within an individual paradigm and only a few later evolved to fit a family

nursing focus (Berkey & Hanson, 1991). The importance of this work in family nursing is the rich understanding it brings to describing the human responses and relationships between client, health, environment, and nursing. Nursing theories need to be expanded to include the client system of family to make this work relevant to family nursing practice.

Nursing has recently come to recognize that family nursing theory has a heritage in all three genres (nursing, family social science, family therapy) (Hanson & Boyd, 1996) and that the next generation of family nurses need to further explicate the utility of how these three traditions fit together to formulate concepts and propositions for the nursing of families. We know we have a growing science and art of "family nursing," and we know that it evolves from a rich background emanating from a multitude of disciplines. Just what this theoretical/conceptual background means for the theory, practice, research, and education of family nursing is an emerging phenomena.

In conclusion, family nursing theory is an excellent example of evolving nursing theory in the 21st century. Family nursing already has a rich background of family social science theory, family therapy theory, and nursing theory. Family nursing has been open to the integration of all three genres. Further family nursing theory development will continue to integrate these ideas from different schools of thought. As we recognize the importance of systems interactions in issues involving families, it makes sense that family nursing would integrate care, ideas, and practice to work together with other family-focused disciplines to improve the health of families and their members. The future focus of family nursing theory needs to be on specific health care needs of families. The concrete day-to-day issues faced by family nurses in their practice will be the foundation of family nursing theory development as these issues will be context relevant.

Families are a global phenomena. Many issues that face families around the world need to be explored. We need to unite our global views and share unique ways in which nursing enhances the welfare of families and its members.

Family nursing needs continued theory development to continue to make sense of the whole, to bring more order to the concepts of family nursing, to clearly delineate interventions that help families. Family theory development of the future needs to address those issues experienced by those nurses and families on the front lines of family nursing practice.

► study questions

1. Match the family social science approaches used in studying family on the left with best descriptions in the right-hand column.

Approaches

a. Systems approach
b. Interactional approach
c. Developmental approach
d. Structural–functional approach
e. Change theory

Descriptions

1. Studies family related to present situation—that is, behavior vis-à-vis "triggering" event.
2. Studies family progressing through life cycle.
3. Family viewed as an open social system and has a process orientation.
4. Deals with internal family dynamics.
5. Describes family as focal system within larger suprasystem.
6. Describes family as having predictable natural history common to families and associated with changing ages and member composition.
7. Family viewed as social system with emphasis on purposes family achieves, its internal organization, and its relationship to the wider society.
8. Focuses on first-order and second-order transitions.

Fill in the correct answer to the following question.

2. The interactional approach analyzes the family in respect to _____.

3. Give three important areas the interactionist would assess using the above framework.

4. Nursing theory development has changed in its approach to generating theory. Which statement best reflects this current trend?
    a. Shift from deductive to inductive theory development.
    b. Shift from inductive to deductive theory development.
    c. Shift from linear to circular causation.
    d. Shift from past- to present-oriented theory generation.

5. What advantages do the following genres of theoretical frameworks have?
    a. Nursing theories.
    b. Family therapy theories.
    c. Social science theories.
    d. Theoretical frameworks in general.

6. The several major family therapy theories have the following commonalities (select all correct answers):
    a. They are systems oriented.
    b. They focus on both the past and the present.
    c. They are behaviorally oriented.
    d. They focus on family dynamics/interactions.

7. With respect to the three integrated family nursing models discussed in this chapter, which of these following statement(s) is/are accurate?
    a. Berkey and Hanson's Family Stressor–Strengths Model/Inventory is an extension of Rogers's model.
    b. The Friedman Family Assessment Model is based primarily on family interactional theory and Bowen's family systems theory.
    c. The Calgary Family Assessment and Intervention Models integrate multiple theoretical approaches from both the social sciences and the family therapy genres of theories.

▶ chapter 4 study answers

1. a. 3 and 5.
    b. 4.
    c. 2 and 6.
    d. 7.
    e. 8.

2. Its internal dynamics or the interaction between the family members.

3. Role structure, power structure (decision-making processes), and communication patterns. Family stress and coping, status relations, and socialization problems are also correct.

4. a.

5. a. *Nursing theories:* specify a nursing focus and suggest nursing actions (what areas to assess and with what emphasis, delineation of goals, and intervention).

   b. *Family therapy theories:* Provide clinical application guidelines (assessment and intervention), particularly in family mental health settings.

   c. *Family social science theories:* provide full description of family relationships (inner dynamics and external interactions) and family behavior.

   d. *A theoretical framework* provides the mechanism by which we can organize and more abstractly understand our observations; focus and guide our assessments, diagnoses, and interventions; and communicate our findings.

6. a and d.

7. c.

Structural–Functional Theory

Marilyn M. Friedman

> ► learning objectives

1. Identify the three primary theoretical perspectives used in this text for completing a family assessment.
2. Define the components and basic characteristics of the structural–functional approach as applied to the family.
3. Explain the usefulness of the structural–functional approach to family nursing.

4. Analyze the relationship of family structure to family functions and the system theory approach to the structural–functional approach.
5. List and briefly describe the five basic family functions.
6. Trace major alterations that occurred in family functions during the change from an agrarian, nonindustrialized society to present-day society.

A central assumption of this text is that clinical practice should be guided by theory. I also believe that the decision regarding what theory or theories to use in one's practice—that is, in assessing, planning, intervening, and evaluating—should be based on practical grounds; in other words, what theory(ies) best/most powerfully explain(s) a situation and suggest(s) meaningful and effective nursing goals and actions. I agree with Blau (1977), a noted sociologist and theoretician, who advises us, "a choice between [theoretical] perspectives can only be made on pragmatic grounds: which theory is more useful for clarifying given problems" (p. 3). And I would extend Blau's thought to include—"and guiding nursing actions."

Looking at the potpourri of theories presented in Chapter 4 (nursing theories, family therapy theories,

and family social science theories), several family social science theories appear at this time, because of the state of theory development among the nursing theories, to be the best, most powerful theoretical perspectives to use in family nursing. These, I believe, are structural–functional theory, developmental theory, and general systems theory. Applying three general theoretical models in addition to some less general theories, encourages family nursing practice to be more holistic and comprehensive.

The structural–functional perspective applied to the family is comprehensive and recognizes the important interaction between the family and its internal and particularly its external environment. The developmental approach is needed to provide the information of family development and life cycle tasks, to examine changes in a family's life over time, and to assess how a family is handling its developmental tasks. A general systems approach applied to the family is also needed to assess the adaptational and communications processes within the family. Family developmental and systems theories are needed to guide practice because structural–functional analysis tends to present a static view of the family, while both developmental and general systems theory handle change over time better. In addition, a structural–functional perspective minimizes the importance of growth, change, and disequilibrium in a family, while a general systems theory explains these processes more fully and convincingly. So while structural–functionalism has these apparent biases (and, in fact, has diminished explanatory power in research and practice today), we still need to understand its relevance as a theoretical perspective for family nursing practice.

▶ THE STRUCTURAL–FUNCTIONAL APPROACH

The structural–functional framework is a major theoretical frame of reference in sociology (Leslie & Korman, 1989; Smith, 1995), particularly in the areas of family and medical sociology. Applied to the family, the scope of the framework is very broad. The family is viewed as an open social system and as a subsystem within society for the socialization of children and the stabilization of adult personalities (Doherty, Boss, LaRossa, Schumm, & Steinmetz, 1993). Relationships between the family and other social systems (e.g., the health care system, educational system, and the family within the larger social system [Dickinson & Leming, 1995]) are examined. A description of the family's structural (organizational dimensions) and family functions are at the core of this approach.

According to Eshleman, the structural–functional approach has its origin in the functionalist branch of psychology (particularly Gestalt psychology), in social anthropology (as exhibited in the writings of Malinowski and Radcliffe-Brown), and in sociology (particularly as described by social systems theorists such as Parsons). The Gestalt position emphasizes that one must view the whole and its parts, exploring the interrelationship between the whole and its parts. Along the same line of thinking, social anthropologists have concluded that one cannot understand a particular aspect of social life detached from its general environment (Eshleman, 1974).

Structural–functionalists see the family, one of the social institutions of a society, as being "functional" for or congruent with the society. In the 1950s, theorists (Parsons & Bales, 1955; Parsons, 1951) envisioned a good fit between society and the family, a basic institution functioning to meet society's needs. Today, with such a changing heterogeneous society, this harmonious, stable picture of the relationship between society and the family has changed. Nevertheless, stability and order in systems are viewed as natural and desirable, whereas conflict and disorder are seen as deviant and dysfunctional in systems (Broderick, 1993).

Most of the sociological literature applying the structural–functional approach to the family makes use of a more macroscopic approach, looking at the family as a subsystem of the wider society. From this perspective, structural–functionalism can be considered the earliest form of systems theory (see Chap. 7) (Broderick, 1993). The general assumptions made include the following (Leslie & Korman, 1989; Parsons & Bales, 1955):

1. A family is a social system with functional requirements.

2. A family is a small group possessing certain generic features common to all small groups.

3. The family as a social system accomplishes functions that serve both the individual and society.

4. Individuals act in accordance with a set of internalized norms and values that are learned primarily in the family through socialization.

Family studies using a structural–functional perspective have demonstrated that the economy and technology are important derminants of family structure and function. In addition, ideological and cultural changes related to individualism, autonomy, and gender roles are vitally important in understanding family structural arrangements and dynamics (Smith, 1995).

The structural–functional perspective is a very useful framework for assessing family life because it enables the family system to be examined holistically (as a unit), in parts (as subsystems or dimensions), and interactionally (as a system interacting with other institutions, such as the educational and health systems, the family's reference group(s), and the wider society). Mancini and Orthner (1988), family educators, remind family professionals that both a micro- and macroscopic perspective is needed when working with families. They explain that "to understand families is to know about those internal dynamics, but also to know something about the common habitat, whether it be the values of society, current economic conditions, or governmental support for families" (p. 363). Structural–functional theory provides these two perspectives.

Structural–functional theory, then, has been selected, along with general systems theory and developmental theory, as the organizing framework for the text, because its use provides a comprehensive and holistic perspective for assessment purposes. The essence of family-centered nursing involves understanding the dynamics of the family and all the forces, both internal and external, that affect it. For this understanding, structural–functional theory serves as one primary theoretical perspective guiding both family assessment and practice.

▶ CONCEPT OF STRUCTURE

The structural–functional approach primarily analyzes the family's structural characteristics—the arrangement of the parts that form the whole, and the functions it performs for both society and its subsystems. The structure of the family refers to how the family is organized, the manner in which units are arranged, and how these units relate to each other. The dimensions, or definitions, of this concept of family structure vary considerably. Some theorists base structure on the type of family form (e.g., nuclear versus extended); type of power structure (e.g., matriarchal versus patriarchal); or marital patterns (e.g., exogamy versus endogamy) (Eshleman, 1974). Another way of looking at the family structure is by describing the subsystems as the structural dimension (Minuchin, 1974).

Assuming that the family is a special kind of small group, the structural dimensions identified by small-group theory as being relevant for assessing such groups are used in this text. Parad and Caplan (1965), in analyzing a family under stress, have identified three structural dimensions, which they call the family lifestyle. Family lifestyle refers to "the rea-

sonably stable patterning of family organization, subdivided into three interdependent elements of value system, communication network, and role systems" (Parad & Caplan, 1965, p. 55). In this text a fourth structural dimension has been added to Parad and Caplan's structural elements—the power structure. To repeat, then, the four basic structural dimensions that are subsumed under family structure, and that will be elaborated on in separate chapters, are (1) role structure, (2) value systems, (3) communication processes, and (4) power structure.

These elements are all intimately interrelated and interacting. When one aspect of the internal structure of the family is affected by input from the external environment, the processing of this input within the family system will also affect the other structural dimensions. The family's high degree of interrelatedness and interdependency is seen when a family health care professional observes how certain family behaviors often become indicators of strengths or dysfunction within several or all the structural elements in the family. For instance, a husband, in an authoritarian way, is observed ordering his wife and children on when and what will be served for dinner. The mother is then seen directing the children to each prepare certain assigned parts of the meal. Mother and children carry out father's wishes with no comments or sign of feelings. No other communications are noted. We can see from this one vignette (and this would have to be verified by further observation of the family) that the power figure in this situation is the father; his role is one of a stern, commanding leader of the family, who probably needs and has much control over his family (because even details are controlled). The communication patterns here are one-way (father to mother and children, mother to children) and completely task centered. No feelings or sharing of thoughts are observed. Again speculating on this situation, the events are congruent with the family's value system. One of the values central to this family probably would be male dominance, while another related value might be respect for and obedience to elders.

Family structure is ultimately evaluated by how well the family is able to fulfill its family functions—the goals important to its members and society. The family's structure serves to facilitate the achievement of family functions, because the conservation and allocation of resources is a prime task for the family structure. Because of this important relationship, functions should be viewed in tandem with family structures.

▶ CONCEPT OF FUNCTION

Family functions are commonly defined as outcomes or consequences of the family structure. Although some authors use "function" to mean "consequences of or results of," it is a little easier to think of family functions as being what the family does (Friedman, 1992; Ingoldsby, 1995). Why does it exist? What purposes does it serve? "Social institutions exist because they perform certain valuable functions for their members and for society of which they are a part" (Ingoldsby, 1995, p. 84). As described in detail in Chapter 1, the family's basic functions meet the needs of both individual family members and wider society.

Five family functions* are most germane when assessing and intervening with families.

1. The affective function (personality maintenance function): for stabilization of adult personalities, meeting the psychological needs of family members. (See Chap. 14 for detailed description of the family affective function.)

2. The socialization and social placement function: for the primary socialization of children aimed at making them productive members of their society, as well as the conferring of status on family members. (See Chap. 15 for a detailed description of the family socialization function.)

3. The reproductive function: for maintenance of family continuity over the generations as well as for societal survival.

4. The economic function: for the provision of sufficient economic resources and their effective allocation.

5. The health care function: for the provision of physical necessities—food, clothing, shelter, health care (Fig. 5–1). (See Chap. 16 for a detailed description of the family health care function.)

---

*These functions represent an adaptation or modification of several theorists' descriptions of family functions, including those of Murdock (1949), Ogburn (1933), Parsons and Bales (1955), and Hill (1965).

Affective Function

The affective function is a central basis for both the formation and the continuation of the individual family unit, and it thus constitutes one of the most vital functions of families. Today, when many societal tasks are performed outside the family unit, much of the family's effort is focused on meeting the needs of family members for affection and understanding. The ability to provide for these needs is a key determinant of whether a given family will persist or dissolve. As Duvall (1977) says, family happiness is gauged by the strength of family love. The family must meet the affectional needs of its members because the affectional responses of one family member to another provide the basic rewards of family life.

Primarily a marital and parental role, this function deals with the family's perception and care of the socioemotional needs of all its members. It involves tension reduction and morale maintenance.

The elevation of this function to a high level of importance within the family is a relatively new notion and is found most strongly among middle-class and affluent families, where choice is more feasible. In middle- and upper-class families, personal happiness in the marital relationship based on companionship and love is critical. The importance of this function has a decreased emphasis in many working-class and lower-class families, largely because more basic functions such as providing the physical necessities of life predominate.

Socialization and Social Placement Function

Socialization of family members is a universal, cross-cultural functional requisite for societal survival (Leslie & Korman, 1989). It refers to the myriad of learning experiences provided within the family aimed at teaching children how to function and assume adult social roles such as those of husband–father and wife–mother. The family has the primary responsibility of transforming an infant in a score of years into a social person capable of full participation in society. Furthermore, socialization should not be thought of as pertaining only to infant and child-rearing patterns, but rather as a lifelong process that includes internalizing the appropriate

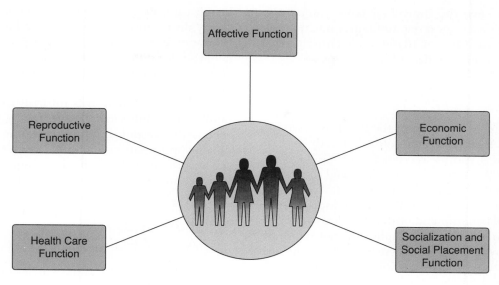

Figure 5–1. The five basic family functions.

sets of norms and values for being a teenager, a spouse, a parent, an employee on a new job, a grandparent, and a retired person (Eshleman, 1974). In short, socialization involves learning the culture.

Because this function is increasingly shared with schools, recreational, and child-care facilities, and other extrafamilial institutions, the family plays a reduced, yet critical, role in socialization. Parents still transmit their cultural heritage to their children.

An integral part of socialization in the family involves the inculcation of controls and values—giving the growing child (and adult) a sense of what is right and wrong. Kohlberg (1970) describes the process of moral development as having its foundations in the family. Moral development is seen as a process similar to the stages of emotional and cognitive development à la Erikson and Piaget, respectively. By identifying with parental figures and being consistently reinforced negatively and positively for their behavior, children develop a personal value system that is greatly influenced by the family's value system.

Social placement or status conferring is the other aspect of the socialization function. Conferring of status on children refers to passing on of the traditions, values, and privileges of the family, although today tradition no longer dictates the patterns of most adult Americans. At birth, a child automatically inherits his or her family's status—ethnic, racial,

national, religious, economic, political, and educational. The family socializes the child into its social class, instilling in him or her relevant aspirations. Additionally, the family has the responsibility of providing necessary socialization and educational experiences that enable family members to assume a vocation and roles in groups that are consistent with status expectations.

Educating parents about child-rearing patterns and ways they may cope with family problems are major components of family health care, beginning with genetic and reproductive counseling, continuing through prenatal and child care, and extending throughout the life cycle of the family. The common health concerns and family problems with which the family nurse can assist families are described within the various stages of the family's life cycle in Chapter 6. Chapter 15 describes the family socialization function more extensively.

Health Care Function: Providing Physical Necessities and Health Care

The physical functions of the family are met by the parents providing food, clothing, shelter, and protection against danger. Health care and health practices (which influence the individual family members' health status) are a most relevant family function for the family nurse. Chapter 16 is devoted entirely to an exploration of this significant function.

Reproductive Function

One of the basic functions of the family is to insure continuity of the intergenerational family and of society—that is, provide recruits for society (Leslie & Korman, 1989). In the past, marriage and the family were designed to regulate and control sexual behavior as well as reproduction. Both these aspects, control of sexual behavior and birth control, are now less important functions of the family; it is not required in this society to limit sexual activity to those who are married or to have children within the confines of the traditional family. Once a child is born, a new family is born—with single-parent families becoming increasingly common. The number of births to unmarried mothers, for example, has continued to rise in the United States as greater acceptability and loosening of sexual mores has occurred (see Chap. 1 for demographic changes in the family).

Along with having children outside of the confines of the traditional family, greater use of birth control measures is another important trend, either within or outside the family context. Moreover, the move toward population control and family planning is affecting the importance of parenthood for both women and men. A shift of cultural priorities and personal values continues to diminish motherhood as a woman's central purpose in life and fatherhood as a man's chief reason to work. Increasingly, public expressions are heard against the bearing of more than two children per couple (as the couple's replacement quota), particularly in developing countries.

Economic Function

The economic function involves the family's provision of sufficient resources—financial, space, and material—and their appropriate allocation by decision-making processes.

An assessment of the family's economic resources provides the nurse with data relevant to the family's ability to allocate resources appropriately to meet family needs such as adequate clothing, food, shelter, and health care. By gaining an understanding of how a family distributes its resources, the family-centered nurse can also obtain a clearer perspective about the family's value system (what is important to the family) and what resources can be accessed to help it meet its needs.

Because this function is difficult for most poor families to fulfill satisfactorily, family nurses must accept the responsibility of assisting families to obtain appropriate community resources where they can secure needed information, employment, vocational counseling, and financial assistance.

► CHANGES IN FAMILY FUNCTIONS

The functions that the family carries out for society and its members have changed over time, as depicted in Table 5–1. Certain functions have changed primarily in response to societal and economic changes. If one examines the American family as it existed before industrialization—when an agrarian lifestyle and culture predominated—and compares the family during that period with the family today, profound changes in family functions become apparent.

It is clear that industrialization and urbanization have intruded forcefully on the family, and its institutions have assumed many functions that were once the family's domain. In addition to changes in family functions, family values and the timing of family transitions have been markedly altered. Demos (1970), in describing the transfer of functions from the family to other social institutions, points out that the preindustrial family served as a workshop, church, reformatory, school, and asylum. Today, many older persons live apart in their own home or in residences for senior citizens. Rather than having to depend on the family for assistance, economic support is now provided to the old, unemployed, disabled, and dependent through Social Security or welfare programs. The young are no longer trained at home, but are educated in schools, and by the mass media, peers, and various other associations and groups.

Activities that traditionally took place within the home or involved the entire family now take place elsewhere and engage only certain family members. For instance, economic activity, which traditionally the family engaged in at home as a whole, has until

CHANGES IN FAMILY FUNCTIONS: PRE- AND POSTINDUSTRIALIZATION PERIODS

Family Function	Family Functions Before Industrialization (Agrarian Setting)	Present-day Family Functions (Urban Setting)
1. Economic	Work and family were not separate spheres. Family served as sole economic unit. It was a self-contained, self-sufficient unit; all family members helped. Family both produced and consumed its products. Family was supported by strong kinship associations (the extended family).	The family's economic function is much more limited. Food and clothes are bought outside of the home. Children are no longer economic assets. Single individuals survive well on their own. Family providers, who in many cases are both spouses, work outside of home, bringing home money to buy outside products and services.
2. Status conferring	Family conferred privilege, honor, and status on people. Family affiliation was crucial in locating and placing someone in society.	Function is still present but much decreased in importance except among upper-class families. People are seen primarily as individuals, not as family members.
3. Education	Education ("schooling") was done primarily in home. Father taught son vocation. Mother taught daughter homemaking and child-rearing skills.	Education is carried on outside of home to a great extent; very formalized and institutionalized, which has a pervasive influence on children in both school and extracurricular activities (e.g., sports, music, school clubs). Economic activities require specialized training. Occupational skills and knowledge are learned outside of home.
4. Socialization of children	Child rearing occurred in the home and was the responsibility of mothers, grandmothers, aunts, and older female children. Parents were fully "in charge" of child rearing.	Socialization function remains as a major function, but is shared with outside institutions (e.g., nursery schools, baby sitters, child-care centers, teachers, counselors). Parents' authority and control is diminished, especially after preschool period.
5. Health care function (care of ill, disabled, and older family members)	Protection, supervision, and care of family members, especially of dependent, disabled, or aged individuals, was entirely family's responsibility. The aged, dependent, and infirm were cared for at home.	This function has decreased greatly, although still present. The family's ethnic background and degree of acculturation to white, middle-class culture influences the family functioning in this area. With older or disabled persons, society takes responsibility when family cannot or will not care for these dependent members. The high proportion of working women and the larger number of elderly in our society have also made home care by family members widespread, but more difficult.
6. Religious	Religious training and practices were carried out in both the home and in religious institutions.	There is increasing secularization within society and religion has a declining influence on everyday behavior. Family religious involvement also declined. Religion is primarily taught in outside agencies.

(Continued)

▶ TABLE 5-1   *(Continued)*

Family Function	Family Functions Before Industrialization (Agrarian Setting)	Present-day Family Functions (Urban Setting)
7. Recreational	Because family was without commercial recreation, family-centered activities predominated.	Commercialization of recreation is ubiquitous. Family-centered activities are greatly curtailed after children are older.
8. Reproduction (procreation)	Marriage and family were necessary for survival.	Having a child creates a family, but marriage or having a family is not necessary. Nevertheless, reproduction remains the one *universal* family function.
9. Affective	Primary group relationships were not as strong; extended family was more important affectively.	This function not only remains, but has increased in importance. The usual American family has weakened extended family ties, whereas emotional relationships between the mates and parent–child are very intense. The result is a great emotional strain in relationships. Historically there existed an economic basis for marriage, which now is usually an affective basis, making divorce more of an acceptable alternative if the affective basis for the marriage fails.

recently been the father's responsibility—one that took him out of the home and away from family life. Today, with the growing number of dual-career/worker families, both spouses are engaged in economic activities. One of the most interesting books in this area is by Christopher Lasch, a social historian. His brilliant book, *Haven in a Heartless World* (1977), expounds on the erosion of family in terms of the loss or partial loss of important family functions.

The affective function of the family is a central family function today. And kinship ties, thought at one time to be "weakened" or "practically absent" because of the demands created by industrialization and urbanization, continue to be "alive and well." Given the urbanized, impersonal character of much public life, people increasingly look to their families for more emotional solace and support than in earlier times.

▶ study questions

1. The text's family assessment tool is based upon three theoretical perspectives. These are:
   a. Orem's, Roy's, and Rogers's nursing theories.
   b. Interactional, structural–functional, and institutional theories.
   c. Structural–functional, developmental, and general systems theories.
   d. Family coping, affective, and economic theories.
   e. Role, communications, and power theories.

2. The interactionist approach analyzes internal family dynamics. The structural–functional approach, which is broader in focus, analyzes what?

3. The following are reasons for using a structural–functional approach for assessing and working with families. Select the most accurate and inclusive reason:
    a. Because it is a microscopic approach, it centers on inner dynamics and provides information for transactional-based diagnoses.
    b. It consists of a comprehensive, holistic perspective by which not only the family can be assessed, but also the family's universe (its inner and outer environments).
    c. It provides the family health worker with an understanding of the forces from within and without that impinge on the family.
    d. Using this framework the common health problems are recognized as the family progresses through the life cycle.

4. The relationship of the family structure to family function is that (select one answer):
    a. The structure provides the organization for family functions to be accomplished.
    b. The functions mandate the family structure.
    c. Structure and function are separate entities and have no direct relationship to each other.

5. The structural–functional approach differs from the systems approach in what way? (Select the correct answers.)
    a. They are two separate frameworks.
    b. The structural–functional approach is in opposition to the systems approach.
    c. The systems theory approach handles change over time better.
    d. The structural–functional approach emanated from theories in psychology (Gestalt), social anthropology (Malinowski), and social systems theory (Parsons).

6. Indicate whether the four descriptions in the left-hand column are structural dimensions or family functions.
    a. Roles of two adult family members   1. Structure
    b. Reproduction   2. Function
    c. Communication patterns
    d. The provision of adequate economic support

▶ family case study

7. *Using the following case study for data, list and then describe how this family is fulfilling each of the five basic family functions.*

Family Composition:

Name	Relationship	Age
Emma	Wife	40
Arthur	Husband	44
Danny	Son	17
Ronny	Son	14
Leonard	Son	11
Sammy	Son	7
Cindy	Daughter	5
Arlie	Son	4
Iris	Daughter	2

All the children appeared in good health and were dressed adequately. Arthur and Emma were rather short and obese.

The house was located in a suburban area, in a neighborhood full of children and pets. The house has three bedrooms, one-and-a-half bathrooms, attached garage, with small front and backyards. The interior is reasonably clean and orderly with bare floors and sparse furniture. The TV is in the living room where there are no pictures, books, or decorations.

This is a Mexican-American family. All the members are bilingual. Arthur completed the 10th grade and served in the army. He has since worked as a maintenance man on refrigeration units of food trucks. He has medical insurance through his company.

Emma has been a housewife since her marriage at 19. She has devoted most of her energies to the family and their care. She spends time cooking and provides hearty, nutritious meals, although overabundant in carbohydrates.

The children are in school with the exception of Iris. They do passable work. The older two boys are involved in athletics, which is a source of pride for the parents.

This is the only marriage for Arthur and Emma, who have been married for 21 years. There has been significant marital discord during the past 11 years.

From Emma's description of home life, she "wears the pants in the family." She describes her husband as a meek, passive man who takes no responsibility in the household. He brings home the check, eats, and sleeps there. She states she finds him "sexually unattractive," and difficult to be "close" to. Emma says she wants to be with her children but that she has no love for her husband.

Arthur says he works and makes a living. "The house is a woman's responsibility," which he has left to his wife.

Emma does all of the disciplining and is the parent children go to for permissions. Emma states that when Arthur tells the children to do something and they disobey, their excuse is they didn't think that he really meant it. The children verified that Emma does the greater part of the disciplining and that when she is home, they really watch their behavior.

Emma prefers her children to her husband. They are the apparent reason the marriage holds together. She seems very fond of all her children, but she mentions Leonard and Iris the most. She seems to favor Leonard because other children tease him for being fat. She tries to give him special attention. She talks about Iris as being her baby.

Arthur appears to love all the children, but makes extra comments about the oldest sons. Arthur says his wife is a wonderful mother and good house-keeper but makes no comments about their personal relationship.

Danny and Ronny seem to pair off because of their ages. Leonard and Iris prefer mother's company, while Sammy cares for and plays with Arlie. Cindy, age 5, appears withdrawn and a loner.

8. Match each family function from the left-hand column with the appropriate description of it in the right-hand column showing how the function has changed (as society changed from an agrarian to industrialized state):

Function	**Description**
a. Affective	1. Continues to be crucial.
b. Socializing	2. Decreased in importance or limited.
c. Economic	3. Increased in importance.
d. Religious	4. Function important; function shared with other institutions in society.
e. Care of disabled family members	
f. Educational	
g. Status conferring	
h. Reproduction	

► chapter 5 study answers

1. c.

2. Both internal family dynamics (structure and functions) and external relationships, i.e., the family system's interface with other systems and suprasystems, such as reference groups and wider society.

3. b.

4. a.

5. c and d.

6. a. 1.
   b. 2.
   c. 1.
   d. 2.

7. *Affective function:* Not being adequately fulfilled for all family members. Minimal data on children, although mother seems quite involved and enjoys her children. Mother is feeling unfulfilled emotionally in her rela-

tionship with her husband. No concrete data on husband's feelings, although it appears he has withdrawn from the family affectively.

Health care function: Food: mother cooks and provides nutritional meals, although excessive carbohydrates; shelter: adequate home provided; clothing: family adequately dressed; health care: children appear in good health. Would need to assess further this area, as it is inadequately described.

Reproductive function: Family has seven children. All living with the family.

Socialization: Emma's central family concern is child rearing; father participates minimally in disciplining and guidance. Family actively fulfills this function via the mother. Social placement: Society will identify family as members of working class.

Economic function: Father employed and provides family with basic necessities for independent living.

8. a. 3.
   b. 4.
   c. 2.
   d. 2.
   e. 2.
   f. 2.
   g. 2.
   h. 1.

Family Developmental Theory

Marilyn M. Friedman with Cynthia D. Connelly, Kim Miller, and Rhea P. Williams

► learning objectives

1. With respect to family developmental theory, discuss three basic assumptions.

2. Discuss the usefulness of the family developmental approach in assessing and working with families.

3. Define the meaning of family developmental tasks and the family life cycle or family career.

4. Identify and describe each of the developmental stages of the two-parent nuclear family.

5. Identify three health promotion needs or health concerns that families commonly experience within each of the two-parent nuclear family's stages of development.

6. Describe developmental tasks of parents and how they relate to the nuclear family's stages of development.

7. Discuss adolescence and its impact on family.

8. Relative to the single-parent and/or divorced family, describe the family life cycle stages.

9. Relative to the stepparent family, describe the family life cycles stages.

10. Identify the primary assessment areas relative to family development and history, as well as two general family nursing interventions appropriate for assisting families developmentally.

One of the more recent frameworks generated for studying and working with families is that of family development. This theoretical approach seeks to explain change over time in the family system, including changes in interactions and relationships among family members over time. It emphasizes members playing roles within and outside the family that affect family interaction. Family development does not cover nonfamily aspects of the life careers of individual or events affecting them that do not impinge on the lives of other family members (Aldous, 1996).

The family developmental approach is based on the observation that families are long-lived groups with a natural history that must be assessed if the dynamics of the group are to be fully and accurately interpreted (Duvall & Miller, 1985). Although each family goes through each stage of development in its own unique way, all families are considered as examples of an overall normative pattern (Rodgers, 1973).

Family development gives a temporal change perspective to the study of families. Time is measured in weeks and years. This theory describes family life over time as divided into a series of stages. A family stage is an interval of time in which the structure and interaction of role relationships in the family are qualitatively and quantitatively distinct from other periods (Klein & White, 1996). Family transitions are shifts from one stage to another and can be viewed over time as consisting of paths taken or not taken (Klein & White, 1996). Family stages cover sizable time spans and, although transitions link one stage to another, there are breaks that give each stage its distinctive character.

The notion of stages rests on the assumption that in families there is high family member interdependence: families are forced to change each time members are added to or subtracted from the family, or each time the oldest child changes his or her developmental stage. For instance, changes in roles, marital adjustment, child rearing, and discipline have been found to change from stage to stage (Klein & White, 1996). The family takes one kind of structure when children are infants or preschool age; another structure when the parents enter into the prime of life and the children reach adolescence; and finally another when the children mature, marry, and go their own ways. Rodgers (1973) describes these changes further:

> The structure of the group changes during its history. . . . As members interact with one another over a variety of matters happening in the group, a whole set of learned and shared experiences develop which become precedents for further interactions. Although many of these experiences are unique, a great many are related to the normal and inevitable issues that arise in living together. Recently married couples must work out a set of relationships which are mutually satisfactory concerning many matters. Once established, however, the relationships do not remain constant, but change subtly or perhaps dramatically because of later events, which may occur in the family or outside of it. . . . Many happenings are anticipated and prepared for, whereas many are unexpected— though not peculiar to that family alone. Thus, though each family's history is unique, it is also common. Furthermore, it has a certain quality of inevitability though not necessarily of predictability as to exact time or circumstance. The developmental approach does not seek to explain family dynamics in terms of its unique elements, but in terms of the common quality of its experience over its history. There exist many more events that are common than are unique. (p. 13)

The historical roots of family developmental theory can be traced to five theoretical legacies. Family developmental framework is eclectic, because it acquired concepts from individual growth and developmental theory and from different approaches to the study of the family. Contributions to family development theory were drawn from symbolic interactionism, structural functionalism, the sociology of work and professions, systems theory, and more recently from family life stress and crisis theory (Mattessich & Hill, 1987). Evelyn Duvall and Reuben Hill, beginning in the 1940s, were the two family scholars who first developed this theoretical perspective (Burr, 1995).

The three basic assumptions of family developmental theory, as outlined by Aldous (1996), are:

1. Family behavior is the sum of the previous experiences of family members as incorporated in the present and in their expectations for the future.
2. Families develop and change over time in similar and consistent ways.
3. Families and their members perform certain time-specific tasks that are set by themselves and by the cultural and societal context.

Family developmental theory is based on the common, general features of family life; it does not address situational or nonnormative stressors (unusual events), and can be criticized for its assumption of homogeneity (its lack of adequate attention to family diversity), its middle-class bias, its assumption of stability within each stage, and its lack of explanation of the processes that occur between stages that allow families to change. Yet the use of this framework for assessment and intervention is exceedingly helpful, because it provides family care health professionals with ways of anticipating what to expect and hence what kinds of teaching and counseling services may be needed. Family developmental theory increases our understanding of families at different points in their life cycle and generates "typical" or "modal" descriptions of family life during the various stages (Duvall & Miller, 1985). Moreover, by assessing the family's developmental stage and its performance of the tasks appropriate to that stage, family health care professionals are provided with guidelines for analyzing family growth and health-promotion needs. The family nurse is better able to provide the support needed for smooth progression from one stage to another.

▶ THE FAMILY CAREER OR FAMILY LIFE CYCLE

Family career is the dynamic process of change that occurs during a family's existence. The concept of family career and family life cycle are used inter-changeably (Aldous, 1996) and will be used as such throughout this chapter. The use of family life cycle, however, is somewhat misleading since a cycle is a repeated sequence of events (Klein & White, 1996). Existence over time does not constitute a cycle. For example, although the family members at the end of the family are the same couple who began the fam-ily's existence, the events of a newlywed couple are not repeated by the aging couple.

A family career includes the diverse paths that unfold during a family's life. It is composed of all the events and periods of time (stages) between events transversed by a family, such as beginning a family, raising and launching children, and experiencing loss of a partner. A reorganization of family roles and tasks as the family progresses through different stages of development and situational events is required (Aldous, 1996).

Duvall's (1977) eight stages of family develop-ment describe the expected changes for the two-parent nuclear family (see Table 6–1). Carter and McGoldrick (1989) generated a similar six-stage model for family therapists. Table 6–2 compares Duvall's stages with those of Carter and McGoldrick.

In Duvall's paradigm, she uses the age and school placement of the oldest child as a guidepost for the life cycle intervals, with the exception of the two last stages of family life, when children are no longer present in the family. When there are several chil-dren in the family, some overlapping of different stages occurs. Carter and McGoldrick (1989), in con-trast, formulated family life cycle stages that focus on the major points at which family members enter or exit the family, thus upsetting the family's equilib-rium. Emphasis here is placed on the altered rela-tionships that are requisite so that the family can move from one life cycle stage to the next.

▶ TABLE 6–1

THE EIGHT-STAGE FAMILY LIFE CYCLE

Stage I	Beginning families (also referred to as married couples or the stage of marriage)
Stage II	Childbearing families (the oldest child is an infant through 30 months)
Stage III	Families with preschool children (oldest child is 2½ to 6 years of age)
Stage IV	Families with school children (oldest child is 6 to 13 years of age)
Stage V	Families with teenagers (oldest child is 13 to 20 years of age)
Stage VI	Families launching young adults (covering the first child who has left through the last child leaving home)
Stage VII	Middle-aged parents (empty nest through retirement)
Stage VIII	Family in retirement and old age (also referred to as aging family members or retirement to death of both spouses)

Adapted from Duvall (1977), Duvall and Miller (1985).

Family Career or Life Cycle Variations

There are predictable stages within the life career of every family; however, they do not necessarily occur linearly. Families vary, as do the family stages. Stages of the family life cycle follow no rigid pattern (Duvall, 1977; Klein & White, 1996). It then goes without saying that many families today do not fit into the traditional two-parent nuclear family stages of Duvall or Carter and McGoldrick. Variations in the traditional family life cycle are seen among fami-lies in which couples do not marry, couples remain childless, and in which there are homosexual unions and single-parent and stepparent families. More peo-ple are choosing various family forms and hence the concept of the family career, covering the two-parent nuclear family, is obviously limited in applicability. For nontraditional families or families that are poor or from minorities, variations in the timing and sequencing of family events exists (Teachman et al., 1987). Current research describes differing career stages and tasks for families not fitting the traditional two-parent nuclear family. The life stages of single

► TABLE 6-2

COMPARISON OF FAMILY LIFE CYCLE STAGES OF DUVALL AND CARTER AND McGOLDRICK

Carter and McGoldrick (Family Therapy Perspective)	Duvall (Sociological Perspective)
1. Between families: the unattached young adult	No stage identified here, although Duvall considers young adult to be in process of "being launched." Because there is often a considerable time period between adolescence and marriage, addition of this "between stage" is indicated.
2. The joining of families through marriage: the newly married couple	1. Beginning families.
3. Families with young children (infancy through school age)	2. Childbearing families (oldest child up to 30 months of age).
	3. Families with preschool children (oldest child, 2½ to 5 years of age).
	4. Families with school-aged children (oldest child, 6 to 12 years of age).
4. Families with adolescents	5. Families with teenagers (oldest child, 13 to 20 years of age).
5. Launching children and moving on	6. Families launching young adults (all children leaving home).
	7. Middle-aged parents (empty nest, up to retirement).
6. Families in later life	8. Families in retirement and old age (retirement to death of both spouses).

Adapted from Carter and McGoldrick (1989), Duvall and Miller (1985).

parent, stepparent, and lesbian/gay families are described later in the chapter.

Even within the traditional two-parent nuclear family there have been changes in the timing of life cycle stages. Increasingly young adults are living with parents, alone, or with other young adults (the "between family life cycle stage" of Carter and McGoldrick). Couples are postponing marriage, shortening the child-rearing period (the result largely of birth control and work), and having fewer children. With these changes and with people living longer, there is a corresponding greater number of years within the last two stages of the family career—the middle years and retirement and old age stages.

Family Developmental Tasks

Just as individuals have developmental tasks* that they must achieve in order to feel satisfied during a

stage of development and to be able to proceed successfully to the following stage, each stage of family development has its specific developmental tasks or role expectations. Family developmental tasks refer to growth responsibilities that must be achieved by a family during each stage of its development so as to meet (1) its biological requirements, (2) its cultural imperatives, and (3) its own aspirations and values (Duvall, 1977; Klein & White, 1996).

How do the developmental tasks of the family differ from those of the individual family member? Although in reality many of them dovetail, family developmental tasks are generated when the family strives as a unit to meet the demands and needs of family members who in turn are striving to meet their individual developmental requisites. Family tasks are also created by community pressures for the family and its members to conform to the expectations of the family's reference group and the wider society.

In addition, family developmental tasks also include the tasks or role expectations specific to each stage inherent in accomplishing the five basic functions of the family, consisting of (1) affective function (personality maintenance function); (2) socialization and social placement function; (3) health care func-

---

*Examples are the developmental tasks that are inherent within the following frames of reference: (1) Erikson's stages of psychosocial development, (2) Piaget's stages of cognitive development, (3) Kohlberg's stages of moral development, and (4) Freud's stages of psychosexual development.

tion—provision and allocation of physical necessities and health care; (4) reproductive function; and (5) economic function (see Chap. 5 for a fuller definition of these functions).

The real challenge for families is to meet each of the members' needs, as well as to meet the general family functions. The meshing of individual developmental needs and family tasks is not always possible. For instance, the adolescent's tasks of developing autonomy includes changes in parental authority that may be in opposition to the family's social control task.

▶ TWO-PARENT NUCLEAR FAMILY CAREER OR LIFE CYCLE STAGES

The following family life cycle stages have been described by Duvall and Miller (1985) and Carter and McGoldrick (1989). The nine stages include the eight stages of Duvall plus the addition of the "between stage" from the Carter and McGoldrick typology to give a more comprehensive depiction of changes in family life (see Table 6–2). These family life cycle stages portray the intact nuclear American family, but are limited in their applicability to single, divorced, and stepparent families. Common health concerns and health-promotion needs are also discussed within each of the respective family life cycle stages.

Transitional Stage: Between Families (the Unattached Young Adult)

This stage refers to the period of time when individuals are in their 20s, are financially independent, and have physically left their family of origin but have not begun their own family of marriage. The between-family stage is not considered a family life cycle stage or career by Duvall and other sociologists. Yet, because this period is such a commonly experienced one (adolescents do not go directly from their family of origin to a family of marriage, as was more frequently seen in the past), and because this period is such a pivotal transition, the stage was added in this text. This stage has also been largely ignored by family health care professionals and family therapists (Aylmer, 1988).

Demographic data support the importance of this stage. Today in the United States more young adults delay marriage while they live in bachelor quarters or cohabitate outside of marriage. First marriage in the United States occurs generally 3 years later than it did a generation ago. Unmarried couples account for 3.7 million of the country's 93 million households, with five times as many young adults cohabiting outside of marriage today than in 1970 (Koeninn, 1997; Saluter, 1994).

The between-family stage is considered by Aylmer (1988) and other family therapists to be the cornerstone for all the successive stages to follow; how the young adult goes through this stage profoundly affects who he or she marries as well as when and how marriage occurs. To complete this stage successfully the young adult must separate from the family of origin without cutting off or attaching reactively to an emotional surrogate.

Developmental Tasks. This stage is "between families"; the development tasks are individual in nature rather than family-oriented. Carter and McGoldrick (1989) explain that the primary developmental task of the unattached young adult is "coming to terms with his or her family of origin" (p. 13). Three developmental tasks are listed by Carter and McGoldrick (1989, p. 15):

1. Differentiation of self in relation to family of origin.
2. Development of intimate peer relationships.
3. Establishment of self relative to work and financial independence.

It is a time for the young adult to form personal life goals and a sense of self before joining with another in marriage (Table 6–3). This is generally a difficult transitional stage, inasmuch as individuating from one's family of origin physically, financially, and emotionally is generally delayed in many families today.

This stage is typically experienced differently depending on one's gender. Carol Gilligan's seminal work, *In a Different Voice* (1982), describes the contrasting orientation of males and females through their socialization. Men generally are taught to pursue their self-identification through self-expression while women pursue theirs through self-sacrifice. As

► TABLE 6–3

THE TRANSITION STAGE: BETWEEN FAMILIES AND CONCOMITANT FAMILY DEVELOPMENTAL TASKS

Family Life Cycle Stage	Family Developmental Tasks
Transition stage: between families	1. Separating from family of origin. 2. Developing intimate peer relationships. 3. Establishing work and financial independence.

Adapted from Carter and McGoldrick (1989).

young men and women go through the unattached young adult period, they have different identity issues to resolve. A balance of both autonomy and attachment is needed in relationships and work, but men generally struggle with issues of attachment and relationships, while women struggle with issues of autonomy.

Most of the above issues involve relationships between the young adult and his or her parents (Aylmer, 1988) and creating a new balance between separatedness and connectedness. How the parents of the young adult interact with their young adult child during this period is therefore vitally important. From a family systems perspective, there are reciprocal or circular effects taking place between the parents and young adults (each mutually influence each other's actions), which enhance or inhibit the process of separation and individuation of the young adult. If parents have an unsatisfying marriage and need the young adult to stay connected to meet their needs, this hinders the young adult's efforts at separating; in turn, if the young adult feels anxious and incompetent about managing independently, he or she will delay separation and attempt to keep the parents involved.

Health Concerns.   Health concerns are both personal and familial during this transitional stage. Family planning and birth control use is a major concern and need. Sexually transmitted diseases are more frequently seen in this group (venereal disease, AIDS, etc.). Accidents and suicides are leading causes of mortality. Mental health problems are also

common, and as explained above, deal primarily with the issue of separating in a functional way from one's family of origin so that healthy, intimate relationships can be formed.

Health promotion needs are similar to subsequent stages. Because young adults are now on their own, typically their lifestyles do not incorporate the recommended health-protective practices such as avoidance of drugs, alcohol, and tobacco; engaging in safe sexual practices; as well as obtaining adequate sleep, nutrition, exercise, and preventive dental and medical examinations and care.

Stage I: Beginning Families

The formation of the couple marks the beginning of a new family with the movement from the former family of origin to the new intimate relationship. This stage is also called the stage of marriage.

Family Developmental Tasks.   Establishing a mutually satisfying marriage relating harmoniously to the kin network, and planning a family constitute the three critical tasks of this period (Table 6–4).

Establishing a Mutually Satisfying Marriage. When two people become united in marriage, their initial concerns are preparing for a new type of life together. The resources of the two people are combined, their roles altered, and new functions

► TABLE 6–4

TWO-PARENT NUCLEAR FAMILY LIFE CYCLE STAGE I AND CONCOMITANT FAMILY DEVELOPMENTAL TASKS

Family Life Cycle Stage	Family Developmental Tasks
Beginning families	1. Establishing a mutually satisfying marriage. 2. Relating harmoniously to the kin network. 3. Planning a family (decisions about parenthood).

Adapted from Carter and McGoldrick (1989), Duvall and Miller (1985).

assumed. Learning to live together while providing for each other's basic personality needs becomes a crucial developmental task. The couple has to mutually accommodate to each other in many small ways. For example, they must develop routines for eating, sleeping, getting up in the morning, cleaning house, sharing the bathroom, recreational pursuits, and going places they both enjoy. In this process of mutual accommodation, a set of patterned transactions are formed and then maintained by the couple, with each spouse triggering and monitoring the behavior of the other.

The success of the evolving relationship depends on the mutual accommodation just discussed and on a complementarity, or the fitting together of the needs and interests of the mates. Just as important, individual differences need to be acknowledged. In healthy relationships differences are seen to enrich the marital relationship. Achieving a satisfying relationship is dependent on the development of satisfactory ways to handle "differentness" (Satir, 1983) and conflicts. A healthy way of resolving problems is related to the mates' ability to empathize, be mutually supportive, be able to communicate openly and honestly (Raush et al., 1969), and approach a conflict with feelings of mutual respect (Jackson & Lederer, 1969).

Moreover, how successful the evolving marital relationship will be depends on how well each of the partners has differentiated or separated from their respective families of origin (the previous developmental task) (Bowen, 1978). A mature person must separate/differentiate from his or her own parents in order to form his or her own self-identity and healthy intimate relationships. An excellent description of this process and psychosocial problems during this period is presented by McGoldrick (1988).

Many couples experience problems in sexual adjustment, often because of ignorance and misinformation leading to unrealistic expectations and disappointment. Moreover, many couples bring their own unresolved needs and desires into the relationship, and these can adversely affect the sexual relationship (Goldenberg & Goldenberg, 1996; Heinrich, 1996).

Relating Harmoniously to Kin Network.   A basic role shift occurs in the first marriage of a couple, as they move from their parental homes to their new setting. Concomitantly, they become members of three families—those of their respective families of origin in addition to the one they have recently created. The couple faces the tasks of separating themselves as a newly formed family from each of their families of origin and working out different relationships with parents, siblings, and in-laws, since their primary loyalty must shift to their marital relationship. For the couple this entails forming a new relationship with each set of parents, one that allows not only for mutual support and enjoyment but also for an autonomy that protects the newly formed family from outside intrusion that might undermine the building of a satisfying marriage.

Planning a Family.   Whether or not to have children and the timing of pregnancies becomes a significant family decision. Littlefield (1977) underscores the importance of considering the whole family pregnant when one is working in maternity care. The type of health care the family as a unit receives during the prenatal period greatly influences the family's ability to cope effectively with the tremendous changes after the baby's birth.

Health Concerns.   The primary areas of concern are sexual and marital role adjustment, family planning education and counseling, prenatal education and counseling, and communication.

It becomes increasingly apparent that counseling should be provided premaritally. Lack of information often results in sexual and emotional problems, fear, guilt feelings, unplanned pregnancies, and venereal disease either before or after marriage. These unfortunate events do not allow the couple to plan their lives and begin their relationship with a stable foundation.

Traditional marriage concepts are being challenged by love relationships, common-law marriages, and homosexual unions. People entering into nonmarriage unions often need as much if not more counsel from health care workers who may be called on to assist such couples. It is perhaps at this point that family nurses may be caught between two "families," the family of orientation and the forming union. In such a situation, family health professionals need not make value judgments but attempt to help each of the two groups to understand themselves and each other (Williams & Leaman, 1973).

Family Planning. Because family planning is such a cardinal responsibility for the nurse working with families, a more detailed discussion of this area follows. The absence of informed, effective family planning affects family health in many ways: maternal–infant morbidity and mortality, child neglect, ill health of parents, child development problems, and marital discord. Informed and intentional family formation involves making decisions regarding the circumstances and timing of marriage, first pregnancy, birth spacing, and family size. Nevertheless, people have the right to make personal decisions about when and/or whether to have children, aside from any family health considerations.

The economic and cultural diversity of families emphasize the need to adapt health promotion activities to the needs of minorities, the impoverished and special ethnic groups. Although the U.S. Bureau of the Census (1992) reports a noticeable trend in delays and declines in childbearing, single-parent families are on the upsurge. Increasingly, mothers are the single-parent family into which the child is born. This family structure results in poverty for 1 out of 5 of all children (National Council of Family Relations, 1993).

One million adolescents become pregnant each year and of those 600,000 give birth (National Center for Health Statistics, 1991). Teenage pregnancy is not a new phenomenon; however, there is a change in the context within which it occurs, pregnancy outside of the context of marriage (Brooks-Gunn & Chase-Landsdale, 1995). Thus, adolescent pregnancy is viewed as particularly problematic because of the vulnerability and lack of resources. Pregnancy is, not surprisingly, the chief cause of women leaving school. Within marriage, early pregnancy (before 2 years) detracts from marital adjustment. All of these are important health factors for children and parents (National Council of Family Relations, 1993).

The physical health of mother and child is a major issue, documented in obstetrical and perinatal studies. Birth intervals of between 2 and 4 years and a maternal age in the 20s are the most favorable factors for reducing maternal and infant mortality and morbidity. Optimal family size, spacing, and timing of births also reduces infant mortality (Cohn & Lieberman, 1974).

The rate of planned pregnancies is growing, as is the number of women or couples who are using contraceptives. Forty-five states, as well as the District of Columbia, have enacted legislation allowing teenage girls under the age of 18 to obtain contraceptives without parental consent. Yet a large proportion of sexually active adolescents and young adult women are not receiving family planning services (Chilman, 1988).

Inconsistent patterns of contraceptive use are attributed to inaccessibility of services and the fractious debate about the role of government in providing such services (Brooks-Gunn & Paikoff, 1993). Religious and sociopolitical factors have interceded to reduce women's and couple's reproductive rights. As of the early 1990s, due to pro-life opposition, the struggle to keep present services available is of growing concern. Public funding for family planning initiatives, as well as abortion, has been cut and services gravely curtailed for the poor and young.

In addition to the need for more health care clinics and permissive legislation for teenagers to receive care, effective sex and family planning health education programs need to be devised and implemented in schools, churches, and health agencies. Such services should be focused not on the general premise that family planning is an end in itself, but on the health benefits of family planning to the individual and to the growth and development of the family.

Forcing birth control on families, however, is not ethical; doing so destroys a family's sense of initiative, integrity, and competence, and violates individuals' rights for self-determination. Teenage girls who want babies need to be counseled on physical and emotional readiness for parenthood and realistic protection from pregnancy along with good health supervision. Little has been done to balance the societal pressures toward sex and marriage with realistic contraception education.

Stage II: Childbearing Families

Stage II begins with the birth of the first child and continues through the infant's 30th month. The transition to parenthood is a key one in the family life cycle. With the birth of the first child the family becomes a threesome, making it a permanent system for the first time, i.e., the system endures regardless of the outcome of the marriage (McGoldrick, Herman, & Carter, 1993).

Although parenthood represents an extremely important goal for most couples, most find it a very stressful life transition. A period of disequilibrium is inevitable as the family moves from one stage to another (Martell & Imle, 1996). Not infrequently, this disequilibrium requires so much change that some researchers find that it can lead to family crisis (Clark, 1966; Hobbs & Cole, 1976; LeMasters, 1957), causing feelings of inadequacy in parenting and a disruption in marital relations.

Miller and Myers-Walls (1983), based on their review of studies of new parents, summarized the specific parenting stressors identified in the literature. The most commonly mentioned stressor appeared to be the loss of personal freedom due to parenting responsibilities; in addition, less time and companionship in marriage were frequently identified.

The adjustment to marriage is usually not as hard as the adjustment to parenthood. Although a very meaningful and gratifying experience to most parents, the advent of the baby calls for a sudden change to an incessantly demanding role. It is especially difficult in the beginning because of the feelings of inadequacy of new parents; the lack of help from family and friends; the conflicting advice of helpful friends, family, and health care professionals; and the frequent awakening of the baby at night—which usually continues for about 3 to 4 weeks. Also, the mother is fatigued psychologically and physiologically. She often feels the burdens of household duties and perhaps also employment responsibilities, in addition to caring for the baby. It is especially difficult if the new mother has been ill or has had a long, difficult labor and delivery or a cesarean section.

Two important factors contribute to the difficulty of assuming the parental role. Most persons today are not prepared to be parents and many deleterious, unrealistic myths romanticizing the rearing of children exist in our society (Szafran, 1996). Parenthood is the only major role for which little preparation is given, and difficulties in role transition adversely affect the quality of the marital and parent–child relationships.

The arrival of a new baby into the home creates changes for every member of the family and for every set of relationships. A stranger has been admitted into a close-knit group, and suddenly the balance of the family shifts—each member takes on new roles and begins new relationships. In addition to a baby being born, a mother, father, and grandparents are born. The wife must now relate to the husband as both a spouse and a father and vice versa. And in families with previous children, the impact of the new baby is as significant on the siblings as on the new parents.

Dramatic social changes in American society since the 1950s have also had a marked effect on new parents. The large proportion of women working outside the home and having careers, the rise in divorce and marital instability, the common use of contraception and abortion, and the large increase in costs of having and caring for children are all factors influencing the passage through the early childbearing life cycle stage (Bradt, 1988; Miller & Myers-Walls, 1983).

Family Developmental Tasks. After the coming of the firstborn, the family has several important developmental tasks (Table 6–5). Husband, wife, and baby must all learn new roles, while the nuclear family unit expands in functions and responsibilities. This involves the simultaneous meshing of the developmental tasks of each family member and the family as a whole (Duvall, 1977).

The birth of a child makes radical changes in family organization. The functions of the couple must differentiate to meet the new demands of the infant for care and nurturance. How these responsibilities are fulfilled varies tremendously with the

---

▶ TABLE 6–5

TWO-PARENT NUCLEAR FAMILY LIFE CYCLE STAGE II AND CONCOMITANT FAMILY DEVELOPMENTAL TASKS

Family Life Cycle Stage	Family Developmental Tasks
Childbearing families	1. Setting up the young family as a stable unit (integrating of new baby into family). 2. Reconciling conflicting developmental tasks and needs of various family members. 3. Maintaining a satisfying marital relationship. 4. Expanding relationships with extended family by adding parenting and grandparenting roles.

Adapted from Carter and McGoldrick (1989), Duvall and Miller (1985).

sociocultural position of the couple. Although most parents continue to assume traditional roles or division of responsibilities, it is not uncommon in contemporary society for both mother and father to share in infant-care tasks (Tiller, 1995).

Relationships with the paternal and maternal extended family must also be realigned during this stage. New roles need to be established with respect to grandparenting and relationships between parents and grandparents (Bradt, 1988).

One of the most important roles for family nurses to assess when working with the childbearing family is the parental role—how both parents interact with and care for the new infant, and how the infant responds. Klaus and Kendall (1976), Kendall (1974), Rubin (1967), and others verify the critical impact of early attachment and a beginning warm, positive parent–child relationship on the future parental relationship with the child. The parents' attitude about themselves as parents, their attitudes about the baby, and the characteristics of parental communication and stimulation of the infant (Davis, 1978) are related areas that need to be assessed.

Role changes and adaptation to new parental responsibilities often are more rapidly learned by the mother than by the father. The child is a reality to the expectant mother much earlier than for the father, who usually begins to feel like a father at the birth, but sometimes even later than that (Minuchin, 1974).

The way in which most fathers have traditionally been left out of the perinatal process has certainly delayed men from taking on this important role change and thereby hindered their emotional involvement. Fortunately, increased awareness of the important role fathers play in child care and the child's development has led to greater involvement of fathers in infant care among the middle class (Hanson & Bozett, 1985; Henderson & Brouse, 1991).

The mother and father grow and develop their parental roles in response to the continually changing demands and developmental tasks of the growing youngster, the family as a whole, and themselves. According to Friedman (1957), parents go through five successive stages of development. The first two stages fall into this phase of family life. First, during the child's infancy, parents learn the meaning of cues their baby expresses in making his or her needs known. With each successive child, parents will go

through this same stage as they adjust to each infant's unique cues.

The second stage of parental development, learning to accept the child's growth and development, occurs in the toddler years. Just prior to and during this stage, parents—particularly parents with their first child—need guidance and support. Parents need to understand tasks the child is attempting to master and the child's needs for safety, limits, and toilet training. They need to understand the concept of developmental readiness, or "the teachable moment." At the same time, parents need guidance in understanding the tasks they themselves are mastering during this stage.

New marital communication patterns evolve with the coming of a child, with mates relating to each other both as mates and as parents. Spouse transactional patterns have been found to change drastically. Feldman (1961) observed that parents of infants talked less with each other and had less fun, less stimulating conversation, and a diminished quality of marital interaction. Some parents feel overwhelmed with the added responsibilities, particularly those in dual-worker families where both parents work full-time. Dalgas-Pelish (1993) found that marital happiness was lower for childbearing families compared to childless couples.

The reestablishment of satisfying communication patterns—including personal, marital, and parental feelings and concerns—is critical. Mates must continue to meet each other's personal adult psychological and sexual needs as well as share and interact with each other about parental responsibilities.

The sexual relationship of the mates generally declines during pregnancy and through the 6-week postpartum period. Sexual difficulties during the later period are common, arising from such factors as the mother's absorption in her new role, fatigue, and feelings of loss of sexual attractiveness, as well as the husband's feeling of being "left or pushed out" by the new baby.

Family communications now include a third member, making for a triad. Parents must learn to perceive and discern the communication cries of the infant. For instance, the baby's cries need to be differentiated into expressions of discomfort, hunger, overstimulation, sickness, or fatigue. And the baby begins responding to cuddles, fondling, and talking, which then are received and reinforced by the parents.

Family planning counseling should begin during the prenatal or early postpartum period since many couples do not wait to resume intercourse until the traditional 6-week postpartum examination. Parents should be encouraged to openly discuss family spacing and planning. Due to the increased personal and family demands new babies bring, parents need to realize that frequent, closely spaced pregnancies can be harmful to the mother, as well as to the father, siblings, and the family unit.

This life cycle stage also requires an adjustment of relationships within the extended family and with friends. When other family members try to support and assist the new parents, tensions may result. Although grandparents, for instance, can be of great help to the new family, the potential for conflict exists because of differences in values and expectations existing between the generations.

Despite the importance of having a social network or social support system for achieving satisfaction with and positive feelings about family life, the young family needs to know when it needs help and from whom to accept it as well as when to depend on its own inner resources and strengths (Duvall, 1977).

A strong, viable marital relationship contributes to the stability and morale of the family. A satisfying husband–wife relationship will give the mates the strength and energy to "give" to the infant and to each other. Conflicting pressures and demands, such as between the mother's loyalty to infant and to husband, are problematic and can be agonizing. This type of conflict can become the central source of unhappiness during this life cycle stage.

Health Concerns. Concerns of families in this stage begin with preparation for parenthood. Family-centered maternity education with a wide variety of prenatal and postnatal classes is available to help prepare young parents for the birth experience and the transition to parenthood (Szafran, 1996). Follow-up home visits after the birth are recommended for meeting the educational and support needs of the child-bearing family in the early days of parenthood (Evans, 1991; Williams & Cooper, 1993). Infant care, well-baby care, early recognition and appropriate handling of physical health problems, immunizations, normal growth and development, safety measures, family planning, family interaction, and general health promotion (lifestyle) are all important areas for discussion.

Other concerns that contribute to the family's health during this period of a family's life are inaccessibility and inadequacy of child-care facilities for working mothers; parent–child relationships; sibling relationships; parenting, including child abuse and neglect; and parent-role transition problems.

Stage III: Families With Preschool Children

The third stage of the family life cycle commences when the firstborn child is about 2½ years old and terminates when he or she is 5. The family now may consist of three to five persons, with the paired positions of husband-father, wife-mother, son-brother, and daughter-sister. The family is becoming more complex and differentiated (Duvall & Miller, 1985).

Family life during this stage is busy and demanding for parents. Both parents have greater demands on their time, as it is probable that the mother is working also, part- or full-time. Nevertheless, realizing that parents are the "architects of the family," designing and directing family development (Satir, 1983), it is critical for them to strengthen their partnership—in short, to keep the marriage alive and well. This is often a problem during this particular stage of family life (Olson, McCubbin et al., 1983).

Preschool children have much to learn at this stage, especially in the area of independence. They must achieve enough autonomy and self-sufficiency to be able to handle themselves without their parents in a variety of places. Experience in nursery school, kindergarten, Project Head Start, a day-care center, or similar programs is a good way to foster this kind of development. Structured preschool programs are especially helpful in assisting parents from inner-city, low-income communities with their preschool children. Although multiple studies have shown the benefit of quality child-care and preschool programs such as Head Start, accessibility of these programs for working poor families is generally poor. Obtaining adequate child care arrangements is a major concern for parents (Kelleher, 1996). Infant and preschool day-care centers that are reasonable and of good quality are difficult if not impossible to locate in most communities. Mothers with careers and adolescent mothers are particularly in need of better child-care facilities and programs (Adams & Adams, 1990).

Many single-parent families exist within this particular life cycle stage. Twenty-one percent of all U.S. children live in single-parent homes (National Council for Family Relations, 1993). Among single-parent families, the role strain of parenting the preschooler, coupled with other roles, is great.

Family Developmental Tasks.   The family is now growing in both numbers and complexity. The need of preschoolers and other young children to explore the world around them, and parents' needs for their own privacy, make housing and adequate space major problems. Equipment and facilities also need to be childproofed, for it is at this stage that accidents become the most common causes of both mortality and disability. Assessing the home for safety hazards is of prime importance for the community health nurse, and health education must then be included so that the parents and children are cognizant of the risks involved and of ways of preventing accidents. (See Table 6–6 for developmental tasks.)

Due to both lack of specific resistance to the many bacterial and viral diseases and increased exposure, preschoolers are frequently sick with one minor infectious illness after another. Infectious diseases often "ping-pong" throughout the family. Frequent visits to the doctor, caring for sick kids, and running home from work to pick up an ill child from the nursery school are common weekly crises. Thus children's contacts with infectious and communicable diseases and their general susceptibility to disease are prime health concerns (Shelov, 1991).

Accidents, falls, burns, and lacerations are also quite common occurrences. These are even more frequently seen where there are large families, families where an adult caretaker is not present (latchkey children), and in low-income families. Environmental safety and adequate child supervision are the keys to reducing accidents (Shelov, 1991).

The husband-father generally assumes more involvement in the household responsibilities during this stage of family development than during any other stage, the largest percentage of this being spent in child-care activities. The father's involvement with child care at this time is especially important, as this relationship with the preschooler assists the child with his or her sexual identification. It is particularly critical for boys in the first 5 years of life to associate closely with a strong, limit-setting, warm father or father substitute so that their masculine role identity can be established (Walters, 1976).

A more mature role is also assumed by the preschooler, who gradually takes on more responsibility for his or her own care, plus helping the mother or father with household jobs. It is not the productivity of the child that is important here, but the learning that is occurring.

Contrary to expectations, research has shown that the advent of the second child into the family has a more deleterious effect on the marital relationship than does the first birth (La Rossa & La Rossa, 1981). Feldman (1971) reports that parental roles make the marital roles difficult, as exhibited by the following observations: couples perceive more negative personality changes in each other; they are less satisfied with their home; there is more task-oriented interaction and fewer personal and child-centered conversations; more warmth is exhibited toward the children and less toward each other; and there is a lower level of sexual satisfaction (Feldman, 1969).

Feldman's well-recognized study parallels reports and observations of family counselors—that the marital relationship is often troubled at this phase of family life. In fact, many divorces occur within these years due to weak or unsatisfactory marital ties. Privacy and time

---

► TABLE 6–6

TWO-PARENT NUCLEAR FAMILY LIFE CYCLE STAGE III AND CONCOMITANT FAMILY DEVELOPMENTAL TASKS

Family Life Cycle Stage	Family Developmental Tasks
Families with pre-school children	1. Meeting family members' needs for adequate housing, space, privacy, and safety. 2. Socializing the children. 3. Integrating new child members while still meeting needs of other children. 4. Maintaining healthy relationships within the family (marital and parent–child) and outside the family (extended family and community).

Adapted from Carter and McGoldrick (1989), Duvall and Miller (1985).

together are prime necessities. Marriage counseling and marriage encounter groups have become important resources among the middle class. For the family without economic resources, however, limited assistance is available for strengthening a salvageable marriage. There is a trend for priests and ministers to become trained as marriage and family counselors and counsel couples who cannot afford private therapy.

A major task of the family is socializing the children. Preschoolers are developing critical self-attitudes (self-concepts) and rapidly learning to express themselves, as seen in their rapid grasp of language.

Another task during this period deals with how to integrate a new family member (second or third child) into the family while still meeting the needs of older child(ren). The displacement of a child by a newborn is psychologically a very traumatic event. Preparation of children for the arrival of a new baby helps ameliorate the situation, especially if the parents are sensitive to the older child's feelings and behavior. Sibling rivalry is often expressed by hitting or negatively relating to the new baby, regressive behaviors, and attention-getting activity. The best way to handle sibling rivalry is for the parents to spend a certain amount of time each day exclusively relating to the older child to give him or her the assurance that he or she is still loved and wanted.

About the time children become preschoolers, parents enter their third parenting stage, one of learning to separate from children as they toddle off to nursery school, a day-care center, or kindergarten. This stage continues during the preschool and early school years. Separation is often difficult for parents and they need support and an explanation of how the preschoolers' mastery of developmental tasks contributes to their child's growth in autonomy.

Separation from parents is also difficult for preschool children. Separation may occur as parents go to work, to the hospital, or on trips or vacations. Family preparation for separation is important in helping the children adjust to change.

Assisting parents to obtain family planning services after the arrival of a new baby, or to continue with contraception if there has been no intervening pregnancy, is also indicated. It is, for instance, not unusual for a woman to have stopped using contraceptives because of a missed period with the belief that she was pregnant, only to find out later that her eventual pregnancy resulted from sexual intercourse during the time she thought she was pregnant and was not using contraception.

Both parents need to have some outside interests and contacts to rejuvenate themselves to carry on the multitude of home tasks and responsibilities. Poor and single parents often do not have this opportunity. These families usually have the least satisfactory associations with the wider community due to their alienated position and the paucity of resources available to them.

Health Concerns. Numerous health concerns have been identified throughout our discussion of the preschool family. As indicated earlier, the major physical health problems concern the frequent communicable diseases of the children and the common falls, burns, poisonings, and other accidents that occur during the preschool age.

The prime psychosocial family health concern is the marital relationship. Studies verify the diminished satisfaction many couples experience during these years and the need for working to strengthen and reinvigorate this vital unit (Olson, McCubbin, and associates, 1983). Other important health concerns involve sibling rivalry, family planning, growth and developmental needs, parenting problems like setting limits (disciplining), child abuse and neglect, home safety, and family communication problems.

General health-promotion strategies continue to be germane during this stage, as lifestyle behaviors learned during childhood can have both short- and long-term consequences. Family health education directed at prevention of major health problems is indicated in the areas of smoking, alcohol and drug misuse, human sexuality, safety, diet and nutrition, exercise, and social support/stress management. "The chief goals for nurses working with the child and family are to assist them in establishing healthy lifestyles and in facilitating the child's optimal physical, intellectual, emotional, and social growth" (Wilson, 1988, p. 177).

Stage IV: Families With School-aged Children

This stage begins when the firstborn child enters school full time, usually at the age of 6 years, and concludes when he or she reaches puberty, around

13 years of age. Families usually reach their maximum number of members, and family relationships at the end of this stage (Duvall & Miller, 1985). Again these are busy years. Now children have their own activities and interests, in addition to the mandatory activities of life and school, and the parents' own activities. Each person is working on his or her own developmental tasks, just as the family attempts to fulfill its tasks (Table 6–7). According to Erikson (1950), parents are struggling with twin demands of finding fulfillment in rearing the next generation (the developmental task of generativity) and being concerned in their own growth; while school-age children are working at developing a sense of industry—the capacity for work enjoyment—and trying to eliminate or ward off a sense of inferiority.

The parental task at this time is that of learning to deal with the child's separation or, more simply, letting the child go. More and more, peer relationships and outside activities play larger roles in the life of the school-age child. These years are filled with family activities, but there are also forces gradually pushing the child to separate from the family in preparation for adolescence. Parents who have interests outside of their children will find it much easier to make the gradual separation. In instances where the mothering role is the central and only significant role in a woman's life, however, this separation

process may be a very painful one and one that is strongly resisted.

During this stage parents feel intense pressure from the outside community via the school system and other extrafamilial associations to have their children conform to the community's standards for children. This tends to influence the middle-class family to stress more traditional values of achievement and productivity, and to cause some working-class families and many poor families to feel alienated from and at conflict with school and/or community values.

Family Developmental Tasks. One of the critical tasks of parents in socializing their children at this time involves promoting school achievement. Another significant family task is maintaining a satisfying marital relationship. Again it has been reported that marital satisfaction is diminished during this stage. Two large studies reinforced these observations (Burr, 1970; Rollins & Feldman, 1970). Promoting open communication and supporting the spousal relationship is vital in working with the school-age family.

Health Concerns. Children's handicaps may come to light during this period of a child's life. School nurses and teachers will detect many visual, hearing, and speech defects, in addition to learning problems, behavior disturbances, inadequate dental care, child abuse, substance abuse, and communicable diseases during this stage (Edelman & Mandle, 1986). Working with the family in the role of health educator and counselor, in addition to initiating appropriate referrals for follow-up screening, assumes much of a school nurse's energies. He or she also acts as a resource person to the school teacher, enabling the teacher to handle the common and more individualized health needs of her or his pupils more effectively.

There are a number of other handicapping conditions occasionally detected during the school years, including epilepsy, cerebral palsy, mental retardation, cancer, and orthopedic conditions. The family health nurse's primary function here—in addition to referral, teaching, and counseling parents regarding these conditions—would be to assist the family in coping so that any adverse impact of the handicap on the family is minimized.

▶ TABLE 6–7

TWO-PARENT NUCLEAR FAMILY LIFE CYCLE STAGE IV AND CONCOMITANT FAMILY DEVELOPMENTAL TASKS

Family Life Cycle Stage	Family Developmental Tasks
Families with school-aged children	1. Socializing the children, including promoting school achievement and fostering of healthy peer relations of children. 2. Maintaining a satisfying marital relationship. 3. Meeting the physical health needs of family members.

Adapted from Carter and McGoldrick (1989), Duvall and Miller (1985).

For children with behavior problems, family nurses in schools, clinics, doctor's offices, and community agencies should seek active parental involvement and provide supportive counseling. Initiating a referral for family counseling/therapy is often very helpful in assisting a family to be aware of some of the family problems that may be adversely affecting the school-age child. When parents are able to reframe the child's behavior problem as a family problem and work toward its resolution with that new focus, more healthy family functioning often results as well as more healthy child behaviors (Bradt, 1988).

Stage V: Families With Teenagers

When the firstborn turns 13 years of age, the fifth stage of the family's life cycle or career commences. It usually lasts about 6 or 7 years, although it can be shorter if the child leaves the family early or longer if the child remains home later than 19 or 20 years of age. Other children in the home are usually of school age. The overarching family goal at the teenage stage is that of loosening family ties to allow greater responsibility and freedom for the teenager in preparation for becoming a young adult (Duvall & Miller, 1985).

Preto (1988), in discussing the transformation of the family system in adolescence, describes the family metamorphosis that takes place. It involves "profound shifts in relationship patterns across the generations, and while it may be signaled initially by the adolescent's physical maturity, it often parallels and coincides with changes in parents as they enter midlife and with major transformations faced by grandparents in old age" (p. 255).

This stage of the family's life is probably the most difficult, or certainly the most discussed and written about (Kidwell et al., 1983). The American family is affected by the tremendous developmental tasks of both the adolescent and parents and the inevitable conflicts and turmoil these create. The family faces new organizational challenges particularly with respect to autonomy and independence (Goldenberg & Goldenberg, 1996). Parents no longer maintain complete authority, nor can they abdicate authority either. Rule changing, limit setting, and role renegotiation are all necessary.

The major challenges in working with a family with teenagers revolve around the developmental changes adolescents undergo in terms of cognitive changes, identity formation, and biological growth (Kidwell et al., 1983) and developmentally based conflicts and crises.

Parental Roles, Responsibilities, and Problems.

Needless to say, parents find it a most difficult task to raise teenagers today. Nonetheless, parents need to stand firm against unreasonable testing of the limits that have been set in the family as they go through the process of gradually "letting go." Duvall (1977) also identifies the critical developmental task of this period to be the balancing of freedom with responsibility as teenagers mature and emancipate themselves. Friedman (1957) similarly defines the parental task during this stage as learning to accept rejection without deserting the child.

When the parents accept themselves as they are, with all their own weaknesses and strengths, and when they accept their several roles at this stage of development without undue conflict or sensitivity, they set the pattern for a similar sort of self-acceptance in their children. Relationships between parents and adolescents should be smoother when parents feel productive, satisfied, and in control of their own lives (Kidwell et al., 1983) and parents/families function flexibly (Preto, 1988).

Schultz (1972) and Elkind (1994) have expressed the view that the increasing complexity of American life has made the role of parents unclear. Parents may feel in competition with a variety of social forces and institutions—from school authorities and counselors to birth control and premarital sex and cohabitation options. Other factors add to their considerably diminished influence. Because of specialization of occupations and professions, parents are no longer able to help children with their vocational plans. The residential mobility and lack of continuing trustworthy adult relationships for both adolescents and parents, in addition to the inability of many parents to discuss personal, sexual, and drug-related concerns openly and nonjudgmentally with their children, has also contributed to parent–adolescent problems. Among immigrant families, generational clashes and value conflicts amplify the common communication problems between parents and children (see Chap. 21).

Family Developmental Tasks. The first and central family developmental task at this stage is balancing of freedom with responsibility as teenagers mature and become increasingly autonomous (Table 6–8). The parents must progressively change their relationship with their teenage son or daughter from the previously established dependent relationship to an increasingly independent one. This evolving shift in the parent–child relationship is typically one fraught with conflicts along the way.

In order for the family to adapt successfully during this stage, the family members, especially the parents, have to make a major "system change"—that is, set up new roles and norms and "let go" of the adolescent. Kidwell and associates (1983) summarize this needed change. "Paradoxically, the [family] system which can let go of its members is the system which will endure and reproduce itself effectively in later generations" (p. 88).

Parents who, in order to meet their own needs, do not let go, often find a major "revolution" by the teenager when separation occurs later. Parents may also thrust forth the adolescent into independence prematurely, ignoring his or her dependency needs. In this case the teenager may fail in attempts to achieve independence (Wright & Leahey, 1994).

As with the last three stages, the marital relationship is also a focus of concern. The second family developmental task is for couples to refocus their marital relationship (Wilson, 1988). Many couples have become so preoccupied with their parental responsibilities that their marriage no longer plays a central role in their lives. The husband usually spends much time away from home working and furthering his career, while the wife is probably also working while trying to keep up with housework and parental responsibilities. Under these conditions little time or energy is left for the marital relationship.

The other side of the coin, however, is that since the children are more responsible for themselves, the couple can more easily leave home to engage in their careers or establish individual and marital postparental interests. They can begin to build a foundation for the future stages of the family career.

A third pressing family developmental task is for family members, particularly the parents and teenager, to openly communicate with each other. Because of the generation gap, open communication is often an ideal rather than a reality. There is often mutual rejection by parents and adolescents of each other's values and lifestyles. Parents in multiproblem families have been found to frequently reject and then to disengage from their older children, thereby reducing whatever open communication channels there might have been.

Maintaining the family's ethical and moral standards is another family developmental task (Duvall & Miller, 1985). Although family rules need to change, family ethical and moral standards need to be maintained by parents. While adolescents are searching for their own beliefs and values, it is of paramount importance for parents to defend and adhere firmly to their own sound principles and standards. Adolescents are very sensitive to incongruities between what is "preached and practiced." Nonetheless, parents and children can learn from each other in the fast-changing and pluralistic society of today. Value transformations of youth are also transforming families. The adoption of a freer and more casual lifestyle symbolizes a value transformation affecting every phase of family life (Aldous, 1996).

Health Concerns. At this stage the physical health of the family members is usually good, but health promotion remains an important concern. Risk factors should be identified and discussed with families, as should the importance of a healthy lifestyle. From age 35 on, the risk of coronary heart

---

► **TABLE 6–8**

TWO-PARENT NUCLEAR FAMILY LIFE CYCLE STAGE V AND CONCOMITANT FAMILY DEVELOPMENTAL TASKS

Family Life Cycle Stage	Family Developmental Tasks
Families with teenagers	1. Balancing of freedom with responsibility as teenagers mature and become increasingly autonomous. 2. Refocusing the marital relationship. 3. Communicating openly between parents and children.

Adapted from Carter and McGoldrick (1989), Duvall and Miller (1985).

disease rises appreciably in males, and at this point both adult members are beginning to feel more vulnerable to ill health as part of their developmental changes and are usually more receptive to health-promotion strategies. With teenagers, accidents—particularly automobile accidents—are a great hazard, and broken bones and athletic injuries are also common.

Drug and alcohol misuse, birth control, unwanted pregnancies, and sex education and counseling are relevant areas of concern. In discussing these topics with families, the nurse may get caught squarely in the middle of a parent–youth dispute or problem. Adolescents often seek health services for pregnancy testing, drug use, AIDS screening, birth control and abortion, and venereal disease diagnosis and care. There has been a legal trend to allow adolescents to receive health care without parental consent. Where parents are involved, separate interviews with the teenager and parents prior to bringing them together are often indicated.

Teenage pregnancy is a critical family problem in many families today. The rate of teenage pregnancy continues to climb. Teenage pregnancy prevention includes both family- and community-based interventions. Family nurses need to assist families with teenage pregnancy prevention. Referrals for family planning services, sexuality counseling and education, encouraging adolescents to participate in after-school leisure time activities, and educational opportunities are basic teenage pregnancy prevention strategies (The Family Connection, 1996).

Another health need is again in the area of support and assistance in strengthening the marital relationship and the adolescent–parent relationships. Direct supportive counseling or initiation of referral to community resources for counseling, as well as recreational, educational, and other services, may be needed.

Stage VI: Families Launching Young Adults

The beginning of this phase of family life is characterized by the first child leaving the parental home and ends with "the empty nest," when the last child has left home. This stage could be quite short or fairly long, depending on how many children are in the family or if any unmarried children remain at home after finishing high school or college. Although the usual length of this stage is 6 or 7 years, in recent years the stage is longer in some families due to more older children living at home after they have finished school and begun working. The motive is often economics—the high cost of living independently. The more widespread trend, however, has been for young adults, who generally delay marriage, to have a period of being unattached during which they live independently in their own households. In a large Canadian survey it was found that children who grow up in stepfamilies and single-parent families leave home earlier than those raised in families with two biological parents. This difference was not seen to be influenced by economic factors, but rather was caused by parent differences and family milieu (Mitchell et al., 1989).

This phase of family life is marked by the culmination of years of preparation of and by the children for an independent adult life. Parents, as they let their children go, are relinquishing 20 years or so of the parenting role and returning to their original marital dyad. Family developmental tasks are critical while the family is shifting from a household with children to a husband–wife pair. The major family goal is the reorganization of the family into a continuing unit while releasing matured young people into lives of their own (Duvall & Miller, 1985). During this stage the marital pair may take on grandparent roles—another change in both roles and their self-image.

Early middle age, which is about the average age of parents during the launching of their oldest child, has been characterized as a "caught" period of life: caught between the demands of youth and the expectations of the elderly and caught between the world of work and the competing demands and involvement of the family, with the often seeming impossibility of meeting the demands of both realms. Studies indicate, however, that while the middle-aged adult may feel squeezed or "sandwiched" between the poles of youth and aging, at least for middle- and upper-class individuals, they can often appreciate their own importance and achievements: "They often know that they are the nation's decision-makers; they set the tone for life in this society. Society depends on middle-aged people's leadership and productivity" (Kerckhoff, 1976).

Family Developmental Tasks. As the family assists the oldest child in his or her launching, the parents are also involved with their younger children, helping them to become independent. And when the "released" son or daughter marries, the family task involves expanding the family circle to include new members by marriage and becoming accepting of the couple's own lifestyle and values (Table 6–9).

With the emptying of the nest, parents have more time to devote to other activities and relationships. Hopefully, they have not grown so far apart from each other that they cannot reinstitute or reestablish the wife and husband roles to the place of primary importance these roles once held. LeShan (1973) views this stage as a challenge to the marital relationship. When the children leave, marriage faces a moment of truth; is there strength enough to sustain it without the excuse of parenthood?

In the past, it was conventional to see this phase as a difficult time for women. The loss of roles related to child care left a feeling of emptiness. Today, far from feeling useless after their children grow up, the majority of women continue to be busy in their job and partner roles (Aldous, 1996). Most women feel satisfaction that their children have taken on adult responsibilities and are still in close contact with them. They now have the time and energy to devote to their own development and to couple intimacies and companionship.

▶ TABLE 6-9

TWO-PARENT NUCLEAR FAMILY LIFE CYCLE STAGE VI AND CONCOMITANT FAMILY DEVELOPMENTAL TASKS

Family Life Cycle Stage	Family Developmental Tasks
Families launching young adults	1. Expanding the family circle to include new family members acquired by marriage of children. 2. Continuing to renew and readjust in the marital relationship. 3. Assisting aging and ill parents of the husband and wife.

Adapted from Carter and McGoldrick (1989), Duvall and Miller (1985).

This period has been associated with menopause, with women historically seen as past their prime, getting old, and unappealing. However, research over the years has documented that many women find this period not only not problematic, but also desirable (N. Woods, personal communications, 1996).

Men in middlescence (the name for middle age in the developmental literature) face potential developmental crises. One potential crisis is the drive to get "ahead" in their careers with the realization that they have not succeeded or have not reached their aspirations. Also, signs of diminished masculinity, such as lower energy levels and lessened potency and sexual excitation, as well as figure, hair, and skin aging signs, and financial worries, are stressors for men during this family life cycle stage. The frequency of extramarital affairs, divorces, mental illness, alcoholism, and suicide all rise among adults of these age groups, underscoring the middle-age developmental crises that occur.

Friedman (1957) reiterates the significance of the marital relationship by characterizing the parental developmental stage at this point in the family as the building of a new life together. Both men and women are looking for married lives that are less hectic than in the child-dependent years (Aldous, 1996).

Another important developmental task of the middle-years family is that of assisting aging and ill parents of the husband and wife. Even though the actual care of aging and/or dependent parents is not an expected function of the American family with the exception of certain ethnic groups, the husband and wife are expected to assist and support elderly family members as much as they feel is feasible. Such activity takes all forms—from frequent telephoning and supportive calls to assisting financially, providing transportation, and visiting and caring for their parent(s) in the home.

In America the family is seen as primarily responsible for the succeeding generation, the offspring, and only secondarily for the previous generation, the parents (Roth, 1996). Currently however, there is a political trend throughout the country for families to assume greater responsibility for all family members, including preceding generations.

Three-generation families, although not the usual pattern, are not uncommon, particularly in "traditional" Asian, Hispanic, Greek, Italian, Middle

Eastern, and Jewish families. Most often in the United States the multigenerational family seems to develop primarily when the nuclear family is disrupted by death or divorce. Financial expediency or child-care needs may also encourage such living arrangements.

Older parents typically desire to live independently so as not to impinge on their children's lives and, more importantly, to retain their own feelings of competence, independence, and privacy (Bengtson et al., 1987; Troll, 1971). Parents may also have to wrestle with the decision to place their parents in a nursing home or retirement or board-and-care facility during these years.

In summary, it can be seen that as children disperse, parents must again learn independence. In readjusting, the marriage must be viable if parents' needs are to continue to be fulfilled. Parents have to readjust their relationship—to relate to each other as marital partners rather than primarily as parents. For this stage to be complete, children must be autonomous, while at the same time maintaining ties and bonds with parents.

Health Concerns. The primary health concerns involve communication problems between young adults and their parents; role-transitional problems for wife and husband; caretaker concerns (for aging parents); and the emergence of chronic health conditions or predisposing factors such as high cholesterol levels, obesity, and high blood pressure. Family planning for the adolescent and young adult members remains important. Menopausal concerns among women is common. The effects associated with prolonged drinking, smoking, and dietary practices become more obvious. Finally, the need for health-promotion strategies and a "wellness lifestyle" become more pressing for the adult members of the launching center family.

Stage VII: Middle-aged Parents

The seventh stage of the family life cycle, the stage of the middle years for parents, begins when the last child departs from the home and ends with retirement or death of one of the spouses. This stage usually starts when parents are about 45 to 55 years of age and ends with the retirement of a spouse, usually

16 to 18 years later. Typically, the marital couple in their middle years constitutes a nuclear family, although still interacting with their aging parent(s) and other members of their own family of origin, as well as with the new families of marriage of their offspring. The postparental couple is not usually isolated today; more middle-aged couples are living out their full life span and spending a greater portion of it in a postparental phase, with extended kin relationships between four generations not being unusual (Roth, 1996).

The middle years include changes in marital adjustment (often better), in the distribution of power between husband and wife (more shared), and in roles (increased marital role differentiation) (Leslie & Korman, 1989). To many families with increased satisfaction and economic status (Rollins & Feldman, 1970), these years are seen as the prime of life. For example, Olson, McCubbin, and associates (1983), in a large, cross-sectional, national survey of predominantly white middle-class, intact families, found that marital and family satisfaction and quality of life increased and peaked during the postparental phase. Middle-aged families, in general, are also better off economically than at other stages of the family career (McCullough and Rutenberg, 1988). Increased labor force participation by women and higher earning power than in previous periods by men account for the greater economic security experienced by most middle-aged families. Mutually enjoyable leisure activities and companionship are mentioned as the prime factors leading to marital happiness. Sexual satisfaction is also positively correlated with both good communication and marital satisfaction (Levin & Levin, 1975), even though middle-aged husbands may experience a decline in sexual adequacy. Intimate husband–wife communication is essential for maintaining understanding and interest in each other throughout these years (Heinrich, 1996).

For some couples, however, these years are generally difficult and onerous ones, because of problems of aging, the loss of children, and a sense of themselves as failures in parenting and work efforts. Some marital satisfaction studies show that marital satisfaction drops soon after marriage and continues to decline through the middle years (Leslie & Korman, 1989).

Family Developmental Tasks. By the time the last child leaves home, many women have rechanneled their energies and lives in preparation for the empty nest. For some women, a middle-age crisis is experienced during the early period of this life cycle. Women work at encouraging their grown children to be independent by redefining their relationship with them (not intruding on their personal and family life). In order to maintain a sense of well-being and health, more women begin to live a healthier lifestyle of weight control, balanced diet, regular exercise program, and adequate rest, as well as to attain and enjoy a career, work, or creative accomplishments.

Occupationally, men may find the same frustrations and disappointments that were present in the previous stage. On the one hand, they may be at the peak of their career and not have to work as hard as previously; or on the other hand, may find their job monotonous after 20 to 30 years at the same type of work. Many middle-class workers suffer from the "plateau phenomenon"—where increased salaries and promotions are no longer available—leaving them to feel in a rut. Career discontent is said to reach alarming proportions under these conditions, with many persons making midlife job changes due to the feelings of discontentment, boredom, and stagnation. On the other hand, in the era of company "downsizing," unemployment during this peak in one's career is often most stressful. Because work has traditionally been a man's central role in life, work discontentment as well as the threat or occurrence of being laid off significantly influence a man's stress level and general health status.

The cultivation of leisure-time activities and interests is significant during this stage, since more time is now available and preparation for retirement must take place in a more planned fashion.

An important developmental task for this stage is the provision of a healthy environment (Table 6–10). It is in this period when taking on a healthier lifestyle becomes more prevalent for couples, despite the fact that they have probably been engaging in self-destructive habits for 45 to 65 years. Although not inadvisable to start now, since "better now than never" is always true, it is largely too late to significantly reverse many of the physiological changes that have already taken place, such as arthritic changes due to inactivity; moderate to severe weight gain;

▶ TABLE 6–10

TWO-PARENT NUCLEAR FAMILY LIFE CYCLE STAGE VII AND CONCOMITANT FAMILY DEVELOPMENTAL TASKS

Family Life Cycle Stage	Family Developmental Tasks
Middle-aged parents	1. Providing a health-promoting environment. 2. Sustaining satisfying and meaningful relationships with aging parents and children. 3. Strengthening the marital relationship.

Adapted from Carter and McGoldrick (1989), Duvall and Miller (1985)

high blood pressure due to lack of exercise, prolonged stress, or poor dietary habits; and vital capacity diminution due to smoking.

The primary motivation of middle-aged persons to improve their lifestyle appears to be a feeling of susceptibility or vulnerability to illness and disease generated when a friend or family member of the same age group has a heart attack, stroke, or cancer. In addition to fear, a belief that regular checkups and healthful living habits are effective ways of reducing susceptibility to various diseases are also powerful motivating forces. Heart disease, cancer, and stroke account for two-thirds of all causes of mortality between the ages of 46 and 64 years of age, with accidents the fourth cause of death (National Center for Health Statistics, 1989).

A second developmental task relates to sustaining satisfying and meaningful relationships with aging parents and children. By accepting and welcoming grandchildren into the family and promoting satisfying intergenerational relationships, this developmental task can be highly rewarding (Duvall & Miller, 1985). It allows the middle-aged couple to continue feeling like a family and brings the joys of grandparenthood without the 24-hour responsibilities of parenthood. With increased life expectancy, being a grandparent typically occurs during this stage (Sprey & Matthews, 1982). Grandparents provide a wide range of support to their children and grandchildren in times of crisis and assist their children in the parent role through their encouragement and support (Bengtson & Robertson, 1985).

More recent research studies on grandparenting suggest that increasing numbers of grandparents (about 3.4 million in the United States) are rearing their grandchildren. Divorce, drugs, alcohol problems, incarceration, and unemployment within the parental generation are contributing to the increase in grandparents who are the primary caregiver (Burton, 1992; Calfie, 1994). Although the great majority of grandparents accept this grandparental responsibility willingly, such caregiving may take a significant toll on them. Minkler and Roe (1995) describe a number of problems experienced by grandparents—ranging from stress-related illness and social isolation to severe financial difficulties. In spite of these potential difficulties, the results of grandparenting are generally not all that negative. Burton and de Vries (1995) report that while providing full-time care for a grandchild may be stressful, grandparent caregivers are likely to obtain certain rewards and informal support from their generational family relations.

The more problematic role is that of relating to and assisting the aging parents and sometimes other older extended family members. Eighty-six percent of middle-aged couples have at least one parent each still alive (Hagestad, 1988). Thus, caregiving responsibilities for aging parents who are frail or ill is a frequent experience. While men are assuming greater caregiving responsibilities than in the past, the majority of caregiving is done by women. Therefore, more women find themselves in a "generational squeeze" in their attempt to balance the needs of their aging parents, their children, and grandchildren. Multiple intergenerational roles and relationships are likely to be more extensive among certain minorities, such as African-American, Asian, and Latino families.

Filial caregiving to disabled elderly parents may lead to physical, emotional, and financial strains for middle-aged persons, who are usually daughters (Brody, Litvin, Hoffman, & Kleban, 1992). Prolonged caregiving may also cause marital relationship strains. According to Brody and associates (1992a), married daughters who had their husband's emotional support fared best in their filial caregiving. The same was true when unmarried daughters had a supportive "significant other," a special male friend whom not-married daughters saw exclusively (Brody et al., 1992b).

The third developmental task to be discussed here is that of strengthening the marital relationship. Now the couple is really alone after many years of being surrounded with other family members and relationships. Although appearing as a welcome relief, for many mates it is a difficult experience to have to relate to each other as marital partners rather than as parents. Wright and Leahey (1994) describe this family developmental task as being "renegotiation of marital system as a dyad" (p. 69). The balance of dependency–independency between couples needs to be reexamined. Often couples develop different arrangements in marriage, such as having greater independent interests, as well as meaningful mutual interests. For couples who experience problems, the reduced pressure of life in postparental years may lead not to marital bliss, but to marital "blahs" and being in a "comfortable rut" (Kerckhoff, 1976).

Health Concerns. The health concerns mentioned throughout the description of the life cycle stage include the following:

1. Health-promotion needs: adequate rest, leisure activities, and sleep; good nutrition; regular exercise program; reduction of weight down to optimum weight; cessation of smoking; reduction or cessation in use of alcohol; and preventive-health screening examination.

2. Marital relationship concerns.

3. Communication with and relating to children, in-laws, grandchildren, and aging parents.

4. Caregiver concerns: assisting in care of aging or disabled parents.

5. Adjusting to physiological changes, such as the hormonal, menopausal changes in women.

Stage VIII: Families in Retirement and Old Age

The last stage of the life cycle of the family begins with the retirement of one or both spouses, continues through the loss of one spouse, and ends with the death of the other spouse (Duvall & Miller, 1985). The number of aging individuals—people 65 and older—in our country has rapidly increased during the last two decades, twice as fast as the rest of the population. In 1970, there were some 19.9 million people age 65 and older, representing about 9.8 percent of the total population. By 1990, according to Census Bureau figures, the elderly population had grown to some 31.7 million (12.7 percent of the total population). By the year 2020, as the baby boom generation joins this age group, 17.3 percent of the nation's population will be age 65 and older (Fig. 6–1). Information on population aging suggest that the "oldest old"—the 85-plus population—is growing especially rapidly. The 85-plus population grew to 2.2 million in 1980. It is projected that in year 2020 this population will increase to 7.1 million (2.7 percent of the population) (Taeuber, 1993). As the result of improved disease prevention and health care, more people are also expected to survive into their tenth decade. Because of the increase in the very old population, it is increasingly possible that older people will themselves have at least one surviving parent (U.S. Bureau of the Census, 1984).

Perceptions of this stage of the life cycle differ significantly among aging families. Some persons are miserable, while others feel these are the best years of their lives. Although much is dependent on the adequacy of financial resources and the ability to maintain a satisfactory home, one's health status has been identified as a primary predictor of the well-being of older persons (Quinn, 1993). The more health difficulties experienced, the more likely the presence of negative feelings toward old age. Those who have lost their independence due to ill health generally have low morale; and poor physical health is often an antecedent to behavioral and psychological problems in the elderly (Chilman, Nunnally, & Cox, 1988). Conversely, those elders who have maintained their health, have kept active, and have adequate economic resources represent a substantial proportion of older people and usually feel positive about this stage of life.

Society's Attitude Toward the Elderly.
Our society emphasizes the achievements of those in the young adult years, glorifying the period of youth.

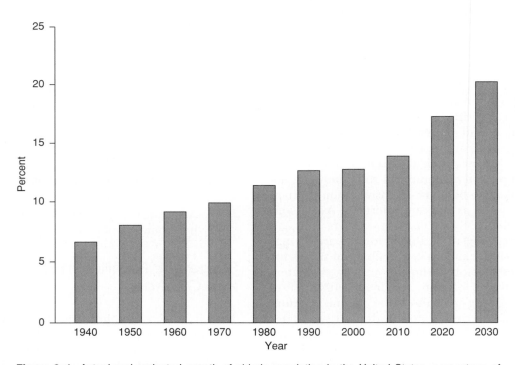

Figure 6–1. Actual and projected growth of elderly population in the United States, percentage of population over 65. *(Source: U.S. Bureau of the Census, 1991a).*

Therefore, adults, through grooming, dress, and styles, try to maintain their youthful appearance as long as possible. Aging has been viewed as an abrupt decline, and the debilitating diseases that affect only a small percentage of the elderly are often viewed as the norm rather than the exception. Normal aging is frequently thought of as a period of sickness, senility, and dependency. For both the community at large and individual families, dealing with the aged has had a negative connotation, one loaded with feelings of being burdened down with imposing problems. Additionally, society has not allowed most aged people to remain productive. Hence, society's negative appraisal of older people has negatively affected their self-image.

Yet today many associations and much of the literature advocate and illustrate the strengths, resources, and other positive aspects of aging. This has begun to diminish the negativism and stereotypical thinking about the aged and help us recognize the assets of the older person and the great diversity of lifestyles among members of this age group.

Our attitudes towards aging and the aged, albeit still negative, appear to be changing. Recent studies conducted on society's attitude toward the elderly have validated that the elderly are being viewed more positively (Austin, 1985; Schonfield, 1982). McCubbin and Dahl (1985) report that "many observers believe that age is regaining respect in the United States. A new generation of old people—better educated, more affluent, healthier and more active than previous elderly generations—is redefining the notion of 'being old'" (p. 276). This change in attitude enhances the elderly's image of themselves.

Losses Common to Aging People and Families.

As aging progresses and retirement becomes a reality, there is a variety of stressors or losses experienced by some older people and couples that confounds their role transition. These may include the following:

- Economic—Adjusting to a substantially reduced income; later perhaps adjusting to economic dependency (depending on family or government for subsidy).

- Housing—Often moving to smaller quarters assisted living facilities, and later perhaps being forced to move to an institutional setting.

- Social—Loss (death) of siblings, friends, and spouse.

- Work—Voluntary or involuntary retirement and loss of the work role and a sense of productivity.

- Health—Declining physical, mental, and cognitive functions; caregiving for the less healthy spouse.

Retirement.

Entry into full retirement is a main life-cycle turning point. It typically means a moderate to significant loss of status and social support and, for many, lifestyle changes, including increased leisure time (Rubin & Neiswiadomy, 1995). This transition involves reorientation of values and goals and a re-direction of energies. What such changes entail, however, is not entirely clear, because the roles and norms for the older person and couple are ambiguous. Clear boundaries may become vague as the retired spouse, especially the husband, is incorporated into domestic activities. This reintegration may not pose problems for some couples, whereas for others it may be difficult (Walsh, 1989).

The retirement years constitute up to a quarter or more of an average person's life. The median retirement ages of both men and women have declined from 66 years of age (1995 through 1990) to about 63 years of age (1985 through 1990) (Gendell & Siegel, 1996). The number of dual-retired couples has been growing steadily in the last two decades and this trend is expected to continue. While some older persons may be fortunate to return to work after retiring from their former position, others may not or cannot, sometimes because of declining health.

Certainly declining health affects adaptation to retirement. Haug, Belgrove, and Jones (1992) also report that the wife's education is a significant variable that influences the retirement transition. Other factors influencing a couple's ability to cope with retirement are their readiness to retire, spouse's expectations, planning for retirement, financial security, and the external support they have (Dorfman & Rubenstein, 1993; Honig, 1996; Knesek, 1992).

Family Developmental Tasks.

Maintaining satisfying living arrangements is a most important task of aging families (Table 6–11). Housing after

▶ TABLE 6–11

TWO-PARENT NUCLEAR FAMILY LIFE CYCLE STAGE VIII AND CONCOMITANT FAMILY DEVELOPMENTAL TASKS

Family Life Cycle Stage	Family Developmental Tasks
Families in the later years	1. Maintaining a satisfying living arrangement. 2. Adjusting to a reduced income. 3. Maintaining marital relationships. 4. Adjusting to loss of spouse. 5. Maintaining intergenerational family ties. 6. Continuing to make sense out of one's existence (life review and integration).

Adapted from Carter and McGoldrick (1989), Duvall and Miller (1985).

retirement may become problematic. In the years immediately following retirement, couples usually remain in the family home until property taxes, neighborhood conditions, size or condition of house, or health forces them to find more modest accommodations. Although a majority of older people own their own homes, a substantial proportion of these are old and often rundown; many are located in high-crime areas where older people are likely to be victims. The elderly often tend to "stay put" despite deteriorating neighborhood conditions (Lawton, 1985). Nonetheless, older persons living in their own homes are generally better adjusted than those who live in their children's homes. According to a study by Day and Day (1993), women living with their spouse and women living alone demonstrated more successful aging than women living with relatives.

A person's living arrangements is a powerful predictor of well-being among the elderly (Berrlesi et al., 1984). Relocation is a traumatic experience for the elderly, whether it is a voluntary or involuntary move. It means leaving behind neighborhood ties and friendships that have provided the elderly with a sense of security and stability. Relocation means separation from one's heritage and the cues that bolster old memories (Lawton, 1980).

Relocation, however, does not affect all of the elderly in the same way. Given adequate preparation and careful planning for the change, the new environment may have positive impact on the elderly. Nevertheless, some research findings suggest that when older people move, some deterioration of their health often results (Lawton, 1985).

The disabled elderly (functionally, physically, or cognitively impaired) are more likely to enter nursing homes because of the lack of assistance in the home. Only about 5 percent of older people live in institutions. This means 95 percent of older people live at home or in other community-based living facilities. Moreover, even among the older people who are disabled, 90 percent live at home with family members, with the care they receive being provided totally or partially by one of their family members.

According to the AARP Report (1993), the oldest old (age 85 and above) are more likely to be in nursing homes (24 percent). Moreover, more women than men will be in nursing homes.

The provision of full-time help in the home or, more feasibly, part-time health and homemaker services through a home health agency or homemaker agency, is protective of the older person's need to remain in his or her own home and retain his or her independence as long as possible. In addition, it is less costly than institutionalization. Albeit difficult, one of the mates and/or grown children of the couple (or the remaining parent) often has to decide what is the best path to take—home health services, retirement home, nursing home, or living with grown children.

Adjusting to a reduced income is a second developmental task for the aging family. When men retire, there is an immediate drop in income, and usually as the years pass by, this income becomes less and less adequate because of the steady rise in cost of living and the depletion of savings. In 1989 one-fifth of the older U.S. population was poor or near poor (AARP, 1990).

Older people have substantially less cash income than those under 65. The elderly rely heavily on Social Security benefits and asset income. More older women tend to be poor; nearly 71.8 percent of the elderly population are women. Women are more likely to delay their career, to work part-time, and to experience disruptions in the work cycle that may lead to lower pay and fewer benefits. They also tend to retire early to assume caregiving responsibilities for their aging parents or spouses (Brody, 1985; Minkler & Stone, 1985). Also due to divorce and death of spouse, women are more likely to be alone after retirement, and may remain poor (Haywood & Liu, 1992). Black and Hispanic elderly have substantially lower money incomes as well as lower median incomes than their white counterparts (U.S. Senate Special Committee on Aging, 1987–1988).

Because of the frequency of long-term health problems, health expenses are a major financial concern. The elderly spend more on health care— both in actual dollars and as a percentage of total expenditure—than the nonelderly. Medicare has certainly alleviated part of this problem, but there are still unpredictable, and many times substantial, out-of-pocket expenses to be paid. For instance, Part B of Medicare covers only 80 percent of "reasonable" costs for medical services. Medicaid is also available to those who are medically indigent and qualify for Supplementary Security Income (SSI). This health insurance program then supplements Medicare coverage.

As average life expectancy increases, more older people will spend more years with severely limiting medical problems. Even though women outlive men by an average of 7 years and the gap in life expectancies between men and women is increasing, more married couples are surviving longer. This means that wives are more likely to be caregivers to their husbands. Stone and colleagues (1987) confirmed this fact in a study they conducted. They found that more wives were caregivers than husbands (23 percent versus 13 percent of all caregiving). Furthermore, according to Montgomery (1989), spouses tend to provide a greater level of assistance for longer periods of time than do their adult children.

Although several studies document the fact that caregiving is uniformly stressful, its impact on individuals who are caring for their ill spouses is not clear. While some researchers report that there are no differences in the level of burden between spouses and adult children (Montgomery, 1989; Montgomery & Kosloski, 1994), other researchers suggest higher levels of burden among spouse caregivers when compared to adult children (George & Gwyther, 1986). Spouse caregivers, as compared to spouses who are not involved with caregiving, tend to

have a lower level of well-being (Sistler, 1989). Also, caregiving spouses are more likely than noncaregiving spouses to be lonely and to experience mild depression, financial worries, and low life satisfaction (Staight & Harvey, 1990). Some researchers report that the physical health of the caregivers suffers, with the negative consequences ranging from a compromised immune system function to undetected hypertension and cardiac problems (Kiecolt-Glaser & Glaser, 1989; Koin, 1989).

Some caregiving literature today describes "the caregiver career," referring to a process or trajectory of caregiving that occurs, particularly in long-term caregiving situations. For example, Lindgren (1993) describes the caregiver career of spouses who are caring for family members with dementia as a "fatalistic" career process. Here Lindgren identifies three stages: (1) the encounter stage, (2) the middle enduring stage, and (3) the final, exit stage. During the encounter stage, the caregivers are adjusting to the impact of the diagnoses, learning new skills, and making lifestyles changes. The enduring stage is characterized by heavy work and disruption of routine work. In this stage of the caregiving career, Lindgren (1993) states that the caregivers are likely to feel hopeless and to have an overwhelming sense of frustration and loss. The third or exit stage is characterized by the caregiver making decisions, taking on activities, and making adjustments associated with total or partial relinquishment of the caregiving role. The caregiving role is relinquished to some degree either through death or institutionalization of the ill spouse.

Maintaining marital relationships, a third developmental task, continues to be paramount to the family's happiness. Marriages perceived as satisfying in the later years usually have a long positive history, and vice versa. Researchers have also shown that marriage contributes greatly to both morale and continued activity of both older spouses (Brubaker, 1985; Lee, 1978). Maintaining a satisfactory marital relationship after one or both spouses retire is also influenced by the support each spouse receives from the other and changes that occur in the health of either or both spouses (Brubaker, 1983; Gilford, 1984; Keating & Cole, 1980). This latter factor often creates caregiving challenges and burdens, which, in turn, influence a couple's marital adjustment (Fitting, Rabins, Lucas, & Eastham, 1986).

One of the myths of old age is that sex drives and sexual activities are no longer possible (or should not exist). Considerable research has shown just the reverse, however. Such studies have found that although there is a slowing down of sexual capacity, the pleasure in sexual activity and interest are consistent with interest and activity during early adulthood (Heinrich, 1996; Starr, 1985). Ill health sometimes diminishes the sex drive, but usually the lack of sexual activity is due to socio-emotional problems.

Adjusting to the loss of spouse, the fourth developmental task, is in general, the most traumatic developmental task. Older women suffer the loss of a spouse more than men. According to statistics for 1986, 75 percent of all older men were living with their spouses while only 38 percent of these older women were living with their spouses. Fifty-one percent of older women were widowed (U.S. Senate Special Committee on Aging, 1987–1988).

In comparison with young groups, the aged are aware that dying is part of the normal process of living. The majority of older persons fear death less than younger persons and are more concerned with the death of their loved ones than of themselves (Butler & Lewis, 1982; Neimeyer, 1988).

The awareness of death does not, however, mean that the spouse left behind will find adjustment to loss easier. Loss of spouse takes its toll—the widowed die earlier than their married counterparts, and the living are more likely to have a serious health problem (social isolation, being suicidal or mentally ill). In addition, the loss of a spouse demands a total reorganization of family functions. This is especially difficult to achieve satisfactorily, since the loss has depleted the emotional and economic resources needed to deal with the change. For women this means a shift from mutual dependency and sharing activities of family living to being alone or associating with a group of unattached older women. For men the loss of spouse means the loss of a companion, as well as of linkages to kin, family, and the social world in general. The aged widower often does not have the same interest in or the ability to perform the homemaker-housekeeper roles as his deceased wife and may need assistance in meal preparation, homemaking, and general care.

How difficult the adjustment is can be seen by the increase in suicides within individuals over 65. Even though there is some increase in suicides among women over 65, the preponderance of suicides is found within the older male population.

Elderly men who commit suicide tend to use more violent methods to kill themselves (Kaplan, Adamek, & Johnson, 1994). According to Kastenbaum (1994), the concerns of older persons that often lead to thoughts of suicide include poor health, loss of mobility and independence, loneliness, isolation, and loss of control. Regardless of the mode of death (a suicide or natural death) the loss of a loved one is a difficult and profound psychological trauma in which depression, confusion, and pervasive feelings of emptiness are often present (Farberow et al., 1992).

Studies of the widowed have consistently verified the difficult living conditions and life of the widowed. The widowed have lower morale and fewer social roles and ties than the married of the same age group. Bild and Havighurst (1976), in a large study of the elderly in Chicago, reported that the loss of a spouse removed the strongest support of the elderly person, although children, when available, usually stepped in to fill the vacuum somewhat. They also found that the childless widowed were even more isolated.

Negative consequences in response to the death of a spouse are many. For instance, widowhood produces negative effects on eating behavior and specific nutrient quality of the elderly widowed person's diet (Rosenbloom & Whittington, 1993). Also, widowed individuals are more likely to have depressive symptoms or even experience a major depressive episode. Zisook and Shuchter (1993) reported that poor health, the use of psychotropic medications, and increased use of alcohol and other nonprescribed substances were associated with postbereavement depression. Fortunately, social support by families, relatives, friends, and/or professionals reduces the likelihood of depression. Mullins and Mushel (1992) suggested that friends, especially close friends, have a positive influence on the emotional well-being of older widowed persons.

A fifth developmental task deals with the maintenance of intergenerational family ties. Although there is a tendency for older persons to disengage from social relationships, the family remains the focus of aging persons' social interactions and their primary source of social support. As the older person withdraws from activities in the surrounding world, relationships with spouse, children, grandchildren, and siblings become more important. The majority of older Americans live close by their extended family members and have frequent contact with them (Harris et al., 1975; Shanas et al., 1968, 1980). Hence, family members are an important source of direct assistance and social interaction. Older families are found generally to reciprocate in the giving of help to the extent to which they are capable.

As people age they must continue to make sense out of their existence. Reminiscing about one's past life, called life review, is a common and vital activity, because it represents a search for the central meaning of life. It is viewed as a sixth "cognitive type" developmental task. Its importance lies in the fact that life review eases the adjustment to difficult situations and provides insight into past events. The elderly are concerned with the quality of their life and being able to live with respect, meaning, and dignity (Duvall, 1977; Roth, 1996).

Health Concerns. According to the 1987 to 1988 report prepared by the U.S. Senate Special Committee on Aging, the elderly are the heaviest users of health services. More than four out of five elderly have at least one chronic condition, and multiple conditions are commonplace among the elderly. In 1990, the elderly made up 12.7 percent of the total population, but they accounted for 33 percent of health care expenditures in the United States.

Advancing age is also highly correlated with functional disability. According to the 1990 U.S. Census data, 15.6 percent of noninstitutionalized older persons report a mobility or self-care limitation (Shrestha & Rosenwaike, 1996). Older women tend to experience greater functional disability, mobility impairment, and chronic illness than older men (Penning & Strain, 1994; Santiago & Muschkin, 1996).

Factors such as diminishing physical vigor and function, inadequate financial resources, social isolation, loneliness, and the many other losses that the older person experiences demonstrate some of the psychophysiological vulnerabilities of human aging. Therefore, multiple chronic health concerns and long-term care needs exist.

Long-term care involves a range of services that address the health, personal care, and social needs of individuals who have self-care limitations. Services may be continuous or intermittent and are delivered for a demonstrated need, usually measured by some index of functional dependency (Kane & Kane,

1989). Services are delivered either in an institutional setting (e.g., a nursing home) or in a community setting (e.g., through a home health care agency with the assistance of a formal caregiver or at home with an informal caregiver). As Figure 6–2 shows, the long-term care needs increase as age advances. Persons 85 years of age and over are at the greatest risk of needing long-term care.

Assisting the aging couple or individual with all phases of a chronic illness, from the acute phase through the rehabilitation phase, is needed. Both medically related functions (physical assessment, reporting untoward reactions) and nursing functions (assessing the client's response to illness and treatment and his or her coping abilities) are relevant here. Health promotion continues to be of critical importance, especially in areas of nutrition, exercise, injury prevention, safe use of medicines, use of preventive services, and smoking cessation. Teaching, counseling, providing encouragement and support, and advocating for families within the

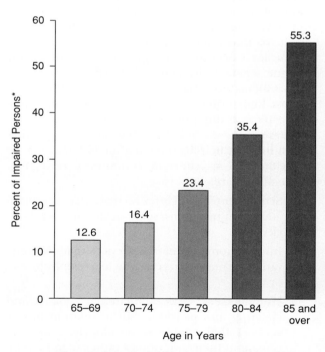

(*Percent with impaired abilities to conduct activities of daily living or to perform basic functions that support those activities.)

Figure 6–2. Age and the need for long-term care. *(Source: Health Care Financing Review, 1988 Annual Supplement; National Sample Survey of Registered Nurses, U.S. Department of Health and Human Services, 1988).*

health care delivery system should be a primary focus of nursing at this stage (Richards, 1996).

Social isolation, depression, cognitive impairment (which may be related to a number of sources including Alzheimer's disease), and other psychological problems are serious health concerns, particularly when combined with physical ill health. Assessment and use of the family's or individual social support system should be an integral part of family health care.

Nutritional deficiencies are extensive among the elderly and contribute to many problems associated with aging (fatigue, confusion, depression, and constipation, to name a few). The older person's nutritional needs may be affected by lifelong eating habits, dietary patterns, socialization, income, transportation, housing, and food dietary knowledge. Nutritionally, the older person has special needs for sufficient fiber, protein, calcium, iron, zinc, and vitamins in the diet (Ebersole & Hess, 1994).

Related problems of housing, a suitable income, adequate recreational and health care facilities adversely affect the elderly's health status. The incidence of falls and other accidents in the home is great, so that environmental safety measures are important. Government programs do not adequately provide secure retirement, as clearly demonstrated in problems concerned with the use of nursing homes, long-term board-and-care facilities, and mental hospitals as dumping grounds for the aged.

Family-centered health professionals can provide much indirect help by referring the older couple or individual to appropriate community resources. Some of these resources are:

1. Senior centers that offer recreation, continuing-education programs, some health and legal services.

2. Information and referral services that give relevant information in response to a telephone call or visit.

3. Homemakers' services, including cooking and cleaning and providing social relationships—services that enable some elderly people to remain in their own homes rather than be relocated in institutions.

4. Geriatric day-care facilities, in which older persons receive supervision and a variety of services during the day—usually restricted to individuals who are not capable of using senior centers.

5. Nutritional programs, some of which transport recipients to a central location to eat and some of which, like the Meals-on-Wheels program, transport food to people who are not ambulatory.

6. The Foster Grandparent program, a federally subsidized program that pays low-income elderly people a small amount to care for, tutor, or play with institutionalized children.

7. The Retired Senior Volunteer Program, also federally subsidized, helping elderly persons to provide community services.

8. Case management services.

► FAMILY LIFE CYCLE OR CAREER STAGES IN DIVORCED FAMILIES

One of the major variations in the family life cycle or career is seen when parents divorce. As mentioned in Chapter 1, one of the most profound changes taking place over the past two decades has been the rise in divorces and female-headed households. About 88 percent of single-parent families are mother–child(ren) families. From 1970 to 1990 the number of one-parent families more than doubled (from 3.4 million in 1970 to 7.4 million in 1990) while the number of divorced couples increased by almost 300 percent (U.S. Bureau of the Census, 1993). Since the early to mid-1980s, the divorce rate, after reaching a peak, has leveled off, even declining slightly (National Center for Health Statistics, 1992). Thirty-seven percent of children in single-parent families are in families where the parent is divorced (Jaluter, 1993). Divorces are so common today (almost 50 percent of all marriages end in divorce) that the event is being viewed as a normative transition.

The single-parent, divorced family passes through the same life cycle stages, with most of the same responsibilities, as the two-parent nuclear family. The basic difference is the absence of the second parent to carry his or her (mostly his) share of the family tasks with respect to support, child rearing, companionship, and gender role modeling for the children. Hill (1986) explains that "the differences in paths of development of single-parent and two-parent families are seen primarily, not in stages encountered, but in the number, timing and length of the critical transitions experienced" (p. 28).

Carter and McGoldrick (1989) conceptualize divorce as an interruption or dislocation of the traditional family life cycle. Divorce, with its losses and shifts in family membership, creates major family destabilization and disequilibrium. Peck and Manocharian (1988) underscore the emotional and physical impact of divorce on the family. "Divorce affects family members at every generational level throughout the nuclear and extended family, thus producing a crisis for the family as a whole as well as for each individual within the family" (p. 335).

As with the two-parent nuclear family, there are crucial changes in roles and relationships and important family developmental tasks to be completed in order for the divorced family to move forward developmentally (Carter & McGoldrick, 1989). As a major disruptive force, divorce compounds the complexity of the developmental tasks the family is experiencing. Each subsequent stage is also affected, so that each postdivorce stage must be viewed within the context of both the stage itself and the consequences of the divorce.

After the divorce, family systems research has found that it takes about 1 to 3 years for the family to restabilize itself. "If a family can negotiate the crisis and the accompanying transitions that must be experienced in order to restabilize, it will have established a more fluid system that will allow a continuation of the normal family developmental process" (Peck & Manocharian, 1988, p. 335). Carter and McGoldrick have summarized the research and writings of Ahrons (1980) on the process of adjustment that divorced families go through. Table 6–12 outlines the pre- and postdivorce adjustment process, including concomitant emotional processes and family developmental issues.

To describe the impact of the divorce on the family life cycle stages, it first should be said that the impact varies depending on what stage the family is in when the divorce occurs. Other factors also make a difference on impact, such as ethnic, social, and economic factors. Divorce is the least disruptive during the first stage of marriage, as there are fewer people involved, fewer traditions established, and fewer couple-based social ties (Peck & Manocharian, 1988). The impact is much greater during the third

and fourth stages in those families with preschool and school-aged children. Moreover, the family is most at risk for divorce during these periods.

Young children are initially most affected by parents' divorce. Children may regress developmentally, making child rearing and separation of parents and children difficult. Single parenthood is often very onerous for the mother, who usually struggles both emotionally and economically. The economic status of female-headed divorced families declines considerably following divorce. Two frequently seen problems are that the father loses his sense of connection to his children and, because of the mother's anger at the father, the mother leaves no room for him. Yet maintaining both the mother–child and father–child relationships is very important for both parents and children. Unfortunately, for both father and children, a large proportion of children virtually lose contact with their fathers after the divorce (Hagestad, 1988).

When divorce occurs among families with school-aged children, the long-term impact of the divorce is even more profound on the school-aged child. Six to eight years of age was the age group that had the hardest time adjusting to divorce in one study (Wallerstein & Kelly, 1980). Children are old enough at that time to realize what is happening, but not old enough to deal effectively with the divorce.

Families with adolescents are often already in turmoil, and divorce only compounds the problem. For the single parent, raising the adolescent alone is difficult. Coparenting is also problematic when the adolescent is having behavior problems. Progressing through the developmental tasks of adolescence and the family life cycle is initially delayed.

In later stages of the family life cycle, children are likely to be affected less profoundly than in the previous family stages because they are older and better able to cope and function more autonomously. In the case of midlife divorce older children may, however, be propelled into filial maturity, accepting of the dependency of a parent, particularly the mother, when a parent turns to a child for support during the divorce crisis.

During these later family life cycle stages, divorce is typically profoundly traumatizing to the divorced partners. Years of shared possessions, memories, and habits have created "a couple identity." Divorce during later years is likened to a death of a partner in some of the divorce literature.

► TABLE 6–12

DISLOCATIONS OF THE FAMILY LIFE CYCLE BY DIVORCE, REQUIRING ADDITIONAL STEPS TO RESTABILIZE AND PROCEED DEVELOPMENTALLY

Phase	Emotional Process of Transition—Prerequisite Attitude	Developmental Issues
■ DIVORCE		
1. The decision to divorce	Acceptance of inability to resolve marital tensions sufficiently to continue relationship.	Acceptance of one's own part in the failure of the marriage.
2. Planning the breakup of the system	Supporting viable arrangements for all parts of the system.	a. Working cooperatively on problems of custody, visitation, and finances. b. Dealing with extended family about the divorce.
3. Separation	a. Willingness to continue cooperative coparental relationship and joint financial support of children. b. Work on resolution of attachment to spouse.	a. Mourning loss of intact family. b. Restructuring marital and parent-child relationships and finances; adaptation to living apart. c. Realignment of relationships with extended family; staying connected with spouse's extended family.
4. The divorce	More work on emotional divorce: Overcoming hurt, anger, guilt, etc.	a. Mourning loss of intact family; giving up fantasies of reunion. b. Retrieval of hopes, dreams, expectations from the marriage. c. Staying connected with extended families.
■ POSTDIVORCE FAMILY		
1. Single-parent (custodial household or primary residence)	Willingness to maintain financial responsibilities, continue parental contact with ex-spouse, and support contact of children with ex-spouse and his or her family.	a. Making flexible visitation arrangements with ex-spouse and his or her family. b. Rebuilding own financial resources. c. Rebuilding own social network.
2. Single-parent (noncustodial)	Willingness to maintain parental contact with ex-spouse and support custodial parent's relationship with children.	a. Finding ways to continue effective parenting relationship with children. b. Maintaining financial responsibilities to ex-spouse and children. c. Rebuilding own social network.

From Carter, B. & McGoldrick, M., eds. The Changing Family Life Cycle, 2nd ed. (1989, p. 22.) Allyn and Bacon. Reprinted by permission.

► LIFE CYCLE OR CAREER STAGES IN STEPPARENT FAMILIES

Divorce is commonly a transitional state, followed by remarriage. Remarriage was so prevalent in the mid-1980s that nearly one-half of all marriages were remarriages (U.S. Bureau of the Census, 1993).

Before age 40, both men and women remarry fairly equally, but after age 40, remarriage is disproportionately a male transition (Hagestad, 1988).

In Table 6–13 Carter and McGoldrick (1989) present a developmental outline of the remarried family formation—the steps involved in the remarriage process, the prerequisite attitudes, and the developmental issues. The family's emotional process at the transition to remarriage is typically one that involves

▶ TABLE 6-13

REMARRIED FAMILY FORMATION: A DEVELOPMENTAL OUTLINE

Steps	Prerequisite Attitude	Developmental Issues
1. Entering the new relationship	Recovery from loss of first marriage (adequate "emotional divorce").	Recommitment to marriage and to forming a family with readiness to deal with the complexity and ambiguity.
2. Conceptualizing and planning new marriage and family	Accepting one's own fears and those of new spouse and children about remarriage and forming a stepfamily. Accepting need for time and patience for adjustment to complexity and ambiguity of: 1. Multiple new roles. 2. Boundaries: space, time, membership, and authority. 3. Affective Issues: guilt, loyalty conflicts, desire of mutuality, unresolvable past hurts.	a. Work on openness in the new relationships to avoid pseudomutuality. b. Plan for maintenance of cooperative financial and coparental relationships with ex-spouses. c. Plan to help children deal with fears, loyalty conflicts, and membership in two systems. d. Realignment of relationships with extended family to include new spouse and children. e. Plan maintenance of connections for children with extended family of ex-spouses(s).
3. Remarriage and reconstitution of family	Final resolution of attachment to previous spouse and ideal of "intact" family; acceptance of a different model of family with permeable boundaries.	a. Restructuring family boundaries to allow for inclusion of new spouse/stepparent. b. Realignment of relationships and arrangements throughout subsystems to permit interweaving of several systems. c. Making room for relationships of all children with biological (noncustodial) parents, grandparents, and other extended family. d. Sharing memories and histories to enhance stepfamily integration.

From: Carter, B. & McGoldrick, M., eds. The Changing Family Life Cycle, 2nd ed. (1989, p. 24.) Allyn & Bacon. Reprinted by permission.

struggling with fears about investment in a new marriage and a new family; dealing with hostile or upset reactions of the children, extended families, and the ex-spouse; worrying about the ambiguous new family situation; feeling guilty and concerned over the welfare of the children; and renewing of attachments (negative or positive) to the ex-spouse. Remarriage, again because it is a disruptive transitional process, impedes the family's movement through and completion of family developmental tasks. Stepparent adjustment and integration, as with divorce adjustment, seems to take a minimum of 2 to 3 years before a new structure allows the family to move on developmentally (Carter & McGoldrick, 1989).

▶ FAMILY LIFE CYCLE STAGES OR FAMILY CAREER IN DOMESTIC PARTNER RELATIONSHIPS

Domestic partnerships refer to gay, lesbian, and heterosexual cohabitants who have an intimate relationship and are financially interdependent (Ames, 1992). U.S. Census figures show there are 6 cohabiting couples for every 100 married heterosexual couples in the early 1990s (Bumpass, Sweet, & Cherlin, 1991). Forty percent of these couples have children.

Lesbian/Gay Family Career Stages

There are estimated to be in the U.S. today 1 to 5 million lesbian mothers, 1 to 3 million gay fathers, and from 6 to 14 million children with homosexual parents (Ames, 1992). The discrimination against same-sex family life within the mainstream culture, however, may lead many families to keep their status secret. Lesbian/gay families, as with other families, change and grow over time.

Lesbians/gays form families based on personal selection of family members. Slater (1995) refers to the lesbian family as the family of creation. It consists of the couple alone or a lesbian/gay couple and their children. Outlining a lesbian/gay family career, however, is complicated by numerous simultaneous influences determining a couple's journey through the stages of their relationship (Slater, 1995). Competing influences of lesbian/gay identity formation, typical lesbian/gay stressors, coping mechanisms, other minority identity development, and the couple's life-long voluntary and required social relationships shape the family career.

Slater's model of the lesbian/gay family career reflects the rich diversity and points of common experience among lesbian/gay families. Slater (1995) describes five stages, which are sequential and with limited duration, some stages enduring far longer than others. The couple's adaptations to the challenges of previous stages become incorporated into their relationship and strengthen or diminish their capacity to confront subsequent obstacles. The layers of partner chronological development, lesbian/gay identity formation, other minority identity formation, and the stage of the life career intersect continually. For an in-depth discussion of lesbian family careers, see Slater's book, *The Lesbian Family Life Cycle*. Table 6–14 outlines the lesbian/gay family career.

▶ IMPACT OF ILLNESS AND DISABILITY ON FAMILY DEVELOPMENTAL STAGES

Serious illness or long-term disability of a family member significantly affects the family and its functioning, just as the behavior of the family and its members simultaneously affects the course and characteristics of the illness or disability (Bahnson, 1987). Given this widely accepted assumption of reciprocity, it is clear that serious illness or disability profoundly influences family development, as well as individual family member development, especially of the sick or disabled member. Often when a family is delayed in meeting its family developmental tasks, it is the interaction of the developmental demands/stressors and a situational demand/stressor that compounds and overloads the family. The added family stress created by the presence of both types of stressors often results in lowered family functioning, whereby mastering of family developmental tasks becomes impeded or retarded.

The extent to which family developmental tasks are affected depends on several factors. One is certainly the family life cycle stage that the family is in; secondly, which family member becomes seriously ill or disabled makes a difference. Some particular stages are already developmentally hazardous, and completing family developmental tasks of a particular stage are more crucial for certain family members. For instance, in a family with a teenager, if the adolescent sustains a serious injury and is left in a dependent state, this will greatly impede the adolescent's own mastery of the developmental task of becoming more independent from the family. Likewise the family developmental task dealing with balancing freedom with responsibility so as to assist the teenager to become increasingly autonomous will also be impeded. The challenge for the family is to attempt to resume working on normal developmental family tasks as soon as possible.

Another major factor that makes a difference in regards to the impact of illness or disability on family development is the formal and informal resources the family is utilizing. A good social support system of extended family and friends, as well as competent, helpful health and psychosocial supports, will augment the family's ability to more quickly get back on track developmentally.

When working with a family with a serious illness or disability, it is useful to compare the "ideal" family developmental tasks within the appropriate family life cycle stage with the family's actual behavior (Friedman, 1987). This type of comparison is useful in evaluating the probable impact of the illness or disability on the family.

► TABLE 6–14

LESBIAN/GAY FAMILY CAREER

Stage	Transition Process	Developmental Tasks
I. Couple formation	Partners need to differentiate when they began to show interest from when they began an actual couple relationship.	a. Building a beginning sense of themselves as a unit. b. Relaxing boundaries around themselves as they tentatively blend aspects of their lives. c. Developing trust between partners. d. Increasing self-disclosure. e. Engaging in empathic responses that encourage further risk. f. Controlling who knows about their relationships.
II. Ongoing couplehood	Couple moves from unbridled passion to beginning of stability, combining passion and dailiness.	a. Recognizing and managing a range of differences that are becoming evident. b. Negotiating conflict. c. Developing relational security and sense of belonging.
III. Middle years	Couple's movement into a permanent or long-range commitment.	a. Diligent reworking of the rewards and disappointments within extended relational commitment. b. Creating security and continuing newness within the relationship.
IV. Generativity	Couple's desire to associate themselves with and provide a sense of identity that will endure beyond their own finite existence.	a. Creating a personal legacy.
V. Couple over 60	Couple facing imposed life changes, some occurring all at once and others emerging, such as retirement, physical illness, and widowhood.	a. Partner renegotiation of interdependence and autonomy. b. Each partner working to secure some power and unique identity for self within the relationship. c. Balancing financial, physical, and emotional independence.

Adapted from Slater (1995).

► ASSESSMENT AREAS: DEVELOPMENTAL STAGE AND HISTORY OF THE FAMILY

Throughout the assessment process, a focus on the family life cycle or family career enhances the family health professional's understanding of the stresses that are impinging on a family and the actual or potential problems of a family. In completing the developmental part of a family assessment, the following areas are suggested:

1. The family's present developmental stage.

2. The extent to which the family is fulfilling the developmental tasks appropriate for the present developmental stage. It is important to note any significant deviations from the norm, as this may serve as an indication of impending or present problems.

3. The family's history from inception through present day, including developmental history and unique health and health-related events and experiences (e.g., divorce, deaths, losses)

that happened in the family's life. Some of this information (divorces, marriages, deaths) can be included on the family genogram (see Chap. 8 for the family genogram).

4. Both parents' families of origin (what life in family of origin was like; present and past relations with parents of parents).

As mentioned, both the family's common and unique experiences and perceptions as they progress through the family career should be assessed to make the developmental history more comprehensive. A description of each parent's family of origin is also useful to include in a family history because of how crucial intergenerational influences are on family life.

It may be more significant to elicit a developmental history from some families than from others. It is important to make sure the family you are working with is open to exploring their past and that your collection of historical data in any of the suggested areas is relevant for understanding and working with the family.

To reiterate, developmental or historical data on a family can be gleaned by (1) asking about common experiences and tasks and how these were accomplished and perceived and (2) asking about special or unique family problems or experiences. The latter include divorces, deaths in nuclear or extended family, separations due to illness or military service, unemployment, and so forth. Asking parents about their present and past relationships with their family of orientation and what life in the original family was like gives the family-centered nurse a better appreciation and understanding of the parents during their formative years.

In order to elicit a family history, Satir (1983) begins by having parents first talk about their own marital relationship, focusing on this relationship because the parents are the family architects. Satir and the parents, with the children present when appropriate, discuss the following areas:

- First meeting of the couple, their relationship before marriage, and how they decided to get married.

- Any obstacles to their marriage. Their responses to getting married.

- Marriage without the children; how they established tasks and roles.

- What life was like in both original family environments, including both parents' families of orientation.

- Any other people who live or have lived with the family.

- Relationships with in-laws.

- Description of each mate's parents and their relationship with them.

- Plans for and arrival of each new child. Were children planned? What was the impact of the arrival of each child?

- How much time the family spends together.

- Daily routine of family life.

Smoyak (1975), in her nursing practice as a family therapist, stresses the significance of assessing the parents' respective families of orientation:

> It is important to know how each present parent was reared and what lessons in childrearing were learned. How the two present parents put together their different backgrounds in childrearing is easier to understand when the background of each has been described. For instance, a German-Jew married to an English Protestant who live as a nuclear unit produce a very different set of mutual expectations than do two Catholic . . . Mexican-Americans living in an extended family. (p. 8)

Satir (1983) also inquires into each parent's ordinal position among their siblings, quoting Toman's (1961) work on family constellation, which showed that siblings' ordinal position greatly influences the type of interactions and relationships one is likely to have with others, as well as one's personality development. For instance, Toman found that firstborn children were more apt to be leaders than followers, while the reverse was more common among last-born children. Another point of inquiry related to the couple's families of origin involves the state of health and marriage of the mates' own parents. Are they still alive, well, married, living together, residing nearby, or geographically distant? (Smoyak, 1975)

One of the ways family nurses obtain a better idea of the progress of the family system over time, as well as the intergenerational family system, is to construct a genogram. The genogram is a type of genealogical chart that traces the kinship history of families. It is widely used by family therapists and family nurses. The advantage to using family genograms is that one can organize a large, unwieldy amount of data in a way that makes it comprehensible and helps reveal important patterns and themes in families (Hartman & Laird, 1983; McGoldrick & Gerson, 1985). Chapter 8 contains both a genogram and instructions for completing this type of family tree.

▶ FAMILY NURSING INTERVENTIONS

One important goal of family nursing is to help families and their members move toward completion of individual and family developmental tasks (Friedman, 1987). Mastery of one set of family developmental tasks allows the family to progress developmentally to the next stage of family development. Family developmental tasks, if unfulfilled, produce dysfunctional families (Mattessich & Hill, 1987).

To accomplish this goal, the family nurse "assists families to achieve and maintain a balance between the personal growth needs of individual family members and optimum family functioning" (family developmental needs) (American Nurses Association Division on Maternal and Child Health Nursing Practice, 1983). The balance between individual and group developmental needs is not easily achieved,

particularly during certain stages, creating dissonance when an imbalance occurs.

When working with troubled families and individuals, family developmental theory helps family health professionals think about life cycle events that establish the context within which family and individual problems occur. Hence, it is important during both the diagnostic and planning phases that a developmental perspective be incorporated into family nursing practice.

It is also significant to incorporate a family developmental perspective into one's family nursing practice when working with healthy families. With healthy families, anticipatory guidance and teaching is often indicated in order to fulfill primary prevention goals (Bobak et al., 1989). Family nursing diagnoses, plans, and interventions should cover potential problems families may encounter because of the need to transform family structures so that family developmental tasks be accomplished. Helping families anticipate and go through different normative transitions in family life is a most germane family nursing goal.

The family nurse and other family clinicians assist families by teaching and counseling modalities. Referral to social support groups, such as a group for parents of infants or older ill parents, is also very helpful. Chapter 18 discusses general family nursing interventions in detail.

▶ study questions

Choose the correct answer(s) to the following questions.

1. Family developmental theory is built on some basic assumptions. What are these? (List at least two.)

2. Usually reliable predictions can be made regarding the common health concerns and forces that are at play within a family if the family nurse knows (select one answer):
   a. The developmental tasks of each member.
   b. The family life cycle or family career stage.
   c. Where the family lives and their social class.
   d. The composition of the family.

3. Which of the following illustrate(s) the value of the developmental approach when assessing and working with families? (Choose all correct responses.)
   a. Gives cues as to the family's past problems and progress.
   b. Forecasts a given family's future needs.
   c. Views the common experiences of families during each of the family career stages.
   d. Highlights critical periods of family and individual growth and development.
   e. Helps to anticipate what to expect in terms of health concerns.
   f. Better able to evaluate the family normatively.

4. The best definition for the family life cycle or family career is:
   a. Predictable stages within the history of the family.
   b. The growth and developmental stages of each family member as he or she progresses throughout life.
   c. Successive stages and commonly experienced events of the family as a unit through its existence.

5. Family developmental tasks have these characteristics (choose all correct answers):
   a. They change in response to cultural imperatives and the family's unique aspirations and values.
   b. They change in response to the developmental needs of its members.
   c. They remain constant throughout the family's existence.
   d. They adapt the family's broad functions to meet the specific tasks of each stage.
   e. They satisfy the biological requirements of the family as a whole.
   f. They avoid clashing with individual needs.
   g. They are growth requirements that must be achieved by the family during each life cycle or family career stage.
   h. Failure to achieve developmental tasks leads to difficulty in achieving later developmental tasks.
   i. Developmental tasks cover only aspects that directly influence psychosocial (interactional) components of family functioning.

6. The developmental approach seeks to explain family dynamics in terms of its:
   a. Unique elements.
   b. Common elements in its history as a family.
   c. Both common and unique elements of family history.

7. The developmental tasks of the family result from a combination of (more than one answer):
   a. Individual developmental tasks of family members.
   b. Sexual norms.
   c. Chronological ages and school placement.
   d. Community pressures for family to conform to societal norms.
   e. General family functions adapted to specific life cycle stages.

8. The stage of the family life cycles are defined by Duvall in terms of (select one answer):
   a. The age and school placement of the oldest child.
   b. The ages of the parents.
   c. The age of the middle child, if present.
   d. Years of marriage.

Complete the following outlines.

9. In the outline below, list the following:
   —The eight phases in the family life cycle for the two-parent nuclear family (excluding the transition stage).
   —A definition for each phase.
   —Three basic health concerns (biopsychosocial and health concerns) frequently present and appropriate for intervention by family nurse.

Family Life Cycle Stage	Definition of Phase	Health Concerns or Needs
I.		1.
		2.
		3.
II.		1.
		2.
		3.
III.		1.
		2.
		3.
IV.		1.
		2.
		3.
V.		1.
		2.
		3.
VI.		1.
		2.
		3.
VII.		1.
		2.
		3.
VIII.		1.
		2.
		3.

10. Within each of the eight life cycle stages of the family, identify the developmental tasks of parents as described by Friedman.

Life Cycle Stage	Developmental Task(s) of Parent
I.	1.
II.	1.
	2.
III.	1.
IV.	1.
V.	1.
	2.
VI.	1.
VII.	1.
VIII.	1.

Choose the correct answer(s) to the following question.

11. When does the marriage relationship, according to studies, appear to be the strongest and most satisfying?
    a. Stage of preschool children.
    b. Stage of childbearing families.
    c. Stage of marriage.
    d. The postparental period (middle-aged parents).
    e. Stage of the contracting family (family in later years).
    f. Stage of families launching young adults.

12. Give the three aspects of the adolescent process that explain the developmental tasks and problems faced in this stage.

13. What is usual impact of adolescent family members on the family as a whole?

*For each question from 14 to 21, select the lettered choice that applies to it.**

    a. Beginning families
    b. Childbearing families
    c. Families with preschool children
    d. Families with school-age children
    e. Families with teenagers
    f. Families as launching centers
    g. Families in the middle years
    h. Families in the later years

14. Beginning of loosening of family ties.

---

*These questions are adapted from Borlick M., et al. *Nursing Examination Review Book,* Vol. 9: *Community Health Nursing.* 2nd ed. Flushing, N.Y.: Medical Examination Publishing Company; 1974.

15. Reaching maximum size in number of members and of interrelationships.

16. Being totally responsible for the first time for another human being.

17. Establishing a home base.

18. Releasing members into lives of their own.

19. Rediscovery of couple as husband and wife.

20. Learning to supply adequate space, facilities, and equipment for a rapidly expanding family.

21. Dealing with death of spouse.

22. Which of the following descriptions apply to the single-parent or divorced family with respect to its development?
    a. The single-parent or divorced family passes through the same family life cycle stages.
    b. The characteristics of the family life cycle—after the divorce—differ because of the absence of a second parent in the family.
    c. The single-parent or divorced family skips one or two of the family life cycle stages, depending on when the divorce occurred.
    d. The timing of the family life cycle transitions will probably be delayed in the immediate postdivorce period.

23. In the stepparent family, remarriage creates initial crisis and destabilization. How generally does remarriage affect the family career stages?

24. What general areas (name three) would you assess to gather information about family development and the family's history?

25. What broad family nursing interventions are appropriate for families having actual or potential developmental problems?

(An assessment question dealing with the developmental stage and history of the family is included in Chapter 9—the case study.)

► chapter 6 study answers

1. Any two:
    a. A family is seen as a long-lived *small group* that changes *over time.*
    b. Families go through *life cycle or family career stages.*
    c. *During each life cycle stage certain developmental tasks* are germane to a family's functioning.
    d. In families there is *high family member interdependency.*

e. Family developmental tasks *are derived from* a combination of individual developmental tasks of each family member and the common family functions.

f. The developmental approach describes *commonalities* in family experiences through time.

2. b.

3. All responses are correct (a–f).

4. c.

5. a, b, d, e, g, and h.

6. b.

7. a, d, and e.

8. a.

9.

Family Life Cycle Stage	Definition of Phase	Health Concerns or Needs
I. Married couple	Couple without children.	1. Generating satisfying marriage (communications, sexual counseling). 2. Planning a family. 3. Prenatal care.
II. Childbearing	Birth of the firstborn until oldest child is 30 months old.	1. Postpartum care, family planning. 2. Sibling rivalry. 3. Infant supervision and education (also family interactions— parental, marital).
III. Preschool	Oldest child is 30 months to 5–6 years old (when child starts school).	1. Preschooler's accidents and infectious illnesses. 2. Adequate child care facilities. 3. Marital relationship problems.
IV. School age	Oldest child is 6 to 13 years old.	1. Marital relationship problems. 2. Learning problems of children. 3. Child-rearing practices.

V. Teenage	Oldest child is 13 to 20 years old.	1. Communication problems (parent–teenager). 2. Discipline and power struggles (parent–teenager).
VI. Families launching young adults	Firstborn through youngest child leave home.	1. Parent–child communication problems. 2. General health promotion. 3. Care of and assistance to aging parents.
VII. Middle-aged parents	Empty nest (no children home) to retirement.	1. Care of and assistance to aging parents. 2. Emergence of chronic illness—need for wellness lifestyle. 3. Grandparent role.
VIII. Family in later years	Retirement to death of both spouses.	1. Declining health status. 2. Retirement. 3. Death of spouse. 4. Adjustment to environmental changes.

10.

Life Cycle Stage	Developmental Task(s) of Parent
I. Married couple	1. None.
II. Childbearing	1. Parents learn cues baby expresses in making needs known. 2. Learning to accept child's growth and development (toddler).
III. Preschool	1. Learning to separate from child.
IV. School age	1. Learning to separate from child continues.
V. Teenage	1. Learning to accept rejection without deserting the child. 2. Learning to build a new life for themselves (marital couple).
VI. Families launching young adults	1. Learning to build a new life for themselves (marital couple) continues.

VII. Middle-aged parents	1. Learning to build a new life for themselves (marital couple) continues.
VIII. Family in later years	1. Learning to adjust/accept dependent role.

11. d.

12. Emancipation, generation gap, and youth culture.

13. The American family is tremendously affected by the developmental tasks of the adolescent. The turmoil and conflicts between parents and teenagers are inevitable as the teenager's assertion of himself or herself and rebellion is part of becoming independent or emancipated.

14. e.

15. d.

16. b.

17. a.

18. f.

19. g.

20. c.

21. h.

22. a, b, and d.

23. Remarriage, because of its disruptive nature, generally impedes the family's movement through and completion of the family developmental tasks for 2 to 3 years after the creation of the new blended (stepparent) family. After the new family is restabilized (with a new structure, roles, rituals, and rules), the family resumes its normal developmental process.

24. The family's present developmental stage, the extent to which the family is fulfilling its family developmental tasks, the family's history from inception to present, and both parents' families of origin.

25. Teaching and counseling modalities.

Systems Theory

Marilyn M. Friedman

► learning objectives

1. Describe the characteristics of the paradigm associated with systems theory.

2. Define the following general systems theory terms: systems, social systems, open versus closed systems, differentiation, wholeness or nonsummativity, and feedback.

3. Relative to the family system, explain either narratively or diagrammatically the family system's relationship to its internal and external environment (the hierarchy of systems).

4. Apply the exchange and processing model (input-flow-output and feedback components) to the family system.

5. Compare the terms self-regulation, steady state, homeostasis, equilibrium, and adaptation.

6. Identify four prime characteristics of a family system.

7. Explain the significance of the family system and family subsystem boundaries.

8. Identify the three family interpersonal subsystems and explain their function.

9. Explain the term differentiation as it applies to the family system.

10. Using systems concepts, name four characteristics of a successfully functioning, healthy family.

Three grand theories—developmental theory, structural–functional theory, and general systems theory—are used in this text to formulate the family assessment areas and questions. These theories also suggest family strengths and problems upon which goals and implementation strategies can be formulated. Structural–functional and systems theory are not mutually exclusive perspectives. Structural–functionalism can be considered the earliest form of systems theory (Broderick, 1993).

Of the three above-mentioned theories, systems theory is clearly the most inclusive and powerful, as is

so convincingly demonstrated by the wide number of fields and substantive areas (including nursing) that have adapted this perspective as foundational to their organizing framework.

General systems theory has received wide usage in such diverse areas as educational systems, game theory, computer science, systems engineering, computer information systems, and communication fields. Growth in the use of systems theory in the health care fields has been especially impressive within the last 30 years, as evidenced by the proliferation of books using this approach to study individuals, the family, nursing and other health care professionals, the health care delivery system, and the community.

Contemporary systems theories about families are derived from general systems theory (Whitchurch & Constantine, 1993). Systems theory then forms the conceptual basis for "thinking systems" or for working with family systems as client rather than the individual client. Systems theory has probably stimulated most of the efforts made to achieve a systematic understanding of the normal and troubled family. As Broderick, a leading family theorist (1990), asserts, systems theory "is one of the most influential and generative of all of the family frameworks" (p. 172).

▶ GENERAL SYSTEMS THEORY: PARADIGM AND ASSOCIATED THEORIES

Von Bertalanffy (1950), an Austrian biologist, is credited with first delineating general systems theory in biology and physics, although sociologists and social anthropologists prior to and concurrent with von Bertalanffy's early publications were also describing systems—social systems (Parsons, 1951). In general systems theory, universal principles were applied to all kinds of groups of phenomena, which von Bertalanffy called "systems." Thus, systems theory can be applied across disciplines whereby universal laws are useful in working with various types of systems (Lee & Lancaster, 1988).

In looking at human behavior, be it of an individual, a family, or a whole community, general systems theory serves as a valuable "umbrella" under which various more middle-range theoretical perspectives may be subsumed (such as the ecological perspective, family communication theory, cybernetics or information processing theory, and adaptation theory). Systems theory constitutes a way of explaining a unit such as the family, as it relates and interacts with other systems. It is an organizational theory that is concerned with studying and describing the way things interrelate together rather than with analyzing the things themselves (Braden, 1984). It explains how each discrete variable affects the whole and how the whole affects each part.

As part of a "systems" revolution (Hartman & Laird, 1983), we have witnessed a shift in thinking from mechanistic, outcome-oriented theories to holistic, process-oriented theories. General systems theory has allowed health care professionals to do this. Systems theories provide us with the concepts and framework to think in terms of facts and events in the *context* of wholes, rather than in a vacuum: "Looking at the world in terms of sets of integrated relations constitutes the systems view" (Lazlo, 1972, p. 19 as cited in Hartman & Laird, 1983, p. 59). Using a systems framework—namely, the organization of knowledge concerning the specific phenomena of interest as a complex system—one focuses on the *interaction among the various parts of the system* rather than on the function of the parts themselves (Buckley, 1967; von Bertalanffy, 1966).

Holistic Paradigm

Some theorists consider general systems theory to be broader than a theory, to be "an alternative *Weltanschauung*"—a unique world view or paradigm that requires "systems thinking" (Whitchurch & Constantine, 1993, p. 325).

Before general systems theory, the tendency was towards reduction and parts analysis (Young, 1982). Those in the holistic health movement labeled that way of looking at things as "the mechanistic paradigm."

The mechanistic paradigm, in seeking to analyze and explain phenomena, reduces them to their parts—in many cases to their smallest parts, to find cause-and-effect relationships. Medical science and most of the sciences tend to operate within this linear (straight-line cause-and-effect or "A leads to B"), atomistic, reductionistic, and highly analytic paradigm. For example, using the mechanistic paradigm and linear thinking, infections in humans are explained in terms of bacterial invasions of certain cells and organs.

In contrast to this traditional paradigm, the systems paradigm, which is holistic (looks at whole systems like individuals or families, with regard to their interconnectedness, rather than separateness), posits circular causality. From a systems perspective, infections in humans would be conceptualized as an imbalance in man's interaction with his environment—where factors in the host (the person) influence the infectious agent and the infectious agent likewise affects the host.

It was Bateson (1972, 1979), a cultural anthropologist who is considered to be the father of the family therapy movement, who stressed this new epistemology, i.e., how one goes about gaining knowledge and making conclusions about the world. He pointed out the limits of linear thinking with respect to living systems. He proposed that in order to understand human behavior a shift to looking at ongoing processes, interrelationships, and circular causality was needed. For instance, applying the systems paradigm to the family, he asserted that there is no true victim and prosecutor in a troubled family. A particular entity (in this case a family member) is focused upon in relation to the things he or she affects and is affected by rather than in relation to his or her individual characteristics. Since both the "victim" and "prosecutor" in a family are serially and simultaneously affecting each other's roles and responses, only circular causality can adequately begin to explain the above situation (Fig. 7–1).*

In the 1950s and 1960s, Parson's (1951) social systems theory was used by sociology, social work, nursing (Johnson's nursing theory grew out of Parson's work) to explain personal and group behavior. Moreover, general systems theory, à la von Bertalanffy (1966), began to filter into nursing's thinking and literature (Rogers's and Roy's nursing models and the family therapy systems models are examples of this influence). Today the systems theoretical perspective and paradigm is widely accepted and utilized in nursing, particularly in family nursing (Richards & Lansberry, 1995).

A broad array of other health-related disciplines have found general systems theory's perspective useful. In medicine, general systems theorys sparked the development of family medicine, in psychology, family psychology, and in social work, the ecological perspective. This latter perspective, derived from general systems theory, focuses primarily on the adaptive balance that exists between living systems and their environments (Hartman & Laird, 1983).

Associated Theories: Cybernetics and Communication Theory

Two other systems-derived theories, again more middle-range in scope, have also revolutionized family-centered practice. These are the theories of cybernetics and family communication processes.

Cybernetics is a science that deals with communication and control theory. Cybernetics focuses on information processing and how feedback mechanisms operate in controlling both simple and complex systems (Goldenberg & Goldenberg, 1996). Cybernetics explains how systems maintain their stability through self-correcting feedback mechanisms. Systems can be self-correcting by reinserting the results of past performance into current functioning (Goldenberg & Goldenberg, 1996). With this focus, a way to change future performance may be generated by modifying feedback information (a strategy used in family counseling). Both parts and wholes are examined in cybernetics relative to their patterns of organization (Keeney, 1982; Weiner, 1948).

Cybernetics and general systems theory provided the legacy for family communication theories (Bateson, 1979; Jackson, 1969; Satir, 1983; Watzlawick, et al., 1967), the theoretical foundations modern-day family therapists most heavily rely on both in terms of assessment and intervention.

In the following discussion of systems theory, only the basic definitions and concepts used in a systems analysis of the family will be presented. Because these concepts are only briefly explained and systems theory is rather abstract, additional sources on this

---

*Circular "systems" thinking applied to families does not mean that abusive, violent family members are absolved of their responsibility for their behavior, as some feminists have feared. Systems analysis, does, however, aid in understanding the underlying dynamics and processes involved in an abusive, violent situation(s).

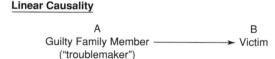

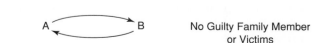

Figure 7–1. Comparison between linear and circular causality in a troubled family.

theory may be useful. The references in this chapter are suggested as supplementary reading to the discussion presented here.

▶ DEFINITIONS OF SYSTEMS CONCEPTS AND PROPOSITIONS

Definitions of the following systems terms are eclectically derived. Three main sources were used: general systems theory, Parsons's (1951) social systems theory, and family systems theory from the family therapy field. Table 7–1 summarizes the main characteristics of systems theory.

System

A **system** is defined as a goal-directed unit made up of interdependent, interacting parts that endure over a period of time. This system, together with its environment, make up a "universe," that is, the totality of what should be studied in a given situation. Systems and their parts have both functional and structural components. *Structure* pertains to the arrangement and organization among the parts of the system, whereas *function* refers to the purposes or goals of the system, such as activities necessary to

---

▶ TABLE 7–1

KEY CHARACTERISTICS OF SYSTEMS THEORY AND THE FAMILY

- Family systems do not exist in a vacuum—the context in which systems function is critical.
- All parts of the family system are interconnected or interrelated.
- The whole is greater than the sum of its parts (nonsummativity).
- Understanding is only possible by viewing the whole family.
- Whatever affects the system as a whole family affects each of its parts (the ripple effect).
- Causes and effects are interchangeable (circular causality notion).
- Family systems are self-reflexive and goal seeking.

---

assure the survival, continuity, and growth of the system. Function in systems analysis also is defined as the result or outcome of the structure.

Holism or Nonsummativity

"No assumption is more fundamental to modern general systems theory than that of holism" (Whitchurch & Constantine, 1993, p. 328). A system is characterized by its property of **wholeness** or **nonsummativity**. The whole is greater than the sum of its parts describes this concept, as first asserted by Aristotle (Broderick, 1993). A system cannot be understood by examining its individual parts in isolation from each other. "Understanding only is possible by viewing the whole" (Klein & White, 1996, p. 156).

Interconnectedness

A vital characteristic of a system is the interconnectedness or interrelatedness of its parts (Klein & White, 1996). This foundational assumption of general systems theory is a basic epistemological statement asserting that systems theory does not believe in isolating behaviors from the environment in which they occur.

Social System

A **social system** is a model of social organization; it is a living system possessing a total unit distinctive from its component parts and distinguishable from its environment by a clearly defined boundary. Parsons and Bales (1955) define a social system as composed of two or more persons or social roles tied together by mutual interaction and interdependence (Anderson & Carter, 1974).

Open System

Systems are characterized on the basis of their degree of interaction with the surrounding environment. An **open system** exists in an environment with which it interacts—from which it derives its inputs and to which it gives its outputs. This environmental interaction is necessary for its survival (Buckley, 1967). By definition, all living systems are open systems.

Closed System

Theoretically, a **closed system**, in contrast to the open system, does not interact with the environment. A closed system would then be a self-contained unit, not dependent on continual environmental interchange for its survival. Because no totally closed system has yet been demonstrated in reality, "closed" denotes a relative lack of energy exchange across a system's boundaries (Parsons & Bales, 1955).

Hierarchy of Systems

No system functions in a vacuum. The system's universe, therefore, needs to be examined to determine its effect on the system under study. The universe—the system and its environment—contains a hierarchy of systems. Each higher-level unit contains lower-level systems. For instance, a hierarchy of systems from higher to lower levels might be as follows: community → family and other interacting systems → parental and other subsystems → individual organism → organ systems → tissues → cells.

When using system theory as a working framework, one must be clear and specific about what system is being assessed. The system under study at a particular time is called *the target or focal system*. After specifying the target system as, for example, the family, one would assess that system, and then its relationship to the interacting systems within its environment, and finally its relationship to suprasystems and subsystems.

In the case of the family focus, one would thus want to study the family *and* both its interacting, internal and external environments. The suprasystems are larger environmental systems of which the focal or target system is a part. The subsystems are smaller subunits or subcomponents of the focal system. For example, if the family is the focal system, then one suprasystem would be the family's cultural reference group and the relational subsystems would consist of the sets of family relationships, such as the spousal, sibling, and parent–child subsystems (Fig. 7–2).

Boundaries

Each system has a boundary that defines the system and demarcates it from its environment. The boundary represents the interface or point of contact between the

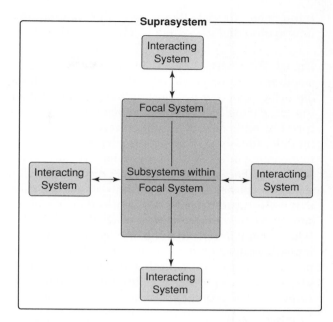

Figure 7–2. Schematic representation of the hierarchy of systems.

system and other systems; that is, between the system and its subsystems and suprasystems (Whitchurch & Constantine, 1993). Auger (1976) explains that

> a boundary may be defined as a more or less open line forming a circle around the system where there is greater interchange of energy within the circle than on the outside. It is helpful to visualize a boundary as a "filter" which permits the constant exchange of elements, information, or energy between the system and its environment. (p. 24)

The more porous or permeable the filter or boundary, the greater the degree of interaction possible between the system and its environment. In contrast, the less porous or permeable the boundary, the more isolated the system is from its environment. The ability of a boundary to control the degree of exchange is of great significance, because it regulates the amount and type of input from the environment at any time, enabling the system to maintain equilibrium or to adapt to new demands.

Input

As mentioned above, all open systems must receive input from their environment in order to survive.

Input refers to such things as energy, matter, and information that the system receives and processes.

Input Processing.

When input is received in a system, it must be processed. This can be done either by accepting or rejecting the incoming input without change (also called assimilation) or by transforming or accommodating, whereby the system modifies the input or alters its structure in response to incoming information. Systems have rules of transformation. For example, a rule of transformation for a marital subsystem might be the *quid pro quo* rule, that is if one spouse acts nasty to the other, the other spouse reacts likewise (Klein & White, 1996). Whether unaltered or transformed, the processed input flows through the system and is released as output. It is by this process that *adaptation* occurs—whereby a social, open system adjusts to demands (inputs) from its outer and inner environments.

Output

The results of the system's processing of the input constitute the output. Output in the form of energy, matter, or information is released into the environment.

Feedback

Feedback refers to the process by which a system monitors the internal and environmental responses to its behavior (output) and accommodates or adjusts itself (Weiner, 1948). Feedback involves receiving and responding to the return of its own output. Information about how a system is functioning is looped back (feedback) from the output to the input, thus altering subsequent input (Goldenberg & Goldenberg, 1996). The system adjusts both internally by modification of subsystems and externally by controlling its boundaries. Thus it is able to control and modify inputs and outputs.

Feedback can be negative or positive feedback. *Positive feedback* refers to the system's output that is returned to the system as information that moves the system away from equilibrium and toward change. It involves amplifying feedback loops. Conversely *negative feedback* is informational output that is returned to the system, promoting equilibrium and stability of the system (Casey, 1989). The use of attenuating feedback loops maintain aspects of the system's func-

tioning within prescribed limits (Goldenberg & Goldenberg, 1996). Figure 7–3 describes these last four terms diagrammatically.

Self-regulation, Homeostasis, Steady State, and Equilibrium

All of these terms are used rather interchangeably in the literature, although there are fine distinctions between terms. Here only two distinctions will be pointed out. System self-regulation is a mechanism within a system that assists the system to balance and control inputs and outputs, via feedback loops. When the system is in balance the result is homeostasis, a steady state, or equilibrium. This balance is not static, however, but dynamic and always changing within certain degrees of variation. Adaptation occurs through system self-regulatory mechanisms. The outcome of this regulation and adaptation is equilibrium, a steady state, or homeostasis (Hazzard, 1971; Klein & White, 1996).

Fishman (1985) asserts that when family members develop symptoms, these symptoms may serve to maintain family homeostasis. For instance, if a child in a family "acts out" (consistently or over some time period), the focus of attention may shift from a conflictual marital relationship to how to manage the rebellious child. With a focus on the acting-out child, the couple may decrease their fighting—a situation the acting-out child prefers.

Differentiation

General systems theory states that the growth and change toward a higher order of organization occur through *differentiation*. This term, then, denotes a liv-

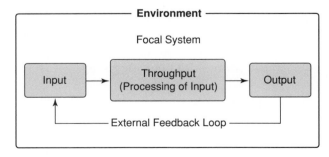

Figure 7–3. Energy, matter, and information exchange and processing model. *(Adapted from Hazzard, 1971.)*

ing system's capability and propensity to progressively and serially advance to a higher order of complexity and organization (referred to also as negentropy). A social system, if acting normally, has a tendency to "grow" (called morphogenesis). The propensity to grow or change is counterbalanced by the tendency of a system to stabilize (return to a state of equilibrium or homeostasis). A balance between stability (called morphostasis) and change is needed for a system to grow or differentiate. Figure 7–4 illustrates the tendency for a system to experience periods of both change and stability. Energy inputs flowing into the system are utilized by the system to grow in complexity and organization (Bowen, 1960).

Energy

"All dynamic, open systems require continuous supplies of energy in sufficient quantity so that demands for system integrity can be met" (Auger, 1976). The most important factor governing the amount of energy needed is the rate of utilization of energy within the system itself. Systems with high levels of activity utilize large quantities of energy, and therefore must receive greater amounts of input from the environment in order to meet their energy demands. This, in turn, implies that the system's boundaries would have to be more open, or porous, to allow a greater input of energy.

The basic systems concepts and propositions will now be applied to the text's focal system, the family.

▶ FAMILY SYSTEMS DEFINITIONS

The following family systems definitions have come primarily from family process or systems theorists who have applied general systems theory, as well as cybernetics and communication theory, to the family system.

Family

The family is defined as a living social system that typically extends over at least three generations (Goldenberg & Goldenberg, 1996). It is a unique small group of closely interrelated and interdependent individuals who are organized into a single unit so as to attain family functions or goals.

> [It] has evolved a set of rules, is replete with assigned and ascribed roles for its members, has an organized power structure, has developed intricate overt and covert forms of communication, and has elaborated ways of negotiating and problem solving that permits various tasks to be performed effectively. The relationship between members of this micro culture is deep and multi-

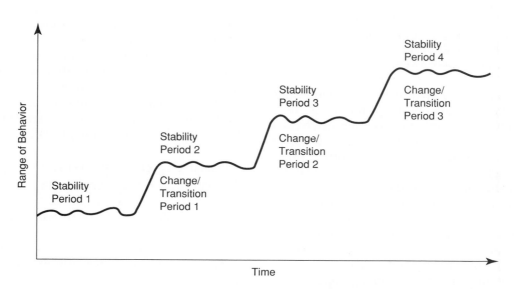

Figure 7–4. A system's tendency toward stability and change.

layered, and is based largely on a shared history, shared internalized perceptions and assumptions about the world, and a shared sense of purpose. Within such a system, individuals are tied to one another by powerful, durable, reciprocal emotional attachments and loyalties that may fluctuate in intensity over time but nevertheless persist over the lifetime of the family. (Goldenberg & Goldenberg, 1996, p. 3)

Reciprocal Determinism or the Ripple Effect

The interrelationships found in a family system are so intricately tied together that a change in any one part inevitably results in changes in the entire system. This reverberating effect is referred to as reciprocal determinism by Goldenberg and Goldenberg (1996), or as a ripple effect by Boss (1988). Each family member and subsystem is affected by transitional and situational stressors that initially impact one or more family members—with the effects on each family member varying in intensity and quality. For example, family health professionals have observed a powerful collective family impact when there is a sick or disabled child in the family. Boss (1988) explains that

> there is a ripple effect when a parent overfocuses on that child in the subsequent reaction of a sibling (or mate) who feels left out. The family member who feels neglected begins to distance himself or herself or to act out for attention. A sibling may run away; a mate may indulge in self-destructive behavior or have an affair. (p. 16)

Forces in the family move in many directions simultaneously, in a *circular* fashion, not in a *lineal* cause-and-effect manner. An example of circular causality is the situation in which parents ask their children, who are fighting with each other, "Who started this fight?" They usually get the same answer from both children, "He/she did!" Both children are right and wrong. From each child's perspective, the other started it, because it all depends on where in the communication loop the investigation begins— each child starting at the point where he or she felt the other one instituted the fight. Circular causality, the language used in systems thinking, suggests that

any search for a "real or ultimate" cause of any interpersonal event is impossible and pointless.

Nonsummativity (Wholeness or Holism)

An essential property of the family as an open system is nonsummativity, which was defined earlier in the context of systems theory. Here it means that the family cannot be considered as merely the sum of its parts. The family viewed as a whole is greater than the sum of its parts. In other words, a family is something more than parent(s), plus child(ren). The assessment of the family unit cannot be based on knowledge about each of the family members or sets of relationships (Wright & Leahey, 1994). "Family systems have emergent properties," state Hartman and Laird (1983, p. 62). By this they mean that the interrelatedness of components in the family system gives rise to new qualities and characteristics that are a function of that interrelatedness.

Self-Reflexivity and Goal Seeking

Family systems are self-reflexive and goal-seeking systems. All cybernetic systems (i.e., systems with feedback) are self-monitoring, although in nonhuman systems this does not require self-awareness. Human systems, including families, are self-reflexive, meaning that they possess the ability and tendency to make themselves and their own behavior the focus of examination and the target of explanation (Whitchurch & Constantine, 1993). Because families are self-reflexive, they examine their own systems and then set goals for themselves (Broderick, 1993). Communication allows for self-reflexivity because it facilitates persons' creation of meaning and their sending and receiving symbolic messages (Whitchurch & Constantine, 1993).

Hierarchy of Systems: Family as Focal System

Figure 7–5 illustrates the relationship of the family to its subsystems, its interacting systems, such as the welfare and educational system, and its suprasystems, e.g., the family's reference group(s), the community, and wider society.

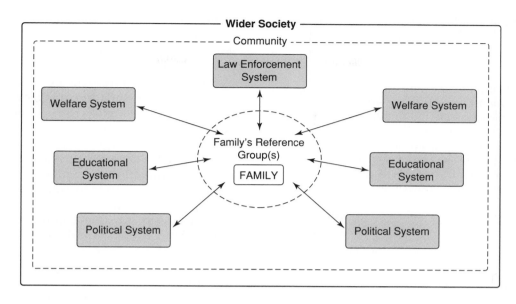

Figure 7–5. Schematic illustration of the family and its external environment.

Relative to the family system's environment, generally speaking, the more immediate the environment, the greater the influence on the system and the greater the input to the family. Conversely, more distant environments generally have less influence on the family. Thus systems with which the family continually interacts, such as the school system, generally have a more potent impact on the family than a remote suprasystem.

Hierarchy of systems means then that systems exist at multiple levels—including the individual as a family subsystem who could be assessed just as other levels could be. These systems, however, are analyzed within the context of their interacting sub- and suprasystems.

Open, Closed, and Random Family Systems

All families are, strictly speaking, open systems, because they must exchange materials, energy, and information with their environment to survive. Families are in constant interaction with their physical, social, and cultural environment. From a clinical perspective, it is possible, however, to identify degrees of openness, closedness, and/or randomness in a family and thus to evaluate a family's ability to change and to maintain stability. Kantor and Lehr (1975), in an in-

depth qualitative study of families, described three types of families: open, closed, and random families.

In *open families* the exchange of information, friends, and activities is extensive. Open families welcome new ideas, information, techniques, opportunities, and resources. Moreover, open families take the initiative by actively seeking out new resources and using these resources to solve their problems. Creative and flexible solutions to problems are sought and are utilized in response to changing and unique needs (Satir, 1972).

Open families are those that perceive change as normal and desirable, and view people as inherently good and helpful and thus to be sought and needed. Open families reach out to the larger community and interact extensively with it. Family boundaries of the open family are much more permeable than in the closed family.

In contrast, *closed families* view change as threatening and are resistant to it. Strangers are perceived as being potentially harmful or at least not to be trusted. Closed families believe that a person's negative qualities are a basic fact of life and that people must therefore be under strict control; thus, relationships have to be regulated by force. Within the family there is extensive social control. These types of families are rigid; as a result, things and events in the closed family remain as constant and predictable as possible. Stability and tradition are core purposes of closed families. Kantor and Lehr (1975) describe the situation existing in the closed family:

> Locked doors, careful scrutiny of strangers in the neighborhood, parental control over the media, supervised excursions, and unlisted telephones are all features of a closed-type family. Closed bounding (boundary) goals include the preservation of territoriality, self-protection, privacy, and, in some families, secretiveness. Perimeter traffic control is never relinquished to outsiders or even to anyone within the family not specifically assigned bounding responsibilities. (p. 120)

The third type of family described by Kantor and Lehr is the *random family*. It is easy to think of this type of family as being the polar opposite of the closed family in terms of family social control and rigidity to change. Whereas time, activities, and family routines are closely regulated and controlled in the closed family, just the reverse is true in the random type family. Individual family members establish their own boundaries, values, activities, routines, and schedules. Traffic in and out of the family is loosely regulated even when strangers are involved. These are high-energy families that value spontaneity, free choice, very fluid norms, and challenge (Mercer, 1989). Here the core purpose of the family is exploration through use of members' sense of intuition (Kantor & Lehr, 1975). In the extreme, this type of family is chaotic and prone to dissolution.

Family Boundaries

Probably the most crucial means families have of facilitating adaptation to outside demands and internal needs is through their effective use of their semipermeable *family boundaries*. The function of metaphoric boundaries is to actively expand (or open) and retract (or close) according to need, thus regulating the amount of input from the environment and output to the environment (Reinhardt & Quinn, 1973). In other words, the key to successful family adaptation is selective permeability of family boundaries. In healthy family functioning, input is screened so that a family takes in what is needed from the environment and assimilates or modifies it to promote its own survival and growth.

When families have boundaries that are too rigid and impermeable, important resources are not forthcoming. These families are deprived of the necessary information and support, as well as, perhaps, the physical resources necessary for family wellness. Family boundary maintenance in information processing determines the openness of the system relative to exchanging information with the external environment. The amount of information a family can handle adequately is limited, and an excess of information or conflicting information from the outer environment amplifies and creates family disequilibrium. Conversely, too little information can also threaten family stability. In the healthy family, boundaries adequately screen information input and output. When an excessive amount of information flows into the family, the boundaries close, and when an underflow of information occurs, boundaries open (Reinhardt & Quinn, 1973).

The family with an underflow of information from the environment relies more heavily on inner familial resources. Relatively closed families may discharge more energy than is constructive, with eventual disorganization the result.

The abused child is frequently found in families that are isolated and have closed boundaries with society. In healthier isolated families, the members tend to believe that all or most of the needs of the members can be met by the family itself or its reference group. Family self-sufficiency may be overemphasized, however, causing family members to view wider society in a distorted or negative way. The children of such families often experience great strain when they are required to interact with the wider society.

On the other hand, families that are indiscriminately open to information tend to become disorganized and chaotic. In this case, ineffective boundary regulation allows information to flow constantly into the family system, with resultant distortion and high levels of anxiety manifested among family members. Children and adults of these families are often forced into the extrafamilial environment of neighbors, community organizations, and state agencies in order to get their needs met. In these cases relationships within and outside of the family are generally shallow, nonrewarding, and frustrating to family members.

Family Adaptation

Family adaptation refers to the capacity of the family and its members to modify their behavior to each other and their outer world as the situation demands. In response to internal or external input, the family adapts by either accepting or rejecting incoming information, energy, or services, or by modifying input to meet its needs.

In an open system the family balances inputs from the external and internal environments by the feedback process. Balanced adequately, this is called *family homeostasis, steady state*, or *equilibrium*. Homeostasis or its synonyms (steady state and equilibrium) should not imply stagnation, however, but the degree of balancing needed while continual change and growth are taking place. Healthy families are flexible, more spontaneous, open to growth and change, responsive to new stimulation, and not status-quo oriented (Beavers & Hampson, 1993).

Because families must change in order to meet both internal and external demands, a sufficient range of behaviors and patterns, plus the flexibility to mobilize these when needed, is essential. Nevertheless, the family system has a tendency to offer resistance to change beyond a certain range and maintains preferred patterns as long as it possibly can. Although alternatives are feasible, the family's threshold of tolerance for change stimulates self-regulatory mechanisms that reestablish the accustomed range. An example of this phenomenon is that when a family member begins to distance himself or herself from the family, it is common for other family members to feel the distancing member is not doing his or her part. Guilt-producing techniques may then be used to return the family member to his or her usual family roles.

A steady state is achieved internally by balancing family members' roles. Family members help to maintain this internal balance either covertly or overtly. The family's repetitive, circular, and predictable communication patterns will reveal this balancing act.

Failure of Adaptive Strategies

As with individuals, the presence of stress in a family initially aids the family to mobilize its resources and work at solving its problems. Stress causes family homeostasis or its steady state to become precarious, in which case family members initially exert considerable effort to regain its balance. However, when initial attempts to resolve problems or to meet demands fail, stress increases. Often a stressor originally affects one individual, followed by one and then the other subsystems—until finally all family subsystems are involved (the ripple effect). For instance, problems in the spouse subsystem can be localized for a while. Then as they continue and intensify, other subsystems, especially the parent–child subsystem, becomes affected. Although stress is experienced by all the subsystems, each subsystem may tolerate and handle the stress differently, as discussed under the ripple effect earlier.

In time, if no solution is found to reduce the stress, the system eventually reaches its limits to respond adaptively, reaching a point of exhaustion. When important familial resources are depleted, family functioning deteriorates, and symptoms of family disorganization set in, such as overt symptoms of an individual family member's distress, economic difficulties, intrafamilial conflicts, or parenting problems. At this point a family crisis is present. If no outside assistance is received, the end result may be the family adapting at a lower level of functioning or perhaps the separation or loss of a family member. In contrast, a stable system under stress will move in the direction that tends to minimize the stress; for example, it will seek help from external sources when its internal resources are inadequate.

Family Subsystems

The family is a system of interacting personalities intricately organized into positions, roles, and norms, which are further organized into subsystems within the family. These subsystems become the basis for the family structure or organization. The family system differentiates and carries out its functions through personal and interpersonal or relational subsystems (Kantor & Lehr, 1975). Interpersonal subsystems are made up of sets of relationships involving two or more family members. Each individual within the family is also a personal subsystem—the smallest of the subsystems in the family. Family subsystems, however, primarily refer to the interpersonal subsystems discussed here. Family members belong to different interpersonal subsystems, where they have different levels of power and learn differentiated roles. An adult female, for example, can be a daughter, wife, or older sister. Each of these roles involves different complementary relationships and the use of a different cluster of behaviors (Minuchin, 1974).

A family contains at least one "control" subsystem that sets the rules for processing input, and compares output with family goals (a cybernetic description). In a two-parent nuclear family, the primary control subsystem is the spouse subsystem.

The two-parent nuclear family has at least three interpersonal subsystems, each of which serves some unique function in addition to common objectives. These subsystems are listed in Table 7–2.

Minuchin (1974), a family therapist and the author of several important books in his field, has worked extensively with families using a systems-based approach in family counseling. He stresses the need to work with and through the several subsystems of the family to effect positive change within the whole family. His approach is to assist in the strengthening of the subsystems so that they function in an effective manner and do not lose their identity or unique contribution to the whole.

Minuchin suggests that in the same way that the family system has a boundary, so does each subsystem, the purpose of which is to protect the differentiation of the system; that is, it is through the growth and evolution of subsystems that the whole family differenti-

ates. Each subsystem has specific functions, which in turn lead to special demands on its members. Thus in the spouse system, the parent is given the child-rearing function. Clear and intact boundaries are required to deter any interference by other subsystems. For example, the spouse subsystem often becomes usurped by the parent–child subsystem because of the overwhelming demands on the adult members (parents) of the parenting role. In another case, the parent–child subsystem cannot function effectively if siblings interfere in the parent–child relationship and compromise the parents' capacity to parent one of their offspring. Minuchin refers to this blurring of subsystem boundaries as "diffuse" boundaries.

A brief explanation of each of the three subsystems will help illuminate their critical functions.

The Spouse Subsystem.

The traditional spouse subsystem is formed when two adults of the opposite sex agree to join together for the primary purposes of mutual support and the meeting of each other's affectional and sexual needs. The couple needs to mutually accommodate and complement each other. The spouse subsystem is vital to the couple, because it acts as a refuge from external stresses and constitutes an avenue for contacting other social systems. It is also the most important subsystem of the family (Goldenberg & Goldenberg, 1996). Utilizing the systems framework, the spouse subsystem boundary needs to be intact and protected from the demands and needs of other systems. Children especially have a tendency to intrude on the spouse subsystem, creating a situation wherein husband and wife have a relationship based not on their own personal relationship with each other but on their parenting functions (Minuchin, 1974).

The Parent–Child Subsystem.

With the birth or adoption of a child by the couple, the original dyadic family grows in complexity as the new subsystem is created. The spouse subsystem now must differentiate itself to perform both mutual support (marital roles) and child-rearing (parental) functions. The parent–child subsystem involves parents and their relationship with each of their children (Minuchin, 1974).

The Sibling Subsystem.

With the advent of additional children, the sibling subsystem comes into

---

► TABLE 7–2

FAMILY SUBSYSTEMS BASED ON SETS OF RELATIONSHIPS IN THE NUCLEAR, TWO-PARENT FAMILY

1. *The Spouse Subsystem.* Here two adult members relate to each other as (a) marital partners and (b) parents of their offspring.
2. *The Parent–Child Subsystem.* This subsystem is composed of the parents and their children. The subsystem has parenting functions (socialization) involving the mother–father roles and the children's roles.
3. *The Sibling Subsystem.* This subsystem is composed of the children and characterized by the children's relationships with each other.
4. *Other Subsystems.* There may also exist, for example, a grandparent–grandchild subsystem or uncle–nephew subsystems in an extended family.

being. As only-children will attest, having a sister or brother is important. These relationships serve as the first social-skills laboratory for children. Here they learn to relate in the peer world. They learn to support, become angry, express feelings, negotiate, cooperate, and imitate each other. In relating to their siblings, children learn to play different roles, which then serve them when they go out into the extrafamilial world. Within these relationships there is an openness and honesty unmatched in outer society; that is, the child obtains constant feedback from siblings concerning his or her behavior.

The significance of the sibling subsystem is underscored by frequent observations made by only-children. Only-children accommodate in the adult world rather than their peer world, often exhibiting precocious development because of extensive parental exposure. Concurrently, they may have difficulty sharing, cooperating, and competing with children of their own age, and are usually more dependent in their behavior (Minuchin, 1974; Toman, 1961).

Differentiation

Differentiation refers to the family's propensity to evolve and grow so that as growth takes place the system becomes more complex, articulate, and discriminate. Developmental studies—studies of families throughout their life cycle—have demonstrated this tendency. Families are dynamic systems that are continually differentiating themselves both functionally and structurally. Because of the family's evolution and growth, there is also a concomitant need for increased numbers of specialized roles. This specialization and increased complexity are direct outcomes of differentiation (Minuchin, 1974).

▶ A SYSTEMS THEORY PERSPECTIVE ON HEALTHY FAMILIES

In concluding an exploration of the basic concepts and definition of systems theory and how these are applied and illustrated within the family system, it is fitting to draw a "composite picture" of the healthy family. According to systems theory, the healthy family is a maximally viable system characterized by complexity of structure; highly flexible organization capable and tolerant of internal changes; highly autonomous subsystems and considerable internal determination; and openness with the outer environment that results in a continual flow of a wide variety of information, experience, and input into the family (Beavers & Hampson, 1993; Lewis et al., 1976). Constantine (1986) adds that healthy family systems succeed at balancing family system needs simultaneously with individual family members' needs. In a well-functioning family all the family subsystems operate in an integrated way to maintain the differentiation and integrity of the family system (Goldenberg & Goldenberg, 1996).

▶ THE RELATIONSHIP BETWEEN THE STRUCTURAL–FUNCTIONAL AND SYSTEMS THEORIES

With regard to the family, apparent similarities between structural–functional and systems theory include the notion that the family (the focal system) interacts with its inner and outer environments and must be examined in context. System theory characterizes the family and other systems as containing a structure and functions. In structural–functionalism, however, these two concepts represent the central thrust of the theory, certainly a much more important emphasis than found in systems theory. Both theories discuss adaptation, with structural–functionalism stressing the tendency toward equilibrium, while systems theory stresses the balance between equilibrium (stability) and change in its analysis.

Systems theory, as noted earlier, is derived from a holistic paradigm, where circular causation and feedback loops are essential elements. Structural–functionalism, counter to some of its assumptions, tends to resort to more "part analysis," linear notions of causation, and a more static view of the family.

Much foundational family theory has been generated within a structural–functional frame, and structural–functional theory technically speaking is the earliest form of systems theory (Broderick, 1993). Both theories converge and diverge at certain points and both are useful in identifying and describing important content areas, explaining family behavior, and providing guidelines for family nursing practice.

▶ study questions

Are the following statements true or false?

1. A system is defined as a unit with distinct parts and boundaries, extending over a period of time and with some identified purpose(s).

2. A social system is either an animate or inanimate system.

3. Open systems depend on the environment for exchange of information, matter, and energy, whereas closed systems do not interact with the environment.

4. Family differentiation occurs when a system bifurcates or splits into smaller subunits or systems.

5. With greater energy use, system boundaries need to be more open.

6. Differentiation, particularly as it applies to the family system, describes the family's tendency to grow and evolve (as time progresses) into a more complex and specialized system.

7. Relative to the family system and its internal and external environments, supply the following information:
    a. Name a focal or target system.
    b. Name a suprasystem.
    c. Give three examples of interacting systems.
    d. Give three examples of family subsystems.

8. Draw a diagram of the energy, matter, and information exchange and process model and show a specific example of this energy exchange and processing pertinent to the family system.

9. Match the correct term from the left-hand column with characteristic from the right-hand column.
    a. Equilibrium
    b. Adaptation
    c. Homeostasis
    d. Steady state
    e. Feedback loop
    f. Self-regulation
    g. Nonsummativity

    1. Synonymous with balancing (used interchangeably)
    2. The result of balancing
    3. A survival mechanism
    4. The whole is greater than its parts

10. Identify which of the following adjectives or terms accurately describe the paradigm used in systems theory.
    a. Reductionistic
    b. Objective
    c. Partial analysis
    d. Atomistic
    e. Linear causality
    f. None of these

Choose the correct answer(s) to the following question.

11. The following elements and characteristics are true of the family system. It is a (an):
    a. Open social system.
    b. Highly organized system.
    c. Highly interdependent system.
    d. System with specified purposes.
    e. System with necessary processes (e.g., integration, adaptation, and decision making).
    f. Independent system.
    g. Undifferentiated system.
    h. Suprasystem to the spouse, parent–child, and sibling systems.
    i. Dynamic system but with little capacity for change.

12. What is the significance of the boundaries of the family system and subsystems?

13. Using the systems approach, explain how family boundaries function to maintain family homeostasis.

14. Match the proper function(s) in the left-hand column with each of the family subsystems in the right-hand column.
    a. A social skills laboratory   1. Spouse subsystem
    b. Mutual support   2. Parent–child subsystem
    c. Meeting of adult affectional   3. Sibling subsystem
       needs
    d. Learning to relate to peers
    e. Socialization function
    f. Disciplining—control and
       guidance function

15. Give four characteristics of a successfully functioning, healthy family according to systems theory.

16. Match the advantages/disadvantages and/or characteristics with "open," "closed," or random families.

    a. Open families   1. Provide for change
    b. Closed families   2. Are stagnated, rigid
    c. Random families   3. Offer choices and flexibility
    d. Does not apply   4. View change as threatening
                          5. Employ greater structuring and control mechanisms
                          6. Stress privacy and territoriality
                          7. See people as good, helpful, and needed
                          8. Seek out new resources
                          9. Family members set their own rules and schedules

17. Sequentially number the events below in terms of their sequencing when a family crisis occurs.
    a. No solution is found to reduce stress—that is, failure of adaptive strategies exists.
    b. Stress and strain are experienced.
    c. A change occurs as stressor presents itself.
    d. Family homeostasis or its steady state becomes precarious and family exerts additional efforts to maintain balance and reduce stress.
    e. Stress spreads from one individual or subsystem to all subsystems of family.
    f. System reaches point of exhaustion.
    g. Family disorganization results.

▶ chapter 7 study answers

1. True.

2. False.

3. True.

4. False.

5. True.

6. True.

7. a. Focal system = family.
   b. Suprasystem = wider community.
   c. Interacting systems = health care system, educational system, law enforcement system, welfare system.
   d. Subsystems = spouse, parent–child, and sibling subsystems.

8. See energy, matter, and information exchange and process model (Fig. 7–3). Various examples could be applied, such as:
   Input (= information): News of risk of inactivity and benefits of exercise program.
   Flow: Spouse subsystem accepts and internalizes this information.
   Output: Spouses begin dance classes weekly for themselves. They also begin hiking with their children on weekends (the energy release—their activity—is the output).
   Feedback: The family members feel better (have more energy, vitality, and strength) plus the parents' figures improve; both then become reinforcers of the exercise program.

9. a. 1.
    b. 2.
    c. 1.
    d. 1.
    e. 3.
    f. 3.
    g. 4.

10. f (see introduction to chapter for relevant discussion).

11. a, b, c, d, e, and h.

12. *Significance of family boundaries*: Boundaries allow for the exchange processes. By controlling the flow in and out of the system, they prevent overload or underload of the system. *Significance of family subsystem boundaries:* They prevent loss of integrity of the personal system and interference with the vital functions individuals in families need to learn and perform.

13. Family boundaries function adaptively by being selectively permeable—that is, actively expanding (opening up) and retracting (closing down) according to need, thus regulating the amounts of input and output.

14. a. 3.
    b. 1, 2, 3.
    c. 1.
    d. 3.
    e. 2.
    f. 2.

15. Any four characteristics of a healthy family: highly organized and differentiated; autonomous integrated subsystems; tolerance and ability to change internally; continual openness to new information and other input; and balancing of family system needs with family members' needs.

16. a. 1, 3, 7, and 8.
    b. 2, 4, 5, and 6.
    c. 9.
    d. None.

17. (1) = c, (2) = b, (3 or 4) = d, (3 or 4) = e, (5) = a, (6) = f, and (7) = g.

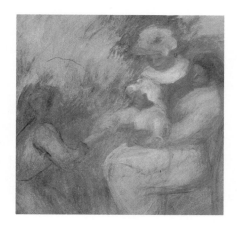

three

FAMILY NURSING PRACTICE: RESEARCH, THEORY, AND PROCESS

In Part III, we now move into more specific applications for working with families. There are five basic areas subsumed under the comprehensive assessment approach used in this text: (1) identifying data, (2) environmental data, (3) family structural dimensions, (4) family functions, and (5) family stress and coping processes.

Chapter 8 covers the identifying sociocultural data and Chapter 9 the environmental data regarding the family. The four dimensions of family structure are discussed in Chapters 10 through 13. Three of the most critical family functions (affective, socialization, and the health care function) are elaborated on in Chapters 14 through 16. Chapter 17 deals with family stress, coping, and adaptation. In each of the chapters, assessment areas related to and part of the broad assessment topic give sufficient detail, in terms of both theory and application, for collecting and interpreting assessment data pertaining to families in a multitude of settings and throughout the family's life cycle. Family nursing diagnoses and interventions appropriate for the area being addressed are also presented. The actual family assessment tool and a suggested care plan form are included as Appendices A and B. Appendix C presents a hypothetical family situation, which is followed by an analysis of the family in Appendix D.

8

Family Identifying Data: Sociocultural Assessment and Intervention

Marilyn M. Friedman

1. Define and describe the following family identifying data, applying content to a written case example:
   a. Family composition
   b. Type of family form
   c. Cultural (ethnic) and religious orientation
   d. Social class status, including occupational, economic, and educational data
   e. Social class mobility
   f. Social supports/network
   g. Recreational activities

2. Diagram a family genogram and family ecomap.

3. Explain why an understanding of a family's ethnic background is crucial for family health practice.

4. Discuss several of the major problems that result when cultural insensitivity and ignorance exist on the part of a health care professional.

5. Define these basic concepts: culture, ethnicity, stereotyping, acculturation, assimilation, biculturalism, cultural relativism, ethnocentrism, cultural imposition, cultural conflicts, cultural shock, indigenous health care system, self-fulfilling prophecy, cultural empathy, and ethclass.

6. Discuss the importance of the cross-cultural/transcultural approach to family health care.

7. Identify some of the differences in values and norms among the social classes.

8. Describe family-oriented interventions appropriate for enhancing/maintaining social supports and financial and economic welfare and providing culturally sensitive services.

9. Differentiate between the concepts of social support, social networks, family social support, and family social networks.

10. Describe two nursing intervention strategies designed to maintain or promote family social support.

11. Summarize basic research findings relative to the impact of social support on health/illness.

12. Identify broad intervention strategies that are effective in working with ethnic families.

13. Identify two strategies for assisting families with their health-related financial difficulties and two strategies for promoting family recreational activity.

▶ IDENTIFYING DATA: GETTING TO KNOW THE FAMILY

As with all assessment tools, it is important to begin by obtaining broad identifying information about the family client. As discussed in Chapter 3, during the initial visit or client contact, the focus is typically on getting to know the family and all its members, as well as attempting to meet their immediate health needs. To learn about the family, a family composition roster or family genogram is an excellent assessment strategy. Duvall and Miller (1985) say that with information about who lives in the home and their relationships, along with knowledge of the time (family life cycle and season, day, and hour) and the family's sociocultural status, one can generally predict current family activities and issues.

Family Composition

Family composition refers to who the family members identify as being part of their family. This may include not only the household inhabitants, but also other extended family or fictive family members who are part of "the family," but do not live in the same household. Obtaining data on the family composition lets family members know of your interest in the whole family rather than solely on an individual client. Completing a family composition roster involves collecting the following information:

- Family name
- Address
- Telephone number
- Family composition

In the family composition form given in Figure 8–1, the adult family members are recorded first, followed by the children in order of their birth beginning with the oldest. Include any other related or unrelated member(s) of the household next. If there are extended family members or friends who act as family members, although not living in the household, also include them at the end of the list. The relationship of each family member, as well as birthdate, birthplace, occupation, and education, are also identified.

The Family Genogram

The second initial assessment strategy for getting to know the family is the family genogram. The family genogram is a diagram that delineates the family constellation or family tree. It is an informative assessment tool used to get to know the family and the family's history and resources.

A genogram interview is seen as one part of a comprehensive clinical assessment of a family (McGoldrick & Gerson, 1985). The diagram maps relationships vertically (across generations) and horizontally (within the same generation) and often helps family nurses think systemically about how events and relationships in the nuclear family members' lives are related to family patterns of health and illness as well as to generate tentative hypotheses about what's going on in the family.

Based on the conventions used in diagraming family trees or genealogical charts and genetics, the family genogram incorporates information about three generations of the family (the two generations within the nuclear family and the family of origin of each parent). Not only are the nuclear and extended fam-

Name (Last, First)	Sex	Relationship	Date/Place of Birth	Occupation	Education
1. (father)					
2. (mother)					
3. (oldest child)					
4.					
5.					
6.					
7.					
8.					

Figure 8–1. Family composition form.

ily members included on the genogram, but also significant nonfamily members who have lived with or played a major role in the family's life. This visual representation of the family consists of information about members' age; gender; significant life events (e.g., birth, marriage, divorce); health/illness status; death; and selected identifying features such as race, social class, ethnicity, religion, occupation, and place of residence.

There has been widespread use of family genograms by family health practitioners and therapists,

and much variety in the way genograms are diagrammed. McGoldrick and Gerson have written an entire book on genograms, *Genograms in Family Assessment* (1985). If a more thorough description of genograms and their application is needed, this excellent reference is suggested.

Constructing Genograms.
Figure 8–2 shows an example of how a genogram is constructed. Symbols used in diagraming are also presented. The example given is relatively uncomplicated, given the

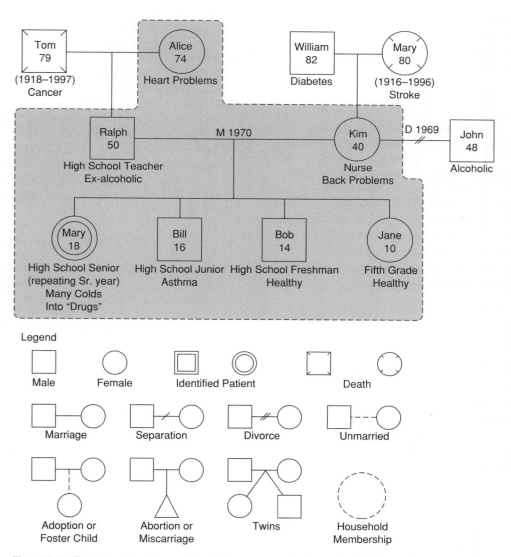

Figure 8–2. Example of family genogram with accompanying legend (symbols used in genograms).

number of families that have experienced multiple significant family transitions and events. Wright and Leahey (1984) explain the basic method involved in recording family data on the family genogram.

> Family members are placed on horizontal rows that signify generational lines. For example, a marriage or common-law relationship is denoted by a horizontal line. Children are denoted by vertical lines. Children are rank-ordered from left to right beginning with the eldest child. Each individual is represented. (p. 30)

Males are designated by squares, females by circles. Horizontal lines that are broken denote a separation or divorce. Household members are identified by encircling all the members of the household with a broken line.

Usually the family genogram is completed on the first visit or interview and revised later as new information becomes available. Letting the family know that background information is needed to more fully understand the specific problems the family is experiencing, coupled with an explanation of the family tree method, usually suffice as explanations to gain family members' participation. It is suggested that questions about the immediate family are asked first (names, ages, sex of household members). Recent life cycle transitions as well as changes in the family situation (additions or deletions of members) may also be inquired about at this time (McGoldrick & Gerson, 1985).

After addressing the immediate family, asking about the parents' families of origin is recommended. Inquiring about the two extended families brings to focus the wider family context. Querying the mother about her side of the family and the father about his side of the family is a way to obtain this information. Moreover, questions should be asked about friends, clergy, caregivers, health care professionals, and others important to the family's functioning; this information may be included on the genogram or used to assess the family's social support system/network. At this point, nonfamily members may also be added as either household members or "family."

Difficult questions about family members' functioning are often saved to later in the interview, when greater trust and rapport has been built. Areas family nurses should ask about include serious medical or psychological problems, work or school changes/problems, drug and alcohol problems, and trouble with the law (McGoldrick & Gerson, 1985).

▶ THE FAMILY'S CULTURAL ORIENTATION

A family's cultural orientation or background may well be the most pertinent variable in understanding the family's behavior, value system, and functions. Because culture permeates and circumscribes our individual, familial, and social actions, its consequences are pervasive and its implication for practice broad.

Because understanding the family's cultural background is so critical in working with families, familial differences among three major ethnic groups in the United States are explored in Chapters 19 through 21. Chapter 13 on the family's value system will also help the family nurse look at cultural patterns, because family values are often a reflection of the value system of the family's reference groups, a major one being the ethnic and religious subculture with which the family identifies.

Importance of Culture for Practice

In a culturally diverse society such as ours, we need to develop cohesiveness as a society and community, while at the same time recognizing and celebrating the uniqueness of our diverse parts. Bringing this notion down to the level of practice, to understand and to be able to work efficaciously with families from cultures different from one's own, health care professionals must be aware of the unique, distinctive qualities and the variety of lifestyles, values, and structures in families' cultures. Hence the importance of culture lies in its vital, unique character. Because cultural differences are often at the root of poor communication, interpersonal tensions, avoidance in working effectively with others, and poor assessment of health problems and their remedies, successful nursing care of clients of various ethnic backgrounds is dependent on the nurse's knowledge of and sensitivity to the clients' culture (Canino & Spurlock, 1994; Lipson, 1996; Ridley & Lingle, 1996).

In counseling families the importance of culture is paramount. Without knowledge of the differences in cultural norms and patterns, behavior that differs from normative patterns is usually labeled as noncompliant, deviant, crazy, immoral, or illegal (depending on the type of prescribed behavior violated). In the absence of cultural data, it then becomes impossible for the health care worker to recognize the possible cultural meaning of the client's behavior or actions. Coddy (1975) identifies four important areas where cultural dissimilarity may permeate and disrupt counseling. These are in the areas of (1) goal expectations, (2) the establishment of rapport, (3) communication styles, and (4) client's acceptance of ideas or recommendations.

The benefit of nurse–client cultural congruence is well documented. Several noted authors have pointed to the greater ease and efficacy when the client and the health care professionals have similar ethnic and religious backgrounds (Flaskerud, 1984). When similar frames of references exist in a relationship, the possibilities of greater freedom of expression, deeper identification, and increased empathy present themselves (Coddy, 1975). However, having a health care worker and client of the same ethnic background is an ideal but usually not a practical situation. In reality ethnic congruency is not often possible, and perhaps may not even be socially desirable. Otherwise, how are we in a multicultural society to learn to live and relate well to one another?

Language is a fundamental aspect of culture/ethnicity. The critical nature of language barriers also deserves mention. In some regions, where a majority or plurality of one's clients are from a different culture and speak a different language, learning the culture's language will not only result in dramatically improved communication but also in a much greater understanding and appreciation of the culture. Padilla (1976) verifies this assertion in his study of lower-class Mexican-Americans who were being seen in therapy in a counseling center in East Los Angeles. He states that it has generally been assumed by therapists that lower-class persons have difficulty benefiting from psychotherapy because of their nonverbalness, inarticulateness, and lack of ability to think abstractly. Padilla reports, however, that in counseling Latino clients, this generalization does not hold true when clients were given the opportunity and encouraged to communicate in Spanish,

English, or a combination of both in order to enhance the meaningfulness of their communication. He concludes that, "It now seems clear that the Chicano poor are quite capable of verbally expressing themselves in the most intensive 'insight' therapy situation, if they are not forced to communicate in English, a language that may be partly or completely foreign to these individuals" (p. 289).

Cultural–Ethnic Pluralism

Our country is truly a matrix of many ethnic groups or subcultures. The United States is experiencing the greatest growth in immigration in 100 years. In 1993 alone, more than one million legal and undocumented immigrants entered the United States (Roberts, 1995). Various geographical regions have felt this influx of immigrants differentially. Examples of cities that have experienced high rates of immigration are Los Angeles and New York. In Los Angeles, 4 out of 10 immigrants are foreign born, while in New York 3 out of 10 are foreign born. The 1990 U.S. Census figures (U.S. Bureau of the Census, 1991) illustrate this trend (Table 8–1).

In the largest state in the Union, California, it is projected that by 2030, whites will be an aging minority within the state's population, while ethnic minority people (Latinos, African-Americans, and Asians/

► TABLE 8–1

PERCENT OF ACTUAL AND PROJECTED U.S. POPULATION OF ETHNIC MINORITIES ACCORDING TO 1980 AND 1990 CENSUS DATA

	Percent of U.S. Population			
Ethnic Group	1980	1990	1996	2050 Projection
Blacks	11.7%	12.1%	12.2%	13.6%
Hispanics[a]	6.4%	9.0%	10.2%	24.5%
Asians and Pacific Islanders	1.5%	3.0%	3.3%	8.2%
Native Americans	0.6%	0.8%	0.8%	0.9%

[a] Hispanics will become the nation's largest minority group by 2009, based on U.S. Census projections.
Sources: Baringer (1991), Rosenblatt (1996), U.S. Bureau of the Census (1991).

Pacific islanders) will be "the emergent majority" (Hayes-Battista, 1990).

Massive waves of immigration have continued to mold and revolutionize the character of the United States throughout the last two centuries. The myth of the American melting pot has been intellectually recognized, although its implications not dissipated. This myth encouraged all diverse ethnic groups immigrating to the United States to succeed in American society by becoming part of the one predominant group. Any differences were typically seen as deviant and inferior. Ethnic variation was perceived as an element of the lower social class and of recent immigrant groups. Moving up the social class ladder to success meant discarding one's ethnic traditions and values and assimilating into the mainstream of society.

The social protests of the 1960s brought about the harsh realization that the society had not, and did not wish to, move toward one homogeneous entity. The civil rights movement and the rise of black consciousness and identity set the model for all other ethnic groups. This model stressed a reaffirmation of cultural differences, a greater demand for equal treatment, and an acceptance of the value of ethnic or cultural diversity in society. This movement was quickly followed by similar demands for ethnic pluralism among white ethnic groups (Jewish, Irish, Italian, and so forth), Asian-Americans, and Mexican-Americans (McAdoo, 1978). Stemming from this push for cultural pluralism and the growing demographic imperative, American values have been changing, reflecting a greater tolerance for diversity. Unfortunately, however, in the mid-1990s the United States has experienced a conservative backlash against immigrants and multiculturalism, as seen in the passing of an anti-immigration proposition (No. 187) in California in 1995.

McGoldrick and Giordano (1996) point out that a ". . . positive sense of ethnic and racial identity is essential for developing a healthy personal and group identity" (p. 4). Trying to assimilate and forget one's heritage may be hazardous to one's health. Several studies agree that "when people are secure in their identity, they act with greater flexibility and openness to those of other cultural backgrounds" (McGoldrick & Giordano, 1996, p. 9).

Kobrin and Goldscheider (1978), researchers of ethnicity, also reaffirm the salience and meaning of ethnicity for society, family, and the individual. The recent reemergence of ethnicity, one's cultural heritage and ethnic identity, has become an even more tangible and acceptable basis for group cohesion in North America. Ethnic identification provides for many persons and families an alternative link to the broader society, partially compensating for the cold, impersonal, and bureaucratic qualities of society today (Kobrin & Goldscheider, 1978). Moreover, ethnicity can be seen as enriching family life and strengthening the bonds of intergenerational continuity.

The reality of the 1990s is that the United States is truly multicultural. A demographic imperative exists for practicing transcultural family nursing.

The Cross-cultural or Transcultural Approach

The cross-cultural approach used in anthropology provides a broad comparative picture of human nature and human behavior (Leininger, 1970). This approach to family nursing care is both a practical necessity and a social reality, due to the awareness of the pervasive part culture plays and also to recognition of the growing numbers of people in the United States from different cultural backgrounds. As we become familiar with other cultures and learn to appreciate why certain values and norms are effective through time in those cultures, it is hoped that health care workers will become more sensitive and effective in providing family health care.

Leininger (1970, 1995) asserts that it is not only sound for nursing to use a cross-cultural or transcultural approach, it is mandatory: clients have a *right* to have their sociocultural backgrounds understood in the same way that they expect their physical and psychological needs to be recognized and understood. The cultural and the social level of analysis and care has been, until only recently, largely ignored. We often pay only lip service to assessing clients' sociocultural factors.

The following concepts or terms are of fundamental importance for understanding cross-cultural principles and processes.

Culture. Foremost among these concepts is that of **culture**. Culture is usually viewed as a blueprint for our way of living, thinking, behaving, and feeling. It circumscribes and guides the ways in which societies and ethnic groups solve their problems and derive meaning from their lives. From a systems perspective, culture is defined as systems of socially transmitted behavioral patterns that link human groups to their environmental settings, as well as systems of social change and organization that act to mediate societal adaptation (Leininger, 1976). Culture denotes patterns of learned behavior and values that are transmitted from one generation to the next.

In other words, culture is a mold from which we all are cast. It constrains and regulates our daily behavior, attitudes, and values in many latent and manifest ways. Because people rely on learned behavior or culture for survival, it is the prime source of our adaptability.

When defining culture, a broad, comprehensive, inclusive definition is needed. With this in mind culture includes:

1. Ethnographic variables, e.g., nationality, ethnicity, language, and religion.
2. Demographic variables, e.g., age, gender, place of residence.
3. Status variables, e.g., social, economic, and education.
4. Affiliation variables, e.g., formal and informal group memberships (Falicov, 1988; Locke, 1992).

The following definition of culture by Falicov (1988) incorporates these components:

> Those sets of shared world views and adaptive behaviors derived from simultaneous membership in a variety of contexts, such as ecological setting (rural, urban, suburban), religious background, nationality and ethnicity, social class, gender-related experiences, minority status, occupation, political leanings, migratory patterns, stages of acculturation or values derived from belonging to the same generation partaking of a single historical moment, or particular ideologies. (p. 336)

Ethnicity.   **Ethnicity** refers to a common ancestry, a sense of "peoplehood" and group identity. From a common ancestry and a shared social and cultural history and national origin have evolved shared values and customs (Giger & Davidhizer, 1995; McGoldrick, 1993; McGoldrick & Giordano, 1996).

Ethnicity is deeply tied to the family as it is the family that transmits this legacy. "A group's sense of commonality is transmitted over generations by the family and reinforced by the surrounding community." (McGoldrick & Giordano, 1996, p. 1).

Race and ethnicity should not be confused with each other. Race denotes biological variation, distinguishing people based on physical characteristics such as skin color, facial features, and hair texture. People of one race can vary in terms of their ethnicity and culture. For example, in the white race there are perhaps a hundred or more different ethnic groups.

Ethnicity is often used interchangeably with culture or subculture, even though ethnicity is defined more narrowly, that is, the term culture includes many more dimensions than just ethnicity. Using the two terms interchangeably leads to confusion. When we speak of a person's or families' "cultural background," we most often are referring to their ethnic background. Therefore, in this text, ethnicity will be used primarily to discuss persons or families from different national origins and different group identities.

Religion is very much intertwined with ethnicity. In some families, the family's religion is a vital shaper of health values, beliefs and practices (Andrews & Boyle, 1995). But in secular families, religion's influence is generally much more muted.

Variation Within Ethnic Groups (Intraethnic Variation).
Just as there are enormous differences in people between ethnic groups, there is also a great variation in people *within* the same ethnic group. Much of the variation we see *in* families with the same ethnic background is a function of the degree to which the family subscribes to the American culture, as well as regional differences in the native culture, social class differences, or simply idiosyncratic variation. It is of utmost importance to take into account the diversity among families within the various ethnic groups (Koshi, 1976).

The Immigration Experience.
Many ethnic minority families are recent immigrants. These immigrant families have experienced the complex stress of immigration and migration and perhaps the even greater stress associated with being a refugee. Although these stressful experiences are often

"buried," they subtly continue to shape a family's outlook and its adjustment (Bullrich, 1989).

Being a refugee is particularly stressful, as most refugees leave their countries of origin involuntarily. They usually enter the United States and other countries to escape from intolerable and chaotic conditions. Leaving one's own country of origin under these conditions causes loss of family, identity, and culture; a lowered socioeconomic and employment status; language problems; dramatic shifts in social, familial, and gender roles; acculturation problems in the new country; and mental health issues (Bemak, Chung, & Bornemann, 1996).

The Dangers of Stereotyping.   Lack of recognition of individual differences or labeling is termed **stereotyping**. Cultural stereotyping involves the nonacceptance or disallowance of individual or group diversity; everyone from a particular culture is viewed as the same and perceived of as fixed in their characteristics. Stereotyping can lead to discrimination such as the widespread "isms" prevalent in our society, i.e., racism, sexism, classism, ethnocentrism, ageism, and heterosexualism (homophobia).

Unfortunately the tendency is to simplify things by labeling people. Kay (1978) discusses the perennial problem of generalizing about a group of people in anthropological–ethnographic descriptions:

> Most ethnographies, or accounts of the life style of people who participate in a specific culture, are like still photographs. They describe people staggered in time and space. We call such fixed images stereotypes. Modal personalities are frozen in a changeless place, and subsequently are supposed to represent millions. But if we try to qualify groups by describing certain differences (e.g., 72 percent of *barrio* women make their own tortillas as compared with 12 percent who buy Rainbo bread), we end up by describing no one. (p. 89)

We need to be able to generalize about an ethnic group in order to learn about and discuss that group of people; but at the same time, remember that cultural characteristics refer to group characteristics only.

Hence the knowledge that the father typically holds primary power in the Mexican-American home, or that the Jewish mother often is "the power behind the throne" in the Jewish culture, serves as a clue about a family's background. However, these culturally derived patterns need to be verified with the particular family the nurse is assessing.

Tripp-Reimer and Lauer (1987) caution family nurses who plan nursing care on the basis of a family's ethnicity. They explain that

> clients may not want traditional beliefs and customs incorporated into their care if alternative approaches are acceptable. Ethnic clients may not wish to remain unassimilated; indeed, it may simply perpetuate another form of stereotype to assume that all members of an ethnic group subscribe to the culture's most conservative position. (p. 96)

Tripp-Reimer and Lauer call this problem the "traditionalist fallacy." We cannot assume we know what the family and its members want simply because we know the family's ethnic background.

Acculturation.   Exposure of persons from one cultural group to another culture leads to a sociocultural process called **acculturation**. As one of the major causative factors of variation within an ethnic group, "acculturation comprises those gradual changes produced in a culture by the influence of another culture which results in an increased similarity of the two" (Kroeber, 1948, p. 425). When ethnic groups immigrate to the United States, the influence is usually overwhelmingly one way—that is, the American culture exerts greater influence on the ethnic group to conform to its cultural patterns than vice versa. The resultant **assimilation** may proceed so far as to practically extinguish the ethnic culture (as occurred with the African culture during slavery) or factors may intervene to counterbalance the forces of assimilation and keep the two cultures isolated from one another. For example, language and religious, economic, and geographic barriers have kept Mexican-Americans and Native Americans fairly separate from American society. The strong cultural traditions of Jews and Armenians have to a large extent limited their assimilation. Assimilation denotes the more complete and one-way process of one culture being absorbed into the other.

Kluckholm (1976) hypothesizes that the rate and degree of acculturation of any ethnic group into the dominant culture depends primarily on the degree of congruency between the group's own basic value orientations with those of the dominant (American) culture. Also, certain groups within a particular ethnic subculture are more receptive to social and cultural change. For instance, among urban residents, the more educated, occupationally successful, or socioeconomically advantaged are more likely to experience assimilatory changes. Hence socioeconomic and class factors are crucial elements to consider in learning about a family's ethnicity.

Acculturation, then, implies that members of cultures other than the dominant culture of the society have internalized to a great extent the norms and values of the dominant culture and, moreover, that the wider society has been influenced to varying degrees by its exposure to each of the ethnic or subcultural groups within its boundaries. Examples of regions where immigrating ethnic groups have greatly influenced the local culture include the border states with Mexico, where the influence of the Latino culture is pervasively seen in many spheres of life, e.g., food, the visual and performing arts, the job/occupational structure, mass media, and neighborhood businesses.

Acculturation does not necessarily suggest the loss of ethnic identity—of a detaching of oneself from an ethnic community (Kobrin & Goldscheider, 1978)— nor does it imply the loss of many of the customs related to that culture. Customs that continue, more or less unscathed, are those that are not stigmatizing or illegal, customs such as those involving food, religion, music, and dance. Many times these become the major tangible cultural difference, remnants of cultures quite different. Price (1976) states that sociocultural groups in America become transformed into ethnic subcultures. Although outright destruction never completely occurs, transformation (acculturation) begins immediately on participation in the American economic system—the adjustments necessitated in order to join the work force produce social change. As elements of the old and new culture intertwine, a unique subculture is formed.

Members of ethnic minorities are inevitably part of two cultures. Most ethnic minority families are then bicultural. **Biculturalism** signifies participation in two cultural systems and often requires two sets of behavior and ways of thinking (Ho, 1987). All ethnic groups have expressed biculturalism as an important adaptive strategy (Harrison et al., 1994).

Real Versus the Ideal. To understand a family's cultural background we need to understand both its values (what family members say is important or *the ideal)* and its actual behavior (*the real).* Often the variance between the two is striking. It is typically due to the pragmatic adaptation of a family to a particular social and historical context (Friedman, 1990). Sheer practical necessity can often distort one's values in everyday life, so that they become unrecognizable (Graedon, 1985). Numerous examples of the distinction between the real and ideal can be seen in the adaptations ethnic families make to poverty and discrimination.

Cultural Relativism. In working with clients from various cultural backgrounds the aim in the health care professions is to eliminate ethnocentric beliefs and substitute instead a relativistic cultural perspective. **Cultural relativism** refers to the perspective that holds that "cultures are neither inferior nor superior to one another and that there is no single scale for measuring the value of a culture. Therefore, customs, beliefs, and practices must be judged or understood relative to the context in which they appear" (Aamodt, 1978, p. 9). To do this, the health care worker must be flexible enough to assume the cultural perspective of those with whom he or she works (Coddy, 1975).

Ethnocentrism. **Ethnocentrism** implies the lack of cultural relativism. There is the tendency for health care professionals to be ethnocentric when working with families from different sociocultural backgrounds. It is then important to become informed about families from other ethnicities to counter the tendency of believing that the way our own family or health system culture operate is the way in which all (normal) families do and should operate.

Cultural Imposition. A result of ethnocentrism is the problem of **cultural imposition**. When health workers feel either consciously or unconsciously that their beliefs and practices are superior and proper, they use subtle and/or apparent ways to force their own values, beliefs, and practices on individuals from different ethnic orientations (Leininger, 1974).

Cultural imposition may then lead to cultural conflicts—situations in which health care professionals have covertly or overtly tried to impose their health practices on their clients and the clients have reacted negatively. As nurses, we can think of many ways in which clients "fight back," many times to their own detriment, because of the health system's lack of recognition of their culturally patterned beliefs and practices. The commonly seen reticence of Hispanic families to place one of their members in a hospital because of being forced to separate from the family member is a case in point. When family visiting and participation rights are relaxed to allow for a flexible consideration of client and family attitudes and patterns, both the client and the health care system benefit.

To counter the frequently experienced problems of cultural imposition and cultural conflicts, Leininger (1976) suggests that "the nurse must truly understand a culture before imposing any changes on the people. Sensitivity and foresight are essential to work in diverse cultural contexts" (p. 40). In order to understand a client's culture and provide *culturally competent* care, one must first be aware of one's own value orientation and the health care patterns in one's own culture (McGoldrick & Giordano, 1996). The family nurse must also discover—through questions we ask and observations of responses we make—the family member's beliefs about health and illness, particularly of the family's perception of the health problems family members are having. We must assume nothing until adequate validation takes place.

Cultural Shock.

Family nurses and students commonly experience feelings of cultural shock when visiting with or interacting with families whose culture is (1) at great variance with their own, (2) one about which they are uninformed, and/or (3) one to which they have had little exposure. **Cultural shock** refers to a condition in which a person, in response to an environment so altered that meaningful objects and experiences have been replaced by those from a different culture, feels confused, immobilized, and "lost" (Aamodt, 1978). Feelings and sensations of discomfort are more pronounced or noticeable when visiting in the home environment, because the family's differences are much more obvious. Discomfort is also more intense because of the fact that the health care worker is in the client's "territory."

Lifestyle and value differences are not easy to deal with. Our own values and attitudes will greatly influence our perceptions and nursing assessments and interventions. Therefore, personal feelings, beliefs, and attitudes must be identified, discussed, and accepted before we can effectively help families seeking assistance (Clemen, 1977).

Indigenous Health Care Systems.

The last of the more general cultural concepts has to do more specifically with health care practices. Every culture has devised its own **indigenous**, or lay, **health care system** as opposed to the Western *scientific or professional health care system*. Some of these systems are well-developed and have been used effectively for centuries to treat certain conditions, such as the Eastern system of health care. The indigenous health care system uses traditional folk care modalities. Practitioners of an indigenous system are often the first-line, primary care practitioners—the first healers to be consulted by unacculturated ethnic families. They also may be contacted for certain "folk" illnesses or when Western medicine fails to be effective. As part of the cross-cultural approach proposed earlier, it is recommended that professional systems need to become more culturally attuned to these systems and to learn ways in which to work cooperatively with non-Western health care practitioners, rather than in opposition to them (Bushy, 1990; Engebretson, 1994; Germain, 1992). Health care professionals tend to downplay the significance and value of folk-health care and practices. These feelings are both inaccurate and detrimental, however, because much folk medicine is effective (Leininger, 1976).

In fact, in most cases the merits of any treatment depend on whether the sick client recovers or not, and indigenous health care does work in many instances. This is particularly true in illnesses where psychogenic factors are prominent and where effective treatment of the disease depends on a knowledge of the context of the person's cultural belief system. Given this, who knows or appreciates the psychogenic and the cultural context better than the folk practitioner?

Minority Families

Minority families are those families that are classified as belonging to ethnic or cultural groups other than white ethnic groups, such as the Irish, Poles, and Jews also called "ethnic people of color," this group comprised about 26.2 percent of our population in 1996 (Rosenblatt, 1996). Minority families, then, in contrast to *all* ethnic families (both white and people of color), have certain common attributes and problems. One major thing they share is that while facing all of the same stressors experienced by all other families, they have the added burdens of the effects of discrimination and racism (McAdoo, 1978, 1993). Vincent and Ransford (1980) remind us that being an ethnic individual in America lowers one's status, just as being of lower social class. These sociologists also note that ethnic groups vary in their status, with some groups, such as blacks and Latinos, suffering more status inequality than white ethnics or Asian-Americans.

Cultural Variation or Deviance? Families
are not isolated groups that exist independently from the society of which they are a part. Thus if a disproportionately large number of families of a particular minority or ethnic group are poor, unemployed, and "dysfunctional to the whole society," a comprehension of their status can be achieved only through an examination of the role played by the larger society. Eshleman (1974) notes that poverty, racism, and/or inferior schools may be due less to an inherent weakness within ethnic groups and families than to:

1. Social and cultural systems which place a higher value on moon walks, military strength, and corporate profit than on human needs;

2. Religious institutions that stress a chosen ingroup as God's people to the exclusion of "nonbelievers" (i.e., anyone who is different);

3. Educational systems that admit and serve those who pass "middle-class" exams, speak the "proper" language, and wear the "acceptable" hair and clothing styles, and, in general,

4. A society that in many ways places higher values on "things" and goods rather than on the needs and social conditions of people. (p. 203)

If we live in a society in which minority families and their members are devalued and seen as inferior, this message and perception very effectively becomes the perception and beliefs of those people. It is a well-known tenet of social psychology that peo-

ple develop their identities and perceptions of their worth in interactions with others (Mead, 1934). As the minority family and individual interacts in a white majority world that encourages feelings of inferiority and degrades self-esteem, they begin to believe what the outer world is saying about them. This trap is termed the **self-fulfilling prophecy**: People will conform to other's expectations and perceptions of them by internalizing their beliefs, even negative ones, and thus seem to fulfill the "prophecies" that were made about them (Eshleman, 1974).

Problems within society set up conditions to which minority families and individuals must adapt. Some of these adaptations—such as going on welfare, dropping out of school, "babies having babies," joining gangs, or selling drugs—are viewed as "dysfunctional." The tendency becomes one of blaming the victim—the welfare mother, the unskilled, unemployed African-American male, the African-American family, the Chicano gangs—instead of looking more broadly at the problem. By seeing the ways in which the entire system is involved (the institutions of society and the individual's interactions within this larger environment), contextual solutions may be identified (Edelman, 1987) and the tendency to blame the already stigmatized individual or group will be curtailed.

Controversies About Minority Family Structures. One way in which social scientists
have unwittingly stereotyped and stigmatized whole ethnic groups is by attempting to describe a particular ethnic group in toto by data actually derived from, and thus only reflective of *poor* segments of that group. In many of these instances, the particular segment of the ethnic group being described is not clearly identified, thereby giving readers an erroneous notion of what that ethnic group is like as a whole.

Casavantes (1970) and others have asserted that this overgeneralization has certainly been true within the social science studies of Mexican-Americans in the period between 1950 and 1970. "The net result of this extraordinary scientific oversight is the perpetuation of very damaging stereotypes of Mexican Americans" (p. 22). Willie (1976) and Billingsley (1968) have pointed out the same criticism of studies about the African-American family and conscientiously differentiate lifestyles and values of the African-American family by the family's social class position. Research has concentrated predominantly on the most oppressed families with findings then generalized to all minority families. In this process, biased attitudes are perpetuated and reinforced. As part of this bias, the majority of stable ethnic families, and the processes by which they have become economically mobile, have largely been ignored (McAdoo, 1978, 1993).

The importance of social class does not mean, however, that the middle class of a particular American ethnic group is like the white middle class. Although ethnic middle-class families are indeed closer to the dominant culture in lifestyles, values, beliefs, and so forth, they are still distinctive from the white middle-class culture because of their ethnic identity and sense of peoplehood. Billingsley (1968) explains that families of the same social class but of a different ethnic group show behavioral and value similarities, but not the same sense of historical identification of peoplehood. And conversely, those of the same ethnic group but of different social class manifest a sense of peoplehood, but dissimilar lifestyles.

▶ THE PROCESS FOR ASSESSING CULTURE

A cultural assessment of a client (individual and/or family) is an essential facet of assessment. Just as a family nurse would not intervene without an assessment of the biopsychosocial aspects of the family and its members, he or she should also not proceed until a cultural assessment has been completed (Leininger, 1976; Tripp-Reimer et al., 1984).

Developing skill in eliciting and recording cultural assessments of the client and the context in which the care is being given (the home, health care setting) is necessary for nurses working in transcultural settings. As part of the broader assessment of families from ethnic groups different than the nurses, we need to become informed about the cultures of the families with whom we interact (Aamodt, 1978; Lipson, 1996). It is extremely important that family nurses try to obtain the perceptions, views, values, and practices of people from the particular ethnic group with which they are working. "It is significant to remember that the ability to work with cultural groups is dependent upon the ability to understand the group in terms of their background as they view it and not in terms of our interpretations of their background" (Clemen, 1977, p. 192).

Ridley and Lingle (1996), cross-cultural counselors, agree that the ability to understand clients in terms of their cultural backgrounds and from their own perspective is essential. They assert that practitioners working with families from cultures different from their own must develop **cultural empathy** in order to be effective. Having cultural empathy should lead to an understanding of clients' culture, which includes the culture's assumptions, values, and patterns of thinking. "Cultural empathy involves the ability of counselors to communicate this understanding effectively with an attitude of concern for culturally different clients" (Ridley & Lingle, 1996, p. 32). Ridley and Lingle believe that before beginning to work with ethnic families, practitioners must understand their own culture, and only after this self-examination can they effectively examine the clients' "cultural self."

When working with ethnic families, it is also important to bring out family strengths, positive adaptations that families have made in dealing with their constraints and vulnerabilities (McAdoo, 1993). Attention to family strengths facilitates positive opinions of families and leads to family nursing approaches that tend to raise a family's sense of competency and empowerment.

Ethnic and Religious Assessment Areas

For many families a thorough cultural or ethnic assessment is not necessary, and yet assessing the family's ethnic background (as identified by the family) and the degree to which they identify with the dominant American culture or their traditional culture (if different from the dominant culture) is basic identifying information needed in any family assessment. Complicating matters, ethnic backgrounds of parents or spouses may differ, and if this is so, it is important to assess how this difference is handled and how it affects family life.

Information on the family's religious beliefs and practices is intimately tied to ethnicity and thus should also be included as part of the assessment (Tripp-Reimer et al., 1984). Religious beliefs often influence a family's conceptions of health and illness and how sick family members are treated. Family roles, rituals, values, and coping patterns are also affected by the family's religious orientation or legacy.

The following specific areas are suggested as part of the identifying data about the family:

1. *The family's ethnic background (self-identified).*
2. *The family's degree of acculturation.* The assessment question posed here is, "To what extent has the family retained its ethnicity or cultural heritage?" Or posed in the reverse fashion, "To what extent has the family assimilated American culture?" Table 8–2 presents overall cultural assessment questions that, when answered, give pertinent information on the family's degree of acculturation. Some of the behavioral clues that indicate that the family still retains traditional (ethnic) practices, values, and beliefs follow:
   a. Recent migration from another country (first generation).
   b. Native culture is very different from American culture.
   c. The family's friends and associations are of the same ethnic group (strong ethnic ties).
   d. Family lives in an ethnically homogeneous neighborhood.
   e. Strong political and religious ties to the ethnic group.
   f. Social, cultural, recreational, and/or educational activities are within the family's cultural group.

► TABLE 8–2

ETHNIC ASSESSMENT GUIDELINES

Assessment Criteria	Questions
Ethnic/racial identity	How does the family identify itself in terms of ethnicity and racial group? Are the parents both from the same ethnic background?
Languages spoken	What language(s) is/are spoken in the home? And by whom? What language is preferred when speaking to outsiders?
Place of birth and immigration history	Where were the parents and children born? If they immigrated from another country, when did they immigrate to the United States and what was their reason for immigrating?
Geographic mobility	Where have the parents lived? When did they move to their present residence?
Family's religion	What is the family's religion? Are both parents from the same religious background? How actively involved is the family in religiously based activities and practices?
Ethnic group affiliation	What are the characteristics of the family's friends and associations? Are they all from the family's ethnic group? Are recreational, political, educational, and other social activities within the ethnic reference group, the wider community, or both? To what extent does the family use services and shop within the family's neighborhood or within the wider community?
Neighborhood affiliation	What are the characteristics of the family's neighborhood? Is it ethnically heterogeneous or homogeneous?
Dietary habits, dress	What are the family's dietary preferences and prohibitions? Do the family members dress in traditional clothing?
Household appearance	Are the family's home decorations, art, and religious objects culturally derived?
Use of folk systems	To what extent does the family use folk healing practices or practitioners? What are the family's health and illness beliefs and practices?
Family life transitions	What are the customs and beliefs about family life transitions such as births, illness, mourning and death, pregnancy and well-baby care?
Acceptance by community	To what extent is the family affected by discrimination?

Adapted partially from Friedman (1990), and Lipson (1996).

g. Dietary habits and dress are traditional.

h. Traditional family roles are carried out.

i. Home decorations, art, and other visual representations congruent with the cultural background.

j. Native language is spoken exclusively or frequently in the home.

k. The territorial complex—the wider community the family frequents—is primarily within the ethnic community.

l. The family uses folk medicine or traditional practitioners, or perhaps a community health worker in whom the ethnic neighborhood has confidence.

m. Community discrimination (and segregation) against the identified ethnic group of the family exists.

n. Family members are nonwhite (creating obvious racial difference making acculturation more difficult).

Not all members of the family may have the same emotional ties to their ethnic background or religion. Older persons and parents who are in or beyond the life cycle stages of raising children are usually more traditional than the children and young adults without children. Those members of the family who work outside the home are more acculturated than those members who work in the home. The poor are generally less acculturated than the more affluent classes.

Within immigrant groups the degree of acculturation into the new culture has generally increased with each succeeding generation. An illustration of this phenomenon is the Japanese acculturation pattern (Matsui, 1996). The first-generation Japanese-Americans, the Issei, who came here from Japan between 1890 and 1920, retained almost all of their former traditions. The second-generation Japanese-Americans, the Nisei, occupied an intermediate position on the assimilation continuum, while the third generation, the Sansei, are quite westernized. Interestingly enough, an opposing trend among the Yonsei, the fourth generation, is also being seen. As with other groups, there is a resurgence of interest in ethnic "roots," particularly among the Yonsei, with whom the learning of the Japanese language and culture has become increasingly popular.

In spite of the tendency for persons from immigrant families to become more acculturated over time and in succeeding generations, some values, practices, and beliefs are retained. In the Mexican-American family the importance of the extended family has not waned over time; in fact, research shows that the extended family has grown in structure and functions when studied across generations (Baca-Zinn, 1981).

3. *The family's religious preference and practices.* The family's religious background should be noted, taking into account how individuals within the family differ in their religious beliefs and practices. How actively involved is the family in a particular church, temple, or other religious organization? As we learned from looking at families historically, the function of religion in family life has diminished (D'Antonio & Aldous, 1983). Nevertheless, we have great cultural diversity in our country and are currently seeing a resurgence of fundamental religion among some sectors of society. Hence, the role and importance of religion in families varies tremendously. In addition, it is suggested that an assessment be made of what religious practices the family engages in and what religiously based beliefs appear centrally important to the family.

In addition to the above general assessment areas, cultural assessment questions/areas are integrated throughout the entire family assessment guidelines. By completing the entire family assessment, one should have culled comprehensive data on cultural influences pertaining to the family organization (role, power, values, and communication facets), child-rearing practices, affective responses, health care practices and beliefs, and coping strategies.

Critical Questions for Nurses in Ambulatory Care.

In ambulatory settings where community-based nurses and nurse practitioners may only see a client or family for a short period of time, a shorter list of critical assessment questions may be needed. Key assessment areas are: (1) the family's self-identified ethnic and religious background; (2) their immigration status (from where and how long they have been here); (3) the language(s) they speak at home and the language they prefer to communicate in; (4) what they believe about their present health problem, such as symptoms and causes, and the appropriate treatment; and (5) the client's use of traditional healing methods (Jiang, 1995).

▶ THE FAMILY'S SOCIAL CLASS

Socioeconomic status, social status, or social class (the terms are used interchangeably) refers to a grouping of persons with relatively similar income, amounts of wealth, life conditions, life changes, and lifestyles (Ropers, 1991). Socioeconomic status, because it has a pervasive effect on families and family members' lives, especially within complex, heterogeneous societies, produces significant differences in a family's culture and lifestyle. Its influence is so pervasive that Oscar Lewis, a noted anthropologist, in 1966 conceptualized poor families as living within a common "culture of poverty." Family lifestyle, structural and functional characteristics, and associations with the external environment of home, neighborhood, and community vary tremendously from social class to social class. According to Kohn (1977), who examined the implications of social class for family life,

> [Social class] is useful because it captures the reality that the intricate interplay of all these variables [education, occupation and income primarily] create. Differing basic conditions of life at different levels of social order are created. Members of different social classes, by virtue of enjoying (or suffering) different conditions of life, come to see the world differently—to develop different conceptions of social reality, different aspirations and hopes and fears, different conceptions of the desirable. (p. 48)

Social class, along with cultural background, exerts the greatest overall influence on family life, influencing family values and priorities, family behavioral patterns, socialization practices, family role expectations, and world experiences. Due to differences in resources, there is also a positive association between socioeconomic status and physical and mental health (Ross, Mirowsky, & Goldstein, 1991), meaning that individuals from families who are poor are more likely to have poorer physical and mental health than those who are socioeconomically better off. Education is the aspect of social status that is most important to health because education is important in shaping knowledge and behavioral patterns.

Occupational position, formal education, and income are used as indicators of social class in American society, with the husband's occupational status being the most used and probably the most powerful indicator of social class (Smith & Graham, 1995). Generally the work deemed to have the greatest value to the society receives the greatest rewards, which include not only money but power, prestige, privilege, and autonomy. It has been frequently assumed that the husband's occupational status is the best single index of family ranking. Currently, however, it is being acknowledged that the wife's occupational level and income also have a major impact on the lifestyle and social class of a family. However, most occupationally based social class scales leave women's occupations out (Smith & Graham, 1995)—given there is a man in the family. Family background can also be a factor for determining social class status among the upper classes.

Social class pertains not only to the family's educational level, occupation status, and income, but also to the intricate interplay of these variables. Persons with different basic conditions of life, by virtue of their varied experience and exposure, come to see the world differently, to develop different conceptions of social reality as well as different aspirations, fears, and values.

Every society differentiates and ranks people, styles of life, automobiles, dress, and work in accordance with what it views as most valuable and important. No society, including American society, is classless, although Americans like to believe theirs is an open society with equal opportunity, where people can pull themselves up by their own bootstraps, American society is stratified into classes. Status consciousness is present even among children who begin very early to recognize their "place" and also the "place" of others in their little world.

By identifying a family's social class, family nurses can better anticipate the family's resources and some of its stressors. A family's structure and functions, moreover, are better understood in the light of its social class background.

Social Classes in the United States

Six discrete classes were described by Warner (1953), Langman (1987), and other sociologists as the upper-upper, lower-upper, upper-middle, lower-middle, working class, and lower class. Gilbert and Kahl (1993) presented another taxonomy of social class and their estimates of what percentage of the population is situated in each of these classes. Their taxonomy is similar to the previous taxonomy but differs in that upper classes are collapsed into one class, the "capitalist class"; the working class is expanded into two classes, working and working poor; and the poorest class is called the underclass (see Table 8–3).

In the American class structure it is the family, not merely the individual, that is ranked. The family is the keystone of the stratification system, the social mechanism by which the social class structure is maintained (Goode, 1964). Presently there is much blurring between the social classes; moreover, within each of the groupings relative to their values and status there is certainly not homogeneity (Kohn, 1969).

Interaction Between Social Class and Ethnicity.
Other factors are also significant in creating diversity within a social class grouping—religion and ethnicity being two prime examples. Intra-ethnic variation, created as a result of the interplay of the family's cultural and social class backgrounds, is called in sociology **ethclass** (Gordon, 1964). Gordon uses this concept to explain the significant role that both the social class membership and ethnicity play in defining the basic conditions of life and simultaneously accounting for differences between ethnic groups situated in the same social class.

Using Warner's schematization of social class in North America, the subsequent section of this chapter will briefly describe some characteristics of each of the six social classes, with an emphasis on value differences. Again, these classes are not precise explanations of reality, but are constructs designed to show the patterned relationships and lifestyle differences between classes.

Upper-class Families.
Upper-class families, according to Warner (1953), are divided into two groupings: the established upper-class family (upper-upper) and the "nouveau riche" or newly rich (lower-upper). Families that have possessed wealth for more than two generations are classified in the established group and probably constitute a small percentage of the wealthy in the United States, while families of more recent affluence are placed in the second group.

The established upper-class family and its members were born into wealth and families try to protect and guard their children from social exposures

---

▶ **TABLE 8–3**

TAXONOMY OF SOCIAL CLASSES IN THE UNITED STATES

Social Class	Occupation and Estimated Percent in Population	Estimated Annual Income Range
Capitalist class	Heirs, top executives, and investors (1% of population)	$750,000 and over
Upper-middle class	University educated, professionals, and managers (14% of population)	$70,000–$749,000
Middle class	White-collar, lower-level professionals, managers and skilled blue-collar workers (30% of working population)	$40,000–$69,999
Working class	Semiskilled blue collar and low-level white collar (30% of population)	$20,000–$39,999
Working poor	Laborers and service workers (20% of population)	$13,000–$19,999
Underclass	Chronically unemployed, underemployed, or erratically employed (5% of population)	$0–$12,999

Adapted from Gilbert & Kahl (1993).

involving other social classes. The upper-upper class is very firmly entrenched in its culture, as well as in an extended family and a patriarchal kinship system. Protestant ethic values are subscribed to, to some extent, but these values do not have to be strictly upheld behaviorally, because the upper-upper class enjoys professional and occupational security and secure monetary resources.

The New Lower-upper-class Family. The "nouveau riche" may lack the financial security provided by the kinship group in the upper-upper-class family. Its members are able to engage in a lifestyle resembling that of the established upper class, but they lack the long history of prestige, power, and family lineage.

In contrast with the upper-upper class, the newly affluent families are less likely to inherit their wealth, and more likely to have a greater cultural diversity. Income is earned rather than inherited, and differences in values (e.g., spending patterns, which are symptomatic of priorities in values) vary between the two upper-class groups. Whereas upper-upper-class members spend more in the areas of culture and philanthropy, the lower-upper class typically spends more on "conspicuous consumption" of goods and products—automobiles, clothes, expensive recreation, and large houses. Because these families are upwardly mobile, they tend to pursue friendships with socially prominent individuals, rather than maintain close ties with their extended family. Thus, the predominant family structure is nuclear and husband dominated, and its members act independently of kin. Both upper classes would be considered "capitalists" according to Gilbert and Kahl's (1993) taxonomy of social class.

Middle-class Families.

The middle class is considered *dominant* numerically (estimated at 44 percent and shrinking) and socially, in the sense that they are most able to disseminate their views on what is right, proper, and expected behavior—whether in the family, school, or health agency. This dominance is due primarily to the key positions of the upper middle class in government, education, and mass communications.

The Upper-middle-class Family. This class is comprised of professionals in law, accounting, and medicine; higher-level businesspeople; middle management in corporations; successful entrepreneurs; service professionals, particularly at the university level; mental health workers; and administrators of social service and governmental organizations (Langman, 1987). Being the career-oriented bearers of the "American success syndrome," most in this class are college graduates and comprise the "solid highly respectable" people in the community. Individualism, rationality, personal achievement, and the other secular Protestant ethic values (mastery, future orientation, work, and so forth) are stressed (Adams, 1980; Schultz, 1972).

The number of dual-career, upper-middle-class families has recently increased. In dual-career families, patterns of traditional sex differentiation have blurred and more egalitarianism is seen between spouses (Perry-Jenkins & Folk, 1994).

Upper-middle-class families are often geographically mobile in pursuit of career goals. But in spite of their mobility, extensive visiting, communication, and aid between generations occurs (Lee, 1979).

The Lower-middle-class Family. The lower-middle class is made up of small businessmen, clerical workers, other low-level white-collar workers, bureaucratic functionaries, and salespersons. This class represents a wide variety of national and ethnic backgrounds. Like those in the class above them, the families are relatively stable in spite of problems connected with their economic security and the education of their children. Frequently students report the conflicts that exist between themselves and their parents. The parents work to provide an education for their children, which in turn introduces the children to a set of values that is often in conflict with those of the parents.

The major distinguishing values of the members of this status group are respectability and achievement. Hard work and honesty are also highly valued.

In the lower-middle-class family today, the power structure is usually egalitarian or mildly husband dominated. The wife defers to the husband's authority, yet maintains control over personal and familial household realms. Socially the kinship group is close, and major social activities often take place with relatives from the husband's or wife's family (Schultz, 1972). Families are generally child-oriented (Langman, 1987).

Working-class Families. Blue-collar or working-class families often came from rural backgrounds. Families moved to the cities as technology progressed and skilled labor was needed. The blue-collar or working class is made up of skilled workers, semiskilled workers in factories, service workers, and a few small tradesmen who usually have steady jobs, even though they often do not pay well. The elite of the working class—electricians, plumbers, and other highly skilled operators—frequently earn more than members of the middle classes and are now in some classifications viewed as part of the lower-middle-class or middle-class group. For members of this class who are in trades that depend on the swings of the business cycle, economic stability is lacking.

A considerable proportion of wives are employed outside of the home. Unlike a sizable proportion of female workers from the upper-middle and upper classes, the upper-lower-class wife takes a job more out of economic necessity than from the desire for a career, but this varies, as some married women work to "expand" their competencies or interact with other adults (Ferree, 1987). Family strains are associated with economic uncertainties.

It is within the less educated blue-collar family more than any other class that one still sees many husbands and wives conforming to the traditional husband and wife roles. The husband is often seen as a patriarchial authority and is generally not very involved in child-care activities (Rubin, 1994). Both of the sexes tend to think that friendship and companionship are more likely to exist between members of the same sex than among marital partners, and see the principal marital ties as involving the sexual union, complementary tasks, and mutual devotion (Adams, 1980; Komarovsky, 1964). Obedience and stricter traditional child-rearing patterns are typically seen in this class (Peterson & Rollins, 1987).

When there is need for assistance, relatives are likely to be called on before turning to a public agency. The extended family, the neighborhood peer group, and the informal work group provide much social interaction as well as actual assistance for blue-collar families.

Lower-class Families. Lower-class families are at the impoverished level of existence, although their degree of impoverishment varies. Gilbert and Kahl (1993) divide the lower class into the working poor and the underclass, estimating that 25 percent of the population fits into this class: 20 percent into the working poor and 5 percent into the underclass. Wide variations also exist in lifestyle, as seen in rural versus urban areas, and in different regional and ethnic/social lower-class communities. Generally, however, the common social characteristics of the lower class include the following:

1. A formal education of 8 years or less.

2. The male's occupation is almost always semiskilled or unskilled. His work pattern is often sporadic, with long periods of unemployment. There is also a strong probability that the woman works in an unskilled or service occupation.

3. Because of unemployment or underemployment and low wages, lower-class families make up a large number of those on the public assistance rolls.

4. If they live in the city, their place of residence is typically in the slum areas of town, often in old, dilapidated homes and buildings converted into small crowded apartments (Bell, 1971).

Poverty in America.   "The story of the 1980s and early 1990s is that the rich got richer and the poor got poorer" (Silverstein, 1996; United Press International, 1990). During the period of the Reagan Administration a significant change in the distribution of income and wealth occurred in the United States. This shift actually began earlier, but accelerated during the 1980s due to the reduction of social programs designed to aid the poor and working and middle classes and certain economic and technological trends such as the competitive globalization of markets and the shift in jobs from goods-producing industries to service-producing industries, which generate many minimally paying jobs (Marshall, 1991). Winnick (1988), a sociologist, calls this a movement toward "two societies, separate and unequal." The gulf in income and resources between rich and poor Americans is wider than at any time since figures were recorded, starting in the 1940s (Kozol, 1990). There is a shrinking of the middle class, with an increasing proportion of the population located in the upper and lower classes (Leeds, 1996).

The effects of certain economic and technological trends, and the last decade of declining domestic and social programs, have had an indelibly harsh impact on poor families. Research findings since the 1930s consistently indicate that economic distress is associated with shorter longevity and poorer health (Carney, 1992), along with lower levels of family stability, marital adjustment, family coping, family cohesion, marital communication, and harmonious family relationships (Voydanoff & Donnelly, 1988).

The lower class is disproportionately composed of ethnic minorities and recent legal immigrants, undocumented workers and families, female-headed households, children, and those with certain personally disorganizing problems: chronic mental illness, alcoholism, and drug abuse. The number of Americans living below the poverty line in 1992 rose to a 30-year high of 39.2 million (Mehren, 1993). In 1995, however, a modest decrease in these very high figures was found. The poverty rate had decreased to 36.4 million (Fulwood, 1996).

Minority status contributes substantially to poverty. Among families, the incidence of poverty is almost three times higher for African-Americans and Hispanics than for whites (Fulwood, 1996). Among children, poverty is widespread (see Table 8–4). The average poor African-American and Hispanic child today appears to be in the middle of a prolonged poverty period in the United States because of cutbacks in social and health benefits and declining family wages (Winnick, 1988; Wright, 1996).

The rate of poverty among female-headed families with children is five times greater than the rate of poverty of married couple families (U.S. Bureau of the Census, 1991b). This disproportionate representation of poor single mother families largely contributes to what is called "the feminization of poverty" (Rodgers, 1990; Starrels, Bould, & Nicholas, 1994).

Both rural and central city areas suffer from high rates of poverty. In 1986, nonmetropolitan (rural) poverty rates were slightly higher than poverty rates in U.S. central cities. The changing economy in farming communities has fueled the growth of poverty in rural America (National Council for Family Relations, 1989).

In summary, current problems of poor families are bleak and almost intractable, according to recent

► TABLE 8–4

FACTS ABOUT CHILDREN AND POVERTY

About 40% of the nation's poor are children.

21% of all children lived below the poverty line in 1995.

Among the world's developed countries, U.S. children have the highest poverty rate and greatest likelihood of living in single-parent homes.

A child in the United States living in a mother-headed home is five times more likely to be poor than a child living in a two-parent home.

65% of African-American mother-headed families with children are poor.

67% of Hispanic mother-headed families with children are poor.

The number of children living in working poor families rose 30% between 1989 and 1994.

African-American and Hispanic children are three times more likely to live in poverty than are white children.

Between 1970 and 1990, the typical Aid to Families with Dependent Children (AFDC) welfare benefit declined 37%, greatly increasing the number of children living in poverty.

Study after study documents the negative effects of poverty on children—on their physical growth, cognitive development, academic achievement, socioemotional functioning, and productivity in later life.

Sources: Ellis (1995), Dodds (1995), Fulwood (1996), Grimes (1996), Leeds (1996), U.S. Bureau of the Census (1991a), Wright (1996).

national reports and surveys. Families are weakened by joblessness, poor and crowded schools, loss of family support systems, family breakdowns, drug and alcohol abuse, crime-ridden neighborhoods, and depression (Ellis, 1995; Family Service America, 1984).

It is difficult for most students and teachers to describe the lifestyle of the lower class without imposing middle-class evaluations. Even the use of the term "lower class" imposes a negative connotation and interpretation to people who occupy this class level. What Rodman (1965) stated over 30 years ago still applies, "It is little wonder that if we describe the lower-class family in terms of illegitimate children, deserting men, and unmarried mothers, we are going to see the situation as disorganized and chockfull of problems" (p. 223).

In observing social conditions of lower-class life from a middle-class perspective, we should not become so engrossed in looking at the victims that we fail to understand the reasons for the problems. Perhaps it is more realistic to think of these conditions as consequences of, or in some instances solutions to, other issues faced by lower-class people as they experience all the social, economic, political, and legal realities of life (Eshleman, 1974). When working with the poor, family nurses need to accord the same respect and regard for them as for all other clients. Identifying the family's strengths and vulnerabilities and seeing the family within its own context are important principles for providing care. Oscar Lewis (1961), a noted anthropologist, termed the lower class "the culture of poverty." He believed that the lower-class lifestyle is the direct result of poverty and that this "culture" is not just an American phenomenon, but represents values and lifestyle patterns that can be found cross-culturally.

In contrast with the working class, the lower class does not have the respect of the larger community. Its existence often becomes a "political football" such as the conflict seen recently over "family values". Its members are likely to be stigmatized and characterized as being lazy, parasitic, dependent, and "those people." The source of the stigma is usually the inability to work or lack thereof. Tacit in public rhetoric is also the assumption that many poor persons "have only themselves to blame" (Grimes, 1996).

Poverty in the Family.   Directly related to the poverty of the lower class is the irregularity of employment, and thus income. Because income is irregular, a considerable amount of insecurity exists in regard to food, clothing, shelter, transportation, health care, and other essentials. Children may be forced or encouraged to contribute to the financial needs of the family, and many drop out of high school.

Lower-class family life, adapting to scarce resources, is based on assumptions and norms that are different from those of the middle class (Staples, 1976). The poor cannot "afford" such values of the middle class as productivity, achievement, work, and long-range planning. The *Chicago Tribune* staff (1986) do a nice job of describing the impact of poverty on family life:

> Poor parents have the same job to do with their children that middle-class parents do; the difference is that poor parents have less money, less education, and less access to resources and

alternatives. Most live under extraordinary stress, facing constant crises centered around food, shelter, and physical illness; these lead to feelings of helplessness, hopelessness and powerlessness. These feelings are based in reality and relate to forces largely beyond the control of the poor family. Much of the time the energy of the poor is focused on getting through a day. Yet tomorrow they expect to have to do more of the same. (p. 95)

It is interesting to note, however, that parents' aspirations for their children are very "middle class," despite their inability to provide the ways and means for achieving such goals.

Many poor families are headed by minority group women who are unemployed or underemployed and dependent on welfare (Langman, 1987). A growing number today, however, are working poor families, that increased 30 percent between 1989 and 1994 (Leeds, 1996).

The American Underclass.   A large portion (about 25 percent) of the poor is now being termed "the American underclass" (Gilbert & Kahl, 1993; Russell, 1977; Wilson, 1987). These are the poor who are in persistent, as compared to temporary, poverty.

These are the people who remain more or less permanently at the bottom of the social ladder, completely removed from "the American Dream." The underclass has become increasingly isolated socially from mainstream patterns and norms of behavior (Wilson, 1987). Although its members come from all races and live throughout the United States, the underclass is made up primarily of (1) impoverished urban African-Americans, who suffer from the heritage of slavery and discrimination as well as the changing economy; (2) Hispanics, primarily Mexican-Americans and Puerto Ricans, who have recently immigrated into cities and rural areas (as migrant workers); and (3) Appalachian migrants who live in dilapidated neighborhoods of some cities (Russell, 1977).

The underclasses' long-term poverty and welfare dependency, plus their bleak environment, nurture values that are often at radical odds with those of the majority—even the majority of the poor. For instance, stable marriages and legal divorces tend to be luxuries in this class. Toughness is a desirable interpersonal trait. Children are frequently taught to defend themselves physically rather than with mental or psychological tactics. Thus the underclass minority is disproportionately represented among the nation's juvenile delinquents, gang members, drug addicts, physically disabled people, and single parents on welfare. They are "responsible," therefore, for a considerable amount of the adult crime, family disruption, urban decay, and need for social expenditures. The underclass remains a nucleus of psychological and material destitution despite some two decades of civil rights gains in the 1960s and 1970s. Federal reductions in domestic social programs, beginning in 1980 and continuing into the mid-1990s, have only magnified the problem.

Even though unemployment decreased in the 1980s somewhat, the underclass is made up of people who lack the necessary education, skills, discipline, and self-esteem to succeed. Long-term unemployment is a common factor here, and large numbers of the underclass are single parents on welfare. The 1996 welfare reform legislation is targeted at the underclass. It hopes to enhance self-sufficiency through work. This is all well and good, but we have to make certain that working will actually enable families to meet the minimum needs of their children (Leeds, 1996).

More jobs that provide for a living wage and a better education are clearly two pressing needs. In our achievement-oriented society, work is more than a source of income. It is also a source of feeling productive, which brings self-esteem, status, a point of identification with the system, and a satisfying social environment. Affordable housing, safety in neighborhoods, and educational and health care reform (universal access to care) must also be addressed if families are to escape from poverty (Allen, 1994).

People from the underclass subculture within our communities, especially our cities, are in the greatest need of our health and social services. In official health agencies, much of the nurse's effort is necessarily concentrated on the very poor. It is only through our understanding and appreciation of some of the major problems and daily realities of the poor that we can even begin to assist these families with a resolution to their health needs.

Impact of Poverty on Health

"Health disparities between poor people and those with higher incomes are almost universal for all dimensions of health," according to the U.S. Public Health Service in their influential and far-reaching publication, *Healthy People 2000* (1990, p. 29). The following list indicates the areas where national survey data show a significant relationship between poverty and particular health problems:

- Poorer self-rated health.
- Increased restricted activity days.
- Increased chronic activity limitations.
- Increased disability.
- Increased work and school absences.
- Increased risk of leading chronic diseases and injuries.
- Increased infant mortality and infectious disease rates.
- Shortened longevity.

Although socioeconomic factors are probably a more powerful determinant of health than medical treatments (Nelson, 1994), no interventions aimed at families' economic status have been proposed by the health community. Furthermore, health disparities by social class will persist as long as inequalities in the fundamental social, economic, and political structure of society remain. Thus, argues Nelson (1994), "socioeconomic conditions that constitute or contribute to health risks must also be targeted in policies and programs to improve the health of populations" (p. 2). Assisting families' economic impoverishment is most essential in working with the disadvantaged and is well within nursing's scope of practice (Nelson, 1994).

Economic Status

Economic status, a component of social class, refers to the family's income level and source of income. Geismar and La Sorte (1964) developed criteria and descriptions for assessing the economically adequate, marginal, and inadequate (poor and very poor/ underclass) family. Income that is sufficient to meet a family's needs is generally derived from the work of family members or from private sources such as pensions and support payments (nonpublic), while income derived partially from welfare or unemployment insurance is generally marginal, unstable, or barely adequate. The family that has inadequate economic resources exhibits these characteristics: (1) income derived entirely from welfare because of failure or inability of adult(s) in the family to work; (2) income derived from welfare by fraudulent means; and (3) amount of income so low or unstable that basic necessities are lacking. Families receiving income from programs such as Aid to the Totally Disabled, Aid to the Blind, Aid to Families of Dependent Children, and Old Age Assistance would fall under the marginal or inadequate category, because the level of funding is so low that basic necessities are barely or inadequately provided for.

One basic family function is the provision of adequate economic support and allocation of resources. Hence, in order to assess economic adequacy, not only income level should be estimated but also expenditures, focusing on the allocation of resources. Assessing expenditures, again a sensitive subject that should be discussed specifically only when needed, consists of asking about regular financial obligations: rent or mortgage payments, insurance, transportation costs or car payments, phone and utility bills, food expenses, and any special bills the family may have incurred.

Social Class Mobility

Another family assessment area related to social class is social class mobility. This refers to vertical mobility upward or downward through the social class strata and is included here because a change in either direction produces considerable stress. Holmes and Rahe (1967), in their social readjustment scale, identify changes of position, status, or prestige, whether positive or negative, as stress producing. Although upward mobility is seen as desirable by most persons, and does often result in new recognition and social prestige, it may also result in rejection and social isolation. The cohesiveness of the extended family most likely decreases. In addition, lower levels of family participation are found in upwardly mobile families. Interpersonal relationships and the degree of personal comfort are also often compromised (Eshleman, 1974).

In America, people have expected a move upward as a natural state of affairs. This is no longer true. Due to structural changes in the economy, frequent recessions, and widespread employment instability,

more and more families will not move up the social class ladder as in previous decades, but will remain stationary or move downward (Voydanoff, 1991). Social mobility was probably never as widespread as generally believed. About 70 percent of families remain in the same social class, and this stability of social class placement can be seen through a number of generations. Examples of the stability of social class status are found among upper-class families, where their wealth or prestige has continued through several generations. A similar continuity is also observed in the lower classes (Cavan, 1969). In the well-known social class study by Hollingshead (1949), he showed that the lower-lower social class of "Elmstown" had retained this position since before the Civil War. Mobility occurs most frequently in the lower-middle, working, and upper-lower classes.

Up until very recently, the majority of the vertical mobility in America has been upward, as evidenced by our large middle class. In some cases, widespread social mobility may result in entire communities or regions as a consequence, for instance, of a prolonged economic depression—producing downward mobility. This process occurred in Texas and Colorado in the 1980s with the collapse of the energy/oil industry. At the other end of the continuum, the full employment and prosperity experienced generally in the 1960s and early 1970s may have carried many families upward. Retirement and becoming disabled often bring downward social class mobility because of the marked reduction in income.

▶ ASSESSMENT QUESTIONS AND AREAS: SOCIOECONOMIC STATUS AND SOCIAL MOBILITY

Social Class Status

Based on the family's income level and source of income, and the adult members' occupation and education, identify the family's social class status.

Economic Status

Asking how much the husband or wife earns can be an invasive question, as income is considered a private matter among most families. A question should be asked only if there is an important reason to do so, such as in determining eligibility for assistance or services. Questions relevant to this area include the following:

- Who is (are) the breadwinner(s) of the family?

- Does the family receive any supplementary funds or assistance? If so, what are they and from where (e.g., retirement fund, Social Security, food stamps, family)?

From this information, plus information on occupations, one can often estimate weekly or monthly income or ask a question regarding approximate income.

- Does the family consider its income adequate? How does it see itself managing financially?

- What financial resources does the family or could the family have (for example, medical insurance, disability insurance, dental insurance, workman's compensation, food stamps, unemployment insurance, crippled children's services, reduced transportation fares)?

Social Class Mobility

Describe the family's social class mobility—the change(s) that occurred to produce downward or upward mobility, when these changes occurred, and how the family has adjusted to the changes.

▶ FAMILY SOCIAL NETWORKS AND SOCIAL SUPPORT: THEORY AND ASSESSMENT

A growing interest by social scientists and health professionals has led to a heightened awareness of the effects of personal and familial social environments and social supports on adaptation and health. Due to the important influence of social support on health outcomes, this concept has emerged as a major variable addressed in health-related research today (Roth, 1996b).

It is widely accepted that people who are in supportive social environments are generally in better condition than their counterparts without this advantage. More specifically, because social supports are thought to attenuate the effects of stress (called a "buffering effect" in research) as well as enhance an individual's or family's mental health directly (called "main or direct effects" in research), social support is a crucial coping strategy for families to have available in times of stress.* Social support also may serve as a preventive strategy to reduce stress and its negative consequences.

Definition of Concepts

In this discussion two closely related key terms are social support and social network. **Social network** (Hall & Wellman, 1985) refers to a weblike structure comprising one's relationships. Network size, density, accessibility, kinship reliance, frequency of contact, and stability are structural areas of assessment. Within a family's social network are friends and work associates, neighbors, and community networks (church and community groups and agencies); professional networks (including health care providers and other professionals); self-help groups; and extended and immediate kin (Pilisuk & Parks, 1983).

In contrast, **social support** "focuses on the nature of the interactions taking place within social relationships as these are evaluated by the individual" (Roth, 1989, p. 91) and their supportive value, as evaluated by the individual or family (Roth, 1996b). Cohen and Syme (1985) further clarify the difference between social support and social networks: "While social network may be defined as the structure of the relationship, social support is the function of the relationship" (p. 11).

Most researchers see social support as including both tangible instrumental support (transactions in which direct aid or assistance is given) and emotional/informational support (House & Kahn, 1985; Thoits, 1982). House and Kahn (1985) include these two components of social support in their four types of support: instrumental, informational, appraisal, and emotional.

In the social support/social network literature these terms refer to individuals, not family groups. To focus on the aggregate level of analysis—the family—these terms need to be modified.

Family social support refers to the social supports that are perceived by family members to be avail-

---

*Family social support is also discussed in Chap. 17 as an external type of family coping.

able/accessible to the family (the social support may or may not be used, but family members perceive that supportive persons are ready to provide aid and assistance if needed). Family social support can either be internal family social support, such as spousal support or sibling support; or external family social support—the social supports external to the nuclear family (within the family's social network). A family's social network is simply that social network of the nuclear family itself.

Although there are voluminous definitions and descriptions of social support and social network, only a few articles discuss family social support (Friedman, 1985; Kane, 1988; Roth, 1996b). Kane defines family social support as a process of relationship between the family and its social environment. The three interactional dimensions of family social support are reciprocity (the nature and frequency of reciprocal relations); advice/feedback (the quality/quantity of communication); and emotional involvement (the extent of intimacy and trust) in the social relationships.

Family social support is a process that occurs over the life span, with the nature and type of social support varying in each of the family life cycle stages. For instance, the types and quantity of social support during the stage of marriage (before a young couple have children) is drastically different than the social support types and amount needed when the family is in the last stage of the life cycle. Nevertheless, in all life cycle stages, family social support enables the family to function with versatility and resourcefulness. As such, it promotes family adaptation and health.

Both the nuclear and extended family serve as support systems to their members. Caplan (1976) explains that the family has eight supportive functions including informational support (the family serves as a collector and disseminator of information about the world); appraisal support (the family acts as a feedback guidance system, guides and mediates problem solving, and is a source and validator of member identity); instrumental support (the family is a source of practical and concrete aid); and emotional support (the family serves as a haven for rest and recuperation and contributes to emotional mastery).

In writing about family social networks, Milardo (1988) states that families live in an elaborate system of interactions where they create ties with a broad array of other individuals, families, and larger groups. "Families are profoundly influenced by this web of ties and they are active agents in modifying and adapting these communities of personal relationships to meet ever-changing circumstances" (p. 14).

A deficit and/or impairment in social support within a person's social network is identified by NANDA as the nursing diagnoses of social isolation and impaired social interaction (McFarland & McFarlane, 1989). These diagnoses could well apply to families, as the nature of the problem and the negative outcomes are similar.

Social Support Research

In summarizing an extensive body of social support and health research, Wills (1985) concluded that both buffering effects (social support buffers the negative effects of stress on health) and main effects (social support directly influences health outcomes) have been found. In fact, the main and buffering effects of social support on health and well-being may function simultaneously. More specifically, the presence of adequate social support has been found to be linked with reduced mortality, more favorable recovery from illness, and among the elderly, better physical and emotional health and cognitive functioning (Ryan & Austin, 1989). In addition, the positive impact of social support on adjustment to stressful life events is most often seen in studies where perceived support versus received support is measured.

Family Social Support

Studies of family social support have conceptualized social support as a type of family coping (Friedman, 1985; Stetz et al., 1986). Both internal and external family social supports were found to be utilized.

Extended families provide critical social support to nuclear families today. Most adults live in communities in which they maintain one or more contacts with a living parent or other close relative (U.S. Bureau of the Census, 1989). Recent U.S. Census data (Table 8–5) validate this point (U.S. Bureau of the Census, 1989). Moreover, most family members are satisfied with the frequency and quality of intergenerational relationships (Shanas, 1980).

► TABLE 8–5

CONTACTS BETWEEN PEOPLE 65 YEARS OLD AND OVER AND CHILDREN WHO DO NOT LIVE IN SAME HOUSEHOLD

■ FREQUENCY OF SEEING OR TALKING WITH CHILD

Daily	=	41%
Two or more times/week	=	21%
Weekly	=	20%
Two or more times/month	=	7%
Monthly	=	5%
Less than monthly	=	6%

■ TRAVELING TIME FOR CHILD TO GET TO PARENTS

Within 10 minutes	=	26%
10 to 29 minutes	=	29%
More than 30 minutes	=	45%

U.S. Bureau of the Census (1989).

In the Latino community, extended family ties have remained particularly strong; extended family ties are also stronger in Asian-American and African-American families than with white American families. In white families typically the strongest supportive tie within the extended family network is between mother and daughter. Litwak (1972) referred to the common American form of family as "the modified extended family," emphasizing that it consists of two or more nuclear families, linked to one another by a web of economic interdependence, mutual aid, and social interaction.

Because we have a large proportion of single parents, blended families, and dual-worker families, the various forms of family life today show a wide range in their ability to access the needed supports during high demand periods. Community resources are often more accessible to the traditional two-parent nuclear family than to the single-parent family or the elderly person living alone (Roth, 1996b). The management of chronic illness is an example of a situation in which the type of family form often makes a difference in terms of the availability of adequate social support. Chronic illness often necessitates substantial economic, social, and psychological resources and having an extended family to call upon is often vital to the

family management of the chronic illness. Although extended kin are reported in research studies to be the preferred source of assistance for long-term crises and more extensive problems such as chronic illness, some families do not have these family ties to fall back on (Pilisuk & Parks, 1983). A good example of the lack of the extended family resources are recent immigrant families, many of whom settle here without extended family members being able to join them. Geographic distance of family does not preclude extended family support (Lee, 1979). If, however, the women in the extended family (the caregivers in our society) work, outside assistance is typically brought in, in areas where support for the dependent relative is not possible (Brody & Schoonover, 1986).

Self-help or mutual aid groups can also be a major source of social support in communities (Pender, 1987). When special problems occur, many family members find they need to share and seek help from others who have the same experiences and concerns. (See the interventions section of this chapter and Chap. 17 for more detail of self-help groups.)

Assessing the Family's Social Support and Social Network

Does the family have meaningful ties with friends, relatives, neighbors, social groups, and community organizations that provide support and assistance when needed? If so, who are they and what is the nature of their relationship? Or does the family have little or no contacts with friends, neighbors, relatives, social groups, or community organizations? If so why? Does the family harbor dissatisfaction or hostility to possible sources of social support?

Hogue (1977) suggests that these types of questions be asked to elicit information on the family's support system. She says that it is more acceptable with clients to move from life events already identified and ask:

> "Who helps you with . . . ? If you had any problems about . . . who would you talk to, get help from?" Asking general, then more specific questions is helpful. For example, "Who helped you through retiring from your job?" (general), "Who or what kind of help have you had with the financial concerns most people have when they retire?" (specific). Another useful question is, "Who has helped you through tough situations in the past?" (p. 77)

To obtain further social support network information, both the genogram and the ecomap are suggested. Figure 8–2, presented earlier in this chapter, depicts the family genogram. The genogram identifies primary kin within the extended family (these are the parents' siblings and parents).

The ecomap graphically depicts the family's relationships and interactions with its immediate external environment. This tool assists the family and family health provider to visualize the family social network and, to some extent, how family members are perceiving and/or receiving social support. Figure 8–3 is a blank ecomap that family members and the nurse may jointly complete.

To complete the ecomap, place the family in the middle circle, and significant people, organizations, and agencies in the outer circles. The nature of the relationships between the family and its various contacts are indicated by lines. Straight lines show strong relationships, dotted lines tenuous relationships, and slashed lines conflictual/stressful relationships. The wider the straight lines, the stronger the relationship. Arrows may be used to show the direction of energy and resources within a particular relationship (Hartman, 1978; Wright & Leahey, 1994). Figure 8–4 shows an example of an ecomap. By using both the family genogram and family ecomap in assessment, the family nurse is able to get a fuller view of the family and its social network and supports.

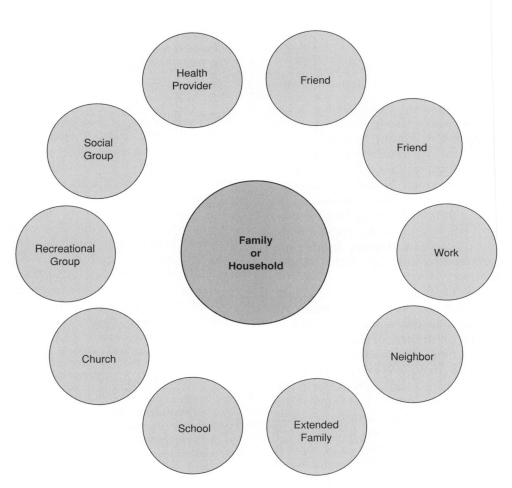

Figure 8–3. Blank family ecomap.

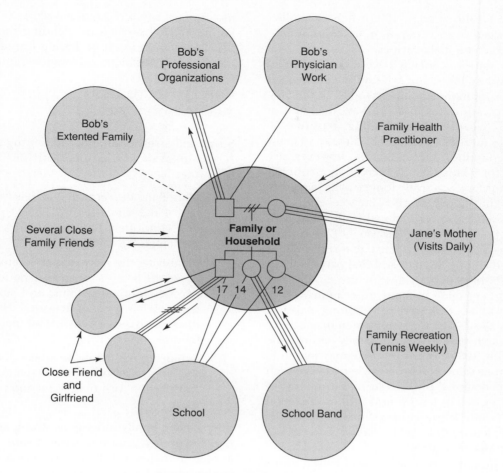

Figure 8–4. Example of family ecomap.

▶ FAMILY RECREATIONAL ACTIVITIES: THEORY AND ASSESSMENT

The importance of family recreation in maintaining healthy family life is consistently recognized in family literature and research. Although each family member has his or her own special leisure-time activities, families also need to have regular family-centered activities in which all members can share and enhance their life together. These activities may be religious, educational, recreational, civic, or cultural in nature. Family rituals and celebrations, most commonly held during holidays or birthdays, are also important times when families come together to renew their ties and sense of continuity as a family and to enjoy each others' company.

Recreational activities refers to those activities that are apart from the obligations of work, family, and society and to which individuals turn at will for relaxation, diversion, self-development, or social participation. Family recreation entails maintaining and strengthening of family bonds, having fun together, sharing feelings, reducing tension, and improving family members' feelings about their family (Geba, 1985; McCown, 1996). Family recreational activities that involve exercise and physical fitness, such as hiking, biking, swimming, and physically active games, also have the benefit of promoting physical fitness in families. Nationwide, only one-fourth of Americans over the age of 18 exercise regularly and sufficiently

(U.S. Public Health Service, 1990); hence, families should be urged to incorporate more exercise into their family recreational activities.

Changing values of society have made quality of life, high-level wellness, and self-fulfillment through work and leisure more prominent today. In the family today recreation has in some ways declined in importance because of competing leisure-time opportunities for individuals and because of so many dual-worker families. Other factors, however, are responsible for making family recreation a continuing significant family activity: longer paid vacations, shorter working hours, more 3-day weekends, and greater accessibility to recreational facilities, at least for more affluent families. Carlsen (1976) reports that there is considerable evidence that recreation is highly valued among families and that parents feel a sense of duty to plan activities for the family. The planning and engaging in family recreational activities appear to be a shared role among parents. Researchers also report that family members believe that not enough time is spent in family leisure time activity (Smith, 1985). It is from the family that individuals learn to value certain lifestyle patterns, such as healthy recreational pursuits such as those involving exercise as well as leisure time and group/team work. The family is the context in which healthy recreational, leisure-time, and exercise patterns are established (McCown, 1996).

Research on family recreation has focused on its positive effect on marital and family satisfaction, family unity, and marital stability (Hill, 1988; Smith, 1985). For instance, Gerson (1960), in studying married college couples, found a positive relationship between a number of leisure-time factors and marital satisfaction. West and Merriam (1969) discovered a positive correlation between outdoor recreation and family solidarity. Hill (1988), applying attachment theory to her study, found that spouses' shared recreational time was predictive of marital stability.

Kelly (1978) concluded that the family is a central social context of leisure. He observed that the home is the most common locale for leisure-time activity and family members are the usual companions for most kinds of weekday, weekend, and vacational leisure. Stinnett (1979), Otto (1973), and McCubbin and McCubbin (1988) validate the important role family leisure-time activity plays in family life by including indicators of family recreational activity in their lists of family strengths—such as spending time together, having common interests, having fun together, and having family traditions, celebrations, and rituals.

Family Recreation Assessment Areas

Suggested assessment areas pertaining to a family's recreational or leisure-time activities include the following:

1. Identifying the recreational/leisure-time activities of the whole family. What types of activities? How often do these activities occur? Who participates in them?

2. Identifying the recreational/leisure-time activities of the family subsystems (spouse subsystem, parent–child subsystems, and sibling subsystems). What types of activities? How often do these activities occur? Who participates in them?

3. Exploring the family members' feelings about the family's leisure-time/recreational activities (satisfaction with time spent and types of activities).

Keeping the family subsystems strong and functioning effectively is crucial to family health. Thus recreational activities involving the subsystems as well as the whole family are viewed as a major family strength.

▶ FAMILY NURSING INTERVENTIONS

This section discusses intervention guidelines associated with the several aspects covered in this chapter—guidelines for working with ethnic minority families, for assisting families with economic difficulties, for promoting adequate social support, and for increasing families' recreational/leisure-time activities.

Sociocultural Family Interventions

Guidelines for providing culturally competent family health care to ethnic families are necessarily broad, because more specific intervention strategies are limited to only certain ethnic groups. Davis and Voegtle (1994) outline five key aspects involved in providing culturally competent health care. These are:

1. Awareness and acceptance of cultural differences.

2. Self-awareness of one's own culture.

3. Understanding the dynamics of cultural differences.

4. Knowledge of the client's family culture.

5. Adaptation of services to support the client's culture.

The first four elements are necessary to be culturally sensitive, but it is the fifth aspect, the adaptation of services to support the client's culture, that makes our services "culturally competent." Seven basic strategies suggested in the cross-cultural literature are outlined and include: (1) selecting the appropriate system to work with, (2) providing more time to work with unacculturated families, (3) dealing with language differences, (4) taking into account the family's interactional norms, (5) focusing on family strengths and families' positive adaptation, (6) promoting positive change, and (7) being aware and utilizing the family's social support system.

Selecting the appropriate family system to work with is a crucial consideration. Which system to work with (a family subsystem such as the marital or parent–child subsystem, the nuclear family, the extended family, or the individual client's self-identified family, which may be composed of unrelated persons) can determine the outcome. Understanding and respecting an ethnic minority family's cultural norms and present social context are perhaps the most important skills in selecting a system for counseling (Dilworth-Anderson & McAdoo, 1988; Ho, 1987). Ho (1987) gives us a good example of this guideline:

> Considering the intense involvement that ethnic minority families have with their extended family, some family problems can be resolved simply by involving the extended family members, especially the spokesperson, who normally is the grandfather (Asian/Hispanic) or grandmother (black and Indian). (p. 258)

Family nurses should be aware of extended kinship networks and should search out significant others to be included in the family assessment and interven-

tion, given, of course, this is mutually agreeable with the family.

A second general intervention guideline deals with the time needed to provide care to ethnic families. If the family is unacculturated, Harwood (1981) stresses the importance of allowing more time for health care interventions. More time is typically required for translation, for assessing relevant health beliefs and practices, for discussion and clarification of health information, for explanation of diagnosis and treatment plans, and for socializing the family members to the health care system.

Language use in clinical encounters with members of ethnic families is a third general consideration. In assessing and intervening, the health practitioner should not assume that a foreign-born client and his or her family wish to carry on an interview in their native language. When the language ability of the individual is not apparent, asking what language he or she prefers to use is indicated. Having translators is not without its problems, but usually is preferable to attempting to use a phrase book or a very limited vocabulary to communicate (Harwood, 1981).

Harwood (1981) gives three recommendations to clinicians working with ethnic minorities that address interactional norms. First, he suggests that in ethnic families that are kin-based or from peasant societies, the elderly are accorded more respect than they are in our society. Moreover, social interaction between sexes is more limited, and standards of modesty more strictly prescribed. As a result, the style of interaction between the family nurse and family members should reflect these interactional norm differences. For example, a younger health care professional should show greater respect and deference to an older family member. Certain potentially embarrassing topics should be discussed only with certain members of the family present. Because the health care professional is usually seen as an authority figure, with Asian and Hispanic families in particular, he or she needs to assume an active, more directive role in the beginning interviews/visits (Ho, 1987).

Secondly, due to professional and class status differences, members of ethnic families are often reticent to ask questions or discuss their concerns. Active encouragement to ask questions and bring up concerns is needed to break down this barrier.

And a third related approach is to listen actively and carefully to what family members have to say.

The family nurse should convey an interest in the client and family, personalizing the encounter such as the folk healer might do.

The fifth general strategy for working with ethnic families is to pay attention to family strengths and families' positive adaptation. This focus facilitates a more positive opinion about ethnic families and their cultural differences (McAdoo, 1993). It also leads to family nursing approaches that tend to raise a family's sense of competency and empowerment. Moreover, focusing on strengths tends to minimize the clinician's tendency to compare an ethnic family to mainstream notions of families and how families should look and act.

The sixth general intervention guideline for working with ethnic families is to promote positive change. This can be done by building on cultural practices. Cultural health practices that are positive should be reinforced and, if possible and practical, incorporated into the plan for care. Promoting changes in health practices should only occur when self-care and health practices are harmful or when additions to a family's self-care or folk remedies are called for. After making recommendations, there is a need to check for client understanding and acceptance. If the recommendation is not accepted, it may be at a later date. For the fit between the family's need and the recommendation may not have been good at that particular time for that particular family.

The seventh general intervention strategy addresses social support systems. Informal social support systems are probably more important for ethnic families to call upon than for white families. Thus, family nurses need to be aware and help families to utilize their natural support systems (McGoldrick & Giordano, 1996). Important social support systems such as extended family, friends, and social and religious groups may not be available or relationships may be strained. In these cases, assisting family members to strengthen clients' connections to family and community resources is indicated.

Ho (1987), a family therapist, discusses culturally relevant techniques and skills in the phases of family therapy. Due to cultural barriers to family mental health services, he stresses the cruciality of developing trust with the family in the beginning phase of family counseling. During the early engagement phase, he suggests that the clinician may need to explore with the family ethnic/cultural differences between the clinician and family.

Family nursing interventions that are culturally appropriate during health care treatment include facilitating access to needed health knowledge, consideration of dietary practices and beliefs, family visiting and participation practices, and understanding preferences for staying home versus obtaining health care in inpatient and long-term care settings.

Unacculturated ethnic minority families generally have poor access to health knowledge (Harwood, 1981). Especially if they do not speak English, are poorly educated, and have a social network composed of families from the same socioeconomic and ethnic background, they have limited access to accurate, up-to-date health knowledge. As a consequence, these families are much more in need of health education than more advantaged majority families. Health knowledge deficits need to be carefully addressed here.

As part of medical regimens, therapeutic diets must incorporate ethnic preferences if they are to be followed; hence, the importance of getting a dietary history before intervening. Ethnically acceptable therapeutic diets should reflect both ethnic food preferences and ethnic food beliefs.

Family visiting and participation in a family member's care while he or she is in the hospital also varies from ethnic group to ethnic group. In many cultures, the family plays a major role in patient care. In ethnic groups with strong familistic orientations, such as in Asian and Hispanic families, sickness is a time when relatives display their support and solidarity. Hence, visiting the hospital and fully participating in care are important family activities for the psychological state of not only the patient but also the family (Harwood, 1981).

There may be a difference in preferences of ethnic minority groups to home care versus hospital care or long-term care. "Many ethnic groups strongly prefer home care over institutionalized care for the incapacitated and terminally ill. . . . Chinese, Haitians, Italians, Mexicans, and Puerto Ricans all manifest this preference, while urban blacks and Navajos do not" (Harwood, 1981, p. 503). Harwood explains that the reasons for this preference among the former groups has to do with their strong extended family ties and the low participation of women caregivers in the work force. The high percentage of urban African-American and white women in the work force is undoubtedly a major barrier to home care in those groups.

Financial Interventions

Interventions that assist families in ameliorating the financial strain of health and illness problems are often overlooked in family nursing. If family nurses are aware of the financial impact of health problems on families, there is often much they can do to help (Millington & Zieball, 1986), particularly if the nurse is in the primary care or community setting. A family that is at high risk medically is also a family that is at high risk financially, given the need for expensive, specialized diagnostic and treatment procedures, personnel, and long-term care.

Financial stress often permeates the family system and results in family disruption. The medical bills may necessitate that the mother work outside the home, the father take on a second job, and vacation and leisure-time activities be eliminated. Strains in the marriage that then "ripple" into the other sets of family relationships are commonplace. Divorce, separation, acting-out children, psychosomatic problems, and substance abuse are symptomatic of the long-term disruptive effects that financial stress may induce (Millington & Zieball, 1986).

For the most part, nurses have tended to leave financial concerns up to the social worker to handle. Yet in many settings there is no available social worker and the nurse is the appropriate health care professional to intervene. Even if there is a social worker available, only when the nurse assesses for financial problems can he or she then become aware of the problem and make the appropriate referral.

Usually nursing interventions in this area center around providing information to families on health care costs and community resources, as well as making referrals—a case management intervention.

Nurses need to be aware of the costs to families when complex problems arise, as well as the family's financial resources and how the family is paying and/or will pay for the needed services, supplies, equipment, and so forth. He or she should be familiar with the types of medical care programs available for the medically needy within the particular target population as well as the community services available free or at reduced costs for all regardless of their ability to pay. Immunizations and screening clinics are examples of these latter types of community resources.

Teaching in the financial area, according to Millington and Zieball (1986) includes teaching families about ways to reduce health care costs, to evaluate their insurance coverage, to determine how their health resources are being allocated, and where costs could safely be reduced. Teaching families how to look at their financial situation objectively and problem solve effectively is also suggested. Table 8–6 summarizes assessment and intervention strategies for assisting families at high risk for financial stress.

Social Support and Social Network Interventions

Because of family nurses' commitment to families and family members, the importance of human relationships and support to families is readily apparent. This places family nurses in an ideal position to assess and intervene to enhance clients' social support and social network.

Social support system interventions are designed to extend or enhance functioning of the client's informal and formal social networks (Stewart, 1993). Of course, interventions should be matched to meet the

---

▶ TABLE 8–6

FINANCIAL ASSESSMENT AND INTERVENTION STRATEGIES

■ **ASSESSMENT STRATEGIES**
Establishing trust and rapport with family.
Assessing family's financial costs, resources, and allocation of resources for health care.
Assessing family's coping efforts and resources.

■ **INTERVENTION STRATEGIES**
Teaching family ways to reduce health care costs by presenting available alternatives/options.
Teaching family to understand and evaluate insurance coverage.
Referring family to appropriate services within and outside health care agency.
Helping family cope with financial stress.

Adapted from Millington and Zieball (1986).

assessed need. In formulating interventions, Stewart (1993) advises nurses to consider not only the stressor(s) causing the need, but also the desired intensity of support, the client's other personal resources, the timing of the intervening, the type of social support desired, the potential drain of resources in support networks, and the appropriate target or level of intervention (i.e., the client, the informal social system, particular key support persons, and groups or community organizations).

Families need to have available social supports to prevent them from entering into crisis when demands on the family increase. When families do face life events and transitions that challenge their coping skills, social support can be mobilized in several ways: (1) by improving the quality of support received by the family's social network, (2) by reanchoring themselves into a network that is more responsive to their present emotional needs or reorienting themselves to sectors of their network containing more appropriate psychosocial resources (Gottlieb, 1983), and (3) by fostering affiliation among people facing similar stressful circumstances (use of self-help groups).

Family nurses are involved in counseling families to cope effectively by using their social supports to share the burden (Venters, 1981) and provide emotional and informational support (House & Kahn, 1985). Reinforcing positive patterns of help-seeking is an excellent preventive intervention strategy. Helping family members access untapped social support, such as mobilizing informal support systems, is another helping strategy aimed at promoting adequate family social support. See Table 8–7 for a listing of social support interventions.

In the social support literature, two specific strategies are described for mobilizing social support. These are (1) the use of self-help groups and (2) the use of social network family therapy principles and strategies.

Use of Self-help Groups.

Nurses are increasingly aware of the value of self-help groups for family members who need support to overcome a stressful handicap or life experience.* Self-help or mutual support groups (the terms are used interchangeably) are defined as small groups of peers who come together to share a common problem

---

* Use of self-help groups is also discussed in Chap. 17 as an external type of family coping.

and through mutual assistance to resolve or ameliorate the problem (Steiger & Lipson, 1985; Trainor, 1983).

Self-help groups have proliferated in the last three decades, and their rapid growth is evidence of their perceived effectiveness. Writers attribute this growth to being a response to a highly technical and mobile society in which ties to naturally occurring support of family, friends, neighbors, fellow church members, and the like are often weakened or absent. Our formal social support systems—the health care and human service systems—also are inadequate in terms of providing accessible, effective assistance to the large number of people who are in need of mutual support mechanisms.

Self-help groups are described as being largely self-governing and self-regulating, emphasizing peer solidarity rather than hierarchical authority. They advocate self-reliance and usually require commitment and responsibility to other members. They generally provide material and emotional support to members, offering a face-to-face or phone-to-phone fellowship network, available and accessible without charge. Groups are self-supporting and usually occur outside the aegis of formal institutions or agencies.

Self-help groups have been established for people and families with almost every conceivable problem. Increasingly, self-help groups are being formed to assist families of those afflicted with a particular illness or disability. Examples of these types of groups are Candlelighters for families with childhood cancer, Al-Anon for families of alcoholics, and Adult Children of Alcoholics. Many groups welcome both the person with the identified problem and family members, such as Make Today Count for clients and family members of persons with life-threatening illness, and Mended Hearts for clients and families of people who have had heart surgery.

Research on the outcomes of self-help group participation has indicated that self-help group participation is useful cognitively, through providing beneficial information, attributing meaning to the problem (Shapiro, 1989) and assisting with problem-solving skills; and emotionally, through providing a network of support for expressing feelings and encouraging grief work. Groups enable its members to pool their experiential knowledge and profit from others' experiences. They provide role models

> ► TABLE 8-7

INTERVENTIONS FOCUSED ON ENHANCING FAMILY'S SOCIAL SUPPORT SYSTEM

Target	Intervention Strategies
Particular significant support persons (e.g., daughter, spouse)	Contacting person(s) and encouraging them to assist if possible. Informing significant support person(s) of need. Providing resources or information on how to seek resources. Correcting inaccurate/inhibiting beliefs about client's need.
Informal social support system (e.g., extended family, neighbors, friends, social groups/organizations)	Informing persons/groups of need. Bringing informal social system members together to provide support collectively. Fostering social network's communication with each other. Referring client/family to self-help group or community organization.
Formal social support system (e.g., health, transportation, welfare, educational, recreational)	Initiating referral to community agency to provide outside assistance and services, e.g., transportation, home health care. Communicating with agency regarding client's need to share information about client with agency and about agency with client; also to coordinate services.
Client(s): family or family members	Targeting negative attitudes and beliefs regarding seeking assistance from others. Helping families identify their strengths and vulnerabilities. Helping families establish new supportive relationships and maintain old relationships. Enhancing support appraisal for families prone to devalue ties. Reinforcing positive efforts family make to reach out for support.

Sources: Pearson (1990), Roth (1996), Stewart (1993), Vaux (1990).

of successful adaptation and reinforcement for successful coping. And lastly, by helping other group members, it is found that those individuals help themselves (Trainor, 1983).

Nursing Interventions. Family nurses are in a key position to encourage family members to mobilize social support by participating in a self-help group. Trainor (1983) summarizes the role of the nurse here by explaining that nurses have a responsibility to:

1. Seek information about groups offering assistance to individuals and families.

2. Collaborate with such groups.

3. Understand how these groups enhance and complement professional services.

4. Refer client and families to appropriate groups.

5. Create new groups or encourage others to do so when there is a lack of a needed self-help group.

In addition family nurses may be engaged in counseling groups of family members who have formed support groups to help themselves with particular problems they are facing.

Social Network Family Therapy. In family therapy, the social network family therapy approach is an innovative strategy aimed at mobilizing family social support. A family in distress is the unit for intervening with this approach. Here the family's social network is mobilized—that network of people with whom the family in crises has a social relationship (extended family, friends, neighbors, and other associates). Healing of the distress is believed to come from within this social unit as it is brought together to support the distressed family (Jones, 1980). Social network family therapy takes place in the home setting with the family and its large social network, which is assembled to create a nurturing and healthy social matrix. More specifically, the family social network is assembled to

> set in motion the forces of healing with the living social fabric of people. . . . We find the energies and talents of people can be focused to provide the essential supports, satisfaction, and controls for one another, and that these potentials are present in the social network of family, neighbors, friends, and associates of the person or family in distress. (Speck & Attneave, 1973, p. 7)

Social network family therapy is a useful strategy for nurses to employ who have more advanced preparation in family systems nursing and who are working with families in crisis. A more limited application of this notion is for family nurses to invite extended family members or close friends to be part of the family unit that is receiving care (Haber, 1987).

Interventions to Promote Family Recreation and Leisure-time Activities

Where nurses, based on a family assessment, find that a family is lacking in cohesiveness or bonding, the fun of being a family, social supports, active recreational activity, or is under stress, promotion of regular, more frequent family recreation and leisure-time activities may be indicated. McCown (1996) identifies the nurse's role in promoting active family recreation as including modeling behaviors, providing education, and contracting for client self-care. Hence, family nurses are urged to be good role models of an active, healthy lifestyle that incorporates family recreation; to act as health educators and counselors for families in need of increasing their recreation and other leisure-time activities; and to use behavior modification and contracting as one mechanism to assist families to acquire additional healthy lifestyle patterns such as family recreation and exercise.

▶ study questions

Choose the correct answers to the following questions.

1. Briefly describe why it is essential to understand a family's ethnic background when providing family health care.

2. One of the assumptions made in dealing with families from different cultures is that we become less judgmental of other people's behavior as we attempt to (select the one best answer):
   a. Give up our values and learn to accept people as they are.
   b. Recognize the origins of our own values and understand why we hold them.
   c. Work purposefully to overlook other people's values that are contrary to our own.
   d. Gradually work to change other's values when we consider them detrimental.

3. Cultural ignorance and insensitivity lead to the following problems (choose all the correct answers):
   a. Poor communication
   b. Interpersonal tensions
   c. Stigmatization
   d. Inadequate assessments
   e. Professional objectivity

4. Ethnicity is an important resource for individuals and families because (choose all the correct answers):
   a. It guides them in occupational choices.
   b. It compensates for the cold impersonality of modern society.

   c. Its traditions enrich family life and strengthen its continuity.
   d. It facilitates upward mobility.

5. The use of a cross-cultural or transcultural approach is vital when providing for family health care because it (select the one best answer):
   a. Provides information about different cultures.
   b. Predicts ethnic minority family behavior.
   c. Provides a broad comparative picture of individual and group behavior.
   d. Assumes a cultural deviant perspective in assessment.

6. Match the proper definition with the corresponding concept.

Concept	Definition
1. Cultural conflict	a. Blueprint for a person's way of living.
2. Acculturation	b. Common ancestry and shared cultural history.
3. Assimilation	c. Nonacceptance of diversity within cultural group.
4. Ethnic identity	d. Gradual changes created as one culture is influenced by another.
5. Ethnocentrism	e. The way individuals see themselves relative to their cultural identity.
6. Stereotyping	f. Denotes the more complete one-way process of acculturation.
7. Cultural relativism	g. Culture is viewed nonjudgmentally and understood within its own context.
8. Ethclass	h. Lack of cultural relativity (seeing one's own culture as superior to others).
9. Cultural imposition	i. Local professional health care system.
10. Culture shock	j. Lay or folk health care system.
11. Indigenous health care system	k. Primary tactic used in cultural anthropology to analyze cultures.
12. Self-fulfilling prophecy	l. Discomfort and confusion created by experiencing cultural differences.
13. Culture	m. The interaction of ethnicity and social class.
14. Ethnicity	n. Forcing one's values and practices on another person because of ethnocentricity.
	o. A degraded person's tendency to conform to the beliefs and expectations others have about him or her.
	p. Negative responses of clients to culturally unacceptable practices of health agencies and health workers.

7. Social class is based generally on three criteria: income, education, and occupational status. Identify which of these is the most important determinant.
   a. Income level
   b. Occupational status
   c. Educational level

8. The primary difference between the "nouveau riche" and the upper-upper class families is:
   a. Wealth.
   b. Spending patterns.
   c. Ethnicity.
   d. Family background.

9. The upper-middle class highly values (choose all the applicable values):
   a. Education.
   b. Productivity.
   c. Materialism.
   d. Community involvement (voluntarism).
   e. Individualism.

10. Lower-middle-class families, in contrast with upper-middle-class families, tend to (choose all correct answers):
    a. Value education highly.
    b. Be more racially and ethnically mixed.
    c. Have closer kinship relations.
    d. Put more emphasis on individualism and productivity values.

11. The blue-collar or working class is often difficult to distinguish from the lower-middle class, especially because there may be little income difference. Nevertheless, the most obvious differences between the two groups are (choose all correct answers):
    a. Wife's employment.
    b. Emphasis on family background.
    c. Spending patterns.
    d. Husband's type of employment—manual versus nonmanual labor.
    e. Education.

12. The lower class consists of the poor. In this social class the following characteristics are prevalent (choose all correct answers):
    a. Most often families live in rural or suburban areas.
    b. Men have unskilled jobs (sporadic and underemployed) or are unemployed.
    c. The family may receive welfare.
    d. Family aspirations and behavior are very similar

13. The poor family's value system is substantially different from the dominant culture values. Identify three examples of these contrasting values.

14. The definition of social support and social network are closely related, but different. The best description of this differences is:
    a. Objective versus subjective perspective.
    b. Micro versus macro perspective.
    c. Family versus individual system analysis.
    d. Perceived quality of support versus quantity of support.

15. Briefly describe two basic family nursing interventions aimed at promoting family social support.

16. Social support research findings show that social support affects the health status of individuals by (choose the correct answer):
    a. Directly influencing health outcomes (main or direct effects).
    b. Acting as a buffer between stress and health outcomes (conditional effects).
    c. Both directly and conditionally affecting health outcomes.

17. Family nursing interventions appropriate for promoting better family financial health and family recreation include the following (complete the sentence):
    a. Health teaching addressing health-related financial problems of families may be in the area of _____.
    b. Initiating referrals addressing health-related financial problems of families may be to _____.
    c. Health teaching aimed at promoting family recreational/leisure-time activities include _____.
    d. A second strategy to help families to increase their family recreation and other leisure-time activities is _____.

18. Broad intervention guidelines for working with families who are ethnically different from the family nurse include (choose all correct answers):
    a. Working with extended family system.
    b. Providing more time to work with unacculturated families.
    c. Using an interpreter to deal with language differences.
    d. Modifying communication after considering family's interaction norms.
    e. Focusing on family strengths and adaptation to adversities.
    f. Promoting positive change by negatively reinforcing families' unscientific health care practices.

19. After reading the following clinical vignette, discuss sociocultural interventions that would be appropriate to incorporate into the care of this family and child.

Nine-year-old Maria was initially seen in the emergency room where she had been brought by both parents and her grandmother. The crisis occurred because a young teenage cousin who was "high on some type of dope" had sexually abused Maria. In the first encounter with Maria and the family, the family nurse practitioner noticed that the Spanish-speaking grandmother had a very supportive impact on her granddaughter, who was very anxious and withdrawn, and on the parents, who were quiet and tense. It was the grandmother who was able to get the family members to explain clearly and fairly calmly what had happened and why they decided to come to the emergency room. She was able to provide comfort and support to Maria and persuade her to allow the nurse practitioner to examine her and ask her some questions about what happened. (Vignette adapted from Canino & Spurlock, 1994, p. 137.)

Now explain what general sociocultural intervention strategies could be used in this situation.

▶ chapter 8 study answers

1. Gaining an understanding of the ethnic background of a family is essential to family health care because without this knowledge, family values and behavior cannot be understood or accurately interpreted. Ethnicity and culture permeate and circumscribe familial actions. In the absence of being able to assess accurately, the health care professional then is not in a position to work with the family to assist it in resolving health problems. It is also imperative to understand a family's culture from their perspective in order to build the rapport and trust necessary to appropriately assess, support, and counsel ethnic families.

2. b.

3. All but e.

4. b and c.

5. c.

6.
1. p.	8. m
2. d.	9. n.
3. f.	10. l.
4. e.	11. j.
5. h.	12. o.
6. c.	13. a.
7. g.	14. b.

7. b (usually of husband, but increasingly of both spouses in dual-career families).

8. d.

9. All (a–e).

10. b and c.

11. c, d, and e.

12. b and c.

13. Any three, with dominant cultural values listed first: productivity versus "getting by"; education versus less value on education; mastery over environment versus fatalism/powerlessness against environment (or harmony with environment); future-oriented, long-range planning versus present-oriented, immediate gratification.

14. a or d.

15. Use of self-help groups and bringing in people from family's social network to be part of the family unit the nurse is working with.

16. c.

17. a. Teaching families how to reduce costs of health care by presenting options. Teaching them about their insurance coverage and community resources for help.
    b. Other services within the health agency, such as the business office or social worker, or community services, such as the Social Security Administration office or the state vocational rehabilitation office.
    c. Teaching about the benefits to the family of having family recreational and other leisure-time activity. Teaching about what types of recreational activity are healthier and more accessible.
    d. Role modeling and behavior modification (contracting).

18. b, d, and e.

19. There are several general intervention strategies that would be appropriate to utilize here.
    a. Select the appropriate system to work with. Include the grandmother with the parents and child in the provision of care. Also provide support to the grandmother and parents and guidance for handling concrete problems (the child's anxieties, immediate child supervision/protection, and referral for crisis intervention and counseling for family and child and abusive cousin). Another system that would be contacted would be the child protective service agency in the community.
    b. Use of an interpreter: Taking into consideration the language difficulties between the grandmother and nurse practitioner and the fact that the grandmother is the key supportive person here, the interpretive process becomes extremely important. Be sure the parent(s) explain carefully and completely to the grandmother what the nurse practitioner says. The nurse practitioner should speak slowly and break up his or her thoughts to make translation easier.

The nurse practitioner should encourage and allow extra time for the grandmother to respond, ask questions, etc.

c. Assessing and utilizing the family's social support system. This should be done as part of the assessment and later intervention. In this family crisis, identifying support for the family and child is critical. In Hispanic families a large extended family usually comes to help in time of crisis. The family should be encouraged to utilize key supportive persons from the extended kin network.

Family Environmental Data

Marilyn M. Friedman

1. Define and describe the following environmental data and apply content to a written case example.
   a. Physical setting: Home (characteristics, safety hazards, spatial adequacy, provision of privacy).
   b. Physical setting: Neighborhood and community, including geographic mobility patterns.
   c. Associations and transactions of the family with the community and the family's perceptions and feelings regarding the neighborhood and community.
2. Explain the territorial concepts and apply to a case example.

3. Discuss housing and the family's habitat relative to its effects on:
   a. Self-perception.
   b. Stress.
   c. Health.
4. Describe the impact that crowding has on health.
5. Summarize research findings relative to the problem of homelessness and its effects on individual and family health.
6. State a family nursing diagnosis within the family environmental area.
7. Propose several nursing interventions aimed at promoting family environmental health.

Families do not exist in isolation, but in constant interaction with the world around them. It is the nature of this family–environment interaction that, in large part, determines the health of the family. Steiger and Lipson (1985) remind us that

> Health and illness are as inextricably connected with environmental factors as they are to social and cultural factors. It has become more and more apparent in recent years that health hazards in the home, on the road, in the work-place, and in the broader environment have striking, if sometimes subtle, effects on health. (p. 276)

There needs to be a good fit between the family's needs and environmental inputs/resources for the maintenance of family wellness (Holman, 1983; Killien, 1985; McCubbin & McCubbin, 1993).

Having an environmental or ecological perspective in family nursing practice is imperative (Wiley, 1996), because families must be viewed within their naturally occurring contexts. Killien (1985) eloquently explains the benefits of incorporating an environmental perspective in nursing assessment and intervention.

> The practice of nursing from an environmental perspective broadens the assessments, diagnoses, interventions, and evaluations made by the nurse to include not only the client but also the environmental systems surrounding the client. As a result, there is increased understanding of client's health behavior, additional intervention strategies become available, and interventions may be more successful than when the focus of practice is exclusively client focused. (p. 259).

Both systems and structural–functional theory, two of the text's organizing theoretical frameworks, stress the vital nature of the family's interaction with its external physical and sociocultural environment.

This chapter presents some of the basic information about the family's environment and discusses the assessment of the home, neighborhood, and community. Family nursing intervention guidelines for promoting family environmental health are also described at the conclusion of the chapter.

The scope of a family's environment is large. "It consists not only of concrete realities such as food, clothing, shelter, medical care, employment, physical safety, education, and recreation, but also includes social realities in terms of interpersonal relationships" (Holman, 1983, p. 40). For the purposes of this chapter, however, the focus is limited to the home, neighborhood, and community, while food, health care, recreation, and social support/social networks are discussed in other chapters (recreation and social support/social networks in Chap. 8 and food and health care in Chap. 16).

▶ THE FAMILY'S ENVIRONMENT

Although the environment is defined in many different ways, the easiest way to think of the family's external environment is anything outside of that particular family, including the immediate physical setting in which the family is situated and the family's social environment. Bronfenbrenner (1979) called the specific places where individuals and families engage in specific activities and roles **microsystems** or behavior settings. In systems language, microsystems are interacting systems. These are the immediate physical contexts where face-to-face encounters between family members and others occur. At a more global level, the family is situated in environmental **macrosystems**. For instance, the macrosystems of a family could be the educational system, work system, social service system, and so forth. In systems language, a macrosystem would be referred to as a suprasystem. Environmental demands and environmental stress (where the demands exceed the family's resources) can exist both within the family's micro- and macrosystems (Melson, 1983).

▶ HOUSING: THE FAMILY'S HOME

Provision of a healthy environment in the form of adequate shelter is an aspect of family functioning that is of special concern to the family-centered community nurse. A family's home is extraordinarily significant for its members because it has a significant impact on both the physical and mental health of the family and its members.

Psychologically, one's home becomes part of the family identity. "Home is that place where things are familiar and unchanging and where people maintain some sense of autonomy and control" (Rauckhorst et al., 1982, p. 159). A home, according to Taylor (1995), who qualitatively looked at "what is a home," says that a home provides a sense of origin and continuity with one's ethnic roots, a sense of privacy, a sense of safety and security, a sense of familiarity, and a sense of behavioral consistency, referring to family rules, and rituals.

Through home visits nurses are able to observe the physical setting of the home and the particular arrangement of family life space, observations that otherwise would be impossible. Such assessment of the home environment provides a most valuable aid in understanding the family and its lifestyle. Because the home is its territory, the family behaves more naturally and comfortably, and health care professionals are able to assess more accurately the particular dimensions of family life. The home's sanitary and safety conditions are also focal assessment areas (Daniel, 1986).

Before describing actual assessment areas relative to the home environment, this chapter reviews salient literature on housing and its effect on families, the concept of territoriality, the impact of crowding and homelessness on families, and safety in the home.

Housing and Its Effects

The effects of housing can be seen in two major areas. First, there are psychological aspects that affect self-perception and life satisfaction; if these are negative, they can serve as stressors and illness-producing factors. Second are the effects of possible physical hazards—due to the house's state of repair, its facilities, and its arrangement (Schorr, 1970; Wiley, 1996). Such physical conditions may influence privacy, child-rearing practices, housekeeping, study habits, as well as contribute to the transmission or exposure to disease and the possibility of accidents and poisonings (Wiley, 1996). Moreover, the placement of houses and apartments in relation to one another and to the larger urban environment clearly influences family and social relationships.

Psychological Effects: Self-perception and Life Satisfaction.

Because house and neighborhood are generally felt to be extensions of one's self, housing is usually a subject of highly charged emotional content, a matter of strong feeling. These feelings about one's habitat are significant factors in determining how individuals and family perceive themselves and are perceived by others. Thus, one evaluates one's surroundings far from objectively. If a person then calls a house a slum, the tenant is likely to hear that he or she is being called a slum dweller (Schorr, 1970)!

To the middle-class resident, the social elements that are involved in self-identification with his or her housing may be quite evident. The following questions are common to the process of deciding where to live: Who is accepted there? Are they my kind of people? Is it a step up or down? What will it do for me and my children? Who will I meet?

Hence self-evaluation and motivation influence where a person selects to live, and conversely, living in poor housing influences a person's self-evaluation and motivation. A good deal has been written about the pessimism that is common to the poor, their readiness to seize the present satisfaction and let the future care for itself, and their feeling that one is controlled *by* rather than in control *of* events. Although there is considerable variability in attitudes, not to say aspiration, among even the very poor, studies of families living in deteriorated neighborhoods make the same point: pessimism and passivity present the most difficult barriers to rehabilitating neighborhoods. Where vigorous effort has gone into the upgrading of neighborhoods, some families have improved their housing and, as a consequence, feel they have improved their situation and status.

Psychological Effects: Stress.

Housing may affect behavior by contributing to or dissipating stress, albeit some people have more effective adjustive mechanisms than others.

Almost any characteristic of housing that negatively affects individuals may be interpreted as stressful—crowding, dilapidation, vermin infestations, or high noise levels are examples. Two further stressful factors are social isolation and inadequate space. There is some evidence that aged people who live alone are more likely to require psychiatric hospitalization than those living with families. Any environment that tends to isolate an individual from others offers a stress that will lead to distinguishable personality changes. The amount of space per person and the way space is arranged to promote or interfere with privacy have also been related to stress (Schorr, 1970).

Effects on Health.

Environments need to be suitable for the development and health of family members as well as for the family as a whole. One of the most difficult problems poor and working-class families face is that their home, neighborhood, and community environments are not conducive to wellness, and yet they do not have the option to move.

Substantial evidence links poor housing with poor health. It is well understood that certain diseases are correlated with poor housing (see Table 9–1 for examples).

Even though family pets provide tremendous psychosocial benefits, they also can cause health problems, either directly from animal bites or through

▶ TABLE 9–1

EXAMPLES OF DISEASES ASSOCIATED WITH POOR HOUSING

1. Acute respiratory infections, related to the multiple use of toilet and water facilities, inadequate heating or ventilation, and inadequate and crowded sleeping arrangements.
2. Minor digestive diseases and enteritis, related to poor facilities for the cold storage of food and to inadequate washing and toilet facilities and sharing of food and drink.
3. Injuries resulting from home accidents related to crowded physical space in home, inadequate kitchens, poor electrical wiring, poorly lighted and unstable stairs, and slippery floors.
4. Infectious and noninfectious diseases of the skin related to crowding and shared or inadequate facilities for washing.
5. Lead poisoning in children who eat scaling paint from typically poor, older homes.

animal-transmitted infections (salmonella from dogs, psittacosis from pet birds, fleas from dogs and cats, allergies—eczema and asthma—from the fur of hairy pets).

Territoriality and Families

Individuals and family groups have a sense of territoriality, also referred to as spatial behavior (Giger & Davidhizar, 1995). We recognize that animals, as part of their innate repertoire of behaviors, lay claim to a specific area and defend this area against intruders, while other animals, in turn, tend to respect their claims. A similar type of instinctual characteristic applies to people and families. The human desire to possess and occupy specified areas is pervasive, even though overt expression of infringement by others is attenuated by socialization. It has been noted that the most sacred prerogative in Western civilization is that of ownership of private property, especially of one's home.

The first home visit by a student nurse may therefore seem quite threatening to him or her, partially due to the feeling of intruding into someone else's territory. Families may also feel uncomfortable about this intrusion, especially when health care workers come unannounced or uninvited.

Home territory is an area where the family has relatively more freedom of behavior and a sense of control and power over both the area and its members. The home is viewed as a "haven in a heartless world," to coin the words of Christopher Lasch (1977) who wrote a book by that name.

When a family member leaves home **personal space** becomes important. Stea (1965) defines personal space as a small circle in physical space, with the individual in its center and a culturally determined radius or "bubble" around the individual. An individual's personal space expands, shrinks, and changes in openness depending on the social situation, the physical context, the culture of the person, and the other persons present (Meisenhelder, 1982). A person's level of comfort is very much related to his or her personal space. If a person's personal space is invaded, discomfort results (Giger & Davidhizar, 1995).

In public health, one will often observe families that are constricted in their movement due to feelings of fear, discomfort, and/or poverty. They are essentially homebound and uncomfortable moving from their neighborhood. Other families may be much more at ease moving in a wider geographic complex. The territory that the family feels comfortable in and moves in may in part be a function of income, physical mobility, cultural or personal values, or a result of socialization. In the Los Angeles area, for example, there are many Mexican immigrants who are more comfortable in visiting Mexico and receiving health care there than going to a new part of the city and attending an Anglo health clinic.

Within families there are both spatial (physical) and behavioral dimensions of territoriality. The feelings of belonging and cohesiveness among family members make up the behavioral component, while the actual physical space of home, yard, family name and address, and frequently visited community systems—school, work, shopping centers, churches, and community agencies with which the family interacts—are the spatial aspects of territoriality (Anderson & Carter, 1974).

Impact of Crowding in the Home

During the 1970s, well over 200 studies researched some facet of crowding (Epstein, 1981). Schorr (1970), in summarizing the results of "crowding studies," commented that fatigue and too little sleep may be consequences of seriously inadequate, crowded housing. School nurses can certainly corroborate these findings, as they observe fatigued children come into their school health offices. The effect of crowding on intrafamily friction has also been observed. One of the results of seriously inadequate space in the home is that family members spend much of their time outside the home. This tendency may be a particularly serious matter in relation to children and adolescents. It has been observed that poor children from crowded, inadequate homes do not study sufficiently and are not within reach of parental control. "Street life" takes on increasing importance for many of these children during grammar school years and by the time the adolescent years begin, peer associations "on the street" are frequently very influential.

There appears to be inconclusive findings with respect to the effects of crowding on family members' actual physical health status. Crowding does, however, make sufficient privacy difficult to achieve. Privacy functions to protect and maintain an individual's need for personal autonomy; to serve as an emotional release; and to provide an opportunity for self-appraisal and protected communication. Having one's own room, bed, possessions, clothes, toys, and pets are assets. Privacy for an adolescent is especially significant in assisting him or her to achieve the developmental needs of independence. Marital privacy is also critical in most families.

Epstein (1981) found that a person's perceived sense of control influences how individuals adjust to crowded conditions. If an individual perceived that he or she was able to maintain adequate personal control over his or her environment, this fostered more favorable adaptation to crowding in the home.

Crowding is very strongly associated with socioeconomic status and ethnic background and is relative to what a person has experienced in the past. If a family has never known anything but "crowded living," then this situation does not seem so intolerable. The percent of ethnic minority families who live in crowded conditions is more than three times greater than that of white families.

Safety in the Home

Two of the most valuable assessment areas for community health and home health nurses relative to the home are the assessment of safety conditions and of potential or real hazards, both inside and outside the home. Especially within the home, accidents are a major threat to a family's health status. Each family member is exposed to certain threats from accidents related to his or her developmental stage (Kandzari & Howard, 1981). "Increasing the family's awareness of the chief accident problems, providing factual information, and suggesting ways for the family to improve its level of safety wellness are the goals" (Kandzari & Howard, 1981, p. 223).

Home accidents kill about 27,000 and injure more than 4.2 million persons in the United States each year. Of the above deaths, 9800 result after falls; 5700 result from fires; and 2500 are the consequence of poisoning. Furthermore, home accidents kill more children between the ages of 1 and 14 years than all the next six causes of death combined. Nearly all of these deaths and injuries could be prevented by proper protection and safety education (Bete, 1976; McFarlane, 1986).

Potential or actual hazards in the home include the possible presence of lead, which adversely affects children's intellectual and emotional growth, and is found in older plumbing and household dust as old paint deteriorates or is chipped away. Approximately 74 percent of dwellings built before 1980 contain lead-based paint (lead-based paint has been prohibited since 1978). Exposure to lead "poses the nation's number 1 environmental health threat to children . . . an enormous number of young Americans will not realize their full potential because of their exposure to lead in their environments" (Lum, 1995, p. 27). Young children who are poor and African-American are disproportionally affected by this health threat.

Other hazardous substances that may be found in homes are indoor air pollution, substances found in some building materials, and radon. Indoor contaminates, especially, may present a widespread pollution threat. Concentrations of some airborne pollutants have been found to be as high as 100 times greater indoors than outdoors (U.S. Environmental Protection Agency, 1988). One major source of indoor air pollution is tobacco smoke. The long-term secondary effects of tobacco smoke are clearly acknowledged as a serious health hazard. The pollutants in smoke caused by improperly maintained or vented wood stoves can be another air pollution hazard in homes.

A wide variety of organic compounds from common household products may contribute to the threat of indoor pollution. According to the Environmental

Protection Agency, benzene, a known human carcinogen, has been found in far higher concentrations indoors than outdoors. Benzene is emitted indoors by synthetic fibers, plastics, some cleaning solutions, and tobacco smoke. Commonly used household products such as air fresheners, shoe polish, paints, cleaners, mothballs, and dry-cleaned clothing contain low levels of chemicals that are known animal carcinogens. Cleaning solutions and powders containing chemicals that are toxic, abrasive, or caustic to eyes and mucous membranes are labeled by most manufacturers with warnings about potential dangers. Families should be encouraged to store such substances properly and out of reach of young children.

Noxious by-products of cigarette, pipe, and cigar smoking such as carbon monoxide and nitrogen dioxide may predispose household occupants, especially children, to pneumonia, other respiratory ailments, and cancer. Formaldehyde, widely used in newer building materials and furnishings, can cause eye, nose, and throat irritation; coughing; skin rashes; headaches; dizziness; nausea; vomiting; and nosebleeds. Products sold to kill household pests may leave pesticide residues, with many of these chemicals having never been tested to determine their health effects.

Building materials in older homes may be a hazard, particularly building materials containing asbestos. Asbestos was used in many types of building materials from about 1950 through the early 1970s to make materials sturdier. Asbestos exposure leads to serious respiratory disease. Radon, an odorless, colorless gas is another home hazard. It is emitted through cracks in basement walls and floors and enters the body through ingestion of contaminated water supplies or in the home, through inhalation of air. Long-term exposure to radon is one cause of lung cancer (Lum, Hibbs, Phillips, & Narkunas, 1996).

Homelessness

Homelessness as a societal problem has risen sharply in the United States since 1980. Particularly in cities and temperate regions, homelessness has been a major community health concern (Taylor, 1995). The problem is much larger than the absence of a home. A family's entire existence is threatened.

Homelessness is a problem that time will not solve. Some studies suggest that the average time being homeless exceeds 3 years (Vernez et al., 1988). Among the most alarming characteristics of this growing population is the rising number of families with children, as well as the increasing proportion of persons who are severely mentally disabled.

Homeless families, in fact, have become the fastest-growing segment of the homeless population (Bassuk, 1990, cited in Taylor, 1995; Jackson & McSwane, 1996). The Children's Defense Fund (Kozol, 1990) recently estimated that 500,000 children in the United States are homeless. A case in point about the rising number of homeless families is the New York City experience. In 1987, nearly one-half of the occupants of homeless shelters in New York City were children. Their average age was only 6 years old (Kozol, 1990).

McChesney (1987), who studied homeless families, found that poverty and unstable/temporary housing arrangements were the major factors leading to homelessness. Personal stressors, family disruption, and unreliable social networks were also factors (Taylor, 1995).

It is accepted that homelessness is a great stress to families and children. But little research has been conducted to document the effects of homelessness on families. Several studies, however, have documented the adverse effects of homelessness on the health of children and mothers. Numerous chronic and acute physical and serious mental health problems have been found (Berne et al., 1990; Bowdler & Barrell, 1987). Homeless children suffer from anxiety, depression, sleep problems, and suicidal ideation (Bassuk & Rubin, 1987), as well as high rates of infectious diseases (Jackson & McSwane, 1996). Harsh environmental conditions and health-damaging responses breed demoralization, hopelessness, despair, mental deterioration, and all the other problems associated with poverty.

Assessment Areas: Home

The following questions are suggested for completing an assessment of the home environment; both Kandzari and Howard (1981) and Rauckhorst and associates (1982) provide more detailed coverage of this area.

1. Describe the dwelling type (home, apartment, or rooming house). Does family own or rent its home?

2. Describe the home's condition (both the interior and exterior of house). House interior would include number of rooms and types of rooms (living room, bedrooms, etc.), their use, and how they are furnished. What is the condition and adequacy of the furniture? Is there adequate heating, cooling, ventilation, and lighting? Are the floors, stairs, railings, and other structures in good repair? Is the water supply adequate? Is there a telephone in the home or accessibility to a phone? What is the condition of the yard?

3. In kitchen, assess the water supply, sanitation, and the adequacy of refrigeration and cooking facilities.

4. In bathrooms, observe sanitation, water supply, toilet facilities, and presence of towels and soap. Does everyone have his or her own towel or are towels shared? In bathtubs, are there grab bars (important to older person's homes)?

5. Assess the sleeping arrangements in the house. Are they adequate for family members, considering their age, relationships, and special needs?

6. Observe the home's general state of cleanliness and sanitation. What are the family's hygiene and cleanliness practices? Are there any infestations of vermin (interior especially)? If there are pets are there any sanitation problems related to their presence?

7. Are there signs of flaking, old paint (possible lead poisoning hazard), which young children might be exposed to?

8. Identify the family's territorial unit. Are family members comfortable driving out of their neighborhood to use resources/services in other parts of the community?

9. Evaluate the privacy arrangements and how the family feels about the adequacy of its privacy.

10. Evaluate the presence or absence of safety hazards in other areas of the home. Ask about the storage of medicines and substances containing toxic substances. Are they stored safely away from children and pets and clearly marked? If family members use poisonous or potentially harmful substances (e.g., cleaning fluids, glues, etc.) do they carefully follow directions on their use? Observe for dangerous objects that might cause safety hazards to children or elderly family members. Are the entry and exits from and into the house barrier free and is there adequate space and lighting to move safely through the house (Daniel, 1986)? Are there any exposed or frayed electrical cords, or loose rugs on the floor? Are there provisions for emergencies (smoke detector, emergency numbers by the phone)? Is there a swimming pool, and if so, is it adequately fenced in and locked if small children are in the home?

11. Evaluate the adequacy of waste and garbage disposal.

12. Assess the family members' overall feelings and satisfaction with their housing arrangements. Does the family consider its home adequate for its needs?

The Omaha System designed by the Visiting Nurses Association of Omaha lists 12 items on their problem rating scale related to the home (see Table 9–2). One beauty of their form is its ease of use.

▶ TABLE 9-2

SIGNS AND SYMPTOMS OF PROBLEM FROM ENVIRONMENTAL DOMAIN, PROBLEM 3: RESIDENCE (FAMILY HOME)

Structurally unsound
Inadequate heating and/or cooling
Steep stairs
Inadequate and/or obstructed exits or entries
Cluttered living space
Unsafe storage of dangerous objects/substances
Unsafe mats or throw rugs
Inadequate safety devices
Presence of lead-based paint
Unsafe gas and/or electrical appliances
Inadequate or crowded living space
Homeless

Adapted from the Omaha System's Data Base/Problem List in Martin & Scheet, 1992, p. 343.

▶ PHYSICAL SETTING: THE NEIGHBORHOOD AND COMMUNITY

The neighborhood and community in which the family lives exerts a tremendous influence on the family. Using a systems and structural–functional frameworks for assessing families, the family nurse needs to examine "the family and its universe." Its universe consists of the inner and outer environments of the family. The outer environment includes the territorial concepts previously described. The territorial unit includes the small "home" circle, while territorial cluster and complex pertain to the family's neighborhood and community.

Impact of Neighborhood and Community on Families

The neighborhood and adjoining community can be described relative to their physical and their psychosocial impact on families. In describing the psychosocial effects of neighborhood on families, the type of social interaction that occurs in different types of neighborhoods has been studied. Substantial social and economic homogeneity has existed in most of the communities that have been studied. In homogeneous neighborhoods, because the families' behavior patterns, values, and interests are alike, neighborhood-based friendships tend to be formed. Homogeneity is found to be more significant in creating a large number of friendships and associations than is proximity (Schorr, 1970).

In stable working-class neighborhoods, family membership is concentrated in the locality, and the most active ties are with other members of the family. Proximity makes for frequent contacts with relatives and other neighbors, casually in passing and less casually on the sidewalk or in the local shops. There is considerable attachment to the place itself. Relationships are identified with locality.

Many middle-class Americans have few neighbor and/or community roots and move from city to city and region to region as their jobs and personal preferences dictate. Mobility is highest among young adults, those in middle-income levels, and those in the military or migrant labor jobs. Hence their support systems within the community may be lacking.

In summarizing social interaction patterns in communities and neighborhoods, it has been consistently found that social class homogeneity, and frequently age, ethnic, racial, and religious similarity, foster social interaction, whereas social class disparity discourages it. People want to live and mix with their neighbors (other families) who share the same, or similar, values and lifestyles (Chilman, 1978).

The neighborhood and wider community that the family lives in have definite effects on family health. Noise, traffic, air, and garbage pollution, of course, produce continual, probably low-level stress. For instances, living near a toxic dump or near stagnant water may adversely affect health. Chronic, low-level exposures to toxic substances in the air, water, and food can produce physical diseases and conditions that have a latency period, an insidious onset, or a diffuse set of symptoms (Wiley, 1996).

Another effect of neighborhood and community is its effect on life satisfaction. Satisfaction with neighborhood and community have been found to be closely associated with satisfaction with life in general (Chilman, 1978). It is also true that people's expectations of neighborhoods and communities by people differ, depending on social class status: The higher the social class, the greater the expectations of the community (Rainwater, 1972). These same differences in expectations are observed in community agencies. The poor demand little, while the affluent have high demands and expectations. The lower expectations are correlated with and result from feelings of powerlessness and learned helplessness.

Rural Families.
It has been noted that rural communities have drastically different effects on individuals and families than do urban areas. Recently there has been extensive interest and concern about the health and other needs of rural families (Bushy, 1990; Weinert & Long, 1987). It seems that the rural environment, in spite of its more personalized social environment and tranquil setting, has some unique, special problems. The rural community is directly affected by the primary economic resources of a region, such as farming, ranching, lumbering, or mining. Inasmuch as farming, lumbering, and mining (three major industries) have experienced recent crises, stressors that rural communities and families face also have amplified. Rural people are described as being self-reliant and traditional in their values and as having a strong work ethic. Increased economic hardships, however, have

markedly eroded the ability of families to uphold these values (DeFrain, LeMasters & Schroff, 1991). Accessibility to health care and other needed services has declined due to geographic remoteless as well as economic hardship (Bushy, 1990).

Assessment Areas: Neighborhood and Community

1. What are the characteristics of the immediate neighborhood and the larger community?

   Type of neighborhood and community (rural, suburban, urban, inner city).

   Types of dwellings in neighborhood (residential, industrial, combined residential and light industry, agrarian).

   Condition of dwellings and streets (well kept up, deteriorating, dilapidated, being revitalized).

   Sanitation of streets and homes (clean, trash and garbage collected, etc.).

   Problems with traffic congestion.

   Presence and types of industry in neighborhood.

2. How exposed are family members to environmental hazards found in the soil, air, and water? Are family members subjected to high levels of noise on a regular basis?

3. What are the demographic characteristics of the neighborhood and community?

   Social class and ethnic characteristics of residents.

   Occupations and interests of families.

   Density of population.

4. What changes have occurred in the neighborhood and community? Is the neighborhood and community in a state of transition or is it demographically stable?

5. What health and other basic services and facilities are available in neighborhood and community?

   Marketing facilities (food, clothing, drug stores, etc.).

   Health agencies (clinics, hospitals, emergency facilities).

   Social service agencies (welfare, counseling, employment).

   Family's church or temple.

   Schools. What is the accessibility and condition of the neighborhood school? Are there problems within the school (e.g., crowdedness, poor quality of education, gangs, racial/ethnic tensions) that affect children's education?

   Recreational facilities (playgrounds, parks).

   Public transportation. How accessible (in terms of distance, suitability, and hours) are these services and facilities to family?

6. How long has the family lived in the neighborhood and/or community? What has been the family's history of geographic mobility? From where did they move or migrate?

7. What is the incidence of crime in the neighborhood and community? Are there other safety problems?

   The rates of certain crimes—robbery, aggravated assault, larceny (pickpocketing), and purse snatching—are much more frequent problems for persons over 65 years of age. More than 60 percent of the elderly live in metropolitan areas, and most of these reside in the central city. For cultural, emotional, and economic reasons, many of the elderly have lived in the same areas for decades. Many cannot afford alternative housing, and they are often dependent on public transportation. Consequently, these poorer urban elderly are close to those most likely to victimize them—the unemployed, the drug addict, and the teenage school dropout (Mallinchak, Wright, & Older, 1978).

▶ ATTRIBUTES OF HEALTHY FAMILIES: THEIR ASSOCIATIONS IN THE COMMUNITY

Healthy families are those that are active and reach out in self-initiating ways to relate to various community groups, according to Lewis and associates (1976). Families who are functioning in a healthy way perceive themselves as being related to and part of the larger community. Part of families' successful coping is their ability to secure compliance from the environment or to maintain a good family–environment fit (Hall & Weaver, 1974; McCubbin & McCubbin, 1993), meaning that within the community the family is able to seek out, receive, and/or accept the appropriate resources to meet its needs for food, services, and information. Passive acceptance of community services, however delivered, may be an indication of an isolated, estranged family or a dependent family that is functioning on a much lower level of health.

Assessment Areas: Community Associations

Completing a family ecomap (see Figure 8–3), as suggested and described in Chapter 8, is quite useful to obtain information about family members' associations and transactions with their social network and community. These specific questions are also suggested to assess this area.

1. *Who* in the family uses *what* community services or is known to which agencies? For example, the family with school-age children might be involved with the public school system, a church group, the welfare department, or a scouting organization.

2. How frequently or to what extent do they use these services or facilities (the area they frequent)?

3. What is the family's territorial cluster and complex?

4. Is the family aware of community services relevant to its needs, such as transportation? Is the family aware of availability of lower transportation fees (monthly card, discount cards for transportation for children and senior citizens) and direct route to health clinics and community resources?

5. How does the family feel about groups/organizations from which it receives assistance? Assess the family's perceptions and feelings regarding association with above community groups and agencies. If the experiences in using community or neighborhood agencies have been positive, these are resources that can be used again and perhaps with even greater success.

6. How does the family view the community? For example, is it a community where the family is worried about having children play outside during the day because of high crime and personal attack rate in the neighborhood? Or is it a neighborhood rich in a sense of common ancestry and cohesion?

▶ NURSING DIAGNOSES: FAMILY ENVIRONMENTAL HEALTH AREA

According to Killien (1985) nursing diagnoses related to an environmental perspective focus on the family–environment fit, "the balance of demands and resources between the client and the environment" (p. 270). The environmental demands can be either actual or potential, making room for preventive, curative, and rehabilitative types of nursing diagnoses. The North American Nursing Diagnosis Association (NANDA) has one family environmental nursing diagnosis listed, that of impaired home maintenance.

This diagnosis is used to describe the array of individual and family environmental problems that result from an individual or family being unable or potentially unable to independently maintain a safe, hygienic, and/or growth-promoting immediate environment (McFarland & McFarlane, 1989).

▶ FAMILY NURSING INTERVENTIONS

McCloskey and Bulechek (1996) in *Nursing Interventions Classification NIC*, the University of Iowa classification project, identify numerous nursing interventions that could assist families with environment safety problems, problems within the family–health care system, and family–formal social support system (see Table 9–3). Safety risk identification, environmental management, and home maintenance assistance are probably the most central of these interventions with respect to family environmental issues.

Many of the strategies for intervention related to environmental health are preventive in nature. Primary prevention should be a primary emphasis here. For instance, working with families to prevent falls in the elderly, poisoning of children in the home, or skin rashes due to vermin infestations,

▶ TABLE 9-3

NURSING INTERVENTIONS RELATED TO FAMILY ENVIRONMENTAL CONCERNS (FROM THE IOWA INTERVENTION PROJECT)

■ **SAFETY DOMAIN: RISK MANAGEMENT**
(INTERVENTIONS TO INITIATE RISK REDUCTION ACTIONS AND MONITOR RISKS OVER TIME)
Environmental management
Fall prevention
Risk identification

■ **HEALTH SYSTEM DOMAIN**
(FACILITATING THE INTERFACE BETWEEN FAMILY AND HEALTH CARE SYSTEM)
Health System Mediation
Culture brokerage
Decision-making support
Health system guidance
Discharge planning
Patient rights protection
Visitation facilitation
Information Management
Health care information exchange
Multidisciplinary care conferencing
Referral
Telephone consultation

■ **FAMILY DOMAIN: LIFE SPAN CARE**
(FACILITATING FAMILY FUNCTIONING THROUGHOUT THE LIFE SPAN)
Caregiver support
Sustenance support
Respite care
Family mobilization
Home maintenance assistance
Social support enhancement

Summarized from McCloskey, J.C. & Bulechek, G.M. (1996). Nursing Interventions Classification. St. Louis, Mo.: C.V. Mosby.

are significant goals of the community-based family nurse.

Primary Prevention: Environmental Health Promotion

Teaching family environmental self-care requires that families accurately perceive their vulnerability to accidents, injuries, or illness and "use self-responsibility to prevent environmental stressors and to protect and promote the family's environmental health and safety" (Wiley, 1989, p. 313). By recognizing and anticipating potential and actual environmental threats to their health, there is much

more families can do to make their home and lifestyle health promoting.

Promoting Safety in the Home. "Increasing the family's awareness of the chief accident problems, providing factual information, and suggesting ways for the family to improve its level of safety wellness are goals for the nurse" (Kandzari & Howard, 1981, p. 223).

Family teaching in the following safety education areas is recommended when potential or actual problems are assessed:

1. How to prevent falls by arranging furniture to avoid obstacles; installing handrails on all stairs; placing cords for electrical equipment away from walking areas; having adequate lighting for all traffic areas, especially the stairs; keeping scatter rugs away from head and foot of stairs; installing handrails for shower and bathtub; using nonskid mats for bathtub and bathroom floor; and placing lights so that they can be turned on from bed and groping around in the dark can be avoided.

2. How to prevent fires by removing rubbish such as old newspapers, wastebaskets, trash cans; never emptying ashtrays or tossing matches into wastebaskets unless one is sure they are out; never smoking in bed; and checking the chimney, fireplace, and furnace to keep them free from fire dangers.

3. How to avoid lifting accidents by using good body mechanics in lifting, reaching, and carrying heavy items.

4. How to avoid poisoning accidents. Most poisonings are due to carelessness, so advise parents to keep medicines locked and away from food if small children are in family; give medicine only as prescribed (never give leftovers to other family members); keep medicines in their original containers (label contains vital information); make sure medicine bottles have safety caps; and store and use household cleaners with the utmost care (they can be lethal if swallowed by children).

5. Make sure the house is tailored to the safety needs of the age(s) of the children and adults

in family. Both the very young and the old have special safety needs. The very young, for instance infants, should never be left unattended on a table or in a tub and should be kept away from the stove. The older person requires excellent lighting, handgrips in bathroom (by toilet, shower, or bath), and stairs that have nonskid surfaces and good, sturdy handrails (Bete, 1976).

6. Point out to families that they should have an emergency plan, so that if an emergency does arise, they will be fully prepared. This includes posting a list of important telephone numbers on a wall by the phone; keeping a first-aid chart accessible and becoming familiar with its instructions; and having on hand in the medicine cabinet the items needed to treat common emergencies.

Secondary Prevention Related to Environmental Problems

Secondary prevention intervention strategies are also indicated. Secondary prevention has to do with early detection and treatment. Teaching families about diagnosis and treatment of common home injuries and exploring with them their proximity to emergency facilities and other needed services are examples of interventions here.

Tertiary Prevention: Environmental Modification Strategies

Tertiary prevention, as you will recall, involves convalescence, rehabilitation, minimization of the effects of the disability, and maximization of the client's functioning. Tertiary prevention in the form of environmental modification is very important for nurses in home health care who care for the disabled and frail elderly. Assisting families in reducing environmental demands and increasing their environmental resources are goals when recommending environmental modifications. Environmental modification or home improvisation is often needed to address the special needs of the disabled and aged. Disabled family members often need modification in their home environment to enable them simply to remain at home. Families

are often not knowledgeable or may not be present to help (unless the nurse or client specifically enlists the aid of extended family members). Environmental modification recommendations for the family with a disabled or elderly member(s) include:

1. Modifying the kitchen to make shelves, cupboards, and drawers more accessible and hence more functional.

2. Clearing hallways and floors of loose rugs and dangerous objects and rearranging furniture for improving home safety.

3. Modifying the bathroom to improve the safety of the toilet, bath, and shower facilities, such as by adding sidebars and handgrips in shower, bath, and toilet areas.

4. Making entrance/exit modifications, such as adding railings to stairs, building ramps, and widening entrances.

Family nurses who work with the disabled should be familiar with the common types of special adaptive equipment needed to make the home safer and more functional. Moreover, the home health family nurse should understand the extent to which these special adaptive devices are covered by Medicaid, Medicare, and other third-party reimbursement sources so that this information can be shared with families.

Interventions to Assist the Homeless

The homeless are in need of a wide variety of services and types of assistance. A comprehensive case management approach (see Chap. 18 for elaboration of this intervention strategy) is suggested due to the complex needs of homeless families. Homeless families need help not only with their multiple primary care needs, but also with subsistence services (shelter, food, and clothing), access to entitlements (welfare, Social Security, etc.), crisis intervention, ongoing mental health services, transportation, and child care. Assisting families to obtain these services, or initiating and monitoring referrals are suggested interventions. Taylor (1995) lists a broad array of intervention roles that are appropriate for family nurses working with homeless families. These include being: a health educator, an interventionist (providing outreach and noninvasive emergency and supportive care for illness/

injuries), an advocate, a counselor, a case manager, a group leader, and a consultant.

Clinicians working with the homeless stress the importance of showing respect toward these clients, being nonthreatening, assuming a low profile, and minimizing reporting and paperwork requirements (Vernez et al., 1988). Political advocacy is urged by nurses who work with the homeless—to exert pressure on government to expand available housing or housing subsidies to poor families.

► study questions

1. "Housing affects a person's self-perception." Discuss in what way this occurs.

2. Housing may affect behavior by contributing to or dissipating stress. Several aspects of housing have been identified as frequently stress producing. Name three.

3. Substantial evidence of linkage between extremely poor housing and physical health exists. Identify three health problems associated with poor housing.

Choose the correct answers to the following questions.

4. The most rapidly growing group within the homeless population is:
   a. The mentally disabled.
   b. Substance abusers.
   c. Children.
   d. Women.

5. Which effect(s) of severe crowding have been described?
   a. Increased intrafamilial stress.
   b. Too little sleep.
   c. Fatigue.
   d. Excessive amount of time spent inside home for all children of all age groups.

6. The number one environmental health threat to children is exposure to:
   a. Radon.
   b. Lead.
   c. Vermin infestation.
   d. Asbestos

Are the following statements true or false?

7. Where families live close to each other in working-class neighborhoods, the most active social ties are with other members of the family.

8. In stable working-class neighborhoods there is considerable attachment to the neighborhood itself.

9. The family–environment interface is a key concept within both systems theory and structural–functional theory.

10. Territoriality as a concept refers to a person's possession of physical land and the resources on that land.

11. Homelessness is associated with acute rather than long-term mental health problems in children and women.

12. Case management is recommended for dealing with the array of complex health and social welfare problems of the homeless.

13–16. Please read the following case study and answer the study questions following this hypothetical case.

► family case study

(Questions are asked here which also relate to Chaps. 6 and 8.)

One year ago, the Juarez family moved to Los Angeles from their birthplace, a small agricultural area in northern Mexico. The husband and wife both worked as migrant workers on a large cooperative farm in Mexico and stated life was "hard" (basic necessities—food and shelter—were a struggle to obtain). Mr. J., age 30, and Mrs. J., age 25, now live with their three children, Maria, age 8, José, age 6, and Pedro, age 4, in an older small wooden house in a low-income Mexican-American district in Los Angeles. The district has a paucity of health and social services, although there is a market and shopping center within walking distance.

Their housing is minimally adequate. There are two bedrooms, with parents sleeping in the larger bedroom, two boys sharing the other, and Maria sleeping on a cot in a small room off the kitchen. The living room is small, with two chairs. The family owns a large old-fashioned radio, an older stove, a refrigerator, a washing machine, and an electric fan without the fan cover. The rooms are clean, but have no carpeting, and few lights. An electrical wall heater warms the living room and hallway. It is minimal but functions. The electric wall heater had a protective screen on it at one time, but it has been removed.

Since the family arrived they have pretty much stayed within their immediate vicinity. Mr. J. is employed in a steady job as a dishwasher for a local Mexican restaurant. Mrs. J. has a part-time janitorial job in a small business nearby.

Because both parents speak very little English and are embarrassed because they did not go beyond the third grade, they have not been to school to talk with the teachers, although the children appear to be having learning problems. The parents and children belong to no community groups, but attend mass at the Spanish-speaking Catholic church in their neighborhood. They have no family recreational activities, except that Mrs. J. occasionally takes the children to a neighborhood park.

In spite of isolation from their extended family, which still resides in Mexico, and their language barrier, they like the community, feel they are starting to get ahead, and that the neighborhood is friendly and its people helpful. They are, however, worried about their children's associations (are they associating with "good" children?) and with the high crime rate in the neighborhood.

Only a limited amount of information was gained about the family's history. Mr. and Mrs. J. were neighbors as children and Mrs. J.'s brother and her husband were friends. Both families felt they would be happy together, so they married when Mr. J. was 20 and Mrs. J. was 15. Maria was conceived 6 months later; both parents were very pleased. Each new child was positively accepted as a natural part of family life. They seem to be quite content in their relationship together, with well-delineated (traditional) roles and functions. Mrs. J. is in the home except for her part-time work; Mr. J. is the breadwinner and "leader" of the family.

Describe the identifying data and appropriate information under these broad headings from the family case study cited.

13. ## Family Identifying Data

    13.1 Composition of family.
    13.2 Type of family form.
    13.3 Religious and ethnic orientation (from Chap. 8).
    13.4 Social class status.
    13.5 Social class mobility.
    13.6 Developmental stage and history of family (from Chap. 6).
    13.7 Social support/social network.
    13.8 Recreational activities.

14. ## Family Environmental Data

    14.1 Home.
    14.2 Neighborhood and community, including geographic mobility.
    14.3 Associations and transactions of family with community.
    14.4 Family's perceptions and feelings about neighborhood and community.

15. State a family nursing diagnosis related to the family's environment.

16. Propose two family nursing interventions aimed at promoting the family's environmental health.

▶ chapter 9 study answers

1. Housing is the symbol of status, of achievement, and of social acceptance. It influences the way in which the individual and family perceive themselves and are perceived by others.

2. Crowding, dilapidation, cockroaches or other insect infestation, and high noise level. Also acceptable answers: social isolation, inadequate space (inadequate internal space of home and arrangement of space in home, lack of privacy).

3. Acute respiratory infections, certain infectious childhood diseases, and infectious gastrointestinal diseases. Also acceptable: home accidents, infectious and noninfectious skin diseases, and lead poisoning.

4. c.

5. a, b, and c.

6. b.

7. True.

8. True.

9. True.

10. False.

11. False.

12. True.

Identifying Data

13.1. Composition of family:

Name	Sex	Relationship	Date/Place of Birth	Occupation	Education
Juarez, Mr.	M	Husband/father	1967 Mexico	Dishwasher (full-time)	3rd grade (Mexico)
Juarez, Mrs.	F	Wife/mother	1972 Mexico	Janitorial work (part-time)	3rd grade (Mexico)
Juarez, Maria	F	Daughter	1989 Mexico	Student	?
Juarez, José	M	Son	1991 Mexico	Student	?
Juarez, Pedro	M	Son	1993 Mexico	Student	?

13.2. Type of family form: two-parent nuclear family.

13.3. Religious and ethnic orientation: Religion—Roman Catholic; attend mass regularly. Ethnicity is Mexican. Family is not acculturated to Anglo culture; evidence: they stay within small ethnically based neighborhood territorial complex. Language is Spanish. Family has no community associations except for Spanish-speaking Catholic church. Live in

Mexican-American neighborhood; friendly with neighbors. Couple has traditional family structure (patriarchal).

13.4. Social class status: Upper-lower social class. Economically independent. Both parents work in unskilled jobs. Father is primary breadwinner. Parents' education limited to third grade. Income very marginal, but work is steady.

13.5. Social class mobility: Have moved upward from state of dire poverty, where basic necessities—food and shelter—were difficult to obtain, to upper-lower class, where family not only has adequate food, but has rented house and both parents have jobs. They are still poor, but relative to their past they have moved upward.

13.6. Developmental stage and history of family: Developmental stage: Family with school-age children. José and Pedro appear to have learning problems and parents have not been to school. By parents not relating to school staff, parents are inadequately promoting school attainment, a developmental task within this stage. Parents were neighbors as children and their families encouraged their marriage. Early marriage (husband was 20, wife 15). They conceived first child 6 months after marriage and felt positive about pregnancy and birth. All of the children were welcomed additions to the family; they were seen as a natural event in family life. Marital relationship—both partners seem content. Family roles are well-delineated along traditional lines.

13.7. Family's support system: Each other (nuclear family members). May have persons at church or neighbors who serve as supports; however, no information available in this area.

13.8. Recreational activities: Very limited. The mother occasionally takes children to the neighborhood park. No books or toys seen in home.

Environmental Data

14.1. Home: Noted to be "minimally adequate." Two-bedroom, old, small wooden house; no carpeting, paucity of furniture, clean. Have a stove, refrigerator, washing machine, and radio. Heating is adequate (electric wall heating). Only unsafe conditions mentioned were that the screen is off the electric wall heater and no fan cover. Inadequate lighting may be safety problem. Types of privacy available: Parents share one bedroom. Have privacy. Boys share another bedroom. Maria does not have the privacy she needs nor a place of her own to play. Family may not perceive themselves as being crowded, since former housing was probably much less spacious. Need to assess for exposure to lead-based paint, since house is old and there are young children in the home.

14.2. Neighborhood and community: Neighborhood is low-income Mexican-American district in Los Angeles. Neighborhood is part of wider Los

Angeles community (a large metropolitan, heterogeneous city). Geographic mobility: Moved here 1 year ago from northern agrarian area in Mexico to the Los Angeles area.

14.3.   Associations and transactions with community: No associations in community except children in school and family attends mass at local Spanish-speaking Catholic church.

14.4.   Family's perceptions and feelings about the community: "Neighbors have been friendly." Family likes community, although worried about children's friends and high crime rate.

15.   Home safety problems: Absence of fan cover and electric wall heater screen are potential problems due to children's age, parents' probable knowledge deficit regarding safety hazards, and poor housing situation.

16.   a. Intervention for actual safety problem: Teach family members about danger of fan's cover and wall heater screen being absent and suggest that they either place fan in inaccessible place (after turning it on) or that they replace fan. They should ask owner to install screen over electric wall heater.

   b. Intervention for potential problems. Teach primary promotion to reduce likelihood of injury or illness due to potential environmental problems. For instance, because of young children in the home, teach about safe storage of medicines and toxic, poisonous substances and where to get emergency care in the neighborhood/community.

Family Communication Patterns and Processes

Marilyn M. Friedman

► learning objectives

1. Define the following systems and communications terms: communication, interaction, punctuation, the redundancy principle, and negative and positive feedback.

2. Identify the content and instruction levels of messages.

3. Compare the effects of negative and positive feedback.

4. Explain the meaning of the six principles of communication.

5. Name two characteristics of both the functional and dysfunctional sender and receiver.

6. Compare women's and men's communication relative to conversation, emotional expressiveness, decision making, and conflict resolution.

7. Identify major ways in which family communication patterns differ across cultures.

8. From hypothetical interactions, identify the use of assumptions, unclear expressions of feelings, judgmental expressions, inability to define needs, and incongruent communication.

9. Given a family case example, use the assessment questions included in this chapter to assess family communication, state a family nursing diagnosis in the area of family communication, and propose two family nursing interventions aimed at promoting more functional communication.

Family communications is conceptualized as one of the four structural dimensions of the family system, along with the power and role structure and the family value system. These dimensions are intimately interrelated and interdependent. Because the family is a social system, there is continual interaction and feedback between its internal and external environments. A change in one part of the family system is generally followed by a compensatory change in the other internal structural dimensions (see Fig. 10–1). Hence, although these dimensions are not separable in real life, they will be dealt with individually in the text for heuristic purposes.

In addition to having an organized scheme or structure, the family must have "system" functions—its purpose(s). Family structure or organization is ultimately evaluated by how well the family is able to fulfill its general functions (the goals important to its members

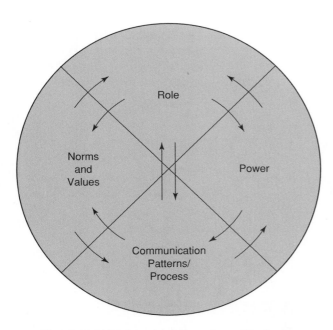

Figure 10–1. The structural dimensions of the family.

and society). The family's structure, especially its communication structure, serves to facilitate the achievement of family functions. For example, adequate family communication makes it possible for the family to socialize children, a basic family function.

Moreover, the communication patterns within the family system have a major impact on the individual members. Individualization, learning about other people, the development and maintenance of self-esteem, and the ability to make choices are all dependent on the information that is passed between members in the family.

▶ DEFINING COMMUNICATION

Communication refers to the process of exchanging feelings, desires, needs, information, and opinions (McCubbin & Dahl, 1985). Galvin and Brommel (1986) in an excellent book titled *Family Communication: Cohesion and Change* define family communication as a symbolic, transactional process of creating and sharing meanings in the family. Just as each person has his or her own distinct style of communication, so too does each family have its unique communication style or pattern.

Family communication can be viewed as both a structural dimension and as a system process. In other words, communication in the family can be considered as patterned content and described as a structural component, and as sequential interactions (as forms) over time and assessed as processes. In this chapter, a systems process oriented perspective is primarily used to discuss family communication. Applying this perspective, behavior is seen as synonymous with communication.

Clear and functional communication among family members is the crucial vehicle for maintaining a nurturing environment through which the necessary feelings regarding self-worth and self-esteem develop and become internalized. Conversely, unclear communications are believed to be a major contributor of poor family functioning (Holman, 1983; Satir, 1983; Satir et al., 1991).

The problem of flawed or problematic communication in families is ubiquitous. Watzlawick and associates (1967), researchers of family communication, estimate that 85 percent of all messages sent in families are misunderstood. With this observation in hand, it is not surprising that in a survey of family therapists 85 percent of couples seeking family therapy reported poor family communication as the primary problem bringing them into therapy (Beck & Jones, 1973, cited in Goldenberg & Goldenberg, 1996).

Ten sections are included in this chapter: elements of communication; communication principles; channels of communication; functional and dysfunctional communication processes; functional and dysfunctional family communication patterns; factors influencing family communication patterns; communication in families with health problems; and family nursing assessment, diagnosis, and intervention guidelines.

▶ ELEMENTS OF COMMUNICATION

As a consequence of using a general systems framework, family communication patterns and processes will be defined in this chapter as the processing of information within the family or its subsystems.

In the language of information processing, communication entails a sender of a message, a form/channel of the message, a receiver, and some interaction between the sender and the receiver. The sender is the person who is attempting to transmit a message to another person; the receiver is the target of the sender's message; forms/channels are the routes of the message. They extend from the cognitions (the thoughts) of the sender, through space, to the cognitions of the receiver.

Interaction is a broader term referring to the sending and receiving of messages, including the response that the message causes in the receiver *and* the sender. Interaction encompasses the dynamic, constantly changing process of communication between people (Watzlawick et al., 1967).

Messages initiated by the sender are always somewhat distorted—either by the sender, through the interaction between sender and receiver, or by the receiver. One primary cause of distortion is anxiety of either interactant; the greater the level of anxiety, the greater the possibility of misunderstanding. Another common cause of message distortion is a difference in the frames of reference of the interactants, due to dissimilarities, such as those created by differences in ages, ethnic background, or gender. In their daily interactions, family members usually assume that other family members have a similar frame of reference; since this is untrue in many cases, misunderstandings inevitably arise.

▶ COMMUNICATION PRINCIPLES

Watzlawick and co-workers (1967), in their seminal text on family communication, *Pragmatics of Human Communication*, delineate six principles of communication that are basic for understanding family communication processes.

First and foremost is the dictum that it is impossible not to communicate, as all behavior is communication. In any situation where two or more persons are present, we may not communicate verbally, but we cannot but help to communicate nonverbally. "All nonverbal communication is meaningful" (Wright & Leahey, 1994, p. 23).

A second principle of communication is that communication not only conveys information or content, but is coupled with a command (instruction). Messages therefore contain *two levels of communication: content and instruction*. Content is the literal definition of what actually is being said (verbal message), while instruc-

tion or the *metamessage* conveys the intent of the message. The content of a message may be a simple statement, but the metamessage or instruction depends on variables such as emotion, intent, and context, and may be expressed nonverbally by the rate and flow of speech, gestures, body position, and tone of voice. If "I am bored" is whispered in a theater to another member of the family, it may be a comment on the quality of the movie. If the "I am bored" message is sent in an emphatic manner during prolonged family discussion, the metamessage probably signifies anger, frustration, and heightened emotionality. Hence emotion, intent, and context have produced very different meanings in a message containing identical content. In the presence of disparity between the two levels of communication, the family member receiver usually "tunes in" more to the instructional level.

A third principle of communication delineated by Watzlawick and associates is what Bateson (1979), another communications researcher and groundbreaking theorist, calls *punctuations* in the sequences of communication. Communications involve a transactional process, and in the interchange each response contains the preceding communication, in addition to the preceding history of the relationship (Hartman & Laird, 1983). Different members of the family will explain interactional events and sequences differently because they impose their own punctuation into the explaining of a situation. Goldenberg and Goldenberg (1996) give a graphic example of this tendency:

> Each [in this case a mother and daughter] arbitrarily believes that what she says is caused by what the other person says. In a sense, such serial punctuations between family members resemble the dialogue of children quarreling: "You started it first!" and so on. . . . It is meaningless to search for a starting point to a conflict between two people because it is a complex repetitive interaction. . . . (p. 210)

In effect there is no beginning (cause) or end (effect) in communication transactions, because a circularity of responses occurs. Family members' interpersonal behaviors (communications) are therefore best understood by taking a circular rather than a linear view of causality (A $\leftrightarrows$ B rather than A $\rightarrow$ B).

To further understand the idea of "punctuations" in communication sequences, the notion of feedback loops needs to be reviewed. Communication serves as an organizing, purposeful, and self-regulating process in families. Self-regulating processes in a system are dependent on two-way communication, termed feedback loops. According to von Bertalanffy (1966), feedback loops are "circular, causal chains." As Figure 10–2 indicates, feedback loops in communication trigger necessary change in the family system that keeps the system "on track." A family member can alter his or her communications (output) based on the information he or she receives regarding the effects of his or her previous outputs on other members. Through feedback mechanisms, a portion of any system's output is reintroduced into the system as input information about the original output (Goldenberg & Goldenberg, 1996). Feedback loops have been likened to home thermostats. Setting the thermostat at 72°F programs a detector device to activate the heating system when the temperature drops below that point. Also a feedback mechanism signals the furnace to cut off the heat once the desired temperature has been obtained.

A continual exchange of communication occurs in families—involving introducing new information, correcting misinformation, problem solving, having and resolving misunderstandings and conflicts, and so forth. The feedback loops entailed in these transactions may be negative or positive.

Negative feedback is "positive." It is the most productive type of feedback because it is corrective; it regulates or modulates communications or information flow so that the system may adjust homeostatically or maintain stability. "Negative" is not a judgmental term, but is simply a reference to the direction in which the information flows (see Fig. 10–2). Self-regulating negative feedback is present when a sender initiates an interaction by sending a message and then, because of a new input received from sender, modifies his or her message before a reply is possible or expected. The problem-solving

and decision-making process depend on negative feedback. This process begins when a problem arises and is identified. In the family problem-solving situation, the sender or initiator of the interaction usually identifies the problem, family members then explore the problem, various solutions are discussed, and a decision is finally made.

Positive feedback, in contrast, is often "negative." It increases instability or deviation from a homeostatic state. In the above case the furnace would continue and the home would get hotter and hotter. Theoretically, if positive feedback continues it has the potential of amplifying deviation to the point that the system self-destructs or no longer functions (Steinglass, 1978, cited in Goldenberg & Goldenberg, 1996). An argument between parent and child that continues to escalate is an example of a common type of family positive feedback interaction.

From these examples positive feedback sounds like it always has adverse consequences. This is not so. Positive feedback needs to occur in families for change and growth to take place. There may be immediate instability and tension created in the family system, but in the long run, selective use of positive feedback is necessary for change and growth to take place.

A fourth principle of communication described by Watzlawick and co-workers (1967) is that *there are two types of communication: digital and analogic*. Digital communication is essentially verbal communication using words with commonly understood meanings. The second kind of communication, analogic, is where the idea or thing being communicated is transmitted nonverbally in a representational manner (Hartman & Laird, 1983). Analogic communication, known commonly as body language, sends messages by means of posture, facial expressions, the rhythm and cadence of the spoken words, "or any other nonverbal manifestation of which the person is capable" (Watzlawick et al., 1967, p. 62). Analogic communication, which conveys the metacommunication, although often ambiguous and imprecise, tends to be a more powerful way to communicate about relationships (Hartman & Laird, 1983).

A fifth communication principle described by the same group of family communication theorists (Jackson, Haley, Bateson, and Watzlawick) is called the **redundancy principle**. It has been consistently observed that a family interacts within a limited range of repetitive behavioral sequences. Hence, if a family observer

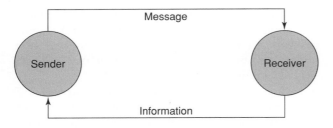

Figure 10–2. Negative feedback loop. *(Adapted from von Bertalanffy, 1968.)*

misses one instance of a behavioral sequence or pattern, according to the redundancy principle, this sequence will soon manifest itself again.

Watzlawick and associates (1967) point out that the repetitive behavioral sequences are circular communication patterns. Repetitive circular communication patterns occur in every family. An example of a repetitive communication pattern in a family is the following scenario. In the Jones family, when the youngest child is angry and has a temper tantrum, the mother rushes to his side to console him. The child then responds by demanding his way, and the mother gives in. Wright and Leahey (1984) suggest diagraming circular communication patterns, as the diagrams tend to "concretize and simplify repetitive sequences noted in a relationship" (p. 56). The basic elements of a circular pattern diagram are shown in Figure 10–3, and an example of a diagram is given in Figure 10–4.

The repetitive interaction patterns in families are evidence that **communication rules** operate in families. They naturally emerge as a consequence of the multiple interactions among family members, as they come to know what is expected of each other. Knapp (1984) asserts that covert and overt rules exist to inform family when and what communication is required, preferred and/or prohibited.

The sixth communication principle described by Bateson and associates (1963) is that all communicational interactions are either *symmetrical or complementary*. In symmetrical communication one interactant's behavior mirrors the behavior of the other interactant (e.g., both mates would equally contribute to the decision about where to go for vacation). In complementary communication, one interactant's behavior

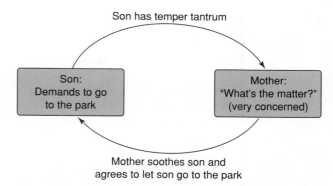

Figure 10–4. Example of circular communication pattern diagram.

supplements the other interactant's behavior (e.g., the husband says he has selected a particular place to go for vacation and the wife nods that she has heard him). When one of these two types of communication is used consistently in family relationships, the communication type is reflective of family values and role and power arrangements.

► CHANNELS OF COMMUNICATION

Channels of information flow are the routes that information may take to reach a receiver. Family communication networks also refer to the flow of messages back and forth among family members (Jenkins, 1995). In the family, these involve the flow of information between the various sets of relationships or members. An example in a patriarchal family would be that a command type communication would go from father to mother to children. This is called a vertical communication network. Families have usual channels of information flow, which reveal the family power structure (the example just described), the closeness of relationships, family roles, and the popularity of individuals within the family. The popularity or centrality of individual members is indicated by a convergence of many channels of information to one person. This person serves as intermediary or "go-between" in families. In contrast, a relative absence of channels to a family member may reveal unpopularity, fear, rejection, or the member's outsider position. Chapter 11 further explains this process.

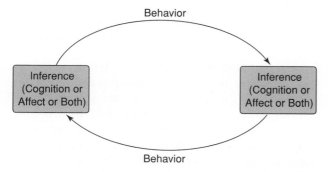

Figure 10–3. Basic elements of a circular communication pattern diagram. *(Wright & Leahey, 1994.)*

▶ FUNCTIONAL COMMUNICATION PROCESSES

Functional communication is viewed as the cornerstone of a successful, healthy family and as such is defined as the clear, direct transmission and reception of both the content and instruction level of any message (Sells, 1973), as well as the congruency between the content and the instruction levels (Satir, 1983; Satir et al., 1991). In other words, functional or healthy communication in the family requires that the intention or meaning of the sender be sent through relatively clear channels and that the receiver of the message have an understanding of its meaning that is similar to that of the sender (Sells, 1973). Effective communication means matching meaning, and attaining consistency and congruence between the intended and the received message. Thus effective communication in the family is a process of constant definition and redefinition that will achieve a matching of the content and instructional levels of messages. Both the sender and the receiver must be actively involved and capable of interchanging positions by becoming either sender or receiver during the process.

In the following two sections descriptions of the specific verbal behaviors the functional sender and functional receiver use when communicating are reviewed. Table 10–1 summarizes these processes.

The Functional Sender

Satir (1967) states that the sender who communicates in a functional way can:

1. Firmly and clearly state his or her case.
2. At the same time clarify and qualify what he or she says.
3. Ask for feedback.
4. Be receptive to feedback when he or she gets it.

Because each of these four elements is basic to understanding healthy communication, each will be briefly discussed.

Firmly and Clearly Stating Case.

Congruent Levels. One of the foundations for firmly stating one's case is the use of communication

---

▶ TABLE 10–1

SPECIFIC FUNCTIONAL AND DYSFUNCTIONAL COMMUNICATION PROCESSES

■ **FUNCTIONAL COMMUNICATION PROCESSES**
Sender
Firmly and clearly states case.
Clarifies and qualifies messages.
Invites feedback.
Is receptive to feedback.
Receiver
Actively and effectively listens.
Gives feedback.
Validates the merit or worth of the message.

■ **DYSFUNCTIONAL COMMUNICATION PROCESSES**
Sender
Makes assumptions.
Expresses feelings unclearly.
Makes judgmental responses.
Is unable to define own needs.
Exhibits incongruent communication.
Receiver
Fails to listen.
Uses disqualification.
Responds offensively and negatively.
Fails to explore sender's message.
Fails to validate messages.
Both Sender and Receiver
Communicate on different wavelengths (parallel talk).
Are unable to focus on one issue.

---

that is congruent on both the content and instruction levels. Satir (1975) calls the person who uses this style of communication a congruent communicator. For example, in the case of a person who is angry, to be congruent not only should the literal message denote anger, but also the tone of voice, body position, and gestures should reflect the same message.

Intensity and Explicitness. When a person communicates, the sender is asking something of the receiver. Such requests include various degrees of intensity and explicitness, both of which involve how firmly the sender states his or her case. Intensity refers to the ability of the sender to effectively communicate internal perceptions of feelings, desires, and needs at the same intensity as he or she is experiencing these perceptions internally.

To be explicit, the functional sender informs the receiver of how serious the message is by stating how the receiver should respond to the message. An example illustrating a high degree of explicitness is: "I want to go home now. I am very tired."

Clarifying and Qualifying Messages.

A second dimension Satir identifies as an essential characteristic of the functional sender is the use of clarifying and qualifying statements in his or her communication. The use of clarifying and qualifying statements enables the sender to be specific and to check out his or her perception of reality against that of the other person. Specific types of clarifying and qualifying statements include those described below.

"I Want" Statements.

A statement that clearly states what the sender wants (Strayhorn, 1977). Example: "Stop contradicting me when I'm disciplining the children."

"I Feel" Statements.

The sender directly states his or her internal perceptions of a specific feeling. These feelings may be internally triggered or may be a reaction to another person's behavior (Strayhorn, 1977). Example of an internally triggered expression: "I sometimes feel frustrated when my hands ache and I'm unable to do the chores around the house" (a patient with arthritis); an externally triggered expression: "When you call me stupid in front of the children, I feel embarrassed and irritated."

"I Intend" Statements.

This type of statement implies a concrete independent action will be initiated by the sender. Example: "I'm still experiencing weakness after my surgery and plan to take a nap this afternoon."

"I Like" and "I Don't Like" Statements.

These are statements in which the sender states precisely what gives him or her pleasure or displeasure, or what the receiver does or does not do that bothers the sender (Strayhorn, 1977). Examples: "I like it when you clean up your room" and "I don't like it when I have to stay in my room by myself when I'm sick."

Self-disclosure Statements.

A self-disclosure statement by an individual refers to an open and honest revelation of an intention, desire, or past action, or a fallibility that is considered private or personal to that individual. Examples: "I'm concerned about my biopsy because my mother died from cancer of the breast" and "I'm scared to show my anger because my husband may leave me."

Direct Questions.

This involves asking concrete questions to elicit specific information. Example: "Are your stitches causing you any pain?"

Open-Ended Questions.

Open-ended questions focus on a general area of interest and encourage the receiver to express his or her own response. Open-ended questions do not structure the receiver's response. Example: "Tell me more about your reluctance to have the surgery."

Inviting Feedback.

A third element of a functional sender is the use of asking for feedback, which enables him or her to verify whether the message was received accurately, as well as enabling the sender to gain information needed to clarify his or her intent. In the following examples the sender seeks feedback to obtain the receiver's perception or reaction to what the sender has communicated: "I keep asking myself, should we tell the children that I have cancer? What do you think?" "Since you're still on limited activities because of your heart condition, I think your parents should visit at another time. What's your reaction?"

Receptivity of Sender to Feedback.

The sender who is receptive to feedback will exhibit a willingness to listen, react nondefensively, and attempt to understand. In order to understand, the sender must not have so narrow a perspective that he or she is unable to comprehend the validity of the receiver's point of view. Thus by asking for more specific criticism or "checking out" statements, the sender demonstrates his or her receptivity and interest in feedback (Strayhorn, 1977).

The Functional Receiver

Functional receivers try to make an accurate assessment of the intent of a message. By doing this they are better able to correctly weigh the message's meaning and can more precisely assess the sender's attitudes, intentions, and feelings as expressed in the metacommunication. According to Anderson (1972), the functional receiver tries to comprehend the material fully before attempting to evaluate. This means that motivations and metacommunication, as well as content, are analyzed. The new information is checked with that which is already known, and the decision to act is carefully weighed. Listening effectively, giving feedback, and validating are three communication techniques which enable the receiver to comprehend and respond more fully to the sender's message.

Listening.

The ability to listen effectively is perhaps the most important quality of a functional receiver. Listening effectively means focusing one's full attention on what is being communicated, thus blocking out all extraneous "noise." The receiver attends to the sender's complete message rather than prejudging the meaning of the communication. Sells (1973) explains:

> To listen is
> to be still
> to expect
> to wait for a response
> to practice restraint. (p. 23)

Many people are passive listeners, responding with blank expressions and a seemingly "couldn't care less" attitude. An active listener responds with gestures that communicate actively listening. Asking questions is a vital part of active listening (Gottman et al., 1977). It is as if the receiver were a student learning a new subject, and as a good student, questions are asked and facts are explored. To listen actively means to be empathetic, to think of the other person's needs and desires, and to not disrupt the sender's flow of communication.

Giving Feedback.

The second major characteristic of the functional receiver involves feedback—

that is feeding information back to the sender that tells how the message was interpreted by the receiver. The following are examples of giving feedback.

Asking Sender to Clarify and Qualify.   These statements encourage the sender to elaborate more fully. Example: "What do you mean when you say I get frustrated too easily with the children?"

Associating.   In the process of associating, the receiver makes a relationship between previous personal experiences (Gottman et al., 1977) or past related incidents and the sender's communication. Example: During her last trimester of pregnancy, Susie comments to the family nurse, "I have been getting upset quite easily and feel more dependent upon my husband. I never felt this way until I got pregnant."

The nurse responds, "I remember when I was pregnant having the same type of feelings. I would frequently ask my husband to do little things for me which I always did for myself before I was pregnant. In the families I visit the women have often shared these same types of feelings with me."

Paraphrasing and Checking Perceptions.   The receiver, by using either a question or a statement, summarizes the sender's message (Gottman et al., 1977). The receiver does this by restating the sender's message in his or her own words. The central purpose of paraphrasing is to clarify the sender's message. Examples: "So you're saying . . ." and "What I understand is. . . ."

Providing Validation.

The third major technique the functional receiver uses is validation. In utilizing validation the receiver conveys the following: "I can see how you think and feel that way" or "It makes sense and is reasonable to feel that way." Validation does not imply that the receiver agrees with the sender's communication, but demonstrates an acceptance of the merit and/or worth of the message (Gottman et al., 1977).

▶ DYSFUNCTIONAL COMMUNICATION PROCESSES

Just as there are functional ways to communicate, there are also dysfunctional ways (see Table 10–1). We all use both, but to various degrees and at various times. The following are descriptions of specific communication behaviors of dysfunctional senders and receivers.

The Dysfunctional Sender

The dysfunctional sender's communication is often ineffective in one or more of the four basic characteristics of the functional sender: in stating case, in clarifying and qualifying, in eliciting, and/or in being receptive to feedback. The receiver is often left confused and has to guess what the sender is thinking or feeling. The communication of the dysfunctional sender is either actively or passively defensive and often negates the possibility of seeking any clear feedback from the receiver. "Unhealthy" sender communication is discussed under five major categories: assumptions, the unclear expression of feelings, judgmental expressions, inability to define needs, and incongruent communication.

Making Assumptions.   When assumptions are made, the sender takes for granted what the receiver is feeling or thinking about an event or person without validating his or her perceptions. The dysfunctional sender is usually not aware of the assumptions he or she is making. He or she rarely clarifies content or intent, thus serving to obscure and distort meaning. When this dysfunction in communication occurs, it elicits anger in the receiver, who is being given the message that his or her own opinions and feelings do not matter much. The following illustrations represent various forms of the use of assumptions.

Speaking for the Other.   The sender acts as a spokesperson for another by telling someone else what the person is thinking or feeling (Gottman et al., 1977). Example: Without checking with spouse, the husband comments to the children, "It is perfectly obvious that your mother never wants to go on walks with us."

What Is Perceived or Evaluated Cannot Be Altered.   The individual assumes that what he or she has perceived or evaluated cannot be changed. Examples: "Jim has always been messy. I've just had to learn to live with that fact." Or, "Joey's so accident prone, but that's life."

Incomplete Messages.   The sender does not finish the sentence or message but assumes that the receiver will complete it. Example: "He said we couldn't agree on . . . you see what I mean?"

Assumes Others Share Same Perceptions, Thoughts, and Feelings.   The sender automatically takes for granted that other people share his or her perceptions, thoughts, and feelings (Satir, 1983). Example: "I dislike going to the free clinic; I know you feel the same way."

Generalizations.   The content of the message describes behavior or events in general terms instead of citing specific behaviors and observations. The sender assumes that the receiver will fill in the specifics. Example: "You're such a poor father," as opposed to, "I wish you would discipline Sarah when she doesn't put away her toys."

One Instance Exemplifies All Instances. The individual, in failing to learn that thoughts, actions, and sentiments change, falls into the error of overgeneralizing and makes an assumption that one situation is an example of all similar situations to follow. Example: "The nurse at the free clinic was impatient and blunt with me. I'm not going there again to get this same treatment from her and the rest of the staff."

Expressing Feelings Unclearly. Another type of dysfunctional communication by the sender is unclear expression of feelings. Due to fear of rejection, the sender's expressions of feelings must go underground or be uttered in such a covert manner that the feelings are not recognizable. In another instance, the sender may express his or her feelings but does so without the same intensity as the feelings were perceived internally, the usual situation being that feelings are understated. Various types of unclear expression of feelings will be presented.

Sarcasm.   Sarcasm denotes the use of humorous or witty statements that enable the sender of a message to avoid taking responsibility for his or her hostile feelings. If confronted, the sender can always reply that he or she was just being humorous. Example: "Fathers were made to play with their sons while mothers were made to take all the responsibility for raising them."

Super-reasonableness.   Satir (1975; Satir et al., 1991) describes being super-reasonable as one of the four modes of dysfunctionally communicating. In this situation the sender's words bear no relationship to how he or she feels. Messages are stated in an unemotional way.

Silent Resentment.   In the case of unclear expression of feeling, the sender feels irritated with the receiver but does not express the anger overtly and/or may displace the resentment onto another person or thing (Satir, 1983). Example: The children have broken a second window in the period of a week. Joan is infuriated but remains silent. When her husband comes home from work, she coldly stares at him and then leaves the room (displacement of anger onto the husband).

Expression of Hurt as Anger.   The sender expresses anger as a defensive maneuver to cover up feelings of hurt, rather than expressing the more basic emotion of hurt. Example: Eileen takes great pride in creating various artistic items for her home. She has just completed a new floral arrangement and made some new drapes for the living room. When her husband comes home from work she proudly shows him the items, at which he only nods his head and seems preoccupied and disinterested. Eileen angrily states, "I'm sick and tired of trying to share my interests with you." This communication technique is extensively used. When hurt (the underlying emotion) is expressed, rather than the cover-up emotion, anger, the receiver then usually reacts in a more appropriate and positive fashion.

Making Judgmental Responses.   This category of dysfunctional communication is characterized by a tendency to constantly evaluate messages in terms of the sender's own value system. Judgmental statements always carry moral overtones where it is clear to the receiver that the sender is evaluating the worth of the other person's message as being "right" or "wrong," "good" or "bad," "normal" or "abnormal." It is not only a message that is being evaluated or judged, but also the sender of a message who is being indirectly evaluated or judged. Two types of judgmental expression are put-down statements or questions and "you should" statements.

Put-down Statements/Questions or Blaming.   These are statements or questions that carry a negative connotation and value judgment. Judgmental expressions may also involve a covert unmet need or an unexpressed dissatisfaction with the other interactant. Examples: "You are really clumsy." (As opposed to, "I want you to be more careful when carrying a glass of milk.") Blaming occurs in families where the blamer wants to let the receiver(s) know who is boss. In families blamers are often called "tyrants" or "dominating husbands or wives" (Satir, 1975; Satir et al., 1991).

"You Should" Statements.   The words "should" or "ought to" imply that the sender is an authority figure who knows what is "good" or "bad." If the sender is a parent and the receiver the child, this type of communication may be functional and necessary in the socialization process, but must generally be held to be a dysfunctional mode of communication. Example: Family health nurse to mother, "Johnny's too fat! You should feed him less."

Inability to Define Own Needs.   The dysfunctional sender is not only unable to express his or her needs, but due to fear of rejection is incapable of defining the behaviors he or she expects from the receiver to fulfill them. Often the dysfunctional sender unconsciously feels unworthy, with no right to express needs or expect that personal needs will be met. Various examples of the sender's inability to express needs follow.

Silent Need for Nurturance. The silent need for nurturance is defined as an unexpressed need for help, empathy, or some aspect of "being taken care of." This may also include an expectation that others should be able to anticipate the sender's needs and that asking for nurturance or assistance renders the response to such requests inauthentic and unsatisfying (Strayhorn, 1977). Example: After her radiation therapy, Jane sometimes experiences nausea. Jack, not realizing his wife's discomfort, does not offer to prepare dinner. When Jane finally asks for Jack's assistance, she feels angry even though he agrees to prepare dinner.

Covert Requests. These types of requests are made without acknowledging "ownership" (the sender does not overtly admit his or her wishes) (Strayhorn, 1977). Example: "It would do you good to spend more time with the children." (The sender does not directly ask the other to spend time with the children.)

Complaints. In this case the sender appears unable or unwilling to describe the desired behavior needed from the receiver, and the sender expresses these needs in terms of a dissatisfaction. Example: the Smiths, a couple in their 70s, typically complain to their children, "You never visit us." (As opposed to, "Please come over for dinner Wednesday evening.")

Exhibiting Incongruent Communication.
In this type of dysfunctional communication, two or more simultaneous and contradictory messages are sent. The receiver is left with the enigma of how to respond.

Verbal–Verbal Incongruency. In this case two or more literal messages sent simultaneously oppose each other. Examples: "Jimmy's such a well-behaved child. Did I tell you last week he had another fight at school?"

Verbal–Nonverbal Incongruency. The sender communicates a message verbally, but the accompanying nonverbal metacommunication contradicts the verbal message (Satir, 1983). This is commonly known as giving "mixed messages." Example: "I'm not angry with you!" spoken in a loud, gruff tone of voice with fists clenched.

The Dysfunctional Receiver

When the receiver is dysfunctional, a breakdown in communication occurs because the message is not received as intended due to the receiver's failure to listen, or the use of disqualification. Responding offensively, failing to explore the sender's message, and failing to validate the message are other dysfunctional characteristics.

Failing to Listen.
In the case of failure to listen, a message is sent, but the receiver does not attend to or hear the message. There may be many reasons for failure to listen, ranging from willfull inattention to a wish but an inability to listen. This is commonly due to concomitant distraction, such as noise, improper timing, or high anxiety (Sells, 1973). A frequently used way in which individuals do not listen is by ignoring messages.

CLIENT: I keep wondering if I will always be this limited in my activities because of my heart condition.

NURSE: Has the swelling in your ankles decreased?

Failure to listen causes distortion and misinterpretation of the message.

Using Disqualification.
A disqualification is an indirect response that allows the receiver to disagree with a message without really disagreeing.

"Yes-Butting." The dysfunctional receiver partially agrees with the intent of the message, yet at the same time finds something wrong with the sender's opinion, feeling, or suggestions (Gottman et al., 1977).

NURSE: When Bobby has temper tantrums, why don't you try going in to see that he's all right, and then leave him alone until he calms down.

BOBBY'S MOTHER: Yes, that's a fine idea, but I'm afraid he would hurt himself.

Evasion. The receiver disqualifies the message by avoiding the crucial issue.

NURSE: Well, how effective was leaving the room when Bobby had a temper tantrum?

HUSBAND: Wouldn't you say it worked, Jean, because the number of tantrums decreased this week?

WIFE: Bobby's constant requests are driving me crazy.

Tangentialization and Distraction.   Here the receiver responds to a peripheral aspect of a message and ignores the central intention or content of the message. He or she "distracts" by responding with words and behavior that are irrelevant or unrelated to the message sent or what is going on (Satir, 1975).

HUSBAND: All of my recreational interests were of a strenuous nature, so all I do now is complain to my wife that I have nothing to do all day.

WIFE: I love strenuous activities myself and have always been interested in tennis.

Responding Offensively and Negatively.
Offensiveness in communication denotes that the receiver of a message reacts negatively, as if being threatened. The receiver seems to react defensively to the message by assuming an oppositional posture and an attacking position. Statements and requests are consistently made in a negative manner or with a negative expectation (Harris, 1975). The family member receiving the consistently negative communication learns to respond with similar statements or behavior. Habitually conflicted couples behave this way.

Attacking With a Different Issue.   Before any progress is made on a threatening issue introduced by the sender, the person receiving the message responds with an extraneous issue that hurts or threatens the sender—that is, the receiver uses a "counterattack."

WIFE: I very rarely see you set any limits on the children.

HUSBAND: After 5 years I keep wondering when you're going to learn to cook a decent meal.

Insulting.   The receiver attributes a negative or insulting characteristic to the sender. In other words, the receiver attacks the sender, not the issue (Gottman et al., 1977).

CHILD: Dad, you never play baseball with me anymore.

FATHER: You're so uncoordinated that you can't even catch the ball.

Rebuff.   In response to requests to clarify or qualify, the receiver conveys disgust by refusing to elaborate or to comply with the sender's request. Examples: "How many times do I have to repeat myself?" And, "You heard me the first time."

Failing to Explore Sender's Message.
In order to clarify the intent or meaning of a message, the functional responder seeks further explanation. In contrast, the dysfunctional receiver uses responses that negate exploration, such as making assumptions (as discussed previously), giving premature advice, or cutting off communication.

Premature Advice.   Premature advice is defined as the offering of a suggestion or solution to a problem before exploring it sufficiently or requesting additional feedback.

PATIENT: This diagnosis of multiple sclerosis has really been a shock.

NURSE: I'd suggest rest periods during the day, and don't overtire yourself by engaging in strenuous activities.

A functional response would have been to explore the emotional impact of the diagnosis on the patient.

Cutoffs in Communication.   When the dysfunctional receiver does not want to continue discussing the issue at hand, he or she makes a statement or uses an action that curtails any further discussion of that issue. This technique is often used to avoid dealing with unpleasant or negative feelings (Strayhorn, 1977). Examples: "Let's just forget it" and "It's not that important." In addition, physical actions are another way of cutting off communication. For example, the receiver could leave the room, engage in busywork, or turn away from the sender.

Failing to Validate Messages.

As stated previously, the receiver in an interaction often has the difficult task of attempting to correctly interpret both the content and the intent of the message. Validation, as previously defined, refers to the receiver's conveyance of acceptance. Therefore, lack of validation implies that the receiver either responds neutrally (shows neither acceptance nor nonacceptance) or distorts and misinterprets the message. Assuming rather than clarifying the thoughts of the sender is one example of a lack of validation.

NEW MOTHER: My mother has just come to stay with us for 3 weeks to take care of the new baby while I get my strength back.

FAMILY NURSE: How wonderful I'm sure that your mother will be a tremendous help to you during this time.

This interaction is dysfunctional because the nurse assumes that the client has positive feelings about her mother's assistance without exploring with the mother her evaluation of her mother's helpfulness.

Dysfunctional Senders and Receivers

Two types of unhealthy communication interactional sequences, involving both senders and receivers, are also widely discussed in the communication literature. These are communications that reflect "parallel" talk and that demonstrate the inability to focus on one issue (see Table 10–1).

Parallel Talk (Communicating on Different Wavelengths).

Each individual in the interaction constantly restates his or her own issues without really listening to the other's point of view or acknowledging the other's needs.

WIFE: To discipline the children, I have them spend 15 minutes in their room. I'm not a believer in severe punishment.

HUSBAND: I believe in stern limits. Last week I took Jody's allowance away for a month and refused to let him play outside for a week.

WIFE: Yes, 15 minutes in their room gets the point across.

HUSBAND: If you dish out stern punishment, the children really listen.

In this situation, each partner continued to restate his or her own viewpoint and did not acknowledge that of the other.

Inability to Focus on One Issue.

Each of the individuals in the interaction rambles from one issue to another instead of resolving any one problem discussed or obtaining closure.

HUSBAND: I'm tired of your mother visiting without calling first.

WIFE: When are you going to take Jack shopping?

HUSBAND: Soon as you balance the checking account correctly.

Notice how each partner introduces a new problem without any attempts of a discussion of one problem at a time.

▶ FUNCTIONAL COMMUNICATION PATTERNS IN THE FAMILY

As distinguished from the discussion of functional communication processes in any context, this section covers family communication rather than specific or discrete interactional exchanges.

Family communication patterns are the characteristic, ongoing, circular interactional patterns of the family, which in addition to influencing and organizing the members of the family, produce the meaning of transactions between family members (Peters, 1974).

Most importantly, it is through interaction that the affective needs of family members are fulfilled. The ability of family members to recognize and respond to nonverbal messages is an important attribute of healthy families. Most family communications take place within the subsystems (the parent–child, spousal–parental, and sibling subsystems), making analysis of subsystem communications in the family a primary locus of interest.

Curran (1983), who extensively studied and described healthy families, writes that the first trait of a healthy family is *clear communication and the ability to listen to each other.* Good communication is necessary for loving relationships to develop and be maintained.

Communicating Clearly and Congruently

In healthy families, family members in most cases communicate congruently. Congruence is a key construct in the Satir growth and communication model. Congruence "is a state of being and a way of communicating with ourselves and others" (Satir et al., 1991, p. 65). When family members communicate congruently there is consistency between the content (the literal message) and the instruction (the metamessage) levels of the communication. What is actually being said is compatible with what the intent of the message is. The words we speak, the affect we express, and the behavior we display are all consistent with each other. With congruency, the receiver is able more clearly to comprehend the sender's message, making communication in the family much healthier. Satir explains the meaning of congruence further when she states that the self (the sender), the other (what the receiver is having conveyed), and the context or situation in which the communication takes place all are in harmony with each other (Satir, 1975).

Satir (1967) emphasizes that in healthy interaction family members recognize each other's *differentness.* Differentness or the acknowledgment of the individuality and uniqueness of each member, is encouraged to the degree that is reciprocally beneficial to the family system and each individual. A sufficient amount of overt openness and honesty exists to enable members to recognize the needs and emotions of one another.

The communication patterns in a functional family demonstrate acceptance of difference, as well as a minimum of judgments and unrealistic criticism of each other. Adjustments that one family member needs to make in his or her behavior (like a mother returning to school) generate healthy adjustments in the whole family; one person is not expected to do all of the changing necessary for the family to continue in a stable manner, and suffi-

cient cohesiveness and flexibility exist for the family to adapt effectively.

Communication in healthy families is an extremely dynamic two-way process. Messages are not simply sent and received by a sender and a receiver. For instance, as the sender begins a message, the receiver may show a facial expression that will, through "negative" feedback, change the sender's message before he or she is finished speaking. As a result, the sender might change the wording of a message in the middle of the sending action so that the receiver will have a similar frame of reference. This dynamic nature of functional communication, however, makes interaction complex and unpredictable. Communication, even in the healthiest of families, many times is still tenuous and problematic. In functional families feelings of family members are also allowed expression. Satir (1983) believes that the acknowledgment of feelings is vital to a family's healthy functioning.

Emotional Communication

Emotional communication deals with the expression of emotions or feelings—from the expression of anger, hurt, sadness, and jealousy to happiness, affection, and tenderness (Wright & Leahey, 1994). Lewis and associates (1976), in carefully studying the differences between dysfunctional and functional white families, found that healthy families displayed a full spectrum of feelings, while more dysfunctional families were emotionally constricted and rigid in their expression of feelings. For instance, in more dysfunctional families anger was permitted from parents to children, but not the reverse. Neither were overt expressions of tenderness and affection permitted in these families. Emotional expression (by both parents and children) in one recent study confirmed the positive impact that emotional expressiveness had on children's social competency (Boyum & Parke, 1995).

Affective communication—the verbal messages of caring and nonverbal, physical gestures of touching, caressing, holding, and looking—is especially important. As Bowlby (1966) demonstrated, physical expressions of affection in early childhood are essential in the development of normal affectional responses. Later in life, verbal affectional communication patterns become more predominant in relaying affectional messages. It should be noted here, however, that cultural background makes a big difference in how much emotional communication is permitted to take place.

As part of healthy affective communications, the family members need to be able to communicate their enjoyment of each other's company. When their responses to each other are fresh and spontaneous, rather than controlled, repetitive, and predictable, this enjoyment can be realized.

Open Areas of Communication and Self-Disclosure

Functional families, those with functional communication patterns, value openness; a mutual respect for each other's feelings, thoughts, and concerns, spontaneity; authenticity; and self-disclosure. It follows that these families would also be able to discuss most areas of life—both personal and social issues and concerns and would not be afraid of conflict. These areas are referred to as "open areas of communication." With respect to self-disclosure, Satir (1972) asserts that family members who *level* with each other are people who feel self-confident enough to risk meaningful interaction. People with good self-esteem tend to be levelers who believe in self-disclosure—a revealing of intimate thoughts and feelings.

Satir and other family therapists assume that complete honesty/self-disclosure is ideal. Contrary to this notion, research in marital relationships demonstrates that total honesty and self-disclosure may not work for many couples. Many satisfied couples report that they do not tell one another everything, for fear it would jeopardize the relationship, hurt the partner's feelings, or create more interpersonal or personal stress (McCubbin & Dahl, 1985; Pearlin & Schooler, 1978). Hawkins, Weisberg, and Ray (1980), family communication researchers, observe that very few marital partners have ideal functional communication styles.

It is generally true, however, that the more functional the family, the fewer areas of closed communication exist, and vice versa. Nevertheless, consideration of a family's culture is also crucial here, because cultural norms concerning modesty, privacy, and sexual roles play a very large part in influencing what areas of communication are open and closed.

Power Hierarchy and Family Rules

Family systems are based on power hierarchies or "pecking orders," wherein communication containing "commands or imperatives" generally flows downward in family communication networks. *Functional* interaction in the power hierarchy occurs when power is distributed according to the developmental needs of the family members (Minuchin, 1974), or when power is assigned according to the abilities and resources of family members and is consonant with the family's cultural prescriptions of family power relationships. (See Chap. 11 for a more complete discussion of the family power structure.)

Power communications have characteristics that are readily apparent. The communication, "Joan, I want you to go upstairs and clean your room now or I will not take you to the show this afternoon" is typical of a coercive power communication. It is a command type message, specifying the action the receiver is to carry out (Miller, 1969).

Family Conflict and Family Conflict Resolution

George Simmel (1858–1918), one of the founding fathers of sociology, was the first scientific observer of the role that conflict plays in human interactions. Simmel's central thesis in writing about human interactions was that conflict is a vital form of social interaction. He believed that social conflict is both ubiquitous and essential for group development and maintenance (Coser, 1956). Conflict functions to maintain family communications and interaction in several important ways (Table 10–2).

Verbal conflict is a routine part of normal family interaction. The literature on family conflict indicates that healthy families seem to be able "to strike a delicate balance between enough conflict to realize the positive benefits, but not too much conflict which would disrupt family relationships" (Vuchinich, 1987, p. 591).

Conflict resolution is a vital task of interaction in the family. Spouses need to learn to have constructive conflicts. Although how marital partners resolve conflict varies, functional conflict resolution occurs when the conflict is openly discussed and strategies to solve the conflict are employed, or when parents

▶ TABLE 10–2

SUMMARY OF SIMMEL'S IDEAS ON CONFLICT

1. Conflict is designed to resolve divergent dualisms; it is a way of achieving some kind of unity.

2. Conflict is often necessary to keep an ongoing relationship going. Without ways of venting hostility toward each other and expressing dissent, family members may feel completely powerless and demoralized, with withdrawal as the usual outcome. By releasing pent-up feelings of hostility, conflicts serve to maintain a relationship.

3. Close, intimate family relationships are likely to contain both converging and diverging motivations, both "love and hatred." In relationships where persons are deeply involved, where they are engaged with their total personalities rather than a segment of it (like their work role only), there arise feelings of both love and hate . . . both attraction and repulsion. This great involvement or investment in a relationship also leads interactants to be likely to suppress hostility to avoid risking their relationship.

4. When conflict does occur, the closer the relationship, the more intense the conflict. The more we have in common with another, as whole people, the more easily will our totality be involved. Therefore, if a quarrel arises between people in such an intimate relationship, it is often so passionately expansive.

5. In marriage and family relationships, the absence of conflict is not functional—it is not an appropriate criterion for judging the vitality, strength, or stability of family interactions. In fact, the very absence of conflict may be an indicator of the existence of underlying strain and insecurity. Closeness in family relationships generates frequent occasions for conflict, but if family members do not feel secure in their relationships, they will avoid conflict, fearing its presence might threaten the continuance of their relationship. In this case, the couple's or family members' disagreements, differences, and hostilities go underground, and their communication becomes more covert and indirect.

Source: Adapted from Simmel (1955).

appropriately utilize their authority to close off conflicts. Parents need to act as role models for their children in terms of expressing conflict/differences and resolving these conflicts.

Research on Marital Interactions

Through observational means, John Gottman (1995) since the late 1970s has been investigating marital interaction in happy and unhappy marriages. He has exploded the myth of earlier researchers who thought that exchange theory explained marital interaction, e.g., if husband sends a sarcastic message, wife responds likewise. The following are some major differences he has found in marital interaction between happy and unhappy couples (Gottman, 1995):

- Happy couples in their interactions exchange higher frequencies of rewards and fewer punishments than unhappy couples.

- Happy couples are generally not reciprocal in their exchange of negative behaviors (negativity).

- Happy couples reduce negativity in interactions by editing their negative responses to their partner's negativity. They attribute his or her negativity to ephemeral, transient factors. Attempts to repair the interaction are made. In these repair attempts, the "repairing" partner develops "sentiment override." He or she respond positively, turning toward, rather than away from, the mate displaying negativity.

- In long-term happy marriages, husbands respect their wives' influence. In fact, it is Gottman's contention (1995) that marriages work to the extent that men accept the positive influence of their wives.

- In happy long-term marriages, one partner is able to have a physiologically soothing effect on the other mate. In other words, he or she (primarily the wife) is able to de-escalate tense interactions by calming down the mate.

▶ DYSFUNCTIONAL COMMUNICATION PATTERNS IN THE FAMILY

In this chapter functional and dysfunctional communication have been separated for discussion purposes. In reality, however, this demarcation does not exist, and communication patterns in families are not all totally healthy or unhealthy. Rather, they should be viewed on a continuum from functional to dysfunctional, with all but a small percentage of families falling somewhere in between these poles.

In contrast to the definition of functional communication, dysfunctional communication is defined as the unclear and/or indirect transmission and reception of either or both the content and instruction (intent) of a message and/or the incongruency between the content and instruction level of the message. Indirect transmission of messages refers to the messages being deflected from their appropriate target(s) to other persons in the family. Direct transmission of messages means the messages "hit" the appropriate target.

In dysfunctional family interaction, two or more family members have established repetitive networks and strategies of dysfunctional communication that attempt to maintain homeostasis and the integration of the family unit. These dysfunctional processes are often subtle, and the intent of the communication is covert or hidden. Thus accurate assessment of this type of unhealthy circular communication patterns becomes more difficult. Satir (1967, 1983) and other family therapists who advocate the use of family communications theory in practice assert that the more dysfunctional the communication, the more dysfunctional the family. This is a primary theoretical proposition within family communication theory. One of the primary factors that generates dysfunctional communication patterns is the presence of low esteem of both the family and its members, especially the parents (Anderson, 1972; Satir, 1972, 1983). Three interrelated types of communication patterns that perpetuate low esteem are self-centeredness, need for total agreement, and lack of empathy. These communication patterns are discussed next.

Self-centeredness

Self-centered communications are characterized by individuals focusing on their own needs to the exclusion of the other person's needs, feelings, or perspectives. In other words, self-centered family members seek to get something from others to meet their own needs. When these individuals must give, they do so reluctantly and then in a hostile, defensive, or self-sacrificing manner. Thus bargaining or negotiating effectively is difficult, because self-centered persons believe they cannot afford to lose what little they have to give (Satir, 1983).

Need for Total Agreement

The family's value of maintaining total agreement and avoiding conflict begins when the marital partners dis-

cover that each is different from the other, although what these exact differences are may be difficult to explain. Differentness—as expressed in opinions, habits, preferences, or expectations—may be seen as a threat because it can and does lead to disagreements and the awareness that they are both separate individuals. If marital partners have low self-esteem and feel that it is absolutely necessary to be loved and approved at all times, they try to constantly please their mate. This need to continually please prohibits them from communicating openly when displeased or acknowledging disagreement. The couple perceives that expressions of their own unique thoughts and feelings might lead to conflicts that could then result in a "catastrophe" (Gottman et al., 1977). Distracting and placating tactics are often used to avoid conflict and act as if there is agreement (Satir, 1972).

Thus unwritten rules come into being that forbid open expression of one's own individuality and differentness as a means of staving off this threat. These rules are often rigid and elude conflict or negotiation, so that there is no consideration of alternatives that would enable each mate to interact differently and yet be accepted. As part of the socialization process, the children learn these same values and ways of relating and thus have difficulty in recognizing and interpreting a variety of feelings and experiences. These values and resultant communication patterns constrict the growth of all family members.

Ruesch and associates (1974), in their research of marital relationships, found that in those marriages where conflict was avoided and negative feelings buried, the negative feelings "poisoned" the relationship. They observed that avoidance of conflict may lead to "devitalized marriages"—marriages in which mates feel emotionally detached and indifferent to each other.

Lack of Empathy

Family members who are self-centered and cannot tolerate differentness also cannot recognize the effect of their own thoughts, feelings, and behavior on other family members; neither can they understand other family members' thoughts, feelings, and behavior. They are so consumed with meeting their own needs that they do not have the ability to be empathetic. Underneath a facade of unconcern, these individuals may suffer feelings of powerlessness. Not only do they devalue themselves, they also devalue others. This leads to an atmosphere of tension, fearfulness, and/or blame. The stage is therefore set for a style of communication that is confusing, vague, indirect, and covert, with defensiveness rather than openness, clarity, and honesty prevailing.

Closed Areas of Communication

While more functional families have more open areas of communication, less functional families often demonstrate more closed areas of communication. Families have unwritten rules about what subjects are approved or disapproved for discussion. These unwritten rules are most overtly seen when a family member breaches the family's rules by bringing up unapproved subjects or expressing forbidden feelings.

Unwritten family rules about what communication is open and closed reveal much about other aspects of a family's structure (their values, norms, power, and roles in the family). Communication restrictions may be limited to certain family subsystems: for example, discussion of sexual habits in front of the children, or a parent's alcoholism. Financial issues may be discussed only between spouses but not with the children. Moreover, an area may be closed in terms of expression of feelings but open in terms of expression of thoughts.

Cultural norms of modesty, privacy, and sexual roles play a large part in influencing the areas where closed and open communication exist. Thus communication patterns must be evaluated in their cultural context.

A common interactional pattern utilized in families for avoiding discussion of meaningful issues and/or expressing salient feelings is termed "chitchat" or "small talk." The family, in using "chitchat" consistently, talks about superficial daily occurrences and avoids the meaningful issues of family life. For example, a mother has been taking her child to a pediatric clinic because of recurrent convulsions. At the clinic the diagnosis of epilepsy was recently confirmed. Since hearing of the diagnosis, the family has never discussed their thoughts or feelings about the diagnosis; their only conversation in this area has dealt with the inconvenient hospital parking arrangements and the long travel time to the clinic.

▶ FACTORS INFLUENCING FAMILY COMMUNICATION PATTERNS

Family communication patterns are influenced by multiple factors—including the immediate context in which the interaction takes place (i.e., the situational variable), the family life cycle stage, the family form, the gender of the interactants, the ethnic background(s) of the family members, and the socioeconomic status of the family (see Table 10–3). As a result, the family develops its own unique mini-culture—although certainly having much in common with families with like characteristics. In this section, five key variables that influence family communication are briefly described—the family's ethnic background, family communication across the family life cycle, gender differences in communication, and differences in communication created by the family form. The family's unique mini-culture, an "idiosyncratic" variable, is also discussed.

Differences in Communication in Families with Different Ethnic Backgrounds

Communication is embedded within a matrix of beliefs and patterns, many of which are culturally derived, particularly in ethnic and immigrant families. Yet in research and in the literature, communication in families is discussed without consideration of the surrounding cultural context—a criticism of the literature that this chapter also reports.

▶ TABLE 10–3

FACTORS INFLUENCING FAMILY COMMUNICATION PATTERNS

The context/situation.
The family's ethnic background.
The family life cycle.
Gender differences.
Family form.
The family's socioeconomic status.
Idiosyncratic factors: The family mini-culture.

Sillars (1995), for example, points out that out of the many studies conducted that examine communication and marital satisfaction, only a few take the mates' cultural orientation into account. And yet in traditionally oriented ethnic families "ethnicity represents a way of living that is fully integrated with individual and family identity. . . . [W]here this sort of ethnicity still persists, the cultural patterns have considerable force" (p. 391). Hence, in traditional ethnic families, family communication patterns vary considerably from the American middle-class, predominantly white family described in the communication sections prior to this section. Communication in families varies in conversation (extent, style, pacing), personal space, eye contact, touch, and time orientation (Lipson, 1996).

A fundamental value orientation that shapes family life and family communication is the prominence in the family of a collectivistic/familistic orientation versus an individualistic orientation value (Gudykunst, 1991). This value and orientation is culturally derived. As discussed in Chapter 13, a familistic orientation is associated with sharing and mutual assistance, high interdependency among family members, and family needs and identity taking precedence over individual needs and identity (Schwartz, 1990; Sillars, 1995). The centrality of the family is the fundamental orientation among ethnic groups, whereas the American mainstream society has a more individualistic orientation. In the United States individual needs and pursuits generally compete on a more equal footing with family needs and obligations (Sillars, 1995; Wilkinson, 1987).

Three areas in which ethnicity particularly affects family communication are talk (the extent and explicitness of information sharing), emotional expression, and tolerance for the expression of conflict.

Talk: Extent and Explicitness of Information Sharing.

In different ethnic groups, communication differs by the "presumed instrumentality of talk" (Sillars, 1995, p. 381). Mainstream Americans tend to believe that it is important to put thoughts into words. Because Americans expect individuals to think and behave uniquely, extensive communication is needed first to know the other person, and then to maintain a relationship and to coordinate actions. Messages are verbally explicit. "Mind reading" is considered ill-advised, presumptuous, and harmful to use in family communications (Sillars, 1995).

In contrast, in cultures that are homogeneous, where roles are "scripted" (very structured and predictable), and roles and messages collectively understood, words are considered as sometimes unnecessary to achieve understanding. In fact, too much talking could be considered "transparent." Messages may appear to be succinct and sparse, with meaningful silences interspersed. For instance, Navajo-Americans, as well as traditional Chinese- and Japanese-Americans view silence as being valuable (Giger & Davidhizar, 1995). Knowledge of the other person's thoughts is taken for granted (Sillars, 1995) and self-disclosure is limited (Draguns, 1996). Marital partners who come from this type of cultural orientation will reflect this type of communication in their families.

The dominant assumption in North America, particularly in the world of psychology, is that talk is good and can heal, hence, "talk therapy." But we can see from the foregoing discussion that different ethnicities place different values on how helpful talk is.

Emotional Expression.

Sillars (1995) states that the expression of emotion versus emotional restraint is the most striking feature with respect to communication differences due to cultural background. In the mental health literature the expression of feelings, both negative and positive, is considered to be vital for healthy family functioning. However, the extent to which emotional expression is tolerated and encouraged varies widely. For instance, in traditional Japanese- and Chinese-American families, emotional expression is muted in comparison to typical Euro-American families.

Expression of Conflict.

Related to emotional expression is the expression of conflict in families. Again, this aspect of communication varies across cultures. Tolerance for the expression of confrontation, dissent, and disharmony dramatically differs. Although in the mental health field the dominant belief is that conflict is ever-present and important to acknowledge and address (resolve), in some traditional ethnic families, this belief may not exist. In family relationships that are homogeneous, structured, and predictable, there is less need for ongoing discussion to maintain coordination. Hence, family members may rely on more passive and indirect conflict strategies. Direct conflicts are much less tolerated and thus are infrequent. However, when they do occur, they are more explosive (Sillars, 1995). In intercultural marriages or families in the midst of cultural change, such as recent immigrant families, conflict is more evident because of the clash of values and acceptable behaviors between the two cultures.

Communication Differences Over the Family Life Cycle

Family communication varies over time. One striking change is in the explicitness and extensiveness of talk over the family life cycle. Family communication patterns often progress "from a maximal reliance on explicit talk in courtship in early marriage to increasing reliance on unspoken understandings later on" (Sillars, 1995, p. 383). In the last family life cycle stage (the aging family), research consistently finds that couples in long-term marriages typically move toward a "disengaged" style of communication, in which extent of talk, conflict, and involvement are relatively low (Mares, 1995). These typical communication patterns are altered, however, during periods of family instability and restructuring.

Gender Differences in Communication

As the women's movement gained momentum, so did the interest in gender differences in communication. It is now widely acknowledged that major differences in interaction exist between the genders. Hence, in marriage and in the family, communication patterns will differ depending on the gender of the family members. Imagine the differences in family communication when the two-parent family is composed of one male—the father—and four females (mother and daughters) versus one female—the mother—and four males (father and sons).

Research has demonstrated differences in attitudes and patterns of conversation (Tannen, 1990), different decision-making approaches (Kolleck, Blumstein, & Schwartz, 1985), different ways of responding to others' concerns (Kollack et al., 1985; Steen & Schwartz, 1995; Tannen, 1990), and differences in conflict recognition and resolution. For instance, women see conversation as a way of building connections, of creating intimacy, whereas men see conversation as a way to demonstrate their status and knowledge (a competitive opportunity to relate information and discuss activities). Women seek consensus, while men seek to make decisions expeditiously (Steen & Schwartz, 1995; Tannen, 1990). When women discuss problems, they want understanding, whereas men want solutions. When working at resolving a conflict, wives tend to take an affiliative, cooperative stance toward their husbands, whereas husbands assume a more coercive, competitive stance toward their wives (White, 1989).

In general, the gender communication research on marital couples has shown that wives are more expressive, send clearer messages than husbands, and are more sensitive and responsive to their husbands' messages during conversations and conflict (Thompson & Walker, 1991).

Communication Differences in Family Forms

"The family" today is defined more broadly to include the diverse forms of families that exist in society (see Chap. 1 for a discussion of the various family forms). Family form refers to the various family structural arrangements, from the traditional two-parent nuclear family to the single-parent and homosexual family.

Family communication is affected by the type of family form under consideration. Most research has been conducted on heterosexual couples and two-parent nuclear families, excluding our understanding of communications in single-parent, dual-career, stepparent, homosexual, and extended families. An example of how communication differs due to family form is presented. The case in point is the stepparent family, where a husband or wife marry into another family (spouse and her or his children).

In the stepparent family, conflict within the family is the most widely cited communication feature. Because two families are joined together, each with its own culture and history, with few guideposts to rely on as to what the stepparent and stepchild role should be, it is no wonder that conflict is a major concern. Stepfamily integration is a process that may take 5 to 6 years or may never fully occur (Burrell, 1995; Visher & Visher, 1990). Authority and boundary issues (who is in and out of the family) are also mentioned by spouses in stepfamilies as pressing concerns (Burrell, 1995). Loyalty issues such as the conflict between divided loyalties, i.e., the conflict between loyalty to one's biological children versus loyalty to the new spouse, and role-oriented issues are other sources of communication conflicts.

Communication Differences Due to the Family Mini-culture

A particular family's communication patterns are a coherent configuration of family traits (Sillars, 1995), which constitute a family's unique mini-culture or family identity. In traditional cultures, ethnicity represents a way of living and valuing, thus the family mini-culture and the larger culture closely resemble each other. However, within modern heterogeneous societies such as ours, individuals are members of different ethnic backgrounds and vary considerably as to the extent to which they are acculturated. In these situations, the family mini-culture might reflect the cultural influence or be almost completely devoid of its influence. In untraditional, modern, secular families, there is much more openness to becoming unique—creating very

particular communication patterns. When couples marry, one of their challenges is creating a shared relational culture, one with its own shared meaning (Jenkins, 1995) and its own family paradigm—the family's fundamental and enduring assumptions about the world in which it lives (Reiss, 1981). Fitzpatrick and Ritchie (1993) refer to the family as "a private miniculture."

▶ COMMUNICATION IN FAMILIES WITH HEALTH PROBLEMS

Findings from research that has examined adaptation of families to chronic and life-threatening illness has consistently demonstrated that a central factor in healthy marital and family functioning is the presence of open, honest, and clear communication in dealing with the stressful health and health-related issues (Kahn, 1990; Spinetta & Deasy-Spinetta, 1981). When families do not discuss the important issues they are faced with, emotional distancing in family relationships results, and family stress increases (Friedman, 1985). Increased stress affects not only family relationships but also the health of the family and its members (Hoffer, 1989).

FAMILY COMMUNICATION: APPLYING THE FAMILY NURSING PROCESS

▶ assessment questions

The following assessment questions should be considered when analyzing a family's communication patterns.

1. In observing the family as a whole and/or the family's set of relationships, how extensively are functional and dysfunctional communication patterns used? Diagram recurring interactional patterns or circular communication patterns. In addition to diagraming circular communication patterns, the following more specific behaviors may be assessed:
   a. How firmly and clearly do members state their needs and feelings?
   b. To what extent do members use clarification and qualification in interaction?

    c. Do members elicit and respond favorably to feedback, or do they generally discourage feedback and exploration of an issue?

    d. How well do members listen and attend when communicating?

    e. Do members seek validation from one another?

    f. To what degree do members use assumptions and judgmental statements in interaction?

    g. Do members interact in an offensive manner to messages?

    h. How frequently is disqualification utilized?

2. How are emotional messages conveyed in the family and within the family subsystems?
    a. How frequently are these emotional messages conveyed?
    b. What types of emotions are transmitted within the family subsystems? Are negative, positive, or both types of emotions transmitted?

3. What is the frequency and quality of communication within the communication network and familial sets of relationships?
    a. Who talks to whom and in what usual manner?
    b. What is the usual pattern of transmitting important messages? Does an intermediary exist?
    c. Are messages appropriate for the developmental age of the members?

4. Are the majority of messages of family members congruent in content and instruction (including observations of nonverbal messages)? If not, who manifests what kind of incongruency?

5. What types of dysfunctional processes are evident in the family communication patterns?

6. What important family/personal issues are open and closed to discussion?

7. How do the following factors influence family communication patterns?
    a. The context/situation.
    b. The family life cycle stage.
    c. The family's ethnic background.
    d. Gender differences in family.
    e. Family form.
    f. The family's socioeconomic status.
    g. The family's unique mini-culture.

▶ FAMILY NURSING DIAGNOSES

Although family communication problems are frequent and very significant family nursing diagnoses, the North American Nursing Diagnosis Association (NANDA) has not identified any family-based communication diagnoses. NANDA does use communication behaviors as part of defining characteristics in some of their diagnoses, such as dysfunctional grieving. The one nursing diagnosis listed by NANDA is "impaired verbal communication," which is focused on the individual client who is unable to verbally communicate (McFarland & McFarlane, 1993). Giger and Davidhizar (1995) assert that "impaired verbal communication" does not take into consideration the client's culture and is, therefore, not a culturally relevant nursing diagnosis.

A broad family nursing communication diagnosis may be used, such as dysfunctional family communication or dysfunctional parent–child, sibling, or marital communication (if the problem is primarily located in the subsystem). Other general family nursing diagnoses in this area are impaired family communication or family communication problems. If broad diagnoses are used, then defining characteristics and related factors should accompany the diagnosis, following the NANDA pattern. Some family nurses may identify a more specific family communication problem as the diagnosis, such as minimal affective or emotional marital communication, or incongruent communication patterns of parents.

► FAMILY NURSING INTERVENTIONS

Family nursing interventions in the area of communication are focused on all three levels of prevention: primary, secondary, and tertiary prevention. Strategies primarily involve teaching and counseling, and secondarily collaboration, contracting, and referrals to self-help groups, community organizations, and family therapy clinics or offices.

General Family Nursing Interventions

Family counselors often remark that one of the major roles they enact in working with families is to teach the members about family dynamics and how to communicate in a more functional way with each other. Much of the teaching that takes place is informal—that which goes on in the spontaneous client–nurse interactions.

Role modeling is also a crucial type of teaching. It is through the family members' observation of the family health professional and how he or she communicates during different interactional situations that they learn to imitate healthy communication behaviors. The nurse in role modeling functional communication should listen intently, deliberately, and empathetically, following up with clarifying questions and encouraging further expression of thoughts and feelings. Role modeling becomes a particularly potent teaching method when family members positively identify with the family nurse.

Counseling in the area of family communication involves encouraging and supporting families in their efforts at improving communication between themselves. In counseling the family nurse is a facilitator of group process and a resource person. His or her presence gives families both permission to try out new ways of communicating and the safety of having "a third person" there when they bring out previously closed areas of communication to discuss or break other unwritten communication rules, such as disagreeing or asserting their view.

Satir, a noted family therapist and role model of superb communication skills, presents tips for clinicians who work with families in a facilitator role (Satir et al., 1991). These tips are equally relevant for family nurses to use when working with families in the communication area (see Table 10–4).

► TABLE 10–4

SATIR'S TIPS FOR BEING A FACILITATOR IN ASSISTING FAMILIES WITH THEIR COMMUNICATION

1. Promote congruent communication.
   Respond with "I" messages.
   Clearly convey ownership for what you say and do.
   Share in descriptive rather than evaluative language, your reactions to what is being said and done by family members.
   In interviews, pay attention to the physical distance or closeness between you and the family members.
   [If culturally acceptable] be at eye level and at a comfortable closeness.
2. Provide alternatives and options for coping.
3. Present opportunities for raising family members' feelings of self-worth.
   Make person-to-person connections with each individual in the family.
   Acknowledge and validate feelings and thoughts of each family member.
   Offer dignity, trust, and respect to family members.

Sources: Satir, Banmen, Gerber, & Gomari (1991), and Schwab (1990).

Specific Family Nursing Interventions

More specific intervention strategies in the area of family communication reflect what we know about functional family communication and how to promote it. Wright and Leahey's (1994) classification of the three types of direct family interventions (those focused upon the cognitive, affective, and behavioral levels of family functioning) aid in organizing specific communication strategies that can be applied. Intervention strategies within each of the three domains include both teaching and counseling.

Cognitive-level Focus.
Family nursing interventions in this area provide new information or ideas about communication. The information is educational and hopefully encourages family problem solving.

Whether family members change their communication behavior is first largely dependent on how they perceive the problem. Wright and Leahey (1994) affirm the crucial role of perception and beliefs. When there are problems, the nurse must help the family to obtain a different view of their problems. Hence, the goal here is to change the family members' perception and beliefs about a specific communication problem.

Helping family members reframe certain messages so that they view more positively a particular situation is very helpful. For instance, helping family members see that when a person in the family gets very angry, this usually means he or she is feeling hurt, pain, and possibly a sense of rejection. Hurt is a much more "acceptable" and positive emotion for family members to respond to than anger and hostility (Satir, 1967).

Another important "lesson" for family members to learn is that there is no one reality. Multiple realities or perceptions exist about a particular situation or event. Each family member will have his or her own perceptions or perspective about a particular situation or event. In order to deal with conflicts or situations requiring decision making, family members' perceptions (and feelings) about the situation should be understood and considered.

Affective-level Focus.
Interventions in this area are directed toward changing the emotional expression of family members—by either increasing or decreasing the level of emotional communication or modifying the quality of the emotional communication. The specific nursing goals here are, within the cultural context of the family, to help the family members express and share their feelings with each other so that (1) their emotional needs can be better conveyed and responded to; (2) more congruent, clear family communication occurs; and (3) family problem-solving efforts are facilitated.

Direct interventions aimed at the affective level of family functioning include urging parents to share their feelings, both positive and negative, with their children. And likewise, supporting parents' efforts at encouraging their children to share the full range of their feelings with their parents, so that children can be better communicators. (Children learn to express themselves as they see their parents expressing themselves.) In addition, family nurses can point out incongruences in family members' levels of communication and encourage them to be more congruent in their content and metamessages (the metamessage or instruction consists of how words are said, including the feelings which accompany the words).

Behavioral-level Focus.
Understanding or having more positive perceptions about a family communication problem is not sufficient for change to occur. There also must be behavioral change (Wright & Leahey, 1994). Rather than search for underlying causes and "whys" to problems, Wright and Leahey suggest that family nurses ask about the "whats" of the problem. For example, when a father decides by himself what movie the family will see, asking what effect that has on the other family members is more helpful than asking why he made that decision himself.

Behavioral changes stimulate changes in perceptions of a family member's "reality" and perceptions stimulate changes in behavior (there is a circular, recursive process involved here). Hence, when the family nurse assists family members to learn new and healthier ways of communicating, he or she is also helping family members to change their perceptions or their construction of reality about a situation.

Some teaching and counseling interventions designed to change family communication (remember, all communication is behavior) or the way family members relate to each other include:

1. Giving the family members instructions on specific behavioral changes. For example, in the case of working with an anxious new mother and her baby who constantly awakens and cries, instruct the mother that when the baby cries to check to make sure his or her needs are met and then leave the infant in the crib alone and let him or her cry for 15 minutes before entering the room again.

2. When family members are exhibiting beginning attempts to communicate clearly and congruently, supporting, and complimenting them for their efforts—so that the positive behaviors are reinforced and will be attempted again.

3. Monitoring behavioral changes that have been suggested at previous meetings. Ask how a particular suggestion worked or if any problems occurred or questions arose when they tried the recommended action.

McCubbin and Dahl (1985), family scholars and educators, recommend communication tactics for couples to use to manage conflict productively. A summary of their guidelines follows.

1. Try not to engage in "kitchen-sink fighting" (throwing all kinds of additional issues into the conflict).

2. Talk in terms of issues, not personalities.

3. Be an active listener (obtain feedback and ask for clarification).

4. Recognize that your mate's unhappiness is not always your responsibility.

5. Find a way for both sides to win (pp. 187–189).

Referring families who are in need of learning new communication skills to appropriate community groups and family counseling facilities is indicated when the available services are not sufficient to deal with the family's problems and the family wishes to seek further assistance. Referral to family mental health clinics as well as to private clinicians may be particularly indicated when working with troubled families. In addition, self-help groups that are emotionally oriented facilitate open group communication, which in turn, assists families in improving their communications. Examples of such groups for troubled families are Alcoholics Anonymous, Al-Anon, and Narcotics Anonymous.

There are numerous community organizations and programs designed to improve marriage and family communication and relationships as well as parenting skills. Parent Effectiveness Training (PET) is probably the most popular of these types of groups in the United States. Marriage Enrichment, Marriage Encounter, and Marriage Communication Lab programs also help spouses enhance their communication skills (Hoffer, 1996).

And finally there are parent and child communication training programs that have assisted parents and children shore up their communications. Particularly during the adolescent years, these types of programs have been found to be quite successful (Riesch et al., 1993).

► study questions

1. From the list below select the four primary characteristics that are *not* representative of a functional sender.
   a. Listens
   b. Receptive to feedback
   c. Elicits feedback
   d. Makes assumptions
   e. Firmly states case
   f. Validates

g. Clarifies and qualifies
h. Generalizes

2. Name two characteristics of both the functional and dysfunctional sender or receiver.

3. Match the five major categories of dysfunctional communication in the left-hand column with the specific illustrations given at the right.

Category	Example
a. Assumptions.	1. "I'm not mad at you," spoken in loud, sharp tone.
b. Unclear expression of feelings.	2. "I dislike patients who are constantly complaining."
c. Judgmental expressions.	3. "I don't understand how you can be so dumb."
d. Inability to define needs.	4. "I just love it when you don't come home for dinner, then I have only a few dishes to wash."
e. Incongruent communication.	5. "If you would like to go out for dinner, so would I."

4. Which of the following situations *best* demonstrates that information has been received from a sender?
   a. A parent tells a child to stop playing with his food and the child continues to play.
   b. A parent tells a child to drink his milk and the child looks at the parent.
   c. A parent shows a child how to butter bread and the child states that she knows a better way to butter her bread.

5. Gender differences in communication are striking. Which of the following is *not* a gender research finding?
   a. Husbands are clearer in their communication than wives.
   b. In decision making, men want expeditious decisions made, while women seek to develop consensus.
   c. Women are more emotionally expressive than men.
   d. Women see conversation as a way to build connections, whereas men do not.

6. Punctuation in interactional sequences means (choose the best definition):
   a. When the beginning of the sequence is perceived to have begun.
   b. How the sequence was ended.
   c. Who, in fact, started the interactional sequence.
   d. A poor grasp of expression of ideas by a family member.

7. Feedback is a term used in systems theory to describe the process of information flow (answer *true* or *false*).

8. In the following situations identify the content and the instructional level of the message.
    a. A newlywed couple is watching a movie. The woman caresses the man's arm and hugs it to her while she whispers, "I'm really not interested in this movie."
    b. A child starts to crawl on his parent's lap. The parent pushes the child away and says, "You know I love you, go play with your new toy."
    c. A child is throwing cereal with a spoon. The mother grabs the spoon and cereal bowl and emphatically states, "Stop it! You may not play with your food!"

9. When a transaction between two family members is repeated over and over again, this tendency is referred to as the _____ principle.

10. A wife, in finding that her husband has not helped with the dishes as he promised to do, expresses her anger at him. He, in turn, yells back that "he will wash the dishes in his own time." She then continues to berate him. What kind of feedback loops are illustrated in this series of transactions?

11. Communication patterns in families very widely according to the family's ethnic background. Noted communication differences are present in these areas:
    a. The extent and explicitness of information conveyed in conversation
    b. The meaning of silence in conversation
    c. The expression of emotion
    d. The expression of conflict
    e. The communication networks in families

► family case study

During the reading of this family case example, jot down your interpretation of the interactions (using the theory presented in chapter), in addition to answering assessment questions at the end of the case description.

A member of the Visiting Nurses' Association is going out to visit Mr. Herman Katz, a Jewish male, age 68, who has suffered a myocardial infarction and has just recently returned home after two weeks of hospitalization. The doctor has requested that the visiting nurse review his dietary and exercise regimen and report back her appraisal of his diet and tolerance to the progressive exercise regimen.

The nurse's notes on the interagency referral form from the hospital state: Mr. Katz was alert, very conscientious about his care, but was quite reluctant to do any of activities—and thus was somewhat demanding and dependent on the nurses. He ate poorly and got up to go to the bathroom by himself. During the last week he has had no pain or dyspnea during self-care activities.

The visiting nurse on her first visit learned that Mr. K. had been a business manager for many years and that he had retired 3 years ago. This was his second heart attack according to his wife (the first occurring 6 months post-retirement). Past recreational interests had been heavy gardening and remodeling of his home prior to his first heart attack.

Mrs. Sylvia Katz is 65 years old and also Jewish. She has been in fairly good health except for being overweight and having osteoarthritis, which has made walking much more difficult for her. She prepares rich Jewish foods for herself and her single daughter, Marian, age 40, who also lives with her and her husband. She or her daughter constantly answer for Mr. K. when the nurse asks questions. Mrs. K. was very talkative and complains of being very tired herself.

The Katz family lives in a nicely furnished three-bedroom house. Mr. K. has a college education and was a certified public accountant for many years. They have two grown sons, who live nearby, and an unmarried daughter, Marian, who is temporarily living with them to help her father out.

On the second visit a week later, the nurse observed the following: Mr. K. continued to be unwilling and afraid to do things for himself and had not increased his level of activity. He appeared short of breath and uncomfortable (as though in pain) when talking about his illness and symptoms, but when distracted he appeared to have no dyspnea or pain. Mr. K. has seen none of his social or work friends since he has been home, according to Mrs. K. He has not been getting dressed or taking care of his personal hygiene adequately.

The following interactional vignettes were extracted as the nurse began to discuss Mr. K.'s rehabilitation program:

NURSE: *(question directed to Mr. K.)* What activities did the doctor recommend for you to do this week?

SYLVIA: *(interceding)* I told Herman that he should take it easy because after all this is his second heart attack and the next one will be his last!

MARIAN: Yes, mother's right. He should be taking it easy. Isn't that right? (Looks at mother for agreement.)

NURSE: I understand both of your concerns for your husband's and father's welfare. But, Mr. Katz, I want to know your understanding and feelings about what activities and the amount of exercise your doctor wants you to get.

HERMAN: Well, my understanding is that I shouldn't do anything that upsets or fatigues me. And up to now I haven't felt like doing anything much.

NURSE: *(again looking at Herman)* What specifically did the doctor say you should do?

Herman looks at his daughter and then wife Marian immediately jumps up to get his written directions on exercises and diet guidelines. Nurse reads these guidelines and explains the concept and importance of the recommended progressive exercise program. As this is being carefully explained,

Mrs. K. looks over to the kitchen as if she is disinterested and then walks out to begin lunch preparation.

As the exercise program continued to be discussed, Herman remarked:

HERMAN: These activities don't use up much of my time and I'm tired of watching TV. I feel restless 'cause I have nothing to do.

NURSE: But, Herman, I understand that you have been refusing to get out of bed or dress yourself every day. We discussed last week that you could go outside and sit on the front porch, socialize, play cards and quiet table games, but you have not been doing any of these things.

MARIAN: Dad, you're just stubborn and unwilling to do anything the doctor says!

MOTHER: *(looking over at her daughter)* Oh, Marian, you're always attacking your father. He's just scared to death to move too much for fear of hurting his heart again.

MARIAN: But you don't help him any by cooking him that rich Jewish food and caring for his every need.

MOTHER: Let's drop it.

From the family case example, answer the following assessment questions involving family communication.

12. How extensively does the family use functional and/or dysfunctional communication?

13. How well do members state feelings and needs?

14. Are qualification, clarification, or feedback techniques used?

15. How well do members listen to each other?

16. Are judgmental statements or assumptions used?

17. What values underlie the family's communication?

18. Are affective messages communicated?

19. Describe the family communication network.

20. What variables influence the family interactions?

21. State one family nursing diagnosis in the area of communication.

22. Propose two family nursing interventions directed toward resolving the above family communication problem.

► chapter 10 study answers

1. d and h.

2. Sender:
   Functional: Message sent through clear and direct channels (firmly and clearly states case, clarifies and qualifies messages, and asks for feedback).
   Dysfunctional: Makes assumptions, unclear expression of feelings, judgmental expressions, and inability to express needs.

   Receiver:
   Functional: Intended message and received message are consistent, congruent, and match in meaning (effective listening, giving feedback, and providing validation).
   Dysfunctional: Failure to listen, disqualification, offensiveness and negativity, lack of exploration, and lack of validation.

3. a. 2.
   b. 4.
   c. 2, 3.
   d. 5.
   e. 1.

4. c.

5. a.

6. a.

7. True.

8. a. *Content level.* Disinterest expressed in movie.
      Instructional level. Expression of warmth, sexual attraction, and interest.
   b. *Content level.* Statement of love and demand that child play with toy.
      Instructional level. Expression of rejection of child's request for closeness and attention.
   c. *Content and instructional level.* Both consonant: Demand to stop behavior.

9. Redundancy.

10. Positive feedback loops.

11. All but e.

> ► family case study

The following interactional vignettes are followed by interpretations in the brackets:

NURSE: *(question directed to husband)* What activities did the doctor recommend for you to do this week?

SYLVIA: *(interceding)* I told Herman that he should take it easy because after all this is his second heart attack and the next one will be his last!
[Speaks for other person; tangentialization and "you should" statement.]

MARIAN: Yes, mother's right. He should be taking it easy. Isn't that right? (Looks at mother for agreement.)
[Short-term, issue-oriented coalition; assumption that father shares their same feelings—lack of exploration or validation with the father.]

NURSE: I understand both of your concerns for your husband's and father's welfare. But, Mr. Katz, I want to know your understanding and feelings about what activities and the amount of exercise your doctor wants you to get.
[Nurse refocuses and paraphrases her question by utilizing an "I want" statement.]

HERMAN: Well, my understanding is that I shouldn't do anything that upsets or fatigues me. And up to now I haven't felt like doing anything much.

NURSE: *(again looking at Herman)* What specifically did the doctor say you should do?

Herman looks at his daughter and then wife, and daughter immediately jumps up to get his written directions on exercises and diet guidelines. Nurse reads these guidelines and explains the concept and importance of the recommended progressive exercise program. As this is being carefully explained, Mrs. K. looks over to the kitchen as if she is disinterested and then walks out to begin lunch preparation.

[Silent disagreement by wife. Perhaps this program violates her need to care for her husband, or maybe she feels it might be too much and is quite concerned over his possible future death. Perhaps Mrs. K. wants to be in charge, to be the spokesperson for her husband, and does not like it when the nurse redirects attention to Mr. K. Also, culturally there is a tendency for family members in Jewish families to greatly assist their sick family members and this often runs counter to "pushing" a patient to be more self-sufficient.]

As the exercise program continued to be discussed, Herman remarked:

HERMAN: These activities don't use up much of my time and I'm tired of watching TV. I feel restless 'cause I have nothing to do.

[This is a case of incongruent behavior—between what he is now saying and what he has been doing and saying.]

NURSE: But, Herman, I understand that you have been refusing to get out of bed or dress yourself every day. We discussed last week that you could go outside and sit on the front porch, socialize, play cards and quiet table games, but you have not been interested in doing any of these things.
[Nurse points out the incongruency.]

MARIAN: Dad, you're just stubborn and unwilling to do anything the doctor says!
[Insulting, judgmental remark.]

MOTHER: *(looking over at her daughter)* Oh, Marian, you're always attacking your father. He's just scared to death to move too much for fear of hurting his heart again.
[She interprets his behavior for him, but neglects to ask for feedback or even to look at him for his reaction.]

MARIAN: But you don't help him any by cooking him that rich Jewish food and caring for his every need.
[Attacks with new issue, as well as changing issues—failure to focus on one problem until closure is reached.]

MOTHER: Let's drop it.
[Cutoff in communication.]

12. Extensive use of dysfunctional communication (from short vignette). Most dysfunctional recurring patterns entail: (a) wife speaking for Mr. K. and daughter and wife assuming that they know his thoughts and feelings; (b) not completing one subject or issue; and (c) not asking for feedback from other family members.

13. They do state some of their fears for and feelings about Mr. K., although they do so indirectly. But none of them state their obvious reticence about the medical regimen.

14. Qualification, clarification, or feedback techniques are not shown in this vignette.

15. The family members sometimes listen to each other. In particular, when they agree, they show they are listening. Mother walks away when she disagrees or doesn't want to hear.

16. In speaking for Mr. K., judgmental statements or assumptions are made; also judgmental statements are made when daughter comments on father's stubbornness and mother's cooking.

17. The values underlying the family's communication include concern over the father and spontaneity of response. Also conflict between family members is tolerated (OK to disagree).

18. Affective are messages are communicated, as in Mrs. K.'s concern for her husband (caring response). However, it was indirectly stated.

19. Nurse asks questions of Mr. K. Both the daughter and wife speak to nurse for Mr. K. and interact among each other. Herman is passive in interaction except for one interaction where he initiated complaint.

20. Cultural influence, as described in the vignette. Home environment is an important variable, because nurse does not have the same influence over the situation. Wife and daughter are the dominant ones here. Situational variable: Recent heart attack of husband, recent hospital discharge, and daughter moving in.

21. The answer for question 13 could be used for a family nursing diagnosis: Extensive use of dysfunctional communication among family members. Defining characteristics: Mr. K. and daughter speaking for Mr. K. and making assumptions that they know his thoughts and feelings (these are dysfunctional sender characteristics). In addition, tangentialization and distraction—jumping to another topic instead of completing discussion on former topic/issue; lack of exploration—messages are sent, but there is a failure of other family members to clarify the meaning of the message or seek further information, such as when Mr. K. explained his restlessness, no one asked him to clarify what he meant (these are dysfunctional receiver characteristics). For related factors see answer 20.

22. Two general nursing interventions. Through teaching and counseling strategies assist family to be more functional in the areas described under defining characteristics. In particular, role modeling clear communication should be used. Directly involving Mr. K. so that he becomes a more active communicator and speaks for himself is vital here. Having the wife and daughter express their own concerns in a more direct and positive manner (so that the daughter doesn't need to blame or attack the mother or father) is also suggested.

11

Family Power Structure

Marilyn M. Friedman

► learning objectives

1. Describe the importance of understanding the family power structure.

2. Define the following concepts: power, authority, decision making, and family power.

3. Distinguish between the various bases for power and recognize some of the major gender, ethnic, age, educational, and socioeconomic differences in the use of power sources.

4. Identify and explain the role each of the following variables plays in influencing family power: power hierarchy, formation of coalitions, family communication network, social class, family developmental stage, situational contingencies, person variables (gender, age, and interpersonal skills), family ethnic/religious background, and spouses' interdependency and commitment to marriage.

5. Describe the most commonly used typology or classification for family and/or conjugal power.

6. Explain briefly how the overall family power structure and marital satisfaction are associated.

7. Discuss the major contemporary change occurring in the family power structure.

8. Using the family power continuum, identify where "healthy" families typically are situated.

9. Apply the following assessment areas in a written case history:
   a. Who makes which decisions? Who has the "last say?"
   b. What are the decision-making techniques utilized?
   c. On what bases of power are decisions made?
   d. What are the significant variables affecting family power?

10. From your assessment of the above areas in a case situation, classify whether the family is dominated by a family member (and if so, who); is egalitarian (syncratic or autonomic); or is leaderless and chaotic.

11. From the written case history, state a family nursing diagnosis within the power domain. Propose two general family nursing interventions to assist the family in dealing with its family power problem.

Numerous authors in the fields of family sociology and family counseling have written of the importance of the power dimension within the family (Balswick & Balswick, 1995; Quinn, 1995). For instance, Cromwell and Olson (1975), researchers of family power, wrote that "power is one of the most fundamental aspects of all social interaction" (p. 3). Haley (1976), a noted family therapist, believed that power is central to all human relations. He portrayed human relationships as an ongoing struggle for status and control.

The family, like all social systems, has structures that determine who wields power and what the family's hierarchy or "pecking order" is. Power, as viewed in this text, is one of the four interdependent structural dimensions of the family, and as such is a reflection of family's unwritten family rules and underlying value system. In addition, it is significant in understanding the interpersonal dynamics within the family and between the family and its external relationships. Power and status dimensions are crucial in the establishment and maintenance of family communication channels and networks. In fact, Blood and Wolfe (1960), who conducted the foundational research in family power, maintain that "the most important aspect of the family structure is the power position of the members." Furthermore, the close interrelationship with family roles is apparent in that a person's roles and positions are basic to his or her capacity to influence others to exercise power.

Power structures vary greatly from family to family, with differences positively related to the overall functioning of the family. Some power arrangements are dysfunctional and thereby contribute to family maladaptation and ill health. Moreover, decision making, as one measure of family power, has been a central concern in family therapy. Satir (1972) notes that "there is probably nothing so vital to maintaining and developing a love relationship (or to killing it) as the decision-making process" (p. 131).

Contemporary changes in the family have created an even greater need for family health professionals to assess the power dimension in families. As part of the rapid changes in family life, families are not rigidly bound by tradition to relationships as they once were. Decision making and family power are generally more shared in families (Scanzoni & Szinovacz, 1980; Szinovacz, 1987). No change in the American family is mentioned more often than the gradual shift from one-sided male authority to the sharing of family power by the husband and wife. Declining sex role traditionalism in the family results in family decision making becoming increasingly complex and conflictual (Scanzoni & Szinovacz, 1980).

A knowledge and an appreciation of a family's power structure may be crucial in providing effective health care, especially when families have problems complying with a health regimen or obtaining needed health services. The family member who acts as health leader (being the recognized authority in the area of health or the overall family leader) must be identified, acknowledged, and consulted. For instance, although the mother may be the person with whom the nurse is usually in contact, some channel of communication with the father or grandparent must be found if he or she in fact has the final decision-making power.

Following a presentation of basic definitions and concepts, this chapter discusses the following basic areas in the assessment of family power: (1) the bases for power, (2) power outcomes, (3) decision-making processes, and (4) variables affecting family power. A discussion then follows of the assessment of overall family power, followed by contemporary trends in family power and a description of the attributes of healthy and unhealthy families relative to the family power structure. In the concluding section we present practice guidelines in the area of family power.

▶ FAMILY POWER: DEFINITIONS AND CONCEPTS

Power has numerous meanings, including the capacity to influence, control, dominance, and make decisions. In other words, **power** is the ability—potential or actual—of an individual(s) to control, influence, or change another person's behavior. Power always involves asymmetrical interpersonal relationships—one interactant exerts greater influence/control in the relationship. Power is also multidimensional in nature, meaning that it includes sociostructural, interactional (process), and outcome components (McDonald, 1980).

Family power, as a characteristic of the family system, is the ability—potential or actual—of individual members to change the behavior of other family members (Olson & Cromwell, 1975). Major components of family power are influence and decision making. The term **influence** is practically synonymous with power, being defined as the degree to which formal and informal pressure exerted by one family member on the other(s) is successful in imposing that person's point of view, despite initial opposition (McDonald, 1977). **Dominance** is also used in the same context. In this chapter power, dominance, and influence will be used interchangeably.

Decision making refers to the process directed toward gaining the assent and commitment of family members to carry out a course of action or to maintain the status quo. In other words, it is the "means of getting things accomplished" (Scanzoni & Szinovacz, 1980). Through decision making, power is manifested.

Authority is another closely associated term referring to the shared beliefs of family members, which are culturally and normatively based and which designate a family member as the rightful person to make decisions and assume the leadership position. In other words, authority is present when the individuals involved believe that it is proper for power to be held by a particular member of the group. Traditional beliefs, values, and roles are largely the basis for these beliefs. **Legitimate power** is a synonymous term.

Power and authority do not always go hand in hand. A family member who has the authority to decide or act may not exercise this power for a variety of reasons. Thus there may be an incongruency between the power and authority elements in a family. Comparing the family to a larger social system, one could equate authority with the formal power structure and power with the informal power structure of a bureaucracy. It has long been recognized that within an organization the formal and informal power structures may be quite different from each other. The same situation applies to families. A family member who nominally holds the power may not be the actual power holder. Although family members might tell the health worker that the father is "in charge," he or she might on observation note that the wife-mother is actually the informal power holder (Pasquali et al., 1985).

Power is an abstract, complex, and multidimensional phenomenon that is not directly observable. It must then be inferred from observable behaviors and/or from self-reports of family members, conducted through goal-directed interviews. What is observed by outsiders and what is reported by family members in terms of family power, however, are often at odds with each other (Szinovacz, 1987).

Power is a dimension of the family *system* or *subsystem*, in that it is not a characteristic of a family member apart from the family system. Thus family power can be assessed only within the context of the system or subsystems, and more specifically within the context of the circular processes of family interaction. Communication patterns reveal family role and power dimensions. Family power can be seen in family processes ranging from daily routine exchanges to negotiation of complicated conflictual issues involving, for example, decision making, problem solving, conflict resolution, and crisis management. Moreover, the power dimension is found in the various subsystems within families (e.g., the sibling subsystem, marital subsystem, and parent–child subsystems); the family as a total system; and the family system's relationship with the external social systems (Olson et al., 1975). Within the family, according to McDonald (1980), there are five different units that can be analyzed in terms of their power characteristics. These are marital power, parental power, offspring power, sibling power, and kinship power. Most research and theoretical writing about family power, however, has focused on marital power (Balswick & Balswick, 1995).

► FAMILY POWER AND RESOURCES

The theoretical literature on family power has been largely informed by conflict theory, a grand sociological theory. One of the basic assumptions of conflict theory is that there is a scarcity of resources in the family and other social systems (Hobbes, 1947). A proposition of this theory is that because of the scarcity of resources, people act primarily out of their own self-interest, which must be regulated in order to maintain social order (Hobbes, 1947). Resources and power are viewed in conflict theory as central to the nature of family interaction, including conflict (Klein & White, 1996).

Although resources and power are closely aligned, resources provide a potential base for the exercise of power. Resources include information, skills, techniques, and materials that are accessible to a person or group. They are personal possessions or qualities that are valued by other persons in the family (Balswick & Balswick, 1995). According to Klein and White (1996), power can only be measured by its outcome—which is control—while resources provide the potential for both power and control. In families where the cultural context permits a more egalitarian distribution of power, the more resources a family member possesses vis-à-vis other members, the greater that person's power.

▶ MEASURING FAMILY POWER

How does one measure or assess power in a family? This is the key question, and one for which there is no consensus concerning the appropriate methodology and focus.

Family Task Allocation: Insufficient Indicator of Family Power

Starting with Blood and Wolfe's large study of 900 families, which was completed in 1955 and reported in 1960, researchers have examined family task allocation on the assumption that a positive relationship existed between whoever was in charge of carrying out a particular task and power in that area. But later investigations of family differences in the allocation of responsibilities for the various decision areas and tasks indicated that such division of responsibility seldom reflected the dominant authority pattern. Reiss (1976) explains:

> We must keep in mind that division of labor does not indicate in any direct way who has power or how a decision was arrived at regarding such division of labor. Rather, such a division of labor indicates that these are the traditional ways that tasks are allocated because of reasons that used to, and in some cases still do, have roots in the differences between the sexes in physical and cultural training. Males are still often trained to be more handy with mechanical tasks and tasks that take muscle power, and females are still trained to know more about cooking and cleaning, and those cultural traditions seem the essential basis of the division of tasks in the family. (p. 254)

Johnson (1975) verified this difference between family power and task and responsibility allocation. She interviewed 104 Japanese-American wives in Honolulu. Part of the interview included specific questions about who was responsible for and made decisions in the major areas of family life. She then asked questions to determine the wives' overall freedom to pursue individual interests, counter to wishes of their husbands.

Interestingly enough, Johnson discovered that by only questioning about specific areas the real source of overall power was often distorted. This is because one partner can be delegated responsibility but ultimate power may lie with the other partner. When wives were queried about specific responsibilities and task allocation, they appeared more influential than the husbands. But when asked broadly stated questions pertaining to the wives' evaluation of their overall power as compared to her husbands' power, the data contradicted the responses to the more specific questions. Relative to their husbands' power, most of these wives placed themselves in a subordinate position, largely attributing this fact to their Japanese heritage and its norms regarding male–female roles. Legitimate power or tradition-derived power appeared to be operating here.

Thus while Japanese-American wives played active roles in decision making, they did so by virtue of a delegation of power from their husbands. In this instance, the husband assigned responsibilities while retaining final authority.

Safilios-Rothschild (1976b) makes a very important distinction between the two types of power demonstrated in the above case of the Japanese family. In some families, one spouse has the "orchestration" power (like the Japanese husbands in the latter study had), while the other has "implementation power" (like the Japanese wives had). She explains:

> Spouses who have "orchestration power" have, in fact, the power to make only the important and infrequent decisions that do not infringe upon their time but that determine the family life style and major characteristics and features of their family. They also have the power to relegate unimportant and time-consuming decisions to their spouse who can then derive a "feeling of power" by implementing those decisions within the limitations set by crucial and pervasive decisions made by the powerful spouse. (p. 359)

Hence, in this type of spousal power arrangement the wife is said to have "implementation power." In spite of the fact that implementation power is, in the last analysis, an inferior type of power, having control over implementation still confers power to the implementor. When a family member, the husband, for example, exerts his influence or control and convinces his nonworking wife that she should maintain more discipline of the children, he depends on the wife's commitment to carry out his wishes, as he is typically not in a position to supervise. In this case, the wife, in her central position, has substantial power, because she will decide how and what to implement. In families where the mother is home most of the time and the father is working long hours, the mother is to a large extent in control of family life (Turner, 1970).

Studies of family power have been under criticism because of disagreement over how to measure family power, as well as other methodological limitations. Researchers in the past have relied heavily on the survey and structured interview schedule, with little direct observation to validate self-reported data. What has been consistently found, however, is that people are notoriously inaccurate in describing their own behavior. A case in point of this tendency is in the area of marital relations. It has been observed that when information has been gathered by interviewing families, a strong tendency has been discovered for couples to report an egalitarian relationship with each other, a characterization that is later not verified by observational study (Cromwell & Olson, 1975). Hence it is suggested that the most accurate way to assess family power is to combine observation of marital, parent–child, sibling, and family interaction with self-reporting by all family members if possible (Szinovacz, 1987).

▶ GENERAL ASSESSMENT AREAS

A comprehensive assessment of family power is provided by Cromwell and Olson (1975), who divide the assessment of power up into three areas: power bases, power outcomes, and power or decision-making processes. The major variables influencing the above three domains of power are also discussed in this section. Using a systems approach, the family system in addition to the conjugal (marital), parent–child, and sibling subsystem contains power elements which are important to assess.

Power Bases

One salient aspect of family power concerns the bases for power within the family and its subsystems—that is, the source from which a family member's power is derived. This information often has to be inferred from observed behavior and by asking relevant questions. The importance of making this determination

lies in the fact that the nature of the particular power base significantly affects interpersonal relationships, marital satisfaction, and family stability.

Raven and associates (1975) and Safilios-Rothschild (1976a) conducted significant studies of family power bases from which they identified the various types of power bases commonly observed in families (Table 11–1). A brief description of these types follows.

Legitimate Power or Authority. Legitimate power (sometimes called primary authority) refers to the shared belief and perceptions of family members that one person has the right to control another member's behavior. By virtue of the roles and positions a person occupies, certain rights and culturally derived privileges exist that are associated with these roles and positions. An example would be the "rightness" of parental control or dominance over children. This is traditionally based authority. Where the husband is traditionally in control of the whole family, a patriarchal pattern exists. When legitimate power is present both the husband and wife accept the husband's dominant role as being "right" and "best," indicating role acceptance. Primary authority has remained the traditional and significant base for power in many families. For authority to be effective, the whole family must accept and support this ideology.

Helpless or Powerless Power. A variant form of legitimate power that is often overlooked is called the "power of the powerless." This type of power is an important form of legitimate power that

---

▶ TABLE 11–1

FAMILY POWER BASES

- Legitimate power/authority
- Helpless or powerless power
- Referent power
- Resource power
- Expert power
- Reward power
- Coercive power
- Informational power
- Affective power
- Tension management power

is based on the generally accepted right of those in need or of the helpless to expect assistance from those in a position to render it. Weeks and Jackson (1982) label the person with this kind of power the victim. They explain that the victim acquires a great deal of quasi-power in families. The victim is able to covertly acquire influence or power from others who often already feel drained of resources. Helpless power may be very effective in families where one member is chronically ill, disabled, or aged. A spouse or a disabled family member may control the family on the basis of his or her frailty or helplessness. This is a commonly seen base for power and, unfortunately, may lead to a situation that makes it difficult for other family members' needs to be adequately met. Children's dependency and helplessness arouse feelings of responsibility in parents and make them susceptible to children's control attempts and use of "helpless power."

Referent Power.

A third source for power is termed referent power and applies to the type of power persons have over others because of family members' positive identification with them, such as in a child's positive identification with a parent. Children imitate behaviors of family members, usually the parents, who serve as their role models.

Resource and Expert Power.

Resource power is the type of power base that comes from having the greater number of valued resources in a relationship. When power is defined as an ability to influence or pressure, resources such as certain attributes, circumstances, or possessions are seen as primary determinants of that ability (Osmond, 1978). The greater resources of one spouse over the other are viewed as the chief alternative source of family power to traditionally based authority (McDonald, 1977). For example, the husband may be dominant because he controls the purse strings, or the wife may be dominant because she is more practical and goal directed than her husband.

One important resource is the use of interpersonal techniques. It is not uncommon to find one family member who has few of the objective resources that ordinarily facilitate dominance actually controlling much of family life through his or her masterful use of a broad repertoire of interpersonal techniques (Turner, 1970).

The person in a relationship who has the least interest in maintaining the relationship (like the wife having less interest in the relationship than the husband) has a very important resource at his or her disposal.

Waller (1938) explains this case by what he calls "the principle of less interest." This principle explains that exploitation is likely to occur in a relationship where the differences in levels of involvement are great. For instance, the principle of less interest states that within a dyadic relationship, the person who cares least about whether the relationship continues or not has the greatest power over the relationship. He or she usually has less interest and involvement in maintaining the relationship because he or she has many more alternatives or resources. With decreased involvement, the less interested person can use manipulative or coercive techniques at the expense of the other. A commonly seen example may help elucidate this principle. In a marital situation, one member may be quite valued and independent, while the other individual feels dependent and inferior. Decisions are then made by the dominant mate, since he or she has many more options open and there is less interest or involvement in the relationship. In middle-class America this principle still operates in favor of the man because of his greater economic resources (Quinn, 1995).

Expert power, a particular type of resource power, exists in a relationship when the person being "influenced" perceives that the other person (the "expert") has some special knowledge, skill, expertise, or experience (Safilios-Rothschild, 1976a).

Reward Power.

Reward power stems from the expectation that the influencing, dominant person will do something positive in response to the other person's compliance. Overt bargaining may accompany the use of reward power. Children, according to Szinovacz (1987), possess an important resource in their compliance. Children's "good" behavior is a source of pleasure and pride to parents, and thus constitutes a basis for power (i.e., children often use "good" behavior in order to obtain desired benefits).

Coercive or Dominance Power.

The effective use of this source of power is based on the perception and belief that the person with power might or will punish through threats, coercion, or violence other individuals if they do not comply.

Coercive power is used with coercive decision making (to be discussed later). (In research of families with adolescents, it has been discovered that the use of this type of power, as well as reward power, is not nearly as effective a base of parental power as is legitimate, referent, or expert power (Gecas & Seff, 1991).

Informational Power.

This power base stems from the content of the persuasive message. An individual is convinced of the "rightness" of the sender's message due to a careful and successful explanation of the necessity for change (Raven et al., 1975). This type of power is similar to but more limited in scope than expert power.

A variation of this direct information power is "indirect" informational power. This occurs when a more subtle dropping of hints, suggestions, and information influences a person to act without the obvious indication of persuasion (Raven et al., 1975). In the traditional sex-role relationship, women often use indirect informational power to gain influence and not to "bruise" men's image in public.

Affective Power.

Affective power refers to the power derived through the manipulation of a family member by bestowing or withdrawing affection and warmth, and, in the case of the spouse, sex. Some couples may be fairly equal in family power because of different resources they bring to the marriage, e.g., the husband brings economic resources, while the wife brings affection and nurturance which is highly valued by the husband (Balswick & Balswick, 1995). Withdrawal of sex has long been discussed in novels as a "woman's hidden weapon." Because women usually lack the socioeconomic weapons of men, affective power historically has been a source of power for women. A woman's affective resource, including being loved by her spouse, if exercised, can be a powerful resource in a marriage.

Tension Management Power.

This type of power base is derived from the control that one spouse achieves by managing the present tensions and conflicts in the family. Using tears, pouting, endless debating, and disagreements to get a family member to "give in" is an example of tension management power, which either child or adult family members may use to obtain power.

Power Outcomes

A second area of assessment relative to family power is the area of power outcomes. Here the focus is on who makes the final decisions or ultimately possesses *control*. In other words, "who wins" or "has the last say" (Cromwell & Olson, 1975; Szinovacz, 1987). Specific questions can be asked of the family to elicit this information. For instance, one might ask who is responsible for making decisions about the areas of major importance in family life. In conjugal relationships power can vary, with role definitions determining who had power in a given area. For example, the wife might have more power in regard to social and kin relationships and household matters, while the husband has more control over the finances. In other families power may be more equally divided, with a pattern of shared power prevailing.

It must be remembered, however, that specific areas of responsibility and of decision making may not coincide with the more general and dominant power pattern in a family. Recall the distinction between implementation and orchestration power described earlier. That is, Johnson's 1975 findings of power within Japanese-American families demonstrated the significance of differentiating implementation from orchestration power. An assessor can easily be misled by the obvious responsibilities and decisions of one mate rather than realize that these are actually delegated, or relegated, to the weaker partner by the dominant member of the family. Thus on the surface it may appear that the wife is responsible for grocery shopping, cooking, and child rearing. But these tasks may only be relegated to her by her husband, and should her actions incur his displeasure, her power may be withdrawn. This is the usual case in authoritarian or patriarchal families. In these types of families, the husband's power may derive not only from a traditional value structure but also from possessing more resources. Economic resources (money) are particularly important in determining marital power (Blumstein & Schwartz, 1983).

A second related question dealing with power outcomes is a more global or general question that can be posed to family members. This question entails asking about whose idea or suggestion is finally adopted when major decisions or choices must be made. In families where decisions are shared and represent the outcome of mutual discussion and exploration, this kind of information is difficult to obtain. But despite the difficulty involved in getting family members to describe the outcome (people remember what decision was made but find it harder to remember who had the last say or made the ultimate decision), assessment of the outcome of an issue, conflict, or argument is helpful to discover in ascertaining the source of power and in whom this resides. Komarovsky (1964) notes that "power is most visible in contested decisions ending in victory of one partner. But power exists irrespective of conflict, because the powerful partner may so influence the wishes and preferences of his mate that a contest of wills does not even arise" (p. 221). Power differentials, then, may function to suppress potential conflictual situations and cause "silent agreement" (McDonald, 1980; Scanzoni & Szinovacz, 1980).

In regard to decisions and their outcomes, discerning what kinds of problems or issues are involved and how important they are to the family is helpful. Does a decision cut across all the major areas of family life or is it limited to a specific area? Komarovsky (1964) underscores the significance of ascertaining the centrality of the issue by observing that "general decision making in one or two areas of family life may not be a good index of general power. It depends upon the importance of such areas for each partner" (p. 221).

Power or Decision-making Processes

In addition to assessing power bases and power outcomes, the process used in arriving at family decisions is also crucial in the assessment of family power (Scanzoni & Szinovacz, 1980; Szinovacz, 1987). Family power has primarily been researched by focusing on decision making. The decision-making process is a principal index of power (Blood & Wolfe, 1960). In fact, power or dominance patterns are the by-product of the decision-making process. Family decision making refers to "the interactional techniques which family members employ in their attempts to gain control in the negotiation or decision-making process" (McDonald, 1980, p. 843).

In assessing this area, the central focus is *how* decisions are made. By understanding the techniques used in family decision making, the assessor will be better able to identify the relative power of each family member and his or her participation in family decision making.

There are three types of decision-making processes discussed in the literature. Families tend to make use of one particular method of decision making over another, although the secondary use of one or both of the other basic techniques of decision making is also seen. Analysis of the family decision-making processes reveals the tremendous interrelationship of these features with the other structural dimensions of the family. For instance, the family that extensively uses democratic methods of decision making (consensus decision making), for example, will generally have an egalitarian role and power structure and a value system in which role sharing and more open communications exist.

Decision Making by Consensus. The first technique of decision making is termed consensus. According to American ideals, this is the healthy way to make decisions. Here a particular course of action is mutually agreed on by all involved. There is equal commitment to the decision, as well as satisfaction with the decision by family members. Consensus decisions are agreed on through discussion and negotiation. Because a substantial degree of interdependence and egalitarianism among family members is needed as well as an ability to discuss and problem solve, this kind of decision making is more difficult, complex, and unpredictable than other kinds.

When there is initial disagreement regarding an issue, negotiation is one of the major techniques used in families to handle a conflictual situation (Klein & White, 1996). Consensus occurs when negotiating members agree to a solution that is seen as meeting their personal or shared values (Turner, 1970). In families with patriarchal or matriarchal (unilateral) authority patterns, there is little room for negotiation. Negotiation is more commonly used in democratic or egalitarian families (Klein & White, 1996).

Decision Making by Accommodation. A second type of decision making is termed accommodation. Here the family members' initial feelings about an issue are discordant. One or more family members then makes concessions, either willingly or unwillingly. Some member(s) assent in order to allow a decision to be reached. Hence it may involve a voluntary compromise in which concessions are made by all persons concerned or a sacrifice, made by one family member so that others may have their own way. Privately or publicly the conceding member(s) will not be convinced, however, that the decision in question was best (Turner, 1970).

Accommodative decisions are made somewhere on a continuum from **coercion** to **compromising**. Differences in the attitudes of participants towards their commitment, as well as differences in the relationship under which the forms of accommodation take place, determine whether the decision making is more coercive or more compromising.

Going from the most functional to the least functional form of accommodating, the several ways (compromising, bargaining, or coercion) in which accommodation occurs are described. **Compromising** refers to the making of concessions by all family members involved so that the decision reached is not reflective of any of the members' original choices, but has some acceptable elements for all concerned. In **bargaining** one or more members make concessions to another/others and expect reciprocity, so that ultimately the sacrifices of each balance out. The use of bargaining in family negotiations demonstrates that a trust exists among the members, along with a belief that others will be fair and honest in keeping up their ends of the bargain. **Coercion** is the least functional technique along the accommodation continuum. It results in an unwilling agreement by one or more family members, whereby commitment is assured only by the continuance of coercive power. The existence of threat of punishment shows the dominance of one member over others.

To summarize, an accommodation is always an agreement to disagree. A common decision is adopted in the face of irreconcilable differences (Turner, 1970).

De-facto Decision Making.

Family members may also arrive at decisions by using a de-facto route. In this case, things are allowed "to just happen" without planning. In the absence of active, voluntary, or effective decision making, decisions just occur. De-facto decisions may also be made when arguments occur to which there was no discernible resolution or when issues were not brought up and discussed. These decisions, then, are made by inaction rather than by deliberate action.

De-facto decision making is seen in many disorganized, multiproblem families, many of whom believe in fate and feel powerless to control their own destiny. Moreover, de facto decision making may be situationally limited or occur when problems in communication exist, as when significant problems or issues are not discussed. Cultural norms are important to consider here, because obstacles to open communication and active decision making may also have a cultural or ethnic basis. For example, among traditional Latino couples, sexual relations and family planning may be an area of closed communication; pregnancies may therefore become the outcome of de-facto decision making.

Variables Affecting Family Power

In addition to the need to assess the above three areas of family power, there are some important contingency variables that significantly influence family power. A listing of these appears in Table 11-2. Each of these factors will now be further discussed.

Family Power Hierarchy.

Each family has a power hierarchy or "pecking order." In the traditional nuclear family and in most nuclear families today, the power structure is clearly hierarchical, meaning that the power structure is tiered and the "pecking occurs downward." Men often develop or maintain power over women, and parents almost always have more power than children (Hoffman, 1981). In the egalitarian family, however, a clear, generationally based power hierarchy may be absent.

► TABLE 11-2

VARIABLES AFFECTING FAMILY POWER STRUCTURE

1. Family power hierarchy
2. Type of family form (single parent, blended family, traditional two-parent nuclear family, etc.)
3. Formation of coalitions
4. Family communication network
5. Social class
6. Family developmental stage
7. Situational contingencies
8. Ethnic and religious influences
9. Person variables (members' gender, ages, and interpersonal skills)
10. Spouses' emotional interdependency and commitment to marriage

Minuchin (1974) and Haley (1976, 1980) place great importance on the lines of authority or hierarchically arranged power structures in families. Minuchin (1974) asserts that parents constitute the executive subsystem and should not forfeit or diminish that responsibility in any way (Minuchin, 1974).

Type of Family Form.

Minuchin (1974) describes variations in the power hierarchy due to differing family forms. In large families, single-parent families, or families where both parents are employed, some allocation of parental power is usually given to an older child(ren). Children may be assigned more rights and responsibilities than is the case in the two-parent nuclear family (Ganong, Coleman, & Fine, 1995). Having older children parent younger children may work well, as younger children are cared for and the parental child can develop responsibility, competence, and autonomy beyond his or her years. The family with a parental child structure may experience problems, however, when the delegation of authority is unclear or if the parents abdicate their authority, leaving the parental child to become the primary source of decision making, control, and guidance. In these situations, the child is given a task that exceeds his or her abilities and that interferes with meeting his or her childhood needs of support and dependency.

In newly formed stepparent families, remarriage puts pressure on the new family to change the power hierarchy that existed in the prior single-parent family. Conflict may occur when stepchildren perceive a loss of power and control within the new stepparent family. Mothers appear to have more decision-making power in their new family than they had in their first marriage, retaining some of the power that they had when they headed the family before they remarried (Ganong, Coleman, & Fine, 1995).

Formation of Family Coalitions.

One of the ways the power structure of the family is altered is by the formation of coalitions. Coalitions are either temporary, issue-based alliances, or long-term alliances made to offset the dominance of one or more other family members. Family members form coalitions based on each person's relative power (Caplow, 1968, cited in Klein & White, 1996). Subgroups within a family band together to support each other and to increase their power position relative to other members of the family (Stachowiak, 1975).

Obviously then, coalitions generate more power for the members who join together.

Coalitions in families are most healthy when they exist within the appropriate power levels (Gorman, 1975). It has been pointed out by family therapists (Lidz, 1963; Minuchin, 1974; Satir, 1972) that a sustaining parental coalition is a healthy and a virtually necessary phenomenon to effectively parent children. In contrast, long-term, extensively used parent–child coalitions are unhealthy, because they disrupt the intact functioning of the parent–child and spouse subsystems (Smoyak, 1975). Nevertheless, mother–child coalitions are especially common in patriarchal families, where the father's power is great and together the mother and an older child can to some degree dilute his power. The child in this case can also expect special favors from the mother. Being in a long-term coalition with one parent may, however, keep the child enmeshed with that parent and inhibit or prevent the child from individuating or separating from the family (Stachowiak, 1975).

Sibling coalitions are also common. Children join forces to oppose more efficaciously or to evade the rules parents establish (Turner, 1970).

Coalition formation most commonly occurs with democratic versus primary (traditional) authority patterns. In addition, over a family's life cycle, the relative power of family members changes and, in turn, potential coalitions change (Caplow, 1968).

One of the difficulties in a single-parent family is the obvious inability to form a parental coalition. Two-parent families tend to have significantly more resources and alternatives available to them than do one-parent families, because partners in the former can support each other and form a coalition. In one-parent families, the strength of primary authority (legitimate power) may be a dominant and necessary factor for the single parent to exercise to control the family situation (Jayaratne, 1978).

Family Communication Network.

Communication is seldom of equal intensity within each of the pairs of relationships in the family. The husband and wife may communicate frequently, intensely, and over a wide area of topics, while the father and youngest son may have very little communication with each other. Two siblings may have a close, confidential type of relationship, while a third sibling communicates only tangentially with her two other siblings. Age and sex characteristics, as well as personality attributes of family members, influence the nature of the family communication network.

When there is unequal communication between family members, intermediaries ("go-betweens") usually exist. The person in the family who serves as an intermediary in communications between others (in many instances the mother), but who is able to interact directly with all family members, holds a central position in the communication network.

Communication networks are mentioned here because of their correlation with the power structure. The greater the centrality of the family member, the greater his or her power, due to his or her control over the outcome of the decision-making process. Because the intermediary understands the attitudes and opinions of most of the family members, he or she can use this information to influence family members. The go-between is also able to censor or screen information from the sender to the other family members. This censorship function and ability to alter messages as seen fit gives the intermediary extensive power, at least in some areas. In larger families one may find a secondary intermediary—such as an older son or daughter—who acts as a link between other children and the mother (Turner, 1970).

Social Class Differences in Family Power

Lower-class Families. Besmer (1967) summarizes the frequently seen power characteristics of poor families in the United States. The husband is more likely to proclaim authority simply because he is a male, although actually having to concede more authority to the wife due to the paucity of his resources. The father most generally loses influence in the family at lower socioeconomic levels as a consequence of his social and occupational inadequacy. An authoritarian theme is a strong underlying factor in the interpersonal relationships of the poor. There is a strong belief in the validity of strength as the source of power and on the rightness of existing patterns. An individual's dominance, rather than expertise and the merit of his or her suggestions, is relied on as the common source of decisions.

The lower-class wife has relatively more responsibilities than either the middle- or upper-class wife or the lower-class husband, and frequently has more influence in the family decision making than house-

wives of the other classes. This is especially true in the financial area, where the lower-class wife may feel that earning money is the man's responsibility and spending it wisely is the woman's.

Working-class Families. In an early influential study by Komarovsky (1964), education was found to be the important determinant as to how authoritarian a family power structure was among working-class families; the higher the education, the more flexible and "middle class" certain ideals and protocols in marriage became. The incidence of dominance by the husband declined with better education of the husband, and in contrast, patriarchal attributes were more prevalent among the less educated.

Middle-class Families. According to Kanter (1978), the most egalitarian or companion-based marriages seem to be found among the lower-middle-class, white-collar workers, perhaps as a result of the greater availability of the husband's time to share chores and act as a companion to his wife. Resource and expert power are more often used as a bases for power in upper-middle-class families (Szinovacz, 1987).

The Family Developmental Stage.
The decisions a family makes are also closely associated with the family's life cycle, as is the distribution of power among the family members. Families tend to evolve from where the major concentration of power is in the hands of the adults when the children are young, to a more shared power arrangement as children move into adolescence. More specifically, during the early years of marriage, before children, couples tend to be syncratic—discussing and mutually deciding on major decisions among themselves, except perhaps decisions about the husband's job and housekeeping matters (Blood, 1969). Later in the family's life cycle, when children are being raised and the system is more complex, each spouse usually has clearly defined areas of power and decision making, although major decisions are still jointly made. Corrales (1975) explains that when the dyad changes to a triad with the addition of a baby, some loss in the wife's power is often seen. Typically, mates discuss most areas less and less as time goes on, a sign that some estrangement from each other may also

be occurring. During adolescence older children assume more power in the family than when they were younger. The shifts in power that take place during the time when adolescents are in the home are never easy, with much of the conflict that arises at this time revolving around the power distribution. In the later years of the family, the marital couple, returning to a dyadic relationship, again typically share in decision making and power.

Situational Contingencies.

Situational changes can also signal changes in the power structure of the family. For example, it has been observed that when a husband is unemployed over a period of time that he usually loses power in the family if resource power has been the basis for his power (Elder, 1974; McCubbin & Dahl, 1985). The chronically ill or alcoholic spouse is often shut out of the family decision-making process.

Other situational contingencies also affect family power. Time pressure is one factor that has been studied. Under high time pressure, there is greater likelihood of agreement (the converse is also true). The presence of others when power is being exercised also influences the power processes utilized. More "acceptable" power or control tactics are used in the presence of others. And finally, family stress affects family members' behaviors in negotiating or bargaining situations. Increased stress tends to decrease interactants' tolerance for ambiguity, cognitive flexibility, and ability to problem-solve (Szinovacz, 1987).

Ethnic and Religious Influences.

Ethnic and religious differences among families also dictate different power arrangements. For instance, male dominance is commonly seen in unacculturated immigrant families from Europe, Asia, and Latin America. In traditional immigrant Asian families in which strong Confucian values are present, the male is ascribed the ultimate authority in the family. It is believed that men, having more important responsibilities, should be relieved of the mundane concerns of everyday life. "Thus, the wife is usually in charge of the budget and makes most of the economic decisions for the family. Although the husband is the head of the family, the wife is in charge of domestic life . . . the husband has orchestration power and the wife, implementation power" (Balswick & Balswick, 1995, p. 301).

Some of our stereotypes about male dominance in Hispanic families and female dominance in African-American families have come under close scrutiny. They are being seriously questioned today (see Chaps. 19 and 20 for elaboration).

An older matriarch is sometimes present in traditionally oriented ethnic families. In this case, or in cases where grandparents have a strong influence on the family, greater culturally derived power resides in the extended family.

Person Variables (Members' Gender, Age, and Interpersonal Skills).

Several variables that reside within the individual family member also influence his or her relative power in the family. The primary ones are the members' gender, age, and interpersonal skills. Of these variables, gender differences are the most widely cited.

Gender Differences. There is wide consensus in the literature, particularly the feminist literature, that gender relations are based on power (Ellman & Taggart, 1993) and that women typically have less power in the family than men. Much of the power differential in the family is based on economic inequality. Women, if they work outside the home, are paid less and thus have fewer economic resources than men to bring into the marital relationship. If women work inside the home, their work is unpaid and often devalued (Goldner, 1985; Okin, 1989). Moreover, our societal notions of what constitutes "masculinity" and "femininity" maintain these gender-based power inequities. Even when women have a considerable amount of resources, they often are inhibited from using them fully because of the cultural norms that support male superiority and power (Blumstein & Schwartz, 1991). Goldner (1985), a feminist, considers power to be a key to understanding family interactions. She explains that since the power of women is considerably less than that of men, the way in which women interact with their spouses is quite different. For instance, it has been observed that men who lack material or personal resources use manipulation and intimidation to gain control. In contrast, women who lack material or personal resources tend to "give in" or gain influence by acting weak, dependent, or manipulative (Balswick & Balswick, 1995).

In comparison to the preceding feminist interpretations of gender and power inequalities, Kranichfield

(1987) gives a more positive view of women's power in the family. She points out that in the family domain women in fact have a great deal of overlooked power. Women's power is pervasive when power is defined as the ability to bear, educate, and determine the personality, values, and beliefs of each new human being in society. Women's lives are far more involved in the family than are men's. Women exert more intergenerational influence than do men and hold the position of "kinkeeper" in most families. This situation has not changed, even with the increased participation of women in the work force.

Age Differences.   As one would expect, as children in a family grow older, their power and ability to influence and make decisions grows. In other words, as children develop social skills and resources, their power correspondingly increases. At the other end of the life span continuum, elderly persons in families often experience a decline in power, as they lose resources (Klein & White, 1996).

Interpersonal Skills of Family Members. One important person variable is the resource of interpersonal skills. This includes the ability to argue convincingly, negotiate or bargain successfully, as well as manipulate, lie, and cajole. It is not uncommon to find a family member who has few of the objective resources that ordinarily facilitate dominance, but who actually controls much of family life through his or her masterful use of a broad repertoire of interpersonal skills (Turner, 1970).

Spouses' Emotional Interdependency and Commitment to Marriage.
Research by Godwin and Scanzoni (1989) demonstrated that partners' emotional dependency (the love and caring for their spouse that each spouse reports) and the degree of commitment to their marital relationship influence the decision-making processes that are used in the family. Data were collected via observation and self-reports from 188 married couples. The study found that the more wives report loving their husbands, the less coercive tactics are used and the more consensus in decision making is likely. And husbands indicate that the more committed they are to the marriage, the more control the wife has.

▶ OVERALL FAMILY POWER

One of the purposes in analyzing the assessment areas (bases for power, power outcomes and decision-making processes, and the variables affecting power) is to be able to classify a family as to its overall power structure. This involves being able to state whether a family is dominated by one member (usually one spouse), has an egalitarian power structure, or has no effective leadership (is chaotic). Some authors point out that most of the classifications used to describe families are too simplistic and do not adequately reflect the dynamic qualities of family power or its complexity. Although we should be aware that an overall labeling of family power may neither be possible nor entirely accurate, we cannot overlook the value of classification: namely, that it permits a lot to be said in a few words. If a family displays an overall dysfunctional power structure, a statement of this conclusion may serve as a family nursing diagnosis.

Historically, the literature has described generalized, pure types of families—in particular (1) the patriarchal, traditional family and (2) the democratic, egalitarian, or modern family. In the patriarchal, traditional family, the father is the head of the family, with family power vested in his hands; and his wife, his sons, and their wives and children, and his unmarried daughters, are subordinated to his power. In contrast, the democratic modern, egalitarian family is based on the equality of husband and wife, with consensus in making decisions and increasing participation by children as they grow older (Burgess et al., 1963; Scanzoni & Szinovacz, 1980).

A frequently used typology today for classifying power in the marital subsystem or family was developed by Herbst (1954). It divides marital power into autocratic, syncratic, and autonomic patterns. **Autocratic** power patterns exist when the family is dominated by a single family member. In these families, decisions on marital activities, and usually family activities also, are made solely by this individual. **Syncratic** power patterns exist when decisions involving the marriage, as well as the family, are made by both members of the marital dyad. In this case there is a greater mutual commitment and shared involvement in the marriage. An **autonomic** power structure is present when the two partners share power but do this by functioning independently of one another in both decision making and their activities. Other authors refer to this pattern at the family attribute as "atomistic."

One of the problems with Herbst's (1954) original typology is that he assumed that the power always rested with one or the other parents (or was shared). This is a constricting approach, because the dominant individual may be a child, grandparent, or another family member if the family is other than a traditional two-parent nuclear family. Most research into family power has, in fact, dealt with conjugal power rather than family power, focusing on only husband–wife interactions to the exclusion of the child's role in the decision-making processes. The relative power of children in families has been found to be substantial, especially in families with older children. For instance, Strodtbeck (1978) found that the power of an adolescent son in a family was almost as great as that of the mother. Thus an adequate assessment must include consideration of the children's power (McDonald, 1977).

In contrast with the analysis and classification of marital power relationships, the categorization of the parent–child subsystem has usually been quite simple: for example, on a continuum from high to low parental control.

In family process literature, which derives largely from family therapy, the categories most widely used are symmetrical (balanced) and complementary (submissive–dominant) relationships. Symmetrical and complementary role relationships are discussed in Chapter 12.

Lewis and associates (1976) developed a comprehensive model for summarizing a family's power structure that includes the chaotic or leaderless family not identified in the former models. Figure 11–1 modifies the model by Lewis and associates, incorporating the various types of power commonly observed in families. This continuum is suggested for use in assessing overall family power dimensions. Subsystem power (marital, parent–child, and sibling) is also important to consider.

Marital Satisfaction and Family Power Type

Research carried out from 1950 through 1990 consistently demonstrates that family power is significantly related to marital satisfaction. Higher levels of

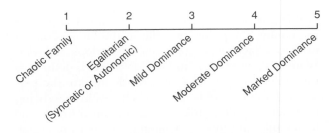

Figure 11–1. The family power continuum. The chaotic family (1) refers to a leaderless family, wherein no member has adequate power to make decisions effectively. In egalitarian syncratic and autonomic families (2), decisions and power are shared. In the syncratic form the decisions are made together; in the autonomic form the decisions are made independently. Dominance or power (3–5) ranges from marked, where there is practically absolute control by an individual and no negotiation, to mild, where there is a tendency for dominance and submissiveness, but most decisions are reached through respectful, mutual negotiation.

satisfaction are found most frequently among egalitarian couples and couples where the husband is dominant versus when the wife is dominant. Wife-dominated couples have generally been found to rate their marriages as less satisfying (McDonald, 1980; Szinovacz, 1987). It is curious that women who were dominant classified themselves as the least maritally satisfied, far below their husbands' satisfaction. The tentative conclusion that may be drawn is that the wife is dominant by default, not choice, being forced to fill the vacuum created by a weak, passive, or incompetent husband. Wife dominance also goes against normative expectations, that is, the cultural prescriptions of either the traditional (husband-dominated) or the modern (egalitarian) marriage. It is interesting to note, however, that husbands in these marriages are not also unhappy. Corrales (1975) speculates that the reason might be because the wife not only makes most of the decisions, but also assumes most family roles.

▶ CONTEMPORARY TRENDS IN FAMILY POWER

There has been a gradual shift from the traditional, patriarchal family structure toward a more democratic, egalitarian family structure. Nevertheless, because male and female roles in the family are socioculturally defined and mediated, family structure is not that easily changed (Ellman & Taggart, 1993). As egalitarianism in the family becomes more prominent, changes in women's base for power are occurring, albeit slowly. Men are often more likely to use expert power or direct informational power as a base for influence in the family rather than primary authority. Women, however, still use referent power, "helpless" power, and indirect informational power much more prominently. These bases for power are selected by women because of their greater acceptability to their mates. When women use expert power and direct informational power, they are sometimes seen as being "masculine" and "aggressive." While the common use of helpless power by women, however, is more acceptable to their spouses, it is not to their own self-esteem. As noted, women also have implementation power, but often not orchestration power. Research findings agree that work force participation and achievement of higher education have given women more power in the family (Balswick & Balwick, 1995; Leslie & Korman, 1989).

► HEALTHY AND UNHEALTHY FAMILY POWER ATTRIBUTES

Lewis and associates (1976) conducted in-depth interviews with a group of middle-class families to determine their psychosocial health status and the family structural characteristics with which health status was correlated. From their analysis of interviews and observations, they grouped families into three categories of health, from the severely dysfunctional to optimally healthy. It was generally found that the most severely dysfunctional families presented chaotic family structures (see Fig. 11–1), and the most competent of families presented flexible structures. These researchers emphasized that "the most direct measure of structure concerned the distribution of power or influence within the family" (Lewis et al., 1976, p. 209).

The power attributes of healthy families were seen to reflect the following:

> . . . the parental coalition played a crucial role in the determination of overall family competence. . . . Leadership was provided by the parental coalition as was a model of relating

which appeared to be of great learning value to the children. Leadership was shared by the parents. . . . This trend toward an egalitarian marriage was in striking contrast to both the more distant marriages of the adequate families and the marital pattern of dominance and submission that so often was seen in the dysfunctional families. (p. 210)

In the healthy families, the parents, acting as a coalition, did not exercise their power in an authoritarian or rigid way but, within their style of leadership, left room for options and negotiation. Nevertheless, power and boundaries were clear; there was no confusion as to the position and power of family members. Generally the father held the most power, the mother somewhat less, and the child distinctly the least power (Lewis et al., 1976). In contrast, all the severely disturbed families showed that none of the family members had much power. The most inept families, the authors reported, had a powerless father and a strong coalition between mother and child. In families labeled as midrange, a strong, healthy parental–marital coalition did not exist. These families characteristically maintained rigid, authoritarian structures via dominance by one mate.

Family control processes, such as rigid authoritarian structures, affect children in the family. Through modeling, children learn power-relevant behaviors such as coercive, Machiavellian, and/or violent behaviors (Straus et al., 1980).

Minuchin (1974) agrees with Lewis and associates' findings when he asserts that the most important aspect of power within a family is the presence of a clear and functioning hierarchy in which the parents function as the executive subsystem and children have different levels of authority. For a family to function effectively, there must also be complementarity of functions, with the husband and wife accepting interdependency and working as a team.

Family Violence: Power Characteristics

Three major theoretical perspectives used to explain the dynamics of family violence (the intraindividual, the sociocultural, and the social–psychological perspective) address unhealthy power characteristics in violent families (Table 11–3). In the **intraindividual** (within the individual) **perspective**, personality attributes of the abusive husband and the victimized wife are believed to "cause" abuse to occur and continue. Bolton and Bolton (1987) summarize research findings relative to the personality characteristics of the conjugal violence perpetrator:

> The need to control pervades the conjugal violence perpetrator's behavioral style. Although capable of controlling very little outside the home, his control in the home is absolute, extending through financial decisions, child care, sexual relationships, leisure time activities, and even menu. Domineering and hostile, this perpetrator acts out his dislike for authority figures through those who cannot exert authority over him: the weaker members of the family. (p. 126)

Abusive spouses can offer occasional warmth and protectiveness on their best days. It is this intermittent positive reinforcement that "locks" the victim(s) into the relationship. In other words, family relationships in abusive families are maintained through the abuse of power by the perpetrator and the dynamics of love, connectedness, and loyalty (Miller, 1989).

Abusive husbands may abuse, threaten, and intimidate women in such a way that they feel powerless to change the relationship or to leave. Sometime they believe that they are to blame for

their spouse's violent outbursts (Murray & Leigh, 1995). Women are more likely to be victims of spouse abuse when they display characteristics of being a weak, vulnerable woman, as well as being an isolated person who is overcome by anxiety, guilt, and shame (Steinmetz, 1995).

In child abuse, parents (both fathers and mothers) also misuse their parental power to sexually or physically abuse their children (Murray & Leigh, 1995). Abusive parents have been found to be socially and psychologically troubled individuals who are less nurturant and have excessive authority and power needs (Steinmetz, 1995).

Sociocultural theories of violence focus on the macrolevel conditions of society that create a tendency for family violence (Steinmetz, 1995). Sexism, racism, ageism, poverty, inadequate housing, unemployment or underemployment, and opportunity disparities are societal conditions that create frustrations that are brought home to the family. They set up significant preconditions for violence to occur. Some family violence theorists believe that a society's general attitudes toward the use of physical aggression to resolve social problems is reflected in families' use of physical aggression. In any case, the impact of society's attitudes and norms on the family is always considerable.

The concept of the children being the property of parents—who are free to discipline as they see fit—is an ancient concept that only recently has been constrained (Steinmetz, 1995). Even today, the introduction of parental rights legislation in some states is evidence that some conservative parents still believe that they should have practically absolute power over how their children are cared for, educated, and disciplined.

Social–psychological perspectives about family violence examine the interface between the individual and society. Issues of power, control, social class, employment opportunities, and transfer of property are central to the analysis of family violence using this theoretical perspective. Steinmetz (1995) and others believe that *power* is a critical component of violence because: (1) it characterizes and legitimates intrafamilial interactions between spouses and between parents and children; (2) it provides an indication of the value society places on each family member (for example, the value of men over women); and (3) the power that is available to a specific family is based on the value that family is seen to have in the family's

► TABLE 11–3

THEORIES OF FAMILY VIOLENCE

- *The Intraindividual Perspective:* This perspective focuses on the personality characteristics of the perpetrator and victim as "causing" family violence.
- *The Sociocultural Perspective:* Sociocultural factors, related to societal or cultural differences in viewing violence as a way to resolve family problems, are described and analyzed.
- *The Social–Psychological Perspective:* This perspective explains family violence as a function of the interface between the individual and society with respect to issues of power, control, social class (poverty), employment opportunities, and transfer of property.

Adapted from Steinmetz (1995).

community (e.g., a prominent family has more value to the community than a poor family). *Control*, the outcome of having greater power, is also a crucial aspect of family violence according to this theoretical perspective. Control includes direct control over another person, as well as control of resources, with poor and working-class families having fewer resources and, hence, less power and control.

One of the interesting suggestions of family violence researchers is that family violence may actually be increasing as women become more educated, obtain better jobs, and make a better income. Because these advances provide them with more power and control, men may react more aggressively and violently to try to maintain their declining power and control (Steinmetz, 1995).

FAMILY POWER STRUCTURE: APPLYING THE FAMILY NURSING PROCESS

▶ assessment questions

In this chapter the various major areas germane to family power are described. Family power is obviously not an easily inferred dimension to assess. In spite of these difficulties, the following summary of the primary facets of power, the areas to observe, and the questions to ask will hopefully make the assessment process more concrete and clear.

Power Outcomes

Who has the "last say" or "who wins"? Who makes what decisions? And how important are these decisions or issues to the family? More specific questions may be asked to elicit this information (validating what you can with observations). General questions followed by more specific questions in these areas may be helpful:

a. Financial: Who budgets, pays bills, decides on how money is spent?
b. Social: Who decides on how to spend an evening or which friends or relatives to see?
c. Major decisions: Who decides on changes in jobs or residence?
d. Child rearing: Who disciplines and decides on children's activities? (Johnson, 1975)

It must be remembered, though, when asking these questions, that *overall* power in the family often does not correlate well with specific task responsibilities (the issue of orchestration power versus implementation power).

Decision-making Processes

What specific techniques are utilized for making decisions in the family and to what extent are these utilized?

a. Consensus decision making
b. Accommodation decision making
   1. Bargaining
   2. Compromising
   3. Coercion
c. De-facto decision making

Specific questions eliciting decision-making techniques used focuses on *how* the family makes decisions.

Power Bases

This area deals with the source from which the power of various family members is derived. To enumerate again, these sources are:

1. Legitimate power/authority.

2. Helpless or powerless power.

3. Referent power.

4. Resource and expert power.

5. Reward power.

6. Coercive power.

7. Informational power—direct and indirect.

8. Affective power.

9. Tension management power.

Questions asked to elicit information on the source or bases of power might be either specific questions about who makes certain decisions and how (sometimes how also reveals the bases for power). For example, in speaking to the husband-father: "On what basis was it decided to send the children to summer camp?" Or you may suggest choices, such as, "Was your wife's suggestion agreed on because of her greater knowledge in that area, because of the children's positive feelings and respect for her, or for some other reason?"

Variables Affecting Family Power

Multiple variables were discussed that affect family power. These are:

1. The family power hierarchy.

2. Type of family form.

3. Formation of coalitions.

4. The family communication network.

5. Social class status.

6. Family life cycle stage.

7. Ethnic and religious background.

8. Situational contingencies.

9. Person variables (members' ages, gender, interpersonal skills).

10. Spouses' emotional interdependency and commitment to the marriage.

Recognizing the influence of other assessment areas as listed above will assist the family nurse in more fully appraising and interpreting family power attributes.

Overall Family System and Subsystem Power

From your assessment of all the above broad areas, are you able to deduce whether the overall family power can be characterized as dominated by wife, husband, child, or grandparent; as egalitarian-syncratic or autonomic; as leaderless or chaotic? The family power continuum presented in this chapter can be used for a visual representation of the analysis.

If dominance is found, who is the dominant person? Power arrangements on this continuum in the 2 to 4 range have been found to be healthy and satisfying patterns (if mild dominance is by husband).

To determine the overall power pattern, asking a broad, open-ended question is often illuminating. For example, the family nurse could ask both spouse and children if feasible: "Who usually has the last say about important issues? Who makes the important decisions involving the family? Who runs the family? Who wins the important arguments on issues? Who usually wins out if there is a disagreement? Who gets their way when parents/spouses disagree?"

Another significant follow-up question is, "Are you satisfied with how decisions are made and with who makes the decisions (i.e., the present power structure)?"

Subsystem power also needs to be assessed. Observation of marital and parent–child interactions and sibling interactions as well as interview data gathered from family members are used to assess subsystem power characteristics (Olson & Cromwell, 1975).

▶ FAMILY NURSING DIAGNOSES AND INTERVENTION GUIDELINES

Understanding the power structure in the family is essential in formulating nursing diagnoses and effective nursing interventions. Several prime examples illustrate the importance of including this facet of the family assessment. When health care actions/decisions need to be made by the family, knowing who holds the power for this type of decision and for overall decisions, coupled with knowledge of how decisions are made, will guide the family nurse to speak to the appropriate persons with sensitivity as to how decisions take place.

Where families have a clear, intact power hierarchy that functions well for them, the nurse may want to support or reinforce this healthy structure (this is important in fostering confidence in parents). In this case, a family strength relative to family power could serve as a health promotional family nursing diagnosis, such as "family consistently uses consensual decision making." Where the parental executive subsystem is weak, the nurse may want to identify this as a family nursing diagnosis and plan ways to assist spouses/parents to strengthen this subsystem.

Turning to a third area where nurses can be instrumental, decisional conflicts and other power conflicts, including potential or actual family violence, need to be identified (McFarland & McFarlane, 1993). If family members are interested in pursuing this problem area, assistance may be provided in helping the family resolve their conflict(s) or in protecting family members in the case of family violence. McFarland and McFarlane (1993), in describing the NANDA diagnosis "decisional conflict," present cogent guidelines for assisting nurses to help family members resolve this problem. Chapter 10 also has suggestions for helping families resolve conflictual communication, and Chapter 17 discusses family violence and its application to family nursing practice.

The Empowerment Model: Promoting Its Use

For the family nurse involved in counseling marital couples, promoting the use of the *empowerment model* is recommended. This model is often appropriate to encourage when one spouse is more powerful than the other and the less powerful spouse would like to increase her or his resources and power. The empowerment model advocates that each spouse can use his or her resources to move the other from a position of weakness to greater strength. Balswick & Balswick (1995) elaborate on this notion:

> Empowering is not merely one spouse yielding to the wishes of the other. It does not involve giving up one's power to empower others. Rather, empowering is the active and intentional process of each spouse developing and affirming power in the other. Each spouse is encouraged to reach full personal potential. (p. 311)

Hence, empowerment in this context means that each spouse desires and assists the other to become all that he or she can be. Focusing on spousal autonomy rather than "control over" someone is a key thrust in the empowerment model. In empowering one's spouse, the consequences are a stronger but healthier interdependency in the marital relationship, as well as a greater sense of autonomy and mutual respect (Balswick & Balswick, 1995).

► study questions

1. Power is an important dimension in human relationships and groups because (select all appropriate answers):
   a. It is critical in understanding role relationships.
   b. It greatly influences the establishment and the maintenance of communication channels.
   c. It is the sole determinant upon which an intimate relationship is formed and maintained.

2. Demonstrate your knowledge of several basic power concepts by matching the correct synonyms or definitions with the concepts in the left-hand column.

Concepts	Synonym/Definition
_____ a. Power	1. Influence.
	2. Legitimate power.
	3. Primary authority.
	4. Dominance.

_____b. Authority
    5. The outcome is control.
    6. Family group dominance patterns.
    7. One facet is decision making.
_____ c. Family power
    8. Process whereby things get accomplished.
_____d. Decision making
    9. Assessed within context of family interaction.

3. Identify three limitations cited relative to studies of family power.

4. Match up the appropriate definition with the specific bases for power.

Bases for Power

_____ a. Authority
_____ b. Referent power
_____ c. Reward power
_____ d. Coercive power
_____ e. Helpless power
_____ f. Expert or resource power
_____ g. Informational power (direct)
_____ h. Informational power (indirect)
_____ i. Affective power
_____ j. Tension management power

Definition

1. Dominant person's obligation to assist the needy.
2. Dominant person's greater knowledge regarding issue.
3. Legitimate power.
4. Tradition-based power.
5. Based upon positive identification with influencing individual.
6. Belief in ability to inflict punishment.
7. Based on belief in the ability to grant privileges.
8. Way of controlling by managing present stress level in family.
9. Based upon having greater competency in a matter.
10. Hinting or "putting suggestions into another's mouth."
11. The giving or withholding of care warmth, love (affection), and sex.

Are the following statements in questions 5 through 7 true or false?

5. In cases where power is maintained by the husband because of his control over money, this type of power is called expert authority.

6. Among traditional patriarchal families, reliance on direct informational power is quite common.

7. Primary authority is based on tradition and family members' acceptance of culturally based roles.

8. Identify and describe the three techniques used in making decisions.

9. Describe how each of the following variables affects family power.
    a. Family communication network

    b. Situational changes

    c. Ethnic influences

    d. Coalition formation

    e. Social class

    f. Developmental or life cycle changes

Choose the correct answers to the following questions.

10. The most commonly used and well accepted typology of family power is:
    a. Democratic–patriarchal.
    b. Companionship–authoritarian.
    c. Husband-dominated, egalitarian, wife-dominated.
    d. Autocratic, syncratic, autonomic.
    e. Familistic–atomistic.

11. Which type of overall power structure seems to be the least satisfying to both spouses?
    a. Husband dominated
    b. Wife dominated
    c. Syncratic
    d. Autonomic

12. What is the most outstanding contemporary trend relative to family power?
    a. The upsurge in traditionalism and conservatism.
    b. The atomistic trend in the family.
    c. The rise of the egalitarian, democratic family.
    d. The rise of the matrifocal, matriarchal family.

13. The healthy family, as described by Lewis and associates and Minuchin, is characterized by:
    a. A strong parent–child coalition.
    b. A clear power hierarchy.
    c. Husband having more power than wife.
    d. A strong parental coalition.

14. The following family roles and power relationships are frequently observed in poor families:
    a. Division of marital responsibilities is informal.
    b. Joint planning predominates.
    c. Father is bestowed titular authority.
    d. Father often plays a more passive, minimal role in the home.

15. Komarovsky found that the following factor played a significant role in the type of power structure present in working-class families:
    a. Occupational status.
    b. Residence (city or rural).
    c. Education.
    d. Ethnicity.

▶ family case study 1

From the following example, answer the two questions below.

Mr. G. walked in the door while Mrs. G. was discussing child rearing with the community health nurse. Mr. G. immediately "took over" the conversation, voicing his opinion about every parenting comment made by the nurse or Mrs. G. The children were heard to giggle about a couple of their father's assertions. Toward the end of the visit he shouted to the children to get up and clean the kitchen. The children did not respond, but looked at their mother. She paused and then said, "Children, please go clean the dishes." With this request the children left for the kitchen.

16. In this situation, which one of the following most clearly describes the power and role relationships of the father and mother?
   a. Male dominance.
   b. Children actually manipulate parents, playing one against the other.
   c. Insufficient data to clearly define roles.
   d. Mother acts as final arbiter and is dominant in parenting area.

17. Data substantiating the above interpretation include:
   a. Father asserting role in an exaggerated manner.
   b. His assertions being responded to by giggles from the children.
   c. Need to show he is "leader."
   d. Children looking toward mother and responding to her request.
   e. No response to father's requests.

▶ family case study 2

Read the family history and then complete an assessment of family power from data presented in vignette by answering questions that follow.

The Simpsons are a middle-class white stepparent family living in a suburban area. John Simpson, age 37, recently (8 months ago) married Sylvia, who had been divorced for 4 years. Sylvia (age 42) has three children, ages 13 (Joe), 10 (Mary), and 8 (Jimmie) from her former marriage. Mr. Simpson had no children from his former marriage. Mr. Simpson is a businessman; he owns and manages a hardware store. Mrs. Simpson is a registered nurse and works at a local hospital. Both have baccalaureate degrees from local colleges and their income level, due to their double income, is "quite comfortable." They live in a lovely, well-kept residential neighborhood. Their home is large and well furnished, containing four bedrooms, a living and family room, and a large, spacious kitchen. They moved to this particular community from the nearby city when they married and formed their new family.

The Simpsons are bringing their 8-year-old child, Jimmie, to the family health center because of bedwetting (enuresis), hyperactivity, and inattention at school. He is being examined and interviewed by a pediatric nurse practitioner who is in the process of completing a family assessment and comprehensive history of Jimmie.

Sylvia, the mother, relates that things in the family have been difficult since John "moved in." "First we had to move and the children lost all their friends. And even though John used to come and take me out for the evening and visit with us—so that the children were able to get to know him—they now resent him terribly and I feel I'm in between the devil and the deep blue sea!"

When asked what seems to be the major area of family conflict and concerns, she mentions disciplining of the children. "John doesn't discipline them, which I wish he did, and when he does set some limits, due to my nagging, the children don't listen to him. Then, I have to come in and settle things myself. I married John because I felt the children needed a father to relate to. Their own natural father lives far away now and seldom keeps in contact with them. The children don't seem to respect John, and the only way he is able to manage them is by promising them something or threatening to punish them."

She says that she never fights or disagrees with her husband in front of the children (believing children should not hear such unpleasant things). But after the children go to bed, she finds herself berating John for not following through with his family obligations—paying bills, repairing house, yard work, and so on. Sylvia sees herself as in charge of the children (primarily), housework, social affairs, cooking, and shopping, and feels that the rest is up to her husband. She does her work, in addition to a full-time job, and expects him to do his.

According to Mrs. Simpson, Joe, the 13-year-old, likes caring for his younger siblings, and Mary and Jimmie turn to him for help and advice if she is not home. She also comments that Joe is the child who really seems to resent John, and he speaks to her husband only when necessary, with most messages pertaining to the step-father going through the mother.

When the nurse asks Sylvia about how the family arrives at the major decisions they have made since she and John became involved with each other—such as marriage, moving, and buying the house—Sylvia says that she initiated all three of these conversations. "I'm a practical person. I could see that marriage would be good for all of us, and so suggested it to John!" The nurse then asks, "And what was his answer?" Sylvia replies, "I don't remember exactly. I think he kind of hemmed and hawed around, and then, anyway, agreed, and I started making plans. He didn't want to move from the city or into such a big house, but I convinced him that it would be better economically and that the commuting time was reasonable for him. And I agreed to let him buy a more comfortable car to commute in, in return."

The pediatric nurse practitioner met with the whole family twice more to discuss their "identified" problem (Jimmie) and the family dynamics and family problems. At these meetings she notices that twice when she speaks to the parents and the children become noisy or disruptive, the older son, Joe, takes over, scolding them. In their discussion she observes that this is a family in which there is a proliferation of "do's" and "don'ts" about everything—from the time they get up in the morning until the time they go to bed at night. Feelings are not openly expressed, and the two youngest children directly answered the nurse's questions in a short, incomplete manner, looking to the mother for approval. The mother appears quite committed to a particular home schedule. John mentions that it is hard to fit into someone else's schedule and way of doing things. Joe confirms this point with the nurse in his statement, "We all know the rules better than he does, so why do we need him to tell us what to do?" (Mr. Simpson just sits quietly, and neither parent responds to Joe's hostile statement.)

In discussing his own feelings and thoughts about the family, Mr. Simpson perceives that Jimmie may feel confused and insecure because of moving, their marriage, and the new school. He alludes to the difficulty he has faced in parenting his wife's children and to their negative reactions toward him. He also finds disciplining very hard because he never had children before and when he was growing up, was treated very permissively ("anything at all seemed to be okay with my parents"). He comments that "he tries to stay out of child rearing as much as possible."

Mr. Simpson appears to be passive and easygoing with his wife. In contrast, Mrs. Simpson initiates topics, leads discussions, and is quite "definite" and opinionated in her statements.

18. Assess the family power patterns described in the above case.
    a. Who makes what decisions?
    b. What decision-making techniques are utilized?
    c. On what basis is family power derived?
    d. What variables affect family power?
    e. Using the family power continuum (see Fig. 11–1), where would you place this family?
    f. If dominance, indicate dominant family member.

19. State a family nursing diagnosis for this family that focuses on the power dimension.

20. Propose two general family nursing interventions to assist the family with a family nursing problem in the power dimension area.

▶ chapter 11 study answers

1. a and b.

2. a. 1, 4, 5, and 7.
    b. 2 and 3.
    c. 6 and 9.
    d. 8.

3. Limitations of family power studies (any three):
   a. Lack of a good correlation between task allocation and decision making and overall dominance patterns in family.
   b. Focusing on the outcome of decision making, which family members have difficulty reporting, rather than the process, which gives much greater information regarding family interaction and dynamics.
   c. Methodological: interviewing wife, rather than whole family.
   d. Methodological: solely depending on the self-reporting of family member (interviews), rather than combining self-reports with actual observations.

4. a. 3 and 4.   f. 9.
   b. 5.   g. 2.
   c. 7.   h. 10.
   d. 6.   i. 11.
   e. 1.   j. 8.

5. False.

6. False.

7. True.

8. a. *Consensus.* Both parties discuss and mutually decide.
   b. *Accommodation.* One partner "convinces" others to adjust or all parties decide to make concessions.
   c. *De facto.* No conscious, overt decision made; "things just happen."

9. Description of how each of the following variables affects family power:
   a. *Family communication network.* The unequal intensity of family relationships influences power, especially the centrality of one or more members in the network of interactions (an intermediary or go-between). Family members who hold these intermediary positions can screen information as they see fit and can use more intimate knowledge of family members' attitudes and opinions to influence them and obtain more control over decisions.
   b. *Situational changes.* A family life change that is nonnormative may cause the allocation of power to be redistributed. For example, if the mother becomes physically handicapped and can no longer carry out her parenting functions she may lose implementation power.
   c. *Ethnic differences.* Ethnic differences dictate what power arrangements are seen as "right" and acceptable to the family members.
   d. *Coalition formation.* By forming coalitions, the members of the coalition increase their power relative to other family members.
   e. *Social class.* Social class affects family power by setting up family life conditions that influence the resources each spouse brings to their relationship, the role that tradition plays over contemporary trends, and more generally, the basic conditions under which the family lives.

f. *Developmental or life cycle changes.* During the life cycle of the family, demands on the family unit vary, and in response to both internal and external demands, power patterns are altered. For example, couples when first married tend to share decisions more than after children arrive because there is usually more emotional involvement at the start of their relationship.

10. d.

11. b.

12. c.

13. b and d.

14. c and d.

15. c.

16. d.

17. All(a–e).

18.   a. Who makes what decisions?

Husband-father. Expected to pay bills, carry out home-maintenance work, garden (his degree of involvement and decision making here is in question).

Wife-mother. She initiates and convinces her husband of the "rightness" of her proposals in areas of major decisions. Also assumes responsibility and decision making in areas of child care, household management, and social activities.

Joe (oldest son). In charge of child-care activity in absence of mother.

b. What decision-making techniques are utilized?

No strong evidence of consensus used. (They may not have the communication ability to negotiate and discuss alternatives so that consensual decision making can take place.)

Accommodation: Use of bargaining seen in moving to suburbs and in purchase of home and car.

No use of de-facto technique noted (wife is probably too task oriented and too much of a planner for this to happen very often).

c. On what basis is family power derived?

Referent power. The children listen to mother, and although it is not clear if this is out of positive identification or primary authority, they seem to "mind" when she is not there to enforce the rules (which would also indicate use of reward–coercive power).

Reward–coercive power. The stepfather appears forced to use this type of power base, although ineffectively, because he does not have children's respect, they do not recognize his authority, and he seems not to have expert or informational power to use.

Expert and informational power. It appears that Mrs. Simpson is perceived by Mr. Simpson as having some special competencies or resources that he needs, or greater information on which to base decisions, because he seems to concede to her wishes. Perhaps the "principle of less interest" is operating here.

d. What variables affect family power?

Family communication network. Mrs. Simpson definitely is in a central position as go-between or intermediary between her husband and children. This increases her dominance.

Interpersonal skills. Mr. Simpson lacks confidence in his parenting skills and is passive, thus decreasing his effectiveness in this area. Mrs. Simpson undermines his parenting by taking over when the children do not listen to him. Also, he may need her more than she needs him (Could he be seeking leadership, a mothering figure?).

Social class variables. Family is obviously middle class, and even though the wife "takes over," she is dissatisfied in her husband's role performance. This may be an indication of the disparity between her expectations (the cultural norm of a husband being either a leader or sharing responsibility with wife) and her reality, or her feeling that he is incompetent.

Developmental variable. During this cycle of the family's life, there are many tasks to be fulfilled, and thus the strain is seen in Mrs. Simpson's feeling that she has to assume too much responsibility. Usually there is more division of role responsibilities and decision making.

Cultural variable. The role of the stepfather is not crystalized in our society, making it unclear as to the extent of legitimate authority Mr. Simpson has over his stepchildren.

e. Overall family power typology:

Family power continuum:

f. Moderate dominance by Mrs. Simpson.

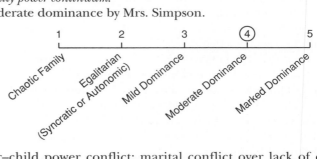

19. Father–child power conflict; marital conflict over lack of exertion of power by stepfather in parenting; marital dissatisfaction in area of husband's exercise of parental authority.

20. Counseling of family members, involving the exploration of each family members' feelings about the impact of becoming a new family. ("What was it like for you when your new family was formed?") Their perceptions of difficulties (goal: development of empathy for each other's feelings and concerns), would be important to discuss, also. Referral to a marriage and family counseling center may be helpful so that the couple can explore their own marital concerns and how to deal with them.

12

Family Role Structure

Marilyn M. Friedman with Susan A. Heady

► learning objectives

1. Define and describe relative to the family:
   Role.
   Position or status.
   Role behavior.
   Normative dimensions of roles.
   Role sharing.
   Role taking.
   Reciprocal roles.
   Principle of complementarity.
   Role conflict.
   Role strain/stress.
   Family homeostasis.

2. From the family role studies presented, summarize the findings of these with respect to the basic roles making up the wife-mother and husband-father positions and which roles are shared and not shared according to present trends.

3. Summarize research findings relative to the role of father, mother, and grandparent in the United States.

4. Describe three types of marital relationships.

5. Describe the common role conflict experienced by the working wife-mother and her husband in dual-career families.

6. Define and give examples of informal roles that often exist in families (both healthy and detrimental roles). Describe why both formal and informal roles are assessed in the family, as well as the purposes that informal roles serve.

7. Explain the process and effects of labeling on individuals in the family.

8. Describe the frequently observed role characteristics in lower- and middle-class families, the single-parent family, the stepparent family, and the family during health and illness, including the caregiver role.

9. Identify some of the primary variables that affect how difficult the family caregiver role is on the caregiver.

10. With the use of a family case example, complete an assessment of the family role structure, state a family nursing diagnosis in the area of family roles, and propose two family nursing interventions directed toward ameliorating or resolving the above role problem.

In all known societies almost everyone lives his or her life enmeshed in a network of family rights and obligations called role relations (Goode, 1964). Family roles are critical, central roles an individual must learn to enact successfully, for adequate role functioning is crucial not only for the individual, but also for the family. It is through the performance of family roles that the functions of the family are fulfilled. In fact, family sociologists have often described the family as an interacting, interdependent set of roles that are in a state of dynamic equilibrium (Turner, 1970).

Because of the critical nature that family roles play in the organization of the family, it is imperative for the family nurse to understand role relationships and, from this, be able to promote healthy role behaviors and identify role problems.

▶ ROLE THEORY AND DEFINITIONS

Because role concepts and terms are fundamental to the discussion that follows, a number of basic terms are first defined. The reader is also directed to the works by Hardy and Hardy (1988) and Biddle and Thomas (1966) for further explanation of these concepts.

Role

Role is referred to as more or less homogeneous sets of behaviors that are normatively defined and expected of an occupant of a given social position. Roles are based on role expectations or prescriptions defining what individuals in a particular situation should do in order to meet their own or another's expectations of them (Nye, 1976, p. 7).

Position or Status

Position or status is defined as a person's location in a social system. Role is subsumed under the notion of position (Merton, 1957). While roles are the behaviors associated with one who holds a particular position, position identifies a person's status or place in a social system. Every individual occupies multiple positions—adult, male, husband, farmer, Elks member, and so on (Biddle & Thomas, 1966; Hardy & Hardy, 1988). Associated with each of these positions are a number of roles. In the case of the mother position, some of the associated roles are housekeeper, child caretaker, family health leader, cook, and companion or playmate. Merton (1957) explains:

> A particular social status involves, not a single associated role, but an array of associated roles. This is a basic characteristic of social structure. This fact of structure can be registered by a distinctive

term, *role-set*, by which I mean that complement of role relationships which persons have by virtue of occupying a particular social status. (p. 3)

Thus for each position a number of roles exist, each of which is composed of a more or less related homogeneous set of behaviors culturally defined as expected of those in that position or status. They might, however, be shared with other members of a group; in the family, for example, the child-care role is now usually a shared responsibility of both the mother and father position (Nye, 1976).

Role Behavior, Role Performance, or Role Enactment

Role behavior, role performance, and role enactment are all interchangeable terms that denote what a person actually does within a position in response to role expectations. Expectations and/or prescriptions for the sets of behavior appropriate for the basic social positions and their associated roles (family roles, occupational roles, etc.) evolve and are developed by society. These expectations are modified in some cases by particular reference groups, such as ethnic associations.

Many of the roles associated with our basic social positions are learned within the family context. Societal role expectations are modified or refined as a result of an individual's exposure to role models and his or her individual personality—that is, his or her capacities, temperament, attitudes, and interests. In other words, an individual enacts particular roles based on societal expectations but modified by his or her identification with role models and individual personality characteristics. The outcome of an individual's role modification is the person's actual role behavior or performance. Figure 12–1 illustrates the process by which role behavior actually develops.

Normative Dimensions of Roles.   Roles are normatively or culturally defined; that is, the culture in which one participates and/or with which one identifies prescribes and proscribes the behavior of the occupants of various positions. However, "not all the family roles are equally normative" (Nye, 1976, p. 15). Jackson (1966) notes that some family roles are more "crystallized"—more clearly spelled

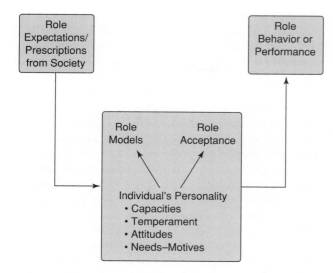

Figure 12–1. Development of role behavior.

out as expected behavior—than others. For instance, in the past in the middle-class white American family the affective (Nye calls it therapeutic) role of the spouses was not crystallized; that is, it was not *expected* of mates to listen to each other's problems. Today, however, spouses see therapeutic support not as optional behavior but as an obligation, because it is a duty to help one's spouse. Thus the therapeutic role for middle-class white American spouses has been "crystallized."

One can infer the strength of a role (whether it is a strong norm or not) in a specific position by assessing the sanction(s) applied when the role is not performed. Certainly social ostracism as a sanction against lack of role fulfillment, as in the case where the wife-mother is not carrying out her housekeeper role, is less strong or intense than imprisonment, as might result from failure to carry out the child-care role when it reaches the point of child neglect or desertion. Sanctions provide evidence that the society or parts of the society perceive a particular role to be sufficiently important that conformity to the norm be enforced.

Role Sharing

Role sharing refers to participation of two or more people in the same roles even though they hold dif-

ferent positions. There is extensive role sharing in most families today. Sharply segregated role structures are unusual. An example of normative role sharing in the family is the case of the child-socialization role where both mother and father usually jointly participate, in addition to school teachers, youth leaders, ministers, and so on. Another example is in the older family, where the housekeeper and shopping roles are often shared by the retired couple.

Role Taking

Another essential concept within role theory is that of role taking. In order for family members to play roles, they must be able to imagine themselves in the role of a counterpart, or role partner; in this way they are able to assign a role to the other and also better understand how they should behave in their own roles (Turner, 1970). Through socialization family members acquire a repertoire of roles through which they can act and interact with others. "Roles are never learned singly, but always as pairs or sets of interacting roles. Because the individual learns the role of alter [his role partner] while playing his own role, he is able to play the role of the alter when others in the situation are playing his usual role" (Turner, 1970 p. 215). Over a period of time, however, the self-conception incorporates certain roles and denies others, so that the individual no longer plays past roles.

Reciprocal or Complementary Roles

A basic concept in role theory is that of the complementarity of roles. A role is interdependent with and patterned to mesh with that of a role partner. In other words, a role is always paired with a **reciprocal role** of another person. One can never look at a role in isolation. To use a teacher as an example, one must look at the teacher's role together with the student's role, because both are necessary for either to function. Society specifies behaviors for each person in these reciprocal arrangements so that each will know what is expected of the role partner. Both role partners are constantly influencing each other's role behavior through their many interactions with one another. For instance, if students become more verbal and assertive with teachers, the teacher responds by modifying his or her expectations and behaviors toward the students. Likewise, as society changes and family systems evolve, changes in social and family roles become necessary. Thus if a wife begins working, she may become more instrumental in financial decisions and the husband may become more involved with household tasks and child rearing.

Parsons and associates (1953) coined the concept of "**the principle of complementarity**," referring to the functional adequacy of roles in social situations that are based on the match between the performances and the expectations of partners in a relationship. The principle of complementarity is of great significance because it is chiefly responsible for that degree of harmony and stability that occurs in interpersonal relations (Spiegel, 1957).

Whenever there is dissimilarity in expectations and performances of family roles—due to cultural, social class, or individual differences—the potential for lack of role complementarity and possible conflict and stress exists.

Role Stress/Strain

Role stress occurs when a social structure, such as the family, creates very difficult, conflicting, or impossible demands for occupants of positions within that social structure (Hardy & Hardy, 1988). It is a characteristic of the social system, rather than of the person in the system. Role stress results in **role strain**—subjective feelings of frustration and tension. Role strain is also perceived and felt by the associated role partners (Hardy & Hardy, 1988).

Role Conflict

Role conflict occurs when the occupant of a position perceives that he or she is confronted with incompatible expectations (Hardy & Hardy, 1988). The source of the incompatibility may be due to changes in expectations within the actor, others, or the environment.

Several types of role conflict are discussed in the literature. *Interrole conflict* is when the norms or behavioral patterns of one role are incongruent with another role that the same individual simultaneously plays. Interrole conflict occurs when an individual's role complex—that is, the group of roles he or she

enacts—involves several roles that are incompatible (Hardy & Hardy, 1988). This type of conflict is due either to the incompatibility of the behaviors associated with the various roles or the excessive amount of energy these roles demand, such as the familiar case of performing the student, housekeeper, cook, marital, and child-care roles simultaneously.

The second type of role conflict, *intersender role conflict* (LaRocca, 1978), occurs when two or more people hold conflicting expectations concerning the enactment of a role. An illustration of this second type of role conflict is the presence of conflicting expectations on how one's role as a professional nurse should be performed. For example, the head nurse may expect efficiency of actions; the patient may expect patient-centeredness, based on his or her perceived needs; and the nurse may expect to be able to give holistic, individualized care as defined by her or his profession.

A third type of role conflict is called *person–role conflict*. This type involves a conflict between the person's internalized values and the external values communicated to this person by others, throwing him or her into a state of role stress. This type of role conflict is similar to the second type, except in this case there is not a disparity in role expectations between people in the outer environment, but a role disparity with one's "inner" environment. One can think of the person–role conflict that results in families with young teenagers—when the teenager has one internalized notion of his or her role as a teenager and peers prescribe a very different role.

Family Homeostasis

Roles, both formal and informal, serve a homeostatic purpose in families. **Family homeostasis** refers to the family's use of regulatory mechanisms to maintain stability or equilibrium in the family. The family achieves homeostasis through adaptation—by altering the family structure such as family roles, and/or by bringing in outside resources. Turner (1970) remarks that once a system of formal and informal roles is established within the family, family processes proceed laboriously unless the members play their expected roles. This is because families become dependent on the existence of certain informal roles to be enacted so as to maintain family homeostasis.

For example, if the family is used to having the middle daughter act as a mediator in disputes, this enables other family members to be less restrained in their sentiments and assures family members that she will step in to help resolve disagreements. When the mediating daughter is not present, conflicts are handled in a much less effective manner due to her absence, until family members learn new roles.

▶ HEALTHY FAMILY ROLE FUNCTIONING

In regards to role relationships in the family, what does the adequate family look like? If we have an understanding of satisfactory family functioning, we may better be able to understand families that are marginally or inadequately coping. Several family scholars/clinicians underscore the importance of role complementarity; compatibility of family roles and norms with societal and cultural norms; the presence of roles in families that meet the psychological needs of its members; and the ability of the family to respond to change via role flexibility (Ackerman, 1966; Glasser & Glasser, 1970; Messer, 1970). In addition, in a healthy family, role allocation is reasonable and does not overburden one or more members. This results in all the necessary family functions being fulfilled.

▶ FORMAL FAMILY ROLES

Family Positions

There are a limited number of positions defined as normative within the most common type of family form, the two-parent nuclear family. These positions are referred to as *formal* and *paired*, and consist of father-husband; wife-mother; son-brother; and daughter-sister. In the extended family (three-generational) more paired positions would exist and in the single-parent family less paired positions.

Each of the normative positions of the family group is associated with related roles. Husband-fathers are expected to be wage earners, among the other roles they may possess. Wife-mothers are viewed as homemakers. When a wife-mother is employed outside the home, as often occurs in American society, this role is usually not viewed as one of her primary responsibilities unless perhaps she has a career, whereas the wage-earner role of the husband-father is viewed as his primary role.

In the single-parent family the mother often plays the mother-father role with no spousal role. In the stepparent family, the husband will often play husband-father, but because the children are biologically not his own, the father role is a quasi-father role (the role lacks crystallization).

Formal Roles

Associated with each formal family position are related roles or clusters of more or less homogeneous behaviors. The family apportions roles to its family members in a manner similar to the way society apportions its roles: according to how critical the role performance is to the system's functioning. Some roles require special skills and abilities; others are less complex and can be assigned to the less skilled or to those with the least amount of power. Standard formal roles exist in the family (e.g., breadwinner, homemaker, house repairman, chauffeur, child rearer, financial manager, and cook). When there are fewer persons in a family the number of persons to fulfill these roles is limited; thus there will be more demands and opportunities for family members to play several roles at different times. If a member leaves home or becomes unable to fulfill a role, someone else fills this vacuum by taking up his or her role to keep the family functioning (Murray & Zentner, 1985, 1993).

Marital and Parental Roles. Nye and Gecas (1976) have identified eight basic roles making up the husband-father and the wife-mother social positions:

- Provider role.
- Housekeeper role.
- Child-care role.
- Child-socialization role.
- Recreational role.
- Kinship role (maintaining relationships with paternal and maternal families).
- Therapeutic role (meeting the affective needs of spouse).
- Sexual role.

In this scheme the companionship role has been subsumed under the recreational and therapeutic roles.

Many people fail to separate parental roles from marital roles, but in reality the two roles are quite distinct, and marital roles should not be shortchanged due to overinvolvement in the parental roles.* Marital roles are focused on the husband–wife interactions, while parental roles are focused upon the parent–child interactions and the parental responsibilities. In spite of their separateness, performance of marital roles will certainly have an impact on parental roles and vice versa.

Marital Roles and Types of Marriages.

Minuchin (1974) stresses the importance of mates maintaining a strong marital relationship. Children especially can interfere with the marital relationship, creating a situation in which a husband or wife may form a coalition with one of their children, which diminishes the close relationship with each other. Maintaining a satisfying marital relationship is identified as one of the crucial family developmental tasks of the family as it progresses through its life cycle. In the previous discussion of family development in Chapter 6, the stress that children put on the marital relationship was made quite evident.

What are marriages supposed to be like? In the past, behavioral scientists put together a composite picture of the well-functioning marriage that we now think of as biased, simplistic, and rarely found in reality. Two fairly well-conducted studies have shown that a variety of relationships are generally present in marriages (Cline, 1966), particularly in stable, long-standing marriages (Cuber & Harroff, 1965). In both of these studies the researchers found that no one pattern of satisfactory marital adjustment existed. A wide range of behaviors and marital roles were found among persons who felt content with, or at least remained in their marriages.

One of these classic studies was conducted by Cuber and Harroff (1965). They interviewed about 400 upper-middle-class couples who had been married at least 10 years and had a stable marriage. From this data they devised a typology of marital relationships illustrating the diverse types of stable marriages they discovered. These varied from conflict-habituated relationships to devitalized relationships; passive, congenial relationships to vital, total relationships. Cuber and Harroff estimate that roughly 80 percent of the marriages they studied were utilitarian oriented, while only 20 percent were vital or total relationships. Thus it appears that the American ideal of a marriage, where most of one's intimate and social needs are met by a spouse, may be a widespread myth.

Bott (1957), in an excellent analysis of marital relationships, attempted to explain some of the differences found in the extent of involvement and intimacy in marital relationships; she theorized that when marriages were superimposed on a social network of friends, neighbors, and relatives among whom there was frequent and meaningful interaction that met many of the needs of the husband and wife, the impetus for the mates to become deeply involved with each other and share roles was decreased. Thus she speculated that a sharper demarcation of roles would be seen, in addition to a lower value placed on the marital relationship itself. It may well be that the social environment in which the family is embedded influences the nature of the marital relationship. Conversely, the nature of the marital relationship probably affects the extensiveness of the mates' social network.

Types of Marital Relationships.

In addition to studies demonstrating the wide diversity of marriages, efforts have also been made to classify the types of dyadic (two-person) relationships. For assistance in assessing the marital and other dyadic relationship in families, one of these typologies will be explained briefly. Described first by Bateson (1958) and later by Watzlawick and co-workers (1967), two types of basic relationships are found in dyadic relationships. These are termed complementary and symmetrical, with parallel relationships being a combination of the two.

Complementary Relationships.   Mates in this type of dyad exhibit contrasting behavior. One spouse is the leading, dominant personality and decision maker, whereas the other partner is the subservient follower (a typical "one-up and one-down" position). A strong element of dependency exists between spouses who have a complementary relationship.

---

* The reader is referred back to Chap. 7, to the section exploring the vital nature of family subsystems and how these need to be kept intact and strong.

The positive element in this type of relationship is that it allows one to give and the other to receive. The inherent danger lies in its tendency to become increasingly rigid, thus stifling the growth of both people.

It is necessary that both partners of a complementary relationship play their "proper" role. If either mate does not continue to perform his or her respective functions, the relationship will come to an end, with each feeling disconfirmed by the other.

Symmetrical Relationships.   This type of relationship is based on the equality of the partners. The partners demand equality through the character of their mutually exchanged messages and behavior, and each mate has the right to initiate action, to criticize the other's behavior, and to have a voice in family decisions.

The positive aspect of this type of relationship is that it allows for mutual respect, trust, and spontaneity, with the optimal effect being that each partner is free to be himself or herself, knowing that each will be accepted and respected by the other. The danger inherent in this type of relationship is that the competitive aspect of the relationship may become overemphasized. When this happens there is increasing frustration and a decrease in cooperative behaviors (mutual assistance and support). Egocentricity by one or both partners may preclude the mutual accommodation and giving needed to enhance and nurture the intimate, affectional part of a marital relationship.

Parallel Relationships.   This third type of marital relationship was later introduced by Lederer and Jackson (1968). In parallel relationships, the spouses alternate comfortably between symmetrical and complementary relationships as they adapt to changing situations. Depending on the situation and the partner's areas of competence, there is an interchange and flexibility in relationship patterns. This switching from one pattern to the other restores the stabilizing properties when either pattern threatens to break down.

Because of the greater flexibility and individual growth-enhancing properties (each partner being able to contribute according to his or her competencies and the situational needs), this type of relationship is seen as the most mature, healthy, and stable

form of the three types. Developmentally, if maturation is allowed to occur, relationships should evolve in a person's lifetime from being complementary to being symmetrical and then to being parallel. If one visualizes this in terms of the dependency factor, relationships undergo a change from dependency (complementary) to independence (symmetry) to interdependence (parallelism). One qualification needs to be made here, however. The value judgment placed on these types of relationships and their perceived degree of maturity does not take into account the cultural background of the individuals involved. Parallel types of relationships may not be acceptible in some ethnic groups.

Contemporary Family Role Changes.
The roles of family members have become more variable, flexible, and complex. In the past, there was "women's work" and "men's work," and little role sharing existed except under special conditions. The family lived according to relatively rigid, traditionally established rules, which were maintained by the social and moral pressures of the entire society. Today, great variation in the roles of both genders is feasible. Expectations and practices differ tremendously. In one family, both adult members may be expected to work and jointly share in all family affairs and responsibilities; in another family, traditional roles are expected and performed; and in yet another situation, the single-parent family, the adult assumes the roles of both parents.

Because the normative limits of family roles are so broad, a wide range of behaviors are accepted as appropriate depending on the situation. Turner (1970) pointed out that the requirements of the situation and the individuals in it determine specific behaviors found in a role. Thus individuals tentatively construct their roles in response to the cues given by other(s) in the situation (their role partners).

Aldous (1996) notes that role performance in families today is increasingly the result of *rolemaking* due to the lack of prepared scripts in performing family roles. Instead, general norms serve as guides to role performance, but situational demands and interactions with others determine specific behaviors. Although rolemaking allows more flexibility in roles, it may make roles more challenging and may lead to more conflict than if prescribed family roles existed.

Research Addressing Contemporary Family Roles.

Research confirms that a spouse's feelings and perceptions about his or her marriage differ from those of his or her mate. Bernard (1972), a noted feminist sociologist, suggests that there are actually two marriages for each couple: "his" and "hers." The couple's differing reality is evidenced in the wife's more negative appraisal of their marriage. Bernard cites the increased rates of depression and illness among married women (when compared to their husbands) as evidence of these two realities. One probable cause for this considerable marital dissatisfaction by wives is that traditionally wives have been socialized to meet their husbands' and childrens' needs rather than their own.

Women's Roles in the Family.

Research on women's roles in the family has focused primarily on the effects of women's employment on the family and in allocation of roles (Elias, 1987; Spitze, 1988). The extent to which women retain the traditional sex-role obligations (child rearing, housekeeping, and so forth) and simultaneously perform their work role has been analyzed. Role overload, role conflict, and role strain are documented in study after study as women move into the labor force and create careers for themselves. With the widespread advent of dual-earner families there are three full-time jobs: the husband's paid work, the wife's paid work, and the family work. "Wives in all social classes do the bulk of family work" (Walker, 1990, p. 16).

When women work they generally expect their husbands to share in the roles of child rearing and housekeeping (Shaw, 1988). Recent research confirms that the role behavior of husbands with respect to assuming more household activities appears to be changing (Spitze, 1988). Working wives still spend much more time than husbands engaged in work at home (John, Shelton, & Luschen, 1995). In one large study, wives spent 37 hours per week working at home while husbands only spent 20 hours per week (Hawkins, Marshall, & Meiners, 1995). The increased involvement of husbands who have working wives appears to be mainly through increased involvement in child care (Pleck, 1985).

Congruence between beliefs about and enactment of provider and homemaker roles tends to foster marital satisfaction (McHale & Crouter, 1992; Perry-Jenkins & Crouter, 1990; Vannoy-Hiller & Philliber, 1992). In one study, gender-role identities and expectations were more important than socioeconomic, life cycle, educational, or occupational status in determining marital quality (Vannoy-Hiller & Philliber, 1992). In another study, both husbands and wives reported that the division of family labor was the issue most likely to cause marital conflict (Cowan, Cowan, Heming, & Miller, 1991).

Cronkite (1977) discusses common dilemmas of the dual-career family and stresses generated by role changes. She describes how couples see the benefit of the additional income outweighing their objections and reluctance to the wife's working. But at the same time, the husband is described as being anxious about his diminished power in the role of breadwinner, and the wife—though enjoying the challenge of work and adult social interaction—often feels guilty about not spending enough time with her children and fulfilling other "traditional" wife-mother functions.

Men's Roles in the Family.

During the last 25 years a great deal of literature has appeared about fatherhood. An impetus for much of the research has been the women's movement and the realization that, as women move from the home into the workplace, their roles have changed, and correspondingly, their role partners' behavior has changed. Research shows changes in men's roles in the family are occurring, but at a slower pace than women's employment and family roles. Two other factors that have created concern, and thus research efforts, are the increased numbers of single-parent families created by mothers and fathers not marrying and by divorce, with many children being separated from their fathers.

Fatherhood.   How these fathers maintain their fatherhood role with their biological children when separated from them is a major concern. Data by Furstenberg & Nord, 1985, show that almost one-half of children had not seen their nonresidential parent in the past year. In 40 percent of all families in the United States, children are not living in the same home with their biological fathers (Stolberg, 1996). How the father role is enacted when men remarry a woman with children is often problematic.

Kennedy (1989), in his review of the fatherhood literature, reports that the fatherhood role is described as the moral overseer, the distance breadwinner, and the sex role model. The moral overseer role predominated during colonial times. The prime role of moral overseer fathers is to exert moral leadership in the family. In contrast, the distant breadwinner is a provider who is uninvolved with child care. The father is a good provider, but does not have a direct influence on the life of the child. After World War II a new theory of gender identity began to emphasize the crucial role that fathers play in molding children's identity, particularly the son's identity. The "new father" began to be advocated in the 1980s and is viewed as an extension of the gender identity theory, modified by changes in the woman's role in the family. Kennedy (1989) describes "the new father's" role as:

> He is present at the birth; he is involved with his children as infants, not just when they are older; he participates in the actual day-to-day work of child care, and not just play; he is involved with his daughters as much as his sons. (p. 364)

Research on the new father role has focused on fatherhood in the family life stages, satisfaction with the new father role, and rural/urban, cultural differences (Bronstein & Cowan, 1988; Kennedy, 1989; Lamb, 1987), and child consequences with and without father involvement (Snarey, 1993). Based on several literature reviews (Bronstein & Cowan, 1988; Hanson & Bozett, 1987; Kennedy, 1989; Lamb, 1987; Snarey, 1993) some interesting research findings in this area emerge.

1. Findings from multiple studies agree that attitudes toward family roles are moving in the direction of egalitarianism and that child care and socialization roles are becoming the shared responsibility of both spouses (Araji, 1977; Hanson & Bozett, 1987; Lamb, 1987).

2. Today's fathers are expected to be more actively involved in child rearing with children of all ages than in the past, and to a modest extent this is evidenced in studies. Lamb (1987) points out, however, that paternal involvement may not be beneficial in all family circumstances.

3. There is no evidence that maternal employment status affects levels of paternal involvement in child care.

4. Fathers spend more time on child care when children are younger; they are more involved and interested in child care with their sons than with their daughters.

5. There are variations in the type of interaction fathers versus mothers have with their children. Mothers' interactions are dominated by caretaking activities, while fathers' interactions are more play-oriented.

6. If both parents are equally involved in infant care, there are no differences in parenting skills between mothers and fathers during the newborn period.

7. In a 40-year longitudinal study examining father involvement practices (Snarey, 1993), father involvement was positively linked to positive marital outcomes and children's educational and occupational mobility.

Health care professionals are increasingly recognizing that pregnancy, delivery, and child care at all ages are family events. As such, the informed father should be an active, involved participant (Hanson & Bozett, 1987).

The Marital Sexual Role.

Another apparent change in roles within the spouse positions involves the sexual role. In the past men had the right to regular sexual activity with their wives, but felt under no obligation to be concerned about the wives' feelings of satisfaction. Today the wife's right to sexual enjoyment and equality is growing in importance, changing the nature of the sexual role for both mates (Napier, 1988).

The Kinship or Kinkeeping Role.

There is a rather extensive body of literature that shows that women are the kinkeepers in the family. Kinkeeping, or the kinship role, involves maintaining communication, facilitating contact and the exchange of goods and services, and monitoring family relationships (Hagestad, 1988). Women function as kinkeepers for both sides of the family.

With this added family responsibility "the superwoman squeeze"—the overload experienced by middle-aged women who provide assistance to both children and two sets of parents in addition to working—is a real possibility.

Being the "sandwiched" generation and the "sandwiched" sex, middle-aged women are caught between the needs of parents with increasing life expectancies and children who remain dependent for a longer period of time and need extra help during periods of marital and other personal disruption (Spitze, 1988). Just as many middle-aged women think they are getting off the "mommy track," they are finding themselves, due to the aging of their parents, getting back on "the daughter track." Data support this phenomenon. In a U.S. House of Representatives report of 1988 (Beck et al., 1990) it is estimated that the average American woman spends 17 years raising children and 18 years helping aged parents.

The Grandparent Role.

The roles of grandparent and even great grandparent are becoming growing objects of interest. Certainly the growing number of individuals who are grandparents and great grandparents is a potent factor for this increased interest. The empirical research describes grandparenthood as a heterogeneous experience, with wide variation in how the grandparent role is enacted. The historical context, age, ethnicity, social class, and gender tend to produce significant differences in terms of what the grandparent role is like.

There is no consensus on whether grandparental involvement has direct positive effects on grandchildren's behavior. In most instances, indirect effects (through helping the child's parents) and symbolic influences play a greater role.

The symbolic expressions of the grandparent role—the functions the role fulfills—are equally diverse and varied. Bengtson (1985) divides these symbolic functions of grandparenthood into (1) simply "being there" (simple presence); (2) acting as the national guard or family watchdog (being there to protect and give care if needed); (3) being an arbitrator (negotiator between parents and children); and (4) being an active participant in the family's social construction of its history (making connections between the families' past, present, and future).

In a study of 510 grandparents, Cherlin and Furstenberg (1985, 1986) identified three styles of grandparenting: "the detached" (26 percent), who were low in both exchange and influence and saw their grandchild(ren) less than once a month; "the

passive" (29 percent), who also scored low on both the above criteria but had seen their grandchild(ren) at least once or twice a month; and "the active" (45 percent), who scored high on exchange and influence regardless of their frequency of visiting. Many grandparents developed companionship relationships with their grandchildren—relationships that were easygoing and lighthearted.

Most of the research has been on grandmothers. Relatively little research has focused on grandfathers and virtually none on the growing number of great grandfathers (Hanson & Bozett, 1987). One of the crucial elements that has been found in terms of the grandchild–grandparent relationship is the relationships between the grandparents and their children. The child's parents are found to determine the frequency of visits and encourage or discourage the development of a positive grandparent–grandchild relationship. Several researchers have observed that grandparents are more involved with grandchildren when parents are divorced or never-married, especially when the grandparents are younger (Burton & de Vries, 1995). Moreover, African-American children have been observed to profit when grandparents play a more active role in their upbringing (Cherlin & Furstenberg, 1986). The grandparent role is also discussed in Chapter 6 in the section on the aging family.

Role Change Problems

The status and associated family roles of individuals change in many ways throughout a person's life cycle. The change in role relationships, expectations, and abilities is referred to as **role transition** (Meleis, 1975). Role transitions occur at clear demarcations of the family life, such as at marriage, divorce, and the death of a parent or spouse, as well as more subtly as an ongoing response to life experience. A role change experienced by one family member necessitates complementary role changes by other family members.*

The advent of role changes in families does not come without a cost to the individuals involved. Families often experience significant stress during

---

*The changes in family roles throughout the family life cycle are explored in Chap. 6.

role transitions. It is well recognized that when individuals deviate from normative role expectations and/or take on new roles, they may lack the role preparation or previous socialization needed to perform these new roles comfortably and adequately. In addition to lacking the necessary training, a family member may not feel that the new roles meet his or her interests or needs. Role changes such as those brought on by having a new baby, a wife's employment, a husband's unemployment, divorce, or family relocation, may create role confusion, anxiety, and unhappiness in the family and may heighten familial conflict (Aldous, 1974, 1996).

The role change necessitated because of having a new baby illustrates the difficulty in making role transitions. Ventura (1987), in a qualitative study of middle-class couples, found that 35 percent of first-time mothers and 65 percent of fathers reported feeling stressed because of multiple role demands. At the third month postpartum, mothers described juggling parenting roles with home and work schedules and having very little time for themselves. Fathers portrayed stresses too, but these were linked to career and work responsibilities.

▶ INFORMAL FAMILY ROLES

As stated previously, there are specific explicit *formal* family roles operating in families, such as husband-father, wife-mother, and child-sibling in the two-parent nuclear family. Within each of these positions are associated roles and clusters of expected, homogeneous behaviors. Family roles can be classified into two categories: formal or overt roles and informal or covert ones. Whereas formal roles are explicit roles that each family role structure contains (father-husband, etc.), informal roles are implicit, often not apparent on the surface, and are played to meet the emotional needs of individuals (Satir, 1967) and/or to maintain the family's equilibrium.

Feldman and Scherz (1967) underscore the salience of looking at both types of roles within a family:

> The family operates through roles that shift and alter during the course of the family's life. Roles can be explicit or instrumental; they can be implicit or emotional. . . . The healthy family carries out explicit and implicit roles. . . . according

to age, competence and needs during all the different stages of family life. (p. 67)

A family member will play many roles in a family, both covert and overt, with some of these roles being shared. The existence of informal roles is necessary to fulfill the integrative and adaptive requirements of the family group. Kievit (1968) explains that:

> Informal roles have different requirements, less likely based on age or sex and more likely based upon the personality attributes of individual members. Thus, one member may be the mediator, seeking possible compromises when the other family members are engaged in conflict. Another may be the family jester, who provides gaiety and mirth on happy occasions, and a much needed sense of humor in times of crisis and distress. Other informal roles may exist and emerge, as the needs of the family unit shift and change. In working with families, awareness of the informal roles may facilitate insight into the specific nature of problems faced and in turn possible solutions. Effective performance of informal roles can facilitate the adequate performance of the formal roles. (p. 7)

The following are some examples of other informal or covert roles described in the literature (Benne & Sheats, 1948; Hartman & Laird, 1983; Kantor & Lehr, 1975; Satir, 1972; Vogel & Bell, 1960). These informal roles may or may not contribute to the stability of the family—some of them are adaptive and others detrimental to the ultimate well-being of the family.

- *Encourager.* The encourager praises, agrees with, and accepts the contribution of others. In effect he or she is able to draw out other people and make them feel that their ideas are important and worth listening to.

- *Harmonizer.* The harmonizer mediates the differences that exist between other members by jesting or smoothing over disagreements.

- *Initiator–contributor.* The initiator–contributor suggests or proposes to the group new ideas or changed ways of regarding group problems or goals. Kantor and Lehr (1975) refer to this type of role as a "mover" role characterized by the initiation of action.

- *Compromiser.* The compromiser is one of the parties to the conflict or disagreement. The compromiser yields his or her position, admits error, or offers to come "halfway."

- *Blocker.* The blocker tends to be negative to all ideas, rejecting without and beyond reason. Kantor and Lehr (1975) label this role the opposer.

- *Dominator.* The dominator tries to assert authority or superiority by manipulating the group or certain members, flaunting his or her power and acting as if he or she knows everything and is the paragon of virtue.

- *The Blamer.* This role is similar to the blocker and the dominator. The blamer is a fault-finder, a dictator, a bossy "know it all."

- *Follower.* The follower goes along with the movement of the group, more or less passively accepting the ideas of others, serving as an audience in group discussion and decision.

- *Recognition Seeker.* The recognition seeker attempts in whatever way possible to call attention to self and his or her deeds, accomplishments, and/or problems.

- *Martyr.* The martyr wants nothing for self but sacrifices everything for the sake of other family members.

- *The Great Stone Face.* The person playing this role lectures incessantly and impassively on all the "right" things to do, just like a computer. Satir (1975) calls this informal role the super-reasonable.

- *Pal.* The pal is a family playmate who indulges self and excuses family members' behavior or his or her own regardless of the consequences. He or she usually seems irrelevant when family issues are discussed.

- *The Family Scapegoat.* The family scapegoat is the identified problem member in the family. As a victim or receptacle for the overt and covert family tensions and hostilities, the scapegoat serves as a safety valve.

- *The Placator.* The placator is ingratiating, always trying to please, never disagreeing, talking out of both sides of his or her mouth—in short, a "yes person."

- *The Family Caretaker.* The family caretaker is the member who is called upon to nurture and care for other members in need.

- *The Family Pioneer.* The family pioneer moves the family into unknown territory, into new experiences.

- *The Irrelevant One or Distractor.* The distractor is irrelevant; by exhibiting attention-getting behavior he or she helps the family avoid or ignore painful or difficult matters.

- *The Family Coordinator.* The family coordinator organizes and plans family activities, thereby fostering cohesiveness and combating family separateness.

- *The Family Go-between.* The family go-between is the family "switchboard"—he or she (often the mother) transmits and monitors communication throughout the family.

- *The Bystander.* The bystander role is similar to "the follower" except in some cases more passive. The bystander observes but does not involve himself or herself; he or she acts like an outsider.

Two informal roles that warrant further discussion are the scapegoat and the go-between roles. The first of these is the scapegoat role, a role adopted by a member to preserve the family and maintain homeostasis. The family member who is constantly scapegoated usually serves to divert attention from a disturbance between the spouses. As described by Ackerman (1966), when the marital pair is in conflict, the attention is focused on the scapegoat and the system is preserved.*

The second informal role that is common in families is that of the go-between (Zuk, 1966). The go-between or intermediary role is usually taken by the mother. In this role the person acts as a "switchboard" between family members, relaying communication from one member to another. In so doing, the direct communication between other family members is blocked. As the switchboard through which all communication must go, the go-between assumes a covert position of power, and by passing along only those messages considered suitable, the go-between acts as a censor. She or he thus becomes a central figure in the family, acting as a confidant to its members. And as the center of the family communication network, the go-between is typically in charge of settling disputes and insuring fairness to all sides. However, when dis-

---

* Chap. 17 discusses this problem in greater detail.

putes or conflicts do not become resolved, the go-between often gets blamed. Consistently having one person act as an intermediary is dysfunctional in that it is an emotional distancing mechanism and promotes estrangement between the other members of the family, because they are discouraged from communicating directly with each other. Satir (1972) discusses the consequences of communicating via a third person.

> If the family habitually transacts business without all the members present, and also has little spare time, then family members get to know each other through a third person. I call it *acquaintance by rumor*. The problem is that most people forget about the rumor part and treat whatever it is as fact. (p. 266)

The presence of a go-between role is revealed in the family's communication patterns. In interviews, it will be observed that the go-between answers for the children or other spouse when not directly questioned. In addition to talking for other family members, he or she usually gets in the way of messages sent or received by family members.

Learning Informal Roles

How do family members come to play these various informal roles within the family? Most learning of these roles occurs through (1) role modeling; (2) filling in "vacuums" where they exist in the family (if there is no leader or decision maker playing the instrumental role, a member of the group will naturally emerge to fill this role); and (3) selective reinforcement that a child receives to behaviors he or she exhibits in the family. The child experiments with various roles in play, receives selective reinforcement for certain roles, and eventually finds informal roles that are comfortable.

Through selective reinforcement of certain behaviors by parents and significant others, children are molded to play specific informal, covert roles. This selective parental reinforcement may occur because of early *labeling* of the child; this labeling leads to a self-fulfilling prophecy. Parents label children for a variety of reasons: projection, comparison with siblings, past unresolved personal needs, and so on. A classic study of large families (Bossard & Boll, 1956) found that there were a number of specialized roles and labels given to the children. Eight informal roles, which

result in or from labels, existed: (1) the responsible one, (2) the popular one, (3) the socially ambitious one, (4) the studious one, (5) the family isolate, (6) the irresponsible one, (7) the sickly one, and (8) the spoiled one. These labels are likely to exist in complementary pairs in a family. Thus if a "sickly" child is identified in a family, the family usually labels another as the "healthy one"; if a "dumb one" is present, there is usually a "smart one." Parents are continually comparing their children with each other.

All labeling limits the way an individual may act or develop. True negative labeling—where adverse adjectives are consistently used—occurs when parents and/or significant others label a child according to an attribute or behavior that indicates the child is inferior or unlovable. Because the parents see these labels as bad, the child sees himself or herself in the same light. Initially parents condemn the child; later the child, through identification with parental labels, internalizes the parental label and condemns himself or herself. Negative labeling has been identified as an antecedent to both depression and lowered self-esteem (Mishel, 1974).

As a result of early negative labeling and the internalization of these labels, individuals often develop certain limited ways of perceiving themselves and of reacting to others called "life games" or "scripts"; these restrict and limit a person's adaptability and repertoire of interpersonal skills (Lange, 1970). In other words, a script is written in early childhood based on messages and labels (both verbal and non-verbal) that a child receives from parents, such as parental perceptions of the child related to his or her worth, lovableness, sexual status, work, responsibility, and dependency. "Life patterns," which include suicide, obesity, and recurrent physical illness—especially when treatable and preventable—are all examples of tragic scripts (Lange, 1970).

▶ VARIABLES AFFECTING ROLE STRUCTURE

As with the family power structure, there are major factors that influence both formal and informal roles. These factors include (1) social class, (2) family forms, (3) ethnic background, (4) family developmental stage, (5) role models, and (6) situational events—in particular health/illness problems.

Social Class Differences

Lower-class Families.   The functions of family life in terms of family roles is, of course, greatly influenced by the demands and necessities put upon the family by the larger social structure. Thus, in response to our society's "benign neglect" of poor families of all ethnic groups, a variety of family role adaptations have evolved as a means of solving the recurrent problems and issues arising from being poor. Single-parent families are the most numerous type of family form that is poor, although the proportion of working poor families is at a 30-year high (Leeds, 1996). Poverty is a predominant feature of many single-parent families. Thirty-five percent of all single-parent families live in poverty (Gelman et al., 1985).

Marital Roles in Lower-class Families.   Marital stability in the lower class is far more precarious than in other social classes, with divorces being two to six times greater among the unskilled labor group than among the professional middle class. The high rate of unemployment among the very poor is a major stressor in the marital relationship and a significant cause of its dissolution.

Several studies have found that lower-class marriages tend to provide less companionship than middle-class marriages. The marital therapeutic role is usually attenuated and marital emotional isolation is common. In studying marriages among the lower class, Bradburn (1970) found that a strong relationship existed between personal happiness and marital satisfaction in all social classes, and that the marital relationship was much less satisfying to mates among the lower social class.

The lower-class family is a relatively loose-knit structure, although the roles of the marital partners and their division of responsibilities are formal. In many poor families there is a sharp demarcation of family roles based on whether the jobs are located inside or outside the home. These firm lines of authority serve to reinforce the emotional distance of the mates. The husband generally plays a minimal role in the low-income family, often conceiving of his role as being simply the provider of money to meet material needs.

Parental Roles in Lower-class Families. Because typically the affective and social needs of women are not met by their husbands, they develop greater emotional attachment to children as compensation for the emotional distance and lack of communication with their husbands. A peer relationship often develops between the mother and her children of either sex. A son may be expected to contribute economically at an early age and become the man of the family (Besmer, 1967).

In the poor family, the parenting role is of central importance to the mother, with mother being more traditional in her outlook toward child rearing (e.g., a greater emphasis on respectability, obedience, cleanliness, and discipline of young children) when compared with the middle-class parent, who centers more on developing self-reliance and independence in children and takes more cognizance of developmental and psychological principles in the parent–child relationship (Kohn, 1977). In other words, the focus of parenting in the poor family is on fulfillment of maintenance functions—providing food for the children, making sure they eat, have adequate rest, bathe, get to school on time—and on the maintenance of order and discipline in the home.

Sibling Roles in Lower-class Families.   When the children are older, the sibling roles acquire significance as a socializing agent far beyond that seen in the middle class. Peer groups are also very important, especially for boys who seek masculine models, given the central role of the mother and the more passive or "missing" role of the father in child rearing.

Working- and Middle-class Families. Komarovsky (1964) and Rubin (1976) found in their qualitative studies of blue-collar workers and their families that the more educated the husband, the greater the degree of companionship in marriage. This was confirmed by later studies. In contrast to working-class marriages where a high degree of "gender segregation" exists within the family, companionship is a strong reason for the initiation and continuance of a marriage in middle-class families.

Working-class families generally tend to have more traditionally based family roles than middle-class families—the husband being more authoritarian in his role as head of the household (Dickinson & Leming, 1995). "The husband's world revolves around the provider role, while the wife has primary responsibility for the home and children in addition to working outside the home" (Dickinson & Leming, 1995, p. 185).

Child rearing is now generally a shared role of middle-class parents, and their role behavior toward their children differs qualitatively from the lower-class family. It has been pointed out that one major reason for this may be the unconscious molding of a child to survive in the world as experienced by the parents. For instance, if a family is poor, parents expect that their boys will probably have to work in a menial position where obedience, respect for authority, and conformity are stressed. Hence, training that promotes creativity, questioning, and independence would be counterproductive to what the child needs when he matures and has to relate and survive in society. In contrast, middle-class parents are more concerned with psychological growth, individual differences, independence, and self-reliance in their children. These traits, encouraged by middle-class parents, are functional to success in the middle-class occupational life (Kohn, 1969, 1977).

Family Forms

The majority of the families we serve are not the typical "idealized" two-parent traditional nuclear families. The 1990 National Census (U.S. Bureau of the Census, 1991a) confirmed the decline of the two-parent family household. In March 1990, 26 percent of all U.S. households consisted of married-couple families with children under 18 years of age. Another 30 percent of married couples had either adult children or no children living with them. About 12 percent of family households were maintained by women alone. Twenty-nine percent of households were non-family units, one-third of these consisted of persons living alone. The type of family form, as explained in more detail in Chapter 1, greatly influences the family's role structure. Because single-parent and stepparent families are probably the two most common nonnuclear family forms, these two types of family forms will be described in terms of their unique role arrangements and role stresses.

Roles in the Single-parent Family.   The number of single-parent families has swelled rapidly in the last 15 years. Twenty-nine percent of all families in the United States in 1990 were single-parent families (U.S. Bureau of the Census, 1993b). The three primary streams swelling this number are divorces, births out of wedlock, and desertions of spouses. Most single-parent families are headed by mothers, although fathers are increasingly heading single-parent families. About 20 percent of single-parent families are headed by men (U.S. Bureau of the Census, Feb. 1991a). Fathers as single parents are much better situated economically than mothers. One reason for this is the father's higher educational attainment (Nortan & Glick, 1986).

Two prominent role features of these families are (1) role overload and role conflicts, and (2) role changes of the single parent. The parent must fulfill both mother and father roles, in addition to lacking the support of a marital relationship. Single parents tend to be either overloaded with roles or in conflict over their various role commitments, because they have double tasks to assume. With a spouse to depend on, there is some role flexibility (if the child-care and housekeeping roles are shared). And even though the single parent is freed from the responsibilities of marital roles, other adult relationships often enter in and create demands on the single parent's precious time. About 80 to 90 percent of the mothers who are single parents will eventually remarry, necessitating another role change—relinquishing the father's role and forming new marital and parental roles (Macklin, 1988). Because most single parents also work, high job/family role strain and reduced levels of wellness were found in a study conducted by Burden (1986).

Significant research has been generated by behavioral scientists who have studied the single-parent family relative to its long-term impact on children. Accumulated evidence from multiple studies consistently shows that children in single-parent families have greater problems (emotionally and behaviorally, than children from two-parent nuclear families (income level was controlled for in these studies). They are also twice as likely to drop out of high school and become teenage mothers (Popenoe, 1995).

Roles in the Stepparent Family.   With the tremendous increase in the number of divorces and remarriages (80 percent of the divorced remarry, one-half within 3 years) there has been a tremendous increase in stepparent families (Glick, 1994). In 75 percent of these cases, this type of family form denotes the entry of a new husband and surrogate father (stepfather), rather than stepmother, into a previously established female-headed single-parent family.

Stepparent families are at higher risk of serious problems than families of "first marrieds" or "second marrieds" with no children: 60 percent of all second marriages end in divorce (Kantrowitz & Wingert, 1990). One of the primary reasons for this is the greater complexity involved with integrating the stepfather into an already established family, coupled with the mixed allegiance the wife-mother experiences—to her new husband on the one hand and to her children on the other.

There has been growing research interest about the stepparent family and the adjustments and the roles of its members. In a groundbreaking study, Fast and Cain (1966) identified role confusion as a major familial problem. The stepfather and mother were both uncertain about whether the stepfather should assume the role of parent or nonparent.

Role confusion, or role ambiguity, is a major source of stress for both stepparents and stepchildren (Crosbie-Burnett, 1994). Perhaps the underlying issues creating role confusion for the stepfather and the resultant family disequilibrium are the issues of child rearing and disciplining of children. As discussed in Chapter 15, the diversity in child-rearing practices and values is great. Each parent draws on his or her own family background when defining child-rearing beliefs, practices, and discipline. And it is difficult to compromise in these values and beliefs, because many of them are not objectively based. When parents enter into a relationship in which the stepfather heads the household but is not really the parent, synthesis of these values and rules is problematic. Furthermore, the children, through exposure to their natural parents' child-rearing practices, have developed their own behaviors and expectations of what is acceptable or unacceptable behavior, for both themselves and their parents. In the stepparent family the stepfather has no biological rights over the children, and whatever parental rights he may have must be granted to him by his wife. This places the stepfather into a rather untenable position. When conflict arises over the disciplining of a child, the mother feels a natural right to decide the issue. If the stepfather goes ahead and disciplines the child, the mother will often either directly become angry, or more often, indirectly strike back by undermining him. This latter course is particularly devastating to the entire family and often exacerbates the conflict, with the mother being torn between the loyalty to her children and to her husband. In addition, integrating the noncustodial biological parent, the kinship system of the stepparent, and the stepparent's children from a previous marriage may require further alterations in family roles (Bray, Berger, & Boethel, 1994).

Children in stepparent families also have difficulties in adjusting to their new households. They are unsure of how to relate to both the stepparent and the biological parent of the same sex and experience loyalty conflicts (Crosbie-Burnett, 1994).

Ethnic Variation

Ethnically derived norms and values strongly influence how roles are carried out within a given family system. Knowledge of the core values, customs, and traditions are important for interpreting whether family roles in a family are appropriate (Holman, 1983).

In some cultures, formal family roles are performed by extended family members who hold other family positions. A common example of this situation is when an uncle acts as a father surrogate in a single-parent family. Members of the extended family (such as a grandfather, uncle, or older brother) may, in some cultures, act as surrogate fathers even though the father is present, without causing any conflict or strained relationships. The maternal grandmother may also perform formal family roles, especially in African-American single-parent families (Burton & deVries, 1995).

Because so many married couples today are from different ethnic backgrounds, a major problem in these types of marriages is often one of role incongruency. Because of the couple's dissimilar cultural backgrounds, the expectations the spouses have of their roles and their spouse's roles differ. Each marital partner may criticize the other for failure to carry out the marital or parental role as expected, while at the same time feeling guilty for not meeting the other's expectations (Hartman & Laird, 1983).

Family Developmental Stage

It is quite clear that the way in which family roles are enacted substantially differs from one life cycle stage of the family to another. The parental roles are a blatant example of this change. Being a parent to an infant requires 24-hour care of a totally dependent baby, while parenting an adolescent requires letting go of the adolescent while still providing guidance and support, as the adolescent differentiates from the family.

Role Models

When a family member is exhibiting or experiencing role problems (role transitions or role conflicts), assessing the role models of the troubled family member is helpful. This analysis is aimed at finding out about the early life of the family, when the individual was learning both his or her role and the counterpart's role (such as learning the role of a daughter, as well as a mother), and how those early experiences have affected his or her present role behaviors and difficulties. Our role behavior as parent or marital partner often imitates the roles we observed our parents playing. For example, it is not uncommon to find people tending to treat their children as their parents treated them in the past. With this observation in mind, family therapists have placed great importance on looking at the intergenerational aspects of clients' marital and parental roles.

Situational Events

Major situational life events confronting families unavoidably affect their role functioning. These situations are usually stressful events such as natural disasters, unemployment, the wife-mother returning to work, or health problems. The one situational factor to be described here is that of the impact of health–illness problems on family roles.

▶ FAMILY ROLES DURING HEALTH AND ILLNESS

Although Chapter 16 elaborates on the entire area of the family's involvement in health care and health practices, one aspect of this broad area is what happens to family roles when family members are sick or disabled, and what factors influence the family role structure during illness. When a family member acquires a chronic, disabling illness and is taken care of at home, another role becomes primary—that of the caregiver. Summarization of these issues are addressed in this section.

Role of Mother in Health and Illness

It has become increasingly clear that in most families an important role subsumed under the mother-wife position is that of health leader and caregiver. Whatever criteria have been used in studies to measure health decision making and roles—including such measures as illnesses incurred and treated, medical and health services used, and primary source of family assistance—the pervasive and central role of the mother as prime health decision maker, educator, counselor, and caregiver within the family matrix has remained a constant finding (Finley, 1989; Litman, 1974). In this role, the mother defines symptoms and decides the "proper" disposition of resources. She also exerts substantial control over whether the children will receive preventive and curative services (Aday & Eichhorn, 1972; Diosy, 1956; Rayner, 1970), and acts as the main source of comfort and assistance in times of illness (Litman, 1974).

One of the ways one can surmise the importance of the mother's health leader role is by observing what happens to her and the family when she is ill and unable to carry on her roles. First of all, the mother-wife has been observed to assume the sick role only when it is absolutely mandatory, and then only reluctantly. Because her role performance is considered essential to family functioning, her illness tends to be quite disruptive and disorganizing (Mechanic, 1964). Usually, severe illness or prolonged incapacitation of the mother-wife is seen as a more serious blow to the family's functioning than is the incapacitation of the husband-father (although if his illness is prolonged, adverse economic reverberations are felt) (Litman, 1974).

If the mother becomes ill, often the oldest female child is expected to help the family carry on (Kahana et al., 1994). Families need to understand the course of a health problem to facilitate flexibility of roles that involve children in caregiving and child-rearing responsibilities when a parent is ill (Rolland, 1994).

The Family Caregiver Role

Family members, and women in particular, play a vital role as primary caregivers not only for the frail elderly, but for many family members of all ages who are dependent due to chronic physical and/or mental illness. Their ability and willingness to provide care is often a critical factor in determining whether or not a disabled or ill member can avoid institutionalization.

Trends in family caregiving include increases in the numbers of: caregivers with multiple caregiving responsibilities; grandchildren responsible for helping one or two older generations; and aging women without caregiver husbands due to high divorce rates (Brody, 1995). The consequences of caregiving may be negative or may include potential benefits. Previously caregiver research has focused on the negative outcomes—caregiver stress or burden—and more recently on physical and mental outcomes (Biegel, Sales, & Schulz, 1991).

Biegel, Sales, and Schulz (1991) summarize caregiver problems:

> Significant caregiving problems identified by researchers include: coping with the increased needs of the dependent family member caused by physical and/or mental illnesses; coping with disruptive behaviors . . . ; restrictions on social and leisure activities; infringement of privacy; disruption of household and work routines; conflicting multiple role demands . . . ; lack of support and assistance from other family members; disruption of family relationships; and lack of sufficient assistance from human service agencies and agency professionals. (p. 7)

Different types of caregiving demands are associated with different types of role strain. Objective stressors, or patient characteristics, that are consistently associated with family caregiver strain include greater illness severity, suddenness of onset, and greater changes in preexisting patient behaviors (Biegel et al., 1991).

In a study of caregivers of older persons, the management of behavior problems was found to be a more powerful predictor of role strain than the management of physical problems (Harvath, Stewart, & Archibold, 1994). Reinhard and Horwitz's (1995) findings substantiate the burden which caregivers of mentally ill relatives experience as the consequence of dealing with disruptive behaviors and having to provide instrumental and emotional assistance.

In a large study of primary caregivers providing care to a spouse or parent with Alzheimer's disease or a related dementia (Aneshensel et al., 1995), one stressor experienced by caregivers was role overload, i.e., feeling overwhelmed by tasks and responsibilities. Role captivity, or feeling involuntarily trapped in the role of caregiver, and the loss of intimate exchange in the caregiver–patient relationship because one of the role partners had "become someone else" were also noted. Relationships of the caregiver to other family members, as well as work and other social roles, were often adversely affected.

Rolland (1994) presents a psychosocial categorization of illness that identifies onset, course, outcome, and degree of incapacitation as four major variables of illness and disability that have an impact on both patient and family performance. These characteristics can be used to anticipate the demands placed on caregivers.

Biegel and co-workers (1991) have diagramed the variables that, according to research findings, predict caregiver strain (see Fig. 12–2). In their diagram, contextual variables that mediate the caregiver's reaction include caregiver demographic factors (gender, type of role relationship with patient, age, and socioeconomic status); preexisting psychological factors, relationship quality, family life stage, and social support. Some of these factors such as gender (female) and role relationship (spouses and parents) are consistently associated with greater caregiving burden whereas other variables show contradictory or more complex patterns. Although most caregivers are women who are socialized to the caregiving role, they exhibit greater adverse effects of caregiving than male caregivers (Pruchno & Resch, 1989).

The contributions of men to caregiving should not be overlooked. Men frequently provide support and affection to the primary caregiver. Many elderly husbands assume the role of caregiver if their wives become ill or disabled (Richards, 1996). In a study comparing the parent care experiences of women in different marital statuses (Brody, Litvin, Kleben, & Hoffman, 1990), married women were noted to have several advantages over women who did not have husbands. The husbands provided financial support, socioemotional support, and helped with instrumental tasks. Women who did not have husbands reported loneliness, lack of support, and lack of instrumental help in parental caregiving.

The caregiver's role varies according to his or her position or relationship to the care recipient; that is,

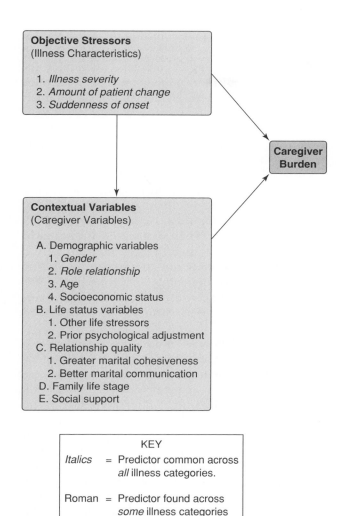

Objective Stressors
(Illness Characteristics)

1. *Illness severity*
2. *Amount of patient change*
3. *Suddenness of onset*

Caregiver Burden

Contextual Variables
(Caregiver Variables)

A. Demographic variables
   1. *Gender*
   2. *Role relationship*
   3. Age
   4. Socioeconomic status
B. Life status variables
   1. Other life stressors
   2. Prior psychological adjustment
C. Relationship quality
   1. Greater marital cohesiveness
   2. Better marital communication
D. Family life stage
E. Social support

KEY

Italics = Predictor common across *all* illness categories.

Roman = Predictor found across *some* illness categories

Figure 12–2. Summary of variables predicting caregiver strain. *(From Biegel, Sales, & Schulz, 1991.)*

the role is significantly altered when the caregiver is a spouse, parent, child, sibling, or friend. Mothers are the primary caregivers of chronically ill children (Shepard & Mahon, 1996). Spouses or adult children are most often the caregivers of the elderly. Parents care for their disabled adult children until they are no longer able to do so. Then a sibling usually becomes the primary caregiver (Roberto, 1993).

Another factor that increases the burden of the caregiving situation is a violation of social norms regarding roles. This often occurs in the following four situations: when children care for parents, when

men or women perform household tasks that are typically performed by the other gender, when parents care for adult disabled children (Litwak et al., 1994), and when siblings care for siblings (Avioli, 1989; Horwitz, 1993).

Although there are numerous caregiving stressors, many positive experiences in caregiving are reported. Some care recipients reciprocate through their expression of affection or appreciation, which may explain why some caregivers do not experience negative consequences despite providing physically demanding care (Carruth, 1996). In studying reciprocity in family caregiving, Walker, Pratt, and Oppy (1992) found that the majority of caregiving daughters perceived that they received valuable aid from their care-receiving mothers in return for their help. The contributions that the daughters received included love, information, advice, and money. Bulger, Wandersman, and Goldman (1993) noted that older parents caring for dependent adult children benefited from companionship and help with physical household work. While the assumption has been that occupying multiple roles, such as employee and caregiver, leads to negative effects such as role conflict and role overload, the emotional impact of combining multiple roles on employed caregivers has more often been found to be positive rather than negative (Neal, Chapman, Ingersoll-Dayton, & Emlen, 1993).

Role Changes During Illness and Hospitalization

In a period of crisis, such as that caused by the serious illness of a family member, the family structure is modified, the extent of modification depending on (1) to what degree the sick member is able to carry out his or her usual family roles and (2) the centrality of the family roles or tasks that are vacated. The roles taken on by the mother are, as discussed previously, a good example of the centrality of a member's roles. When illness results in the vacancy of critical roles, the family often enters a state of disequilibrium in which role and power relationships are altered until new homeostasis is achieved (Fife, 1985; Hill, 1958).

Shared, balanced role functions often become impossible to maintain in couples when one partner becomes disabled. Negotiation of revised roles is often needed to prevent role strain and confusion (Rolland, 1994). In a study of the effects of a critical care illness on family members (Johnson et al., 1995), most family members reported changes in family roles and increased responsibilities as the result of critical care hospitalization.

The role changes that occur due to the loss or incapacitation of a family member may be of two basic types. First, the remaining family members have enough inner and outer resources that they are able to take on the basic and necessary role obligations and tasks that the sick family member is unable to assume—this is the functional way the situation is managed. Or second, they lack the needed inner and outer resources, and as a consequence, certain basic and necessary roles in the family are not performed or are performed unsatisfactorily. In other words, the adequately functioning family can either flexibly modify family roles to meet the demands of the situation or may call in resources and assistance from the outside to fill the vacuum. In dysfunctional families, however, this does not happen.

Because of the role changes necessitated due to the loss or incapacitation of a family member, role conflicts and role strain are often present, especially during the stage of family disequilibrium immediately following the loss or incapacitation, when family structure is in the transitional period. Either interrole or intrarole conflict may exist, as the family members are "forced" to accept new roles and have had little opportunity to learn these roles or to rearrange all their other role responsibilities. Role strain/stress is often the outcome. The family members burdened with the acquisition of new roles may feel worried, anxious, and guilty because of feelings that they are not doing a competent job in their new roles or that with these added responsibilities, their role complex is excessively demanding and unmanageable.

In a recent review of family nursing research regarding the impact of illness on families with a member experiencing ischemic heart disease (Tapp, 1995), spouses frequently reported stress that was related to the need to assume additional household roles, and health monitoring responsibilities (Artinian, 1989; Gillis, 1984; Gilliss et al., 1985; Hilgenberg et al., 1992; McRae, 1991; Nyamathi, 1987b; Stanley & Frantz, 1988). Marital conflict related to role reversal and attempts of the healthy spouse to monitor noncompliance were also consistently reported (Caplin & Sexton, 1988; Hilgenberg et al., 1992; McRae, 1991; Mishel & Murdaugh, 1987; Nyamathi, 1987a).

Once a family has achieved a new equilibrium in response to a sick member's inability to perform his or her roles adequately, a similar reintegration must take place when that member resumes his or her old place in the family unit. Understandably, having once gone through the process of adapting, the other members may well be reluctant to again "reshuffle" family roles and tasks, despite the recovery or reentry of the "lost" member. One sees this reluctance even in the most well-functioning families, because the process of reintegrating a family member entails the difficulties and problems that are part of any disorganization before a new (in this case, renewed) balance is achieved.

FAMILY ROLE STRUCTURE: APPLYING THE FAMILY NURSING PROCESS

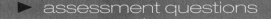

▶ assessment questions

An assessment of family roles primarily focuses on the characteristics of the formal and informal role structure, coupled with a consideration of how sociocultural, situational, and historical factors affect family role structure. There are four broad areas for the assessment of the family role structure:

1. The formal role structure.

2. The informal role structure and types of relationships.

3. Role models.

4. Variables affecting role structure.

Formal Role Structure

Each family member's position and roles are described by addressing the following questions:

1. What formal positions and roles do each of the family members fulfill? Describe how each family member carries out his or her formal roles.

2. Are these roles acceptable and consistent with the family members' and family's expectations? In other words, are there any role conflicts present?

3. How competently do members perceive they perform their respective roles?

4. Is there flexibility in roles when needed?

Informal Role Structure

Questions pertinent to this area include:

1. What informal or covert roles exist in the family, who plays them, and how frequently or consistently are they enacted? Are members of the family covertly playing roles different from those that their position in the family demands that they play?

2. What purposes do the identified covert or informal roles serve?

3. Are any of these informal roles dysfunctional to the family or family members in the long run?

Role Models

The following questions are important when role problems are present:

1. Who were (or are) the models that influenced family members in their early life, who gave feelings and values about, for example, growth, new experiences, roles, and communication techniques?

2. Who specifically acted as role model for the mates in their roles as parents, and as marital partners, and what were they like? From this information a family member can be helped to see how past models influence his or her expectations and behavior (Satir, 1983).

3. If the informal roles are dysfunctional in the family, who enacted these roles in previous generations?

4. What is the impact on the person(s) who play dysfunctional formal or informal family roles?

In analyzing the informal role structure, an important area to describe relates to the types of role relationships within the subsystems of the family. Role relationships can be observed and assessed within each of the family subsystems, thus adding further information on both the adequacy of those sets of relationships and also the informal roles played within the subsystems. In assessing marital, parent–child, and sibling relationships, it is suggested that reference be made to the types of dyadic relationships discussed previously (complementary, symmetrical, and parallel), which will assist in describing the nature of subsystem role relationships.

In identifying formal and informal roles that adult family members play, Satir (1972) questions patients about their roles by asking: "You wear three hats . . . individual, marital partner, and parent. I can see the parent, but where are the other two?" "Before marriage you were Miss So and So. What happened to her?" (pp. 174–175). Satir also explicitly teaches family members about their roles by listing the three basic roles—individual, marital partner, and parent—on a blackboard and explores their responses to interactions in these different roles and what other response options are available.

Variables Affecting Role Structure

- *Social class influences.* How does social class background influence the formal and informal role structure in the family?
- *Ethnic influences.* How is the family's role structure influenced by the family's ethnic and religious background?
- *Developmental or life cycle influences.* Are the present role behaviors of family members developmentally appropriate?
- *Situational events, including health and illness changes.*
  1. How have health problems affected family roles? What reallocation of roles and tasks have occurred?
  2. How have the family members who have had to assume new roles adjusted? Is there evidence of role stress and/or role conflict as a result of these role shifts?
  3. How has the family member with the health problem reacted to her or his change or loss of a role(s)?

▶ FAMILY NURSING DIAGNOSES

Families are continually bombarded with demands for change—either because of normal developmental transitions or because of the various situational stressors families experience. Health stressors are one prime example of demands families face. Stressors/demands require family role changes. If family members do not have the requisite knowledge, skills, or emotional readiness for adjusting to the needed role changes, then numerous types of role problems may result. One important role of the family nurse in this regard is to assist families to identify role transitions so that information about the new role (anticipatory guidance) is provided to prevent role problems.

Role problems are frequently observed by family nurses. They may not, however, be identified as role problems, because there are so many interrelationships and overlaps between problems. Any of the above role problems may be stated as a family nursing diagnosis, remembering that role problems involve at least two people: the role occupant and his or her role partner(s). Because role problems are usually very general, it is also useful to state defining characteristics and related factors.

In reviewing the list of nursing diagnoses approved by the North American Nursing Diagnosis Association (NANDA), the diagnoses given in Table 12–1 relate to role problems. It should be noted here that most of these diagnoses do not mention "role" in the diagnostic title, but actual and potential role problems could be a related nursing diagnosis. In NANDA, included under altered role performance are four more specific role problems: role transition, role distance, role conflict, and role failure. Defining characteristics of each of these types of role problems are seen in Table 12–2, as well as associated, relevant nursing diagnoses.

In *A Pocket Guide to Nursing Diagnoses*, Kim, McFarland, and McFarlane (1995) list nursing diagnoses associated with medical diagnostic categories. For instance, for Alzheimer's type dementia many nursing diagnoses are listed, but in particular five dealing with role problems are identified. They are alteration in family processes, impaired social interaction, altered role performance, caregiver role strain, and risk for caregiver role strain. These diagnoses have been incorporated into the NANDA listing in Table 12–1.

► FAMILY NURSING INTERVENTIONS

Assessment and diagnosis guide health professionals in their planning and implementation strategies. Role transitions and role problems may create substantial disequilibrium and stress throughout the entire family

► TABLE 12–1

NANDA NURSING DIAGNOSES RELATED TO ROLE TRANSITIONS/ROLE PROBLEMS

NANDA Nursing Diagnoses	Related Role Problem(s)[a]
Anticipatory grieving	Role loss
Dysfunctional grieving	Role strain
Social isolation	Role change
Impaired social interaction	Role loss and strain
Alteration in family processes	
Potential alteration in parenting	Role conflicts
Alteration in parenting	Role overload
Potential for violence	Role change
Altered role performance	Role conflict
Caregiver role strain	Role loss and strain
Risk for caregiver role strain	Role strain
Impaired home maintenance management	Role strain
Body image disturbance	Role strain
Family coping diagnoses	Role loss
	Role insufficiency or role ambiguity

[a] These are only samples of role problems that could be associated with the accompanying nursing diagnoses.
From: McFarland & McFarlane (1989), and Kim, McFarland, & McFarlane, (1995).

system, even though on the surface only one or two family members seem to be affected. This is due to the high degree of interdependency between the subsystems and the "ripple effect." Hence, teaching and counseling strategies, as well as coordination/case management and referral strategies, are used to ameliorate role transitions and role problems, and are often directed at the family level.

As seen in Table 12–2, the Nursing Interventions Classification (NIC) Project at the University of Iowa has identified numerous nursing intervention approaches which may be used with families and are associated with actual or potential role problems. These interventions are research-based and well explained in McCloskey and Bulechek's (1996) text, *Nursing Interventions Classification (NIC)*.

Johnson (1986) summarizes general nursing interventions appropriate for role transitions and role problems. She refers to these interventions as "role theory strategies." Johnson's role theory strategies include:

- Helping family members identify significant cues of the other family members (e.g., teaching parents how to distinguish between hunger crying and crying for attention in newborns).
- Clarifying expectations about the needed roles (family members identify their expectations for new roles).
- Strengthening the family members' abilities to enact a new role. Teaching strategies are used here.
- Rewarding the new role-taking behaviors.
- Helping the family member to modify the new role by helping him or her see how the role fits into his or her role complex.
- Reinforcing the feedback of the "relevant others."

Role Supplementation or Role Enhancement Strategies for Role Transitions

Role supplementation or role enhancement consists of a set of interventions to assist family members to improve their role relationships and facilitate their role changes by clarifying and supplementing role behaviors (McCloskey & Bulechek, 1996; Meleis & Swendsen, 1978). Role supplementation strategies can also be preventive, in this case used to clarify role insufficiency (Morehead, 1985).

Role transitions involve adding new roles and dropping others. Role transitions are created because of developmental changes and situational changes including health-related stressors. The result of unsuccessful role transition is role strain, role insufficiency, role failure, and/or role distance. Role transitions involve role loss; hence some reactions to loss or grieving should be expected.

Role supplementation or role enhancement consists of components, strategies, and process. The two components are (1) role clarification, understanding the specific information and cues needed to enact the role; and (2) role taking, being able to imagine yourself in a particular role and assuming the perspective of the other person. Roles are paired and learned in pairs. Hence, if an individual learns the expectations of a parenting role, theoretically he or she should also know the role of the role partner, in this case the child.

▶ TABLE 12-2

TYPES OF ALTERED ROLE PERFORMANCE NURSING DIAGNOSES (NANDA) WITH DEFINING CHARACTERISTICS AND RELEVANT NURSING INTERVENTIONS (NIC)

NANDA Nursing Diagnoses with Defining Characteristics[a]	Nursing Interventions (NIC)[b]
■ ROLE TRANSITION • Change in capacity to perform role. • Change in other's perception or expectations of role. • Change in usual pattern of responsibility. • Feelings of anger and depression. • Inability to achieve desired role. • Refusal to participate in role. ■ ROLE DISTANCE[c] • Uncertainty about role requirements. • Lack of knowledge of role. • Different role perceptions. ■ ROLE CONFLICT • Frustration in role or conflict of roles; intrarole, or interrole conflict. • Ambivalence about role. • Incongruent or incompatible role expectations. • Confusion. • Inadequate problem-solving skills. ■ ROLE FAILURE • Loss of role skills. • Difficulty learning new roles. • Withdrawal. • Inability to achieve desired role. • Refusal to participate in role.	Role enhancement Developmental enhancement Anticipatory guidance Teaching: Individual and family Teaching: Disease process and medical/health regimens Patient education Emotional support Support group Counseling and family therapy Cognitive restructuring Communication enhancement Family involvement and support Active listening Decision-making support Caregiver support Family mobilization Grief work facilitation Home maintenance assistance Respite care Family integrity promotion

[a] NANDA refers to the North American Nursing Diagnosis Association.
[b] NIC refers to Nursing Interventions Classifications developed by McCloskey and Bulechek and associates at the University of Iowa.
[c] Role distance is present when a person's role behavior differs from socially prescribed expectations.
From McCloskey & Bulechek (1996), McFarland & McFarlane (1989).

The strategies used to accomplish role clarification and role taking are role modeling, role rehearsal, and reference group interactions. Role modeling is a very useful and effective teaching strategy (Bandura, 1977). Through modeling, the desired behavior is performed by the health professional for the family member to imitate; the imitation eventually becomes part of the family member's own behavioral repertoire (Goldenberg & Goldenberg, 1996). For example, a family nurse may serve as a role model for a caregiver by showing how to help the stroke patient ambulate and how to praise every small improvement that is made.

Role rehearsal is a second role supplementation strategy suggested by Meleis (1975). Here the role behavior and reactions of significant others are mentally enacted. This strategy is very helpful when a new role can be anticipated. This mental practice prepares the individual for a future role change. The nurse can effectively use role reversal with parents, marital partners, and in parent–child and sibling relationships. Helping family members to rehearse their interactions is good anticipatory guidance. For instance, this may be a useful strategy to use when helping a stepfather deal with his stepchildren who are displaying anger and resistance toward his parenting efforts.

The third role supplementation strategy is initiation of referrals to reference groups. Reference groups are groups with which an individual or family identifies. Self-help groups can become powerful reference groups for individuals and families. Self-help groups assist their members to adapt to their new roles by sharing feelings and perceptions in the group and offering practical solutions to vexing issues related to the new role. Nurses often initiate referrals of family members struggling to learn a new role to self-help groups and, in some cases, lead a self-help group or act as a consultant to the group.

The process used in role supplementation is communication. Through communication new information needed to enact the new role or role options can be shared. Feelings can be ventilated—such as feelings of anger, depression and frustration over difficulties in learning the new role. Exploration of family members' perception of what has changed and how the role change has affected them is a vital area to discuss. And lastly, through communication clients should be encouraged to seek out new information and explore role options themselves.

Interventions for Role Strain

Several ways have been suggested to deal with role strain. Family nurses can explore the following options with family members who are experiencing role strain:

1. Redefining the role in terms of what behaviors are considered adequate role performance.

2. Examining an individuals's role complex (the various roles the role occupant plays) and setting priorities within a role and among roles.

3. Role bargaining or role negotiation with role partners so that role occupants achieve a set of roles that collectively are relatively equitable and rewarding. Role negotiation involves influencing the members of one's role set so that they agree to changes in the role and the allocation of resources.

4. Reduced interaction with role partners. If, however, role partners have a high interdependency on each other, this tactic usually leads to unsuccessful role bargaining and role distancing. Partial withdrawal from interaction may relieve role strain when the interdependency is not so great and when diminished interaction is possible (Hardy & Hardy, 1988). This suggestion is often not possible in family relationships.

Interventions for Caregiver Role Fatigue

Respite care and participation in self-care groups are recommended for those primary caregivers who are strained in their caregiver role (Dell Orto, 1988). Studies of caregiving role strain and reports from family support groups indicate that regularly scheduled periods of respite are essential to counter role fatigue and stress (Pallett, 1990). Respite care refers to temporary care of disabled individuals for the purpose of providing relief to the primary caregiver (Dell Orto, 1988). Friends and family sometimes serve as surrogate caregivers. Nurses can assist families in locating community resources for respite care, such as adult day care, temporary nursing home placement, and/or intermittent home care. Unfortunately there is a scarcity of funding for respite services. Pioneering efforts have been made by groups and organizations to implement respite care programs for the developmentally disabled, the physically disabled, and the chronically mentally ill. Some family caregiving situations are very intense, and if left without intervention such as respite or home care, increased family stress and accelerated deterioration in family functioning may result.

Participation in a formal self-help support group for caregivers has proved to be important in boosting morale and preventing social isolation. Family caregiver groups have been found to be very helpful in a number of research studies (Pallett, 1990). Feelings and frustrations, as well as practical solutions, are shared in groups. Additional interventions to reduce caregiver burden include caregiver education and skill training (Schmall, 1994).

Interventions for Role Distance or Role Inadequacy

Role distance or role inadequacy refers to a role occupant not fulfilling the role behaviors that are a part of that role. In this type of role problem, role expectations are set by society and they are in conflict with the role's occupant's behavior.

Support and counseling strategies, as well as teaching, strategies should be used here. Family members need to understand role requirements; they very much need information, because knowledge deficits are usually present. Focusing on clarifying perceptions and fostering awareness of prevailing expectations is recommended. In addition, in working with immigrant families, showing respect for role behaviors that are culturally derived and comparing the role occupant's customs with expected practices in their new country is suggested.

Many fathers in our society have a role distancing problem—that is, they are not undertaking the father role that the culture today expects of them. Hanson and Bozett (1987) and Kunst-Wilson and Cronenwett (1981) recommend several tactics for nurses to use to promote greater active participation by fathers in family health care. These suggestions include:

1. Encourage fathers to attend clinics with their children and to attend prenatal clinics and family planning clinics with their wives.
2. Encourage fathers to join men's support groups and resource centers if they feel they need support to undertake new father roles.
3. Encourage fathers' participation in birthing and parenting classes.
4. Encourage spouses to negotiate infant and child care roles. Role sharing and role negotiation can help reduce role stress. Role negotiation involves an agreement among involved persons regarding the behaviors that are expected in an associated role.
5. Support fathers' active involvement in labor, delivery, and newborn care in the hospital.

Interventions for Role Conflict

Interventions for role conflict cover both intrarole and interrole conflicts. Guidelines for this problem include the following:

1. Before beginning to intervene, plan strategies to reduce or resolve role conflict. To do this, determine the sources of stress and the type of role conflict present.
2. Actively listen, encouraging expression of frustration with role conflict.
3. Encourage role partners who are in conflict to discuss their perceptions and feelings about the roles in question.
4. Encourage family members to discuss their feelings and perceptions together and assist them in problem solving.
5. Assist family to set priorities.
6. Family members should meet together to discuss role incompatibilities. The nurse, acting as a facilitator, encourages the family members to explore role incompatibilities and to come up with a different allocation of roles or perhaps different role expectations.

Interventions for Role Failure

Role failure implies that the client has tried to carry out the role, but has failed. Role failure addresses the lack of knowledge and skills for a particular role and perhaps the needed emotional or developmental readiness (such as "babies having babies"—the teen-mother problem). Strategies are aimed at resolving role failure problems and assisting family members to achieve satisfactory role competence. Here teaching and support are primary strategies. Teaching about role requirements is paramount. Supportive counseling involves encouraging family members to voice their concerns and questions about their new role(s). Because clients are often disappointed and frustrated about the new role, recognizing and praising each successful behavior is important. Strengths and resources that the client possesses should also be recognized and supported. Behavior modification and contracting may be used here. Setting up a behavioral therapy plan involves tasks analysis (defining the tasks within the role), breaking the tasks into small chunks of information or skills, and then consistently reinforcing each small chunk of behavior or information as it is learned.

In conclusion, family nurses are able to effectively assess and intervene to assist families with role transitions and role problems. In assessing family roles (the formal and informal role structure), our understanding of family strengths and resources is also enhanced. This supplies us with important data for planning interventions to resolve health problems.

► study questions

1. Match the correct definition or description with the appropriate term.

Terms	**Definitions**
a. Role	1. Status
b. Position	2. Incompatibility of the role(s) (intrarole or interrole).
c. Role enactment	3. A set of behaviors of an occupant of a particular social position.
d. Socialization	4. The process of learning family and adult roles in preparation for societal responsibilities.
e. Role conflict	5. Balancing in family structure to maintain stability.
f. Reciprocal role	6. Joint participation in fulfilling same role.
g. Role strain	7. Complementary role.
h. Family homeostasis	8. The worry or guilt felt as a result of difficulty with role enactment or presence of role conflict.
i. Role sharing	9. The actual behavior exhibited in a role.

Are the following statements true or false?

2. A most functional way of maintaining equilibrium in a family in the face of change is by use of role flexibility.

3. The principle of complementarity states that there must be a match in expectations and performance of roles by role partners in order for stability and harmony to be present in the relationship.

4. Paired relationships in the family refer to father-son and mother-daughter relationships.

5. For each of the roles making up the wife-mother and husband-father positions listed in the following table, indicate whether in the American family these roles are normatively shared or the primary responsibility of one or the other partner. If the trend is toward sharing or being more or less a single partner's role, indicate this with an arrow pointing up (increasing emphasis) or down (decreasing emphasis). A check (✓) indicates that role remains the same.

Role	Shared Role	Role of Wife-Mother	Role of Husband-Father
Provider			
Housekeeper			
Child care			
Recreational			
Kinship			
Therapeutic			
Sexual			
Companion			
Health leader			

6. From the two studies presented on the observed types of marriages (by Cline, and Cuber and Harroff), which conclusion would be the most accurate and practically significant?
   a. Well-functioning or long-standing marriages are distinguished from poorly functioning marriages.
   b. It was discovered that diverse patterns of marital relationships existed.
   c. A wide range of behaviors and roles existed in the marriages studied.
   d. Because there is no one type of marriage which fits the needs of most couples, acceptance and understanding of this diversity among couples is indicated.

7. When a wife is employed full-time in a two-parent nuclear family with young children, what are common role changes and conflicts experienced by the husband and the wife?

8. Identify three commonly seen differences in role structure between the lower- and middle-class families.

9. List five examples of informal roles seen in the family, indicating which of them could be functional.

10. The maintenance of informal roles is vital to the family because (select the best answer):
    a. It relieves the role overload of some members.
    b. Without covert roles the family could not exist.
    c. Each formal role has an associated informal role.
    d. Through the assumption of informal roles, family homeostasis is maintained and individual socioemotional needs are met.

11. Why are both formal and informal roles important to assess?

12. Give reasons why labeling is restrictive to an individual's growth and development.

13. Identify two role characteristics of single-parent families that act as stressors to the family and its members.

14. What are two prominent role problems within the stepparent family?

Are the following statements true or false?

15. When a family member is ill, the functional way of handling the situation is to leave the roles unfulfilled until he or she returns.

16. Role flexibility suggests that family members have the motivation and capacity to shift and reenact new roles when needed.

17. Middle-class parents are generally more concerned with promoting self-reliance and independence in their child-rearing practices, while lower-class parents stress respect and obedience.

18. Male caregivers experience greater adverse effects of caregiving than female caregivers.

▶ family case study*

After reading the following case study, answer questions 19 through 23.

Mr. and Mrs. G. are a young couple, married for 3 years, with a 2-year-old son. The 23-year-old husband is a garbage collector, earning $18,000 a year. He completed 2 years of high school; his 22-year-old wife is a high school graduate. (But the family nurse commented: "It is hard to believe in view of her poor vocabulary and illiterate handwriting that she had completed high school." The husband said: "She was sort of a dumbbell at school, but people liked her and she got through.")

Mr. G. is a slim tall man, slow moving and soft spoken. When asked what he liked about himself, he replied, "People tell me I'm easygoing but not a chump." The assessor observed his deceptively lazy attitude as the manner of a man who thinks that most people, particularly women, become too excited about things and foolishly so. He reports that he quit school at 14 because he did not like it. Since then he has held a number of unskilled jobs. Concerning

---

*Adapted by permission of Random House, Inc., from *Blue-Collar Marriage*, by Mirra Komarovsky with the collaboration of Jane H. Phillips. Copyright 1962, 1964, 1967 by Random House, Inc.

his present occupation as garbage collector, he stated: "People laugh at you for being in this line of work. I don't know what's so funny about it. It's got to be done. There is no future in it, though, and the pay is terrible. I'm going to make a break for it as soon as I can. Everybody's looking out for me now, and something is bound to turn up pretty soon."

Both Mr. G. and his wife express satisfaction with their sexual relations and with the marriage in general. Mr. G. is in charge of the outside of the house and repairs to their home, and Mrs. G. is in charge of the interior of the home and child.

A good deal of the communication between them is nonverbal. This type of communication pattern began during their courtship. When asked whether her husband had said he loved her when he proposed, Mrs. G. answered, "He just got softer and softer on me and I could tell that he did and we got to necking more and more and he wanted to go all the way and I didn't want to unless we were going to get married." The nurse asked whether he had ever said out and out that he could go for her or wanted her or anything like that. Mrs. G. said, "No, we don't go in for that kind of stuff." When she told him she was pregnant, "He looked a little funny when I told him, but he didn't say much. You know that's what's going to happen. After a while, when I began to show a lot, he asked me sometimes how I felt."

Mrs. G. was asked to describe their quarrels. She said they quarrel little, but when they do, it is about such things as his failure to help move the furniture or her failure to do something he demands. "We just get over it." He might "crab around and then he would know that he had been mean to me and makes it up." There is no conversation about such quarrels, but Mr. G. helps to dry the dishes or asks her if she likes a television program or wants something else. Mrs. G. felt that talking does no good, since it might worsen things.

When asked whether they like to talk about what makes people tick or to discuss the rights and wrongs of things, each said in separate interviews, "No, we don't hash things over." Mr. G. added, "It's either right or wrong—what is there to discuss?"

This "conversation of gestures" between Mrs. G. and her husband contrasts sharply with the communication characterizing her relationships with female relatives and friends. On many counts Mrs. G. reveals her emotional life to the latter. And this extends to spheres of experience beyond the "feminine world" of babies, housework, or gossip.

Mrs. G. sees her sister and her mother daily. "Oh yes," she said about her sister, "we tell each other everything, anything we have on our minds. We don't hold nothing back. We discuss the children, the house, cooking, and 'female things.' " But when asked whether she can talk to her husband, she answered, "Sure, I can talk to him about anything that has to be said." Her view is that "men and women do different things; he don't want to be bothered with my job of cleaning and children and I don't want to be bothered with his. He makes the big decisions and I don't have to bother with it. Sometimes we got to do the same things, something around the house and we have to tell each other."

When asked what helped her when she was in the "dumps," Mrs. G. replied, "Talking to my sister or my mother helps sometimes." When asked directly whether conversations with her husband ever have a similar effect, she replied, "No."

Mr. G. enjoys an active social life with his male friends and relatives, Mr. G. revealed to his father and his brother he fears that Mrs. G. was making a "sissy" out of their son, and he regularly consults with them about his occupational plans. He does not discuss the latter topics with his wife because "there is no need of exciting her for nothing. Wait until it's sure. Women get all excited and talk too much."

Mr. G. thinks the world of the fellows in his own clique whom he sees after supper several times a week and on Saturday afternoons. Mrs. G. does not always know where he meets his "friends" when he leaves in the evenings. Mr. and Mrs. G. testified independently that having a beer with the fellows is the best cure for his depressions.

Select the one best answer referring to the family case study.

19. This marriage was characterized as "happy" by both marital partners. This was because:
    a. Both come from same social class.
    b. Both shared same marital role expectations.
    c. Both were denying how really alienated they were from each other and how unsatisfactory their marriage was.
    d. Their sex life was adequate.

20. This marriage illustrates:
    a. The mates' lack of understanding of one another.
    b. An insufficient amount of communication in meaningful areas of family life.
    c. That marital companionship is not essential to make a satisfactory marriage.
    d. That both mates did not communicate openly with anyone.

21. This type of marriage is frequently seen in:
    a. Lower-class families.
    b. White, skilled working-class families.
    c. Disorganized families.
    d. Middle-class white families.

22. Through the couple's communication we can gather that:
    a. Both mates carry out traditional male–female roles.
    b. Mrs. G. would rather move out and be with her sister and friends.
    c. Mr. G.'s occupational role is of central concern to him.
    d. Mr. G. desires to raise his son to be "a man."

23. Which type of relationship does this marriage most closely fit?
    a. Symmetrical
    b. Parallel
    c. Complementary

24. Complete a brief description of the couple's formal roles from what can be inferred from the narrative.

25. In the above case study, are there any potential or actual role problems manifested?

26. If the wife was going to vocational school and began to question her husband's traditional sex roles in the family, what kind of role problems might result? (Name at least one.)

27. Suggest two strategies to ameliorate or resolve the role problem identified in question 26.

▶ chapter 12 study answers

1. a. 3.   f. 7.
    b. 1.   g. 8.
    c. 9.   h. 5.
    d. 4.   i. 6.
    e. 2.

2. True.

3. True.

4. False.

5. See table below:

Role	Shared Role	Role of Wife-Mother	Role of Husband-Father
Provider	↑	—	✓↓
Housekeeper	—	↓	—
Child care	↑	—	—
Recreational	↑	—	—
Kinship	—	✓	—
Therapeutic	↑	—	—
Sexual	↑	—	—
Companion	↑	—	—
Health leader	—	✓	—

6. d.

7. *Husband:* Feels partial role loss having to share the enacting of provider (breadwinner) role. Necessitates role transitions when he assumes greater (shared) responsibility for child care and perhaps other areas. Usually experiences role changes rather than role conflicts.

Wife: Feels role conflict and strain. Most often still retains the house-keeper role and child-care role (although this is often shared) in addition to working. Her other shared and assumed roles remain also, producing role overload. Commonly feels role strain as a result of role conflict, feeling worried and guilty that she is not spending enough time with children or is hurting husband's pride in being sole provider.

8. *Lower-class Family.* Marital roles: Sexual role less satisfying and diminished in importance, companionship role attenuated, therapeutic role attenuated. Parenting roles: The child-care role is exclusively the mother's domain (and the central role in her life).
   Middle-class Family: Marital roles: Sexual role is shared and more satisfying, companionship and therapeutic roles are strong basis for marriage. Parenting roles: Child-care role is shared.

9. Informal roles in the family (any five):
   a. Integrator (functional).
   b. Mediator (functional).
   c. Scapegoat.
   d. Jester (functional).
   e. Child (when formal role is parent).
   f. Blocker.
   g. The bystander.
   h. The placator.
   i. The family pioneer (functional).
   j. The "great stone face."
   k. The pal (may or may not be functional).
   l. Encourager (functional).
   m. Harmonizer (may or may not be functional).
   n. Initiator-contributor (usually functional).
   o. Compromiser (functional).
   p. Follower.
   q. Dominator.
   r. Recognition seeker.
   s. Martyr.

10. d.

11. They describe how family members have allocated tasks to fulfill family functions; they disclose the socioemotional needs of family member(s) and the family and whether and how these needs are being met.

12. An individual cannot fully develop because he or she is rewarded only for certain behaviors and thus matures only in these rewarded areas.

13. a. Role overload.
    b. Role changes or shifts, which occur if there is remarriage.

14. a. Whether the father (in the case of a stepfather family) is a parent or not (parental role confusion).

        b. The incompatibility of the wife and mother role. She has divided loyalties (to her children and to her husband), and conflict is seen when being supportive as a wife conflicts with being supportive as a mother.

15. False.

16. True.

17. True.

18. False.

19. b.

20. c.

21. a.

22. a.

23. c.

24. *Formal role structure of hypothetical family:* The family was characterized by a sharp demarcation of roles (traditional pattern).
    Husband-father:
        Sole provider—breadwinner role.
        Home repairman and gardener role.
    Wife-mother:
        Child-care role.
        Housekeeper role (inside the house).
        No roles are shared, nor do they wish to share any roles.
        The companionship and therapeutic roles are not present in their marriage.
    Sexual roles are not clear, but probably traditional.

25. None present.

26. The mother feeling role strain and role overload. Marital and parental role conflict and role strain (of marital partners).

27. For role strain: (1) Discuss housekeeper and child-care roles with the mother and help her to redefine these roles in terms of what behaviors are necessary to maintain and which behaviors (tasks) can be eliminated or reduced in frequency. (2) Facilitate a discussion between mates of roles that wife-mother has and help her negotiate roles so that there is a more equitable distribution of role responsibilities.
    For role conflict: (1) Encourage mother to express her feelings and perceptions about her roles and the incompatibility between the roles she is enacting. (2) Help wife-mother to problem-solve to reduce incompatibilities of present roles and to set priorities.

Family Values

Marilyn M. Friedman

► learning objectives

1. Define the terms values, family values, norms, and family rules, and give their significance relative to family assessment.

2. Describe the common outcome of a disparity in values between health worker and client.

3. Identify and briefly explain four recent important changes that have taken place in society related to family values.

4. Discuss the core value orientations of American society in terms of their significance today and their interrelationships with each other.

5. Identify four of the variables that influence the family's value system and that create value conflicts.

6. Given a case situation and, using the value assessment process, identify the salient values operating within the hypothetical family and state a family nursing diagnosis and intervention in the area of values.

7. Describe the meaning and purposes of the value clarification process.

Family health assessment is not complete without an analysis of a family's central values, because the value system is one of the four highly interdependent structural dimensions of a family. Understanding what is important to a particular family is vital in terms of assessment, diagnosis, and health care intervention, for we know that what a family believes and values affects both the family's and its members' behavior. Moreover, when family values and beliefs are identified, we may better understand family dynamics and behavior.

It needs to be recognized that as health care professionals we have the tendency to diagnose or label a family as pathological when they deviate from the dominant cultural values and norms. Most research on families is based on the mainstream or dominant culture (described later), and we must be particularly cautious about extrapolating these findings to all social classes and cultural groups, whose life conditions and traditions differ greatly from those of the dominant culture.

An accurate assessment of a family's value system should help us tailor our nursing interventions to a particular family or groups of similar families. We need to work within the family's value system and relate our services to goals that are important to the family being assisted. For instance, it is well accepted that "ideas and methods which least affect the patient's habits, beliefs, and values meet less resistance than those that attempt to alter existing behavior patterns and values (Dougherty, 1975, p. 441).

In assessing a family's value system it is also imperative for us, as health care providers, to recognize our own priorities and values and to examine carefully how our values and attitudes subtly—and sometimes not so subtly—affect our family-centered care. One ultimate goal in assessing family values is to demonstrate to families our appreciation of and respect for different value systems (Clemen, 1977).

▶ BASIC DEFINITIONS

One of the most developed definitions of **value** is by Rokeach (1973): "A value is an enduring belief that a specific mode of conduct or end-state of existence [such as freedom] is . . . preferable to the opposite or converse mode of conduct or end-state of existence" (p. 5). Values are central features of an individual's belief system due to their enduring quality; they are not short-lived attitudes. Values serve as guides to action (Rokeach, 1973).

Family values are defined as a system of ideas, attitudes, and beliefs about the worth of an entity or concept that consciously and unconsciously bind together the members of a family in a common culture (Parad & Caplan, 1965). The family's cultural heritage is a prime source of a family's value system and norms. In turn, the family group is a prime source of family members' belief systems, value systems, and norms regarding the nature and meaning of the world, their place in it, and how to reach personal goals and aspirations.

Values serve as general guides to behavior. Within families values guide the development of family norms or rules. For instance, if a person values health and feels it is a desirable state, he or she is much more likely to engage in preventive health care and salubrious health habits. In addition, there will be a moral injunction (a norm or family rule) against "bad" health habits.

Values are not static. As the family developmentally evolves over time, and as particular situations in society or the family demand a shift of priorities by the family, the potency or primacy of a family's values change over time.

Furthermore, families and individuals rarely behave according to consistent value patterns. Certain values we hold compete with other values which we simultaneously hold, like the competition between valuing individualism and freedom versus valuing familism (meeting of the family's needs before personal needs).

Also certain values are amenable to conscious identification, whereas others are less susceptible to conscious expression. Simply put, some values are consciously held while others are not.

There is a hierarchical nature to values. Some values are more central, molding or influencing most aspects of our lives, while other values are more peripheral and have less influence, involving only certain aspects of our lifestyle and daily functioning. In other words, certain values have a greater priority or potency than other values, particularly when looking at a family at a given point in time.

A family's configuration of values ascribes meaning to certain critical events and at the same time suggests ways to respond to these situations. This configuration of values provides definitions of the time dimension; contains concepts concerning the responsibility and worth of the individual members of the family; ranks certain commonly held life goals; imposes a framework within which the pursuit of risks connected with the pleasure impulse takes place; defines what messages, thoughts, and feelings should and should not be shared and with whom; and lastly, involves a system of sanctions.

Values are learned from the family of origin, which is the basic transmitter of societal or cultural values from one generation to the next. The family of origin assimilates societal and cultural values and modifies them somewhat to match with its own values. Societal values change, with some values becoming more important than others; these value changes and swings greatly affect the family, profoundly affecting its own family values, norms, and ultimately its behavior.

Family values are not only a reflection of the society in which the individual or family resides, but also of the subculture(s) with which the family identifies. Most persons belong to a number of subcultures based on social class, ethnic background, occupational groups, peer groups, religious affiliation, and so forth. Subcultures exist within the larger, dominant culture, and so aspects of that value system also pervade the subculture. Thus members of a particular subculture respond to both subcultural and dominant value systems, although at different moments the values of one or the other may be more relevant to the individual or family. Obviously the greater the degree of congruence between a family's subcultural values and the community's values, the easier the individual's and family's adjustment, and the greater degree of success the family will meet in relating to the community.

Families will often have values that are not realizable. Sheer practical necessity can often distort a family's values in everyday life so that they become unrecognizable (Graedon, 1985). In assisting families, both their values and actual behaviors need to be understood—for what families say is important may be at striking variance with their actual behavior. In anthropology this is referred to as the *real* or *manifest* (family's actual behavior) versus the *ideal* (the family values espoused) (Leininger, 1978). The variance between the ideal and real is typically due to the family making a pragmatic adaptation to a particular social and historical context. Poor ethnic minority families often have had to compromise their values or ideals due to the harsh realities of their world.

Norms are patterns of behavior considered to be right in a given society and, as such are based on the family's value system. They are also modal behaviors. In other words, norms prescribe the appropriate role behavior for each of the positions in the family and society and specify how reciprocal relations are to be maintained, as well as how role behavior may change with the changing ages of occupants of these positions.

Family rules are an even more specific reflection of the family values than family norms. They refer to the specific regulations the family maintains as to what is acceptable and what is not. The family rules, guided by more abstract values, provide the stability, commonality, and guidance family members need. Holman (1979) suggests that family rules form the family miniculture, the shared meanings that define the individual character of each family as different from all other families.

An example of how family roles express the value system by which the family operates is the case of the Latino family. The high value of familism among Latino families translates to the norm and family rule that members of the extended family are all part of the "familia," and are to be treated as such. Values

are also determinants of family rules about communication—perhaps what is discussed and not discussed and with whom. Recall the high value that respect for elders, especially fathers, has in some families, with a resultant family rule being to not openly challenge the father's decisions or actions.

Family rules are reflective of the family's level of functioning. Whall (1986b) corroborates this association by stating that in general "it is fair to say that dysfunctional families have dysfunctional rules since one begets the other" (p. 100).

▶ DISPARITY IN VALUES SYSTEMS

Between Client and Health Care Professional

One of the primary stressors in relationships between health care workers and family clients is the social distancing created because of social class and/or cultural value differences. When the professional and client do not possess the same basic beliefs and values, the results are often divergent goals, unclear communication, and interactional problems. As professionals working within the mainstream health care systems, we generally uphold the values of the dominant culture of which the health care system is a part. These are generally white, Anglo-Saxon, Protestant (WASP) values. Brink (1976) described the American nurses' value system thusly:

> The American nurse, educated in the United States, falls within the "Old Yankee" classification of value systems. American nurses are future-oriented, belong to a doing-oriented profession, are individualistic in decision-making, but lineally-oriented in the health institution, believe that disease is controllable, and view the human being as neither good nor evil, but ill. (pp. 63–64)

This picture of health providers' having one common value orientation does not negate the reality that many nurses and nursing students come from diverse cultural and social class backgrounds and possess their own configuration of more particular values and goals, although also conforming to the central values of the health care system of which they are a part. Clients, on the other hand, come from all walks of life and more often than not hold different values than the health care worker. Because the class and cultural backgrounds of many clients differ from those of the health care professional, the possibility of value conflicts is present (Lauver, 1980).

▶ VALUE CHANGES IN AMERICAN SOCIETY

Since the 1960s the United States, as well as the world at large, has witnessed a profound revolution in ideas, values, and norms. Most of the literature suggests that the Civil Rights Movement marked the beginning of America's cultural revolution. Because of turbulent events in society and the family, a widening social stratification, a rise in poverty, a growth in consumerism and materialism (Samuelson, 1986), and globalization of our economy, American cultural values are continually being shaped and modified. Although the family has been widely perceived as threatened by multiple societal events and concomitant value shifts, turning the tide back to "the good old traditional days" appears futile, in spite of fervent efforts by some fundamentalist and reactionary groups.

Profound physical and social changes have also taken place. For example, in the last 200 years, the United States quadrupled in physical size and its population grew 52 times greater. We have gone from an overwhelmingly rural society to a highly urbanized nation. Whereas only 1 percent of Americans were high school graduates in 1800, 76 percent of Americans now graduate from high school. And more recently, the country changed from an overwhelmingly white, Anglo-American country to one with increasingly significant Asian, African-American and Hispanic populations.

In recent years a number of authors (Aldous, 1996; Koten, 1987; Glick, 1989; Schwartz, 1987; Yankelovich & Gurin, 1989) have suggested that the vitality of the traditional values (the Protestant ethic, essentially) has declined. Surveys of Americans and their values and lifestyles indicate that Americans, particularly middle-class Americans, are a very heterogeneous group today. There is no one overarching core value orientation today like there was in the 1960s and 1970s. Koten (1987) of the *Wall Street Journal* agrees that there is no longer one set of values to which the

middle class subscribes. "There are fewer things that everybody wants and fewer things that everyone feels compelled to do" (p. 25).

Shifting values have fueled institutional changes throughout society. Both Family Service America (1984) and Scanzoni (1987) describe surveys in which Americans, according to the values they reported, were divided into three groups. At one end of the continuum were the "traditionalists," those who espoused traditional values, such as preserving the good old days, duty, obligation, and hard work. At the other end of the continuum were the "new wave," the "progressives," those espousing emerging values of self-fulfillment, freedom, and individualism over authority. The middle-of-the-continuum group was composed of the vast majority of Americans. They valued some of the old and some of the new values and goals. Scanzoni (1987) reports that in one national survey 20 percent were traditionalists and another 20 percent new wavers or progressives, while 60 percent were middle-of-the-roaders. Most sociologists explain that our values are in a state of flux or transition. The increasing proportion of families that are either single-parent, blended, or cohabiting families, coupled with the widespread practice of divorce, lends evidence to the shifting from traditional, conventional values to individualistic, utilitarian values (Glick, 1989).

Despite the continual clash between the new and traditional values and the resultant modification in values and priorities, a substantial amount of continuity in the American value system has, however, prevailed.

A discussion of American society's core value orientation, coupled with the recent value shifts, provides the foundations for understanding our primary family values today. Some of these values are of lesser importance today and some are of greater importance. A discussion of this shift in priorities follows.

▶ MAJOR VALUE ORIENTATIONS

In spite of the declining state of the secularized Protestant ethic and the existence of other strongly conflicting values, a cluster of core values still molds and shapes, to a varying degree, American society, and thus also shapes family life and the behavior of health care professionals. (See Table 13–1 for a listing of America's core values.)

> ## TABLE 13–1

AMERICA'S CORE VALUES

- Productivity/Individual achievement
- Individualism
- Materialism/The consumption ethic
- The work ethic
- Education
- Equality
- Progress and mastery over the environment
- Future time orientation
- Efficiency, orderliness, and practicality
- Rationality
- Quality of life and maintaining health
- The "doing" orientation
- Tolerance of diversity

Productivity/Individual Achievement

Individual achievement and productivity have been consistently identified as key traditional values in this society (D'Antonio, 1983; McKinley, 1964; Williams, 1960). Success and achievement, the reputed outcomes of being productive, are corollary social values (Stewart & Bennett, 1991). In the middle class, extensive stress is placed on personal achievement, especially occupational achievement.

Because so much apprehension surrounds choice of occupational goals, there is an anxious postponement in selecting one's career. Many Americans also have not learned how to relax and enjoy life, as seen by their anxious preoccupation with activity and productiveness and the enormous numbers of people suffering from stress-related illnesses. Another behavioral consequence of our achievement value is its effects on individuals who do not have the required position and role adequacy for productiveness. For those people, the emphasis on achievement often leads to a lack of goals and/or to alienation.

In order for a value to continue to mold a person's goals and behavior, a powerful system of social sanctions and rewards must be present. According to McKinley (1964), there are four major rewards available to the "successful," which are referred to as the "American Dream": material possessions, interpersonal approval and status, control over others, and control over self (autonomy).

Various types of interpersonal sanctions are employed against those individuals who are "unproductive," including the unemployed, those on welfare, or those who choose values markedly different from society's values. These responses range from gossip, laughter, and ridicule to social ostracism, isolation, or rejection. Members of society will vary their reactions depending on the society's evaluations of where the responsibility for unproductiveness lies and how important the deviation is. As a result of society's disapproval, many times the individual adopts those same attitudes toward himself or herself (i.e., low self-esteem, lack of self-worth), a phenomenon referred to as "the self-fulfilling prophecy."

Individualism

In the numerous writings about value changes in American society and the family, there is agreement about the rising importance of individualism today (Bellah et al., 1986; Glick, 1989; Orthner, 1995; Schwartz, 1987). Individual freedom of choice is one of our central social values in Western societies according to Lesthaeghe (1983). The trend toward more individualism and independence and away from familism and collectivism has weakened but not killed the ideal of permanence in marriage.

Part of individualism and individual freedom of choice is the shift from a child-centered to a self-centered culture (Elkind, 1994). This transformation means that people are becoming less firmly rooted in the traditional institutions of family, community, and church and more committed to individual goal attainment—unfettered by traditional obligations (Orthner, 1995; Rossi, 1986). Other authors, based on demographic trends, also emphasize that people in Western societies are becoming "averse to long-term commitments and increasingly focused on individual autonomy and detachment" (Rossi, 1986, p. 123). Lasch in the *Culture of Narcissism* (1979) talks similarly about the emphasis on personal autonomy and self-centered narcissism. Some authors (Elkind, 1994; Popenoe, 1995) believe that for the good of society, the family, and the individual, the individualistic trend has gone too far. Until recently there has been a balance between helping community and family (collectivism) and helping oneself. This balance has become lopsided as individuals become more focused on their own pursuits.

Individualism is the reverse of the traditional Catholic doctrine of the ethic of reciprocity in which "you are your brother's keeper," or of familism (where family needs take precedence over family members' needs). Individualism suggests that every person has to make it on his or her own merits. A large survey conducted by Bellah and associates (1986) confirmed the centrality of personal autonomy and individualism in the United States.

Individualism also involves the associated values of self-reliance and self-responsibility. The prevalent belief remains that "strong" persons can control their own lives and that lack of such control is evidence of their own weakness. Self-fulfillment is another value closely associated with individualism.

Many ethnic families do not share this same value of individualism (Sillars, 1995). These families have a familistic orientation, whereby there is much sharing and interdependency between extended family members. In highly familistic cultures, an individual's identity and place in society may be defined more by family than by individual achievement (Sillars, 1995).

Materialism/The Consumption Ethic

The possession of money and goods is not only an essential reward for being productive, but is also a central value of society in and of itself. This value is referred to as materialism (Stewart & Bennett, 1991). Materialism declined somewhat in the 1960s, but is again on the rise. Samuelson (1986) writes about "the discovery of money" and society's increasing preoccupation with wealth as a measure of achievement. Money and wealth are both the foundation for power and prestige and the primary symbol of success and achievement. Money has been consecrated as a value over and above its use in procuring goods and services or for its enhancement of power. Society, through its major institutions, reinforces this cultural emphasis except perhaps among the lower class. These institutions join to provide the disciplining and training required for an individual to retain this elusive goal and be properly motivated by the promise of gratification.

Along with materialism has come a relaxation of prohibitions against expressiveness and hedonism (Orthner, 1995). In a society in which the consumption of goods has become a fundamental value, people are enjoined to cease being ascetic and self-denying and to abandon guilt about spending and expressing their pleasure impulses.

The moral values of thriftiness and saving were parts of the Protestant ethic. As with other traditional values, their importance arose partly from the short supply of material goods and money that existed in the past. In fact, often the ability to save and conserve was critical to survival.

In more recent times Americans seem to have entirely disregarded these values (except perhaps by members of the older generation) as evidenced by our wasteful habits of acquiring vast goods and constantly replacing material items. Toffler (1970) calls this "planned obsolescence." We have acted as if there were a limitless supply of goods and resources. This consumption ethic has now largely replaced the thrift ethic, and the "put-away" society has become the "throw-away" society (Inkeles, 1977).

We may now be seeing a modest swing back to "conservation" goals, however. There is a noticeable attitudinal change among some Americans that our habits of waste and enormous consumption of the world's resources must be altered. More concern is voiced about ecology, dwindling resources, and environmental impact (Harris, 1984). In spite of these encouraging signs, however, Americans continue to consume goods and resources at increasingly high levels.

The Work Ethic

The rule of "He who does not work should not eat" expressed the deadly struggle of the early settlement and frontier days and explains the primacy of this ethic as due to the objective conditions of want that existed historically. As part of Puritanism and the Protestant ethic, however, work literally became an end in itself not the means to an end. Americans were obsessive about work, and even today we meet individuals who are "workaholics." Although the work ethic has lost much of its potency today, it is still part of our dominant culture and upheld by our societal institutions (Stewart & Bennett, 1991). The success of modern industrial states remains dependent on work-oriented individuals.

According to Inkeles (1977) and Glick (1989), in the 1960s and 1970s the ethic of hard work was fast eroding. Increasing numbers of Americans during that period considered the most important attributes of a job to be high pay and short hours, not the intrinsic importance or a promise of advancement. Yet Yankelovich and Gurin (1989), surveyors of American values, noted a change in this trend in the 1980s. They observed many Americans returning to the workplace as a site for self-expression of competence, creativity, and satisfaction. A resurgence in entrepreneurship accompanies the resurgence of the work ethic. The scarcity of work and jobs has certainly augmented the return of the work ethic. Even if work is not the central overriding value today that it was in the past, it would be premature to prepare for a demise of the ethic of work.

Education

Education is seen by the middle class as the means by which to achieve productivity and to "get ahead." The value placed on education is closely aligned with the work ethic, materialism, individualism, and progress. Although education is much more emphasized among the middle and upper classes, its value has also become more prominent within the working class (Inkeles, 1977) and many immigrant families.

Equality

The value of equality has become more important in American society (Stewart & Bennett, 1991), although it is only a partially realized value.

The dominant culture values equality in personal relationships much more than many other cultures. Antiauthoritarianism is also still a very important characteristic of present-day American society. Flacks (1971) found that children were dissatisfied about the use of arbitrary or coercive power, feelings that are derived from the family values favoring a power structure based on egalitarianism, as well as expectations resulting from parental fostering of participation, independence, and autonomy.

On the other hand, a strong hierarchical and authoritarian emphasis exists in large-scale organizations. Individual achievement and status are more valued than equality. And running through the whole of our society is the thread of nonequalitarian beliefs and practices concerning interpersonal relations with people of different ethnic groupings and women, recurring manifestations of prejudice and bigotry.

Smelzer and Halpern (1978) clearly point out the clash between individualism/individual achievement and equality. If the priority in the society is on individual achievement, this produces greater inequality and a call for equality. Prioritizing equality generates a counterreaction as well. The fact that these values are inherently "at odds with each other" is not so surprising—what is, however, is the oscillations that have occurred in recent times concerning the saliency of these two competing values or cultural themes (Smelzer & Halpern, 1978). During the 1960s and early 1970s, equality, as seen in the liberal ideas and programs of the "Great Society," the Peace Corps, and affirmative action and civil rights programs, was prioritized. Beginning in the late 1970s, the pendulum swung back again—with a dismantlement of programs that fostered the value of equality, and a return to the more conservative values of achievement and individualism. A return to more conservative values of achievement and individualism can be seen in the recent legislative fights over affirmative action and welfare reform.

In spite of the resurgence of conservativism, individualism, and achievement values, equality still is recognized as a central cultural value. The importance of equality is closely linked with an increasing tolerance of diversity and the growing tendency to pursue individualistic personal goals, where freedom, independence, and autonomy, as well as greater expression of feelings, are paramount.

The rise of egalitarianism is reflected in American family life. According to Toynbee (1955), the noted historian, the most vital revolution of our time has been the emancipation of women, because women's emancipation affects family life, moving marital relationships closer to equality. In addition to the women's movement and the affirmative action programs, there has been considerable progress in protecting the rights of the mentally ill and of children. These legislative trends demonstrate the continued potency of equality as a value.

In the health care field, the value and commitment to equality is seen in the recurring concerns about equal access to health care for all (universal coverage). This value, though, runs into competition with the value of individual freedom of choice. As health care reforms occur, the fight between these two often opposing values becomes evident. We are likely to see many experiments involving managed care and extending access (Pew Health Professions Commission, 1991).

Progress and Mastery Over the Environment

Kluckholm (1976) refers to this value orientation as involving the "man–nature relationship issue"— whether human beings are viewed as subjugated to nature, as part of nature, or as lord over nature. Traditional Spanish-American culture in the American Southwest illustrates the first relationship. To the rural, traditional rancher in the Southwest in the past, there was little or nothing that could be done if a storm damaged range lands or disease destroyed flocks. He or she simply accepted these events as inevitable. This fatalistic attitude may also be found in dealing with illness and death in a statement such as, "if it is the Lord's will that I die, I shall die" (p. 69). The second relationship, in which humans and nature are viewed as aspects of a harmonious whole, is found in many of the North American Indian tribes and traditional Chinese cultures. The dominant American culture, however, views the man–nature relationship in the third way—that of humans against, or over, nature (Stewart & Bennett, 1991). Natural forces are seen as things to be overcome, mastered, and utilized by people. We build bridges, blast through mountains, create lakes and massive dams, and exploit all of nature's resources—all to serve humankind (Kluckholm, 1976).

It is this general attitude of being able to problem solve and overcome seemingly impossible obstacles that is referred to as progressiveness. Change is seen as progress or going forward (Stewart & Bennett, 1991), even though it sometimes seems that the pendulum swings backward. Innovativeness and openness to new experiences is highly valued, as is an optimism or the confidence that striving and change are positive (Inkeles, 1977).

Future Time Orientation

Obviously all societies must deal with three time dimensions—past, present, and future. All cultures have some conception of the past, all have a present, and all give attention to the future time dimension. They vary, however, in the emphasis they place on each dimension. The time orientation in the United States is toward the discernible future (Stewart & Bennett, 1991). For example, Kluckholm (1976) and Murillo (1976) report that in contrast to Americans, unacculturated Mexican-Americans are more present oriented. Historically, China and Japan, on the other hand, were societies that put their main emphasis on the past. Ancestor worship and strong family traditions were both expressions of this time orientation. Many modern European countries, such as England, have also tended to stress the past more than America.

Most middle-class Americans, regardless of ethnic heritage, place their emphasis on the future (Tripp-Reimer & Lively, 1988), which we anticipate optimistically will be "bigger and better." Past ways are considered "old fashioned." The value put on the future correlates closely with the value on change and progress. A Frenchman, Servan-Schreiber, wrote, "We Europeans continue to suffer progress while Americans pursue it, welcome it and adapt to it" (Inkeles, 1977, p. 1).

Efficiency, Orderliness, and Practicality

In frontier society, being practical—learning to improvise and make the best out of one's resources—was tied up with survival. Individuals and families concentrated on obtainable goals in the immediate situation—"If it works, it must be good." Today, this same kind of pragmatism views technical advances with great appreciation, especially those resulting in savings of time and manpower—after all, "time is money."

Science is highly valued as an endeavor through which efficiency, practicality, and progress can be achieved. The way we treat food and the manner in which we consume it are expressions of values we hold. Seventy percent of households today have microwave ovens and 40 percent have personal computers. We have a strong faith in the efficacy of technology.

Rationality

Rationality and reason are highly valued in our society (Herberg, 1995). In order to be efficient, orderly, progressive, productive, and practical, one must be rational and able to react by problem solving and by logically thinking through one's situation and goals. Foresight, deliberate planning, allocation of resources in the most efficient way, and long-term gratification is necessary. Rationality became a prime value during the Enlightenment in the late 1700s and early 1800s. Science was a natural outgrowth of this rational philosophy, because it depends on the same logical cognitive approach to the world and its problems. Applied science is highly esteemed in the dominant culture as a tool for controlling nature and the environment.

This value has led to the "rational scientific man" becoming the exemplar of our society. Women, in contrast, have historically been stereotyped with the opposite of these desirable attributes; women have been deemed irrational, illogical, emotional, and intuitive, albeit this stereotyping is diminishing as women move into cognitively challenging fields and succeed admirably.

Quality of Life and Maintaining Health

People today are becoming increasingly interested in making qualitative changes in their lives. These include such lifestyle improvements among adults as curtailing smoking, making dietary changes, and partaking in self-help stress reduction and other mental health programs*; people are also making environmental alterations such as moving from city and suburbia to small towns and rural environments, and participating in creative and leisure endeavors. All these signify a basic modification of values to a more introspective orientation where personal and familial happiness and personal independence in decision making have greater priority. While it is difficult to measure how highly health is valued and how widespread this shift is, available evidence suggests that maintaining health is becoming a major value within the American hierarchy of values (Harris 1984; Yankelovich & Gurin, 1989). This is especially true when it comes to valuing public health mea-

---

* Since 1975 U.S. mortality figures have shown significant decreases in cardiovascular deaths. This has been largely attributed to a decrease in smoking among those at risk for heart disease (U.S. Department of Health & Human Services, 1993).

sures, such as immunizations and clean, safe water supplies (Stewart & Bennett, 1991). The importance of this value is probably influenced not only by social class, but also by age and ethnicity.

The "Doing" Orientation

Kluckholm (1976) refers to the normative interpersonal behavior valued in American society, or its national character, as being exemplified in the "doing orientation." Its most distinctive feature is its demand for action in terms of accomplishment and in accord with external (societal) standards. The person who "gets things done" is seen as productive. The person who finds ways to do something and is the rational problem solver is much esteemed. Along with "doing" is a dominant value of keeping busy. "Idle hands are the devil's workshop" (Stewart & Bennett, 1991).

Tolerance of Diversity

Although it may be stretching it to be including this value in the central values of Americans, it has been included because of the notable change toward greater tolerance in recent years for diversity in many areas of community life—such increased acceptance for various forms of family, for cohabitation of couples before marriage, and of ethnic peoples and women. Perhaps due to the civil rights and antiwar movements of the 1960s and/or because of the increasing number of minorities in the United States, a greater tolerance of diversity has been noted (Boulding, 1976; Koten, 1987).

Weaver (1976) states that the major and most significant result of the women's movement and growing ethnic consciousness has been the growth of popular questioning of cultural assumptions held by Americans for generations, such as the myth of the melting pot. "Rather than having values of a subcultural group dissipated and absorbed by the dominant culture, these two groups have undermined the values and assumptions of the dominant culture" (p. 123).

Movement away from the value of increased tolerance is also seen. A major backlash is occurring in America today, fueled by a sizeable number of persons who espouse intolerance for diversity and alarm the public about the menace of immigration, welfare and affirmative action programs, and abortion rights.

► FAMILY VALUES

The family's value system is thought to be heavily influenced by the society's core values, as well as by the values of the family's subcultural and other reference groups. Family changes in values and norms are very much connected to and rooted in fundamental shifts in the values and norms in North American society (Orthner, 1995).

Basic family values embedded in our culture have not changed dramatically, according to Orthner (1995), but our family norms and rules guiding family behavior have. Norms are guidelines for behavior and both norms and family rules, particularly those associated with family roles, have been relaxed or lost over the past several decades. Norms related to sexual behavior and marriage, as well as those linking marriage and pregnancy have also changed. Today, with traditional family roles changing, most men and women are uncertain of what is expected of them in their family roles (Orthner, 1995).

David Elkind (1994), a renowned child psychologist, gives a more gloomy view about the shift in values and norms in the American family than does Orthner (1995), a sociologist. In Elkind's analysis of how the family has been impacted by societal changes, he sees that an imbalance in family values has taken place—as society emphasizes the importance of individualism and individual achievement (as seen in descriptions of recent generations being the "me generation"). In this permeable family each family member (as soon is he or she is able) is supposed to be "independent, competent, achievement-oriented and able to go it alone" (Elkind, 1994, p. 75).

Elkind calls the postmodern family of today the "permeable family," a family that is more open, more fluid, more flexible, more vulnerable to outside pressures, and not as protective of children. Although parents in permeable families have more personal freedom and lifestyle choices to pursue their own individual interests, children suffer. Hence, there is an imbalance in values, favoring individualism over family togetherness and familism. The postmodern family is individual-centered, not child-centered. Elkind (1994) points to the change in family forms as evidence of the widespread permeable family. Single-parent families are the fastest growing family structure in American in the 1990s, with more parents choosing divorce or opting not to marry when pregnancy occurs. We are also seeing a growth in blended families.

Nevertheless, because families have their own special functions within the larger societal context, they also subscribe to their own combination of certain values—which guide family life.

Families create their own family miniculture or family paradigm—an enduring structure of shared beliefs, convictions, and assumptions about the social world (Reiss, 1981; Fitzpatrick & Ritchie, 1993). These shared beliefs are largely based on the family's past experiences. Families develop their own paradigm as an extension of how they deal with hardships and crisis. Family belief systems can have a more internal locus of control (mastery over nature) or external locus of control (situations are governed by external factors beyond the family's control) (Rolland, 1988, 1993).

A family's value and belief system shapes its patterns of behavior toward health problems families face. Family values and beliefs shape the views families have of stressors and how they should respond to stressors. In other words, family beliefs and values determine how a family will cope with health and other stressors.

"A family's beliefs about mastery strongly affect the nature of its relationship to an illness and to the health care system" (Rolland, 1993, p. 464). A family with a mastery orientation may believe it can control and solve almost every problem it faces. In this case the family would use more active, assertive coping strategies, like seeking out new information or community resources to resolve or control the problem. Conversely, a family less oriented toward mastery and control and more oriented toward passive acceptance may believe in accepting whatever happens. They may cope by resigning themselves to God's will. Often such families view disease progression and outcomes as a matter of chance and tend to establish marginal relationships with health professionals (Rolland, 1988). These families are often called "fatalistic" (Boss, 1988). Fatalism needs to be distinguished from acceptance according to Boss (1988). Fatalism is the belief that everything is predetermined by a higher power or "powerful others." The family feels powerless to change what is preordained to happen. Families that are fatalistic are those that because of their cultural, socioeconomic, and environmental conditioning, feel a sense of powerlessness to change the course of events.

In situations that are hopeless, with loss inevitable and control impossible, the mastery-oriented and fatalistically oriented families typically behave quite differently. The mastery-oriented family will be less likely to give up hope, even with terminal illness, but will experience much more stress than the fatalistically oriented family, which will passively accept the situation.

▶ MAJOR VARIABLES AFFECTING FAMILY VALUES

There are several important variables or factors that greatly influence whether a family assimilates the "major value orientation" of American society, or whether differences in priorities and values or divergent norms operate. Two important variables are the family's social class and ethnicity, both of which are discussed in Chapter 8. Other important variables include a family's degree of acculturation to the dominant culture; generational differences, geographical location, and familial and personal idiosyncrasies.

Family's Socioeconomic Status

Because a family's socioeconomic status shapes the family lifestyle, it also is a powerful shaper of family values. The dominant American core values are in large part middle-class values. Poor families may share American dominant values such as productivity and work, but be unable to achieve what they value because of their limited resources (the difference between the ideal and the real as previously mentioned).

Relative to the time dimension, poor families are likely to be more present-time oriented than the middle class. Among some poor families, for example, time and appointments are perceived as "flexible"; that is, events will start when everyone involved arrives. Middle-class families, in comparison, hold the dominant time value. They are typically future oriented and are therefore likely to save and plan for the future (Giger & Davidhizar, 1995).

Family's Ethnicity and Acculturation

Ethnic background makes a major difference in how important each of the core American values are to a family. For instance, Irish-American families place a high value on independence. Irish culture is replete with many sayings that illustrate the importance of this value. "You've made your bed, now lie in it" tells a married family member not to bring his or her problems home to the parent. In contrast, the Italian-American family could hardly imagine this being uttered (Foley, 1986, p. 191). Table 13–2 provides a description of core values of several ethnic groups.

A family's degree of acculturation to dominant cultural values also varies widely. The more acculturated the family members, the more they subscribe to modern American core values.

▶ TABLE 13–2

CORE VALUES OF SELECTED CULTURALLY DIVERSE, TRADITIONALLY ORIENTED FAMILIES

- *Irish-Americans:* Independence, strong religious orientation, highly verbal, humor, sociability.
- *American Indian:* Living in harmony with nature; spiritual inspiration; folk healing; respect for elders, authority, and children; collectivism (family and tribe); ethnic pride.
- *Italian-American:* Familism, traditional male–female roles, loyalty through personal relationships.
- *Jewish Americans:* Valuing of education, success, family, and community connections; encouragement of children; democratic principles; highly verbal.
- *African-Americans:* Informal kinship network (more collectivistic); flexibility in family roles; strong religious orientation; commitment to education; commitment to self-help, service to others.
- *Asian-Americans:* Respect for elders; familism; harmony and interdependence in relationships; filial piety; saving face, ancestor worship.
- *Asian Indians:* Purity, sacrifice, passivity, spirituality.
- *Hispanic-Americans:* Familism, respect for authority and elders, strong religious orientation, people valued for their character rather than their success, traditional male–female roles, more present-oriented.

Sources: Billingley (1992), Harrison et al. (1994), Herberg (1995), Ho (1992), McGoldrick (1993, 1996), Stauffer (1995).

Geographical Location (Urban, Suburban, or Rural)

Whether a family resides (or has resided for a long period of time) in a rural, urban, or suburban community also plays a significant role in shaping their values. In terms of country versus city residence, rural dwellers tend to be more traditional and conservative than their urban or suburban counterparts. Suburban communities are primarily residential and middle class, and usually espouse more middle-class urban cultural values. In contrast, urban, inner-city populations are diverse, generally containing families from the whole social class spectrum, as well as families from various ethnic and racial groups; thus urban families usually show a greater diversity of values, although generally tending to hold more liberal social and political views.

Generational Differences

Another variable influencing the values and norms of a family is the generation(s) of its members. There are "generational" value systems in the United States. Most core values are instilled at a early age by parents (Lustig, 1988). Yet, core values are also altered by society's value shifts. For instance, certain values were predominant when persons were in their early adulthood years in the 1950s. These individuals are now most likely in the phase of retirement/aging or the contracting family phase, and they retain many of their traditional work-oriented Protestant ethic values (values that have more potency in their lives than for younger adults today). McLeod and Cooper (1996) and Slater (1970) illustrate the drastic differences in values when they compare the value of the "youth generation," the "me generation," and "generation X" with the old values of the dominant (adult) culture.

▶ VALUE CONFLICTS

Diverse Social Values

Because there are so many factors which serve to alter an individual's or a family's values and norms, conflicts inevitably exist. Issues or unresolved conflicts are present because traditional and emerging sets of norms exist simultaneously, both within and outside of the family. Within communities certain groups and individuals resist emerging norms and cling vehemently to more traditional patterns, whereas other individuals and groups find traditional patterns unacceptable and adhere to new set of norms and values. The result of this social change is that areas of major conflict arise. Although our society values its pluralism, where both traditional and emerging value systems and patterns can exist side by side, this social diversity played out in the family results in conflict and confusion. A very common family value issue is that concerning the meaning of marriage. Whereas traditionally marriage was viewed as sacred and binding, today among those espousing emerging social values, marriage is increasingly viewed as a contract to be voided when either or both parties have legitimate grievances (Eshleman, 1974; Scanzoni, 1987).

Clash of Values Between Dominant Culture and Subculture

Another common source of value conflict is a clash between the values of the dominant culture and a family's cultural reference group. When we consider the family as the mediating agent between the culture (or the wider society) and the individual, it follows that a basic incompatibility in values between the family's reference group and wider society generates certain value conflicts, which increase stress within the family as a system and also negatively affect family members. Larrabee (1973), a Cheyenne Indian, describes this clash of values and one of its effects:

> In trying to teach our young about themselves, we must tell them about the Indian values of compassion, respect for elders, sharing, and wisdom. We want our children to have these values and to know about them. When our children go to school and are told by the teacher that they must learn to be saving instead of sharing, the child becomes confused. This terrible conflict of values contributes to the high suicide rate among our youth.

The same observations about a clash in values is found in the literature about Asian-American families. The clash in values between Asian-American parents who retain their traditional values and their children (particularly adolescents) who take on the American values of independence, individualism, and assertiveness is a commonly cited problem brought to counseling (Hong, 1996; Pedersen et al., 1996).

The findings of Cleveland and Longaker (1972) confirm the disruptive effects value conflicts have on the ethnic family. Based on extensive data collected from interviews, home visits, testing, and therapeutic sessions, they concluded that the emotional problems in family members studied were a function of two processes: (1) a value conflict between the society the family resided in and the family, and (2) a culturally recurrent mode of self-disparagement linked to the failure of individuals to adjust to incompatible value orientations.

Clash of Values Between Generations

A third source of value conflict within families lies in generational differences in values, as mentioned previously. A family may be composed of several generations of individuals, each bringing to the family group his or her generationally based values. When the grandparents hold traditional values, the parents a combination of traditional and emerging (progressive) values, and the children emerging values, value conflicts are inevitable, especially if the family household is an extended family or a family with adolescents. This generational clash of values is magnified among first generation immigrant families from non-Western countries (Hong & Ham, 1992).

FAMILY VALUES: APPLYING THE FAMILY NURSING PROCESS

► assessment questions

An understanding of the prevailing value system of American society and how societal values affect the family, as well as an understanding of some of the variables influencing family values, provide the foundation for assessing family values. We should use this foundational information discretely, however. Studies and descriptions address *group* tendencies not particular families and individuals. Therefore, our assessments must be individualized, recognizing the unique family values and norms of the families we care for. Assessing specific values to which a family adheres and the generational, cultural, and developmental value differences among family members will lead to detection of intrafamilial value conflicts.

Assessment of a family's values is very helpful in motivating a family to take preventive or restorative health action or to make health decisions. Elkins (1984) reminds us that the basis for motivation is derived from a family's value system—what is important and unimportant to it and how important different values are. Although health for its own sake may not be a high value in a family's list of priorities, helping the family see that other very important values will be adversely affected if health actions are not taken (such as a parent not being able to work) may be a way of motivating a family. Elkins (1984) explains this motivational strategy:

> A client's value system can serve as a guide in choosing positive reinforcers for client progress toward goals. The client must believe that the behavior change will result in something of greater value to him—a good return on his investment. The nurse can help the client see the results. Any behavior change requires an investment of self, time, and possibly money, all of which are high on the value scales of most people. In reinforcing newly acquired behavior, the community health nurse, by understanding the client's values, can direct the intrinsic and extrinsic rewards so that the client perceives them as being more valuable than the old behavior patterns. (p. 279)

Values cannot be seen directly, but must be inferred from observations and assessment of family structure, functions, and coping because these dimensions are strongly influenced by the underlying values held by family members. When family values and beliefs are identified, this information will help the family nurse to better understand the reasons for family behavioral patterns.

One way of simplifying the assessment of family values is for nursing students to make use of a "contrast and compare" method. This involves comparing and contrasting a specific family's values with those of the dominant American culture. This enables the assessor to identify various areas that need assessment and to appraise how much conformity or disparity in values exists between the dominant culture and the family under consideration. If an assessor is familiar with the values and norms of a specific ethnic group, then this same comparison process could be applied, using the family's cultural reference group as a basis for comparison (see the assessment areas listed in Table 13–3).

To illustrate the "compare-and-contrast" process more concretely, it is suggested that a list of central values be utilized as a guide for this assessment. Using a list of central values of the dominant culture or of the family's subcultural reference group on one side of the assessment form identify the family's values on the other side. The assessor can then discuss a family's particular values in each of these areas. This listing should help in identifying the specific values to which the family adheres.

▶ TABLE 13–3

ASSESSMENT OF FAMILY VALUES, PRIORITIES, AND VALUE CONGRUENCE WITH REFERENCE GROUP AND/OR WIDER COMMUNITY

1. Identify family's and individual family members' values and beliefs. Are there any significant value differences and clashes between family members?
2. Estimate how important particular key values are to the family and/or individuals within the family.
3. Estimate the extent of compliance and rewards a family is receiving from its reference group and society in general. (Lack of compliance and rewards will be present if there is moderate or marked value disparity, as well as stigmatization of the family by the community.)

American Societal Values

1. Productivity/achievement
2. Work ethic
3. Materialism
4. Individualism
5. Education
6. Consumption ethic
7. Progress and mastery over environment
8. Future time orientation
9. Efficiency, orderliness, and practicality
10. Rationality
11. Democracy, equality, and freedom
12. "Doing orientation"
13. Patriarchal authority
14. Family's interests
15. Family as a haven
16. Health

The Family's Values

Following this listing, the following questions should be addressed:

- Is there congruence between the family's values and the family's reference group and/or interacting systems like the educational and the health care systems and the wider community?

- Is there congruence between the family's values and each family member's values?

- How important are the identified values to the family? (Rank order the family values.)

- Are the values consciously or unconsciously held?

- Are there any value conflicts evident within the family?

- How do the family's social class, cultural background and degree of acculturation, generational differences, and geographical setting (rural, urban, suburban) influence the family's values?

- How do the family's values affect the health status of the family?

▶ FAMILY NURSING DIAGNOSES

Family nursing diagnoses in the area of values are not seen so commonly. This is because family value problems are generally considered to be underlying causes (related factors) of other problem areas that are more behaviorally oriented.

The one family nursing diagnoses that has been identified is "value conflicts." If a value conflict diagnosis is made, then the system in which the problem resides (between "whom") must be specified—such as, "value conflict between grandparents and grandson" —and defining characteristics and related factors

included. Value conflicts are often seen as a contributory factor to family problems in the other structural dimensions (communication, power, and roles) or in the functional areas (affective, socialization, and health care) or in coping.

▶ FAMILY NURSING INTERVENTIONS

Knowledge about family values is important data for the nurse to have in order to establish realistic goals and intervention strategies with the family (Elkins,

1984). In addition, understanding the relationship of the family's values to the values of community agencies will help the nurse suggest more value-appropriate community resources when making a referral.

In the nursing literature only one intervention strategy is specifically discussed in the area of values—that is, value clarification. The family nursing interventions described under role conflict (see Chap. 12) and communication conflicts (Chap. 10), however, with slight modification should also be appropriate for value conflict problems.

Value Clarification

Value clarification is a technique or process used to increase a family's awareness of value priorities as well as the degree of congruency between family member values, attitudes, and behavior. Because values are a basis for decision making and coping, helping families reaffirm their existing values, clarify their values, or reprioritize their values will help them become more autonomous and responsible for their own health (Wilberding, 1985).

In addition to moralizing (telling a person, usually a child, what is right and wrong) and role modeling, the value clarification process assists both children and adults to think critically about their values and undertake the process of valuing (Raths et al., 1978). Value clarification, Kirschenbaum (1977) explains, is an approach that uses questions and activities designed to teach the valuing process. These exercises help people to apply the valuing processes to value-rich areas of their lives. Once values become clearer, it is easier to see dissonance between values and behavior; if an individual values health, the dissonance should be reduced by changing his or her health-related behaviors.

A perplexing issue occurs when value clarification is used and the client's values differ greatly from the nurse's values. Is the nurse able to accept differing values without resorting to moralizing? This is an ethical question that must be addressed before undertaking value clarification. According to Wilberding (1985), the ultimate issue is whether the family nurse can accept the client as being an autonomous self-care agent.

There are numerous value clarification tools mentioned in the literature. Pender (1987) has developed and adapted tools and exercises to help individuals and families clarify their values. Pender believes that the nurse interested in health promotion should assist clients with value clarification and value changes. She explains that

- Value clarification involves increasing personal or group awareness of value priorities and the degree of consistency among values, attitudes, and behavior.
- Value change addresses the reprioritization of values, abandonment of existing values, or acquisition of new values and subsequent attitudes and behavior change.

Assisting family members with value changes is an intervention discussed in rehabilitation nursing. Disabled persons and their families need to reprioritize their values when certain values are no longer possible to operationalize. This process is a crucial one for a disabled client and family to accomplish in adapting to the disability in a functional manner.

Pender (1987) adds one caveat about the use of value clarification. She states that value clarification should be used cautiously with individuals who have emotional problems or with families who are markedly dysfunctional.

Cross-cultural Counseling Approaches

In working with families of various ethnic backgrounds, counseling approaches need to be adapted to make the counseling interventions more culturally relevant and, thus, effective. To vary one's counseling approaches, an understanding of the family's values is essential. For instance, in the traditionally oriented family from a culture that is familistic, counseling should be directed more toward relationships of the collective (the extended family). In collectivistic environments, the paramount concern is the promotion and maintenance of intrafamily and interpersonal harmony and being able to fit into the group (Gudykunst, 1991). For families who are individualistic in their value orientation, counseling could be concentrated more on the individual family members. A basic goal in this case might be to assist family members with their own issues and concerns to raise their self-esteem or self-growth (Draguns, 1996). When dealing with family issues, expression of the individual family members' perceptions and feelings could be sought, while this may not be appropriate in a hierarchical family structure where the father is the head of the family.

Another example of instances in which counseling may need to be adapted to be more culturally appropriate is in the area of the time dimension. Anglo-Americans value punctuality or "being on time," and have the attitude that "time is money" and hence, should not be wasted. In traditional families from present-oriented cultures, time does not have the same meaning or significance. "Things happen when I get there" may be the attitude, causing clients to show up for appointments on the right day, but not at the right time.

▶ study questions

Choose all correct answers to the following questions.

1. It is true that:
   a. Values are defined as a system of ideas and beliefs that bind families together.
   b. Values serve as general guides to behavior.
   c. The family is the basic transmitter of values.
   d. Values are relatively fixed and change very little over time.
   e. All values have the same or similar weight as far as their influence and centrality in a person's life are concerned.

2. The best definition of norms is:
   a. Patterns of personal behaviors.
   b. Patterns of behavior considered "right" in a given society.
   c. Role behaviors or expectations associated with family positions.
   d. Clustering of attitudes and beliefs.

3. Family rules are related to family values in which of the following ways?
   a. Family rules generate family values.
   b. Family rules are specific manifestations of family values.
   c. Family rules and family values are distinct concepts and have no overlapping meaning.

4. List and briefly explain four major, recent value changes that have occurred in society and within families. *Individualism, workethic, tolerance/diversity equality, consumerism, health/quality of life*

5. Individualism is criticized for "going too far." Identify which of the following choice(s) reflect(s) critics' concerns regarding the impact of this trend on the family:
   a. Individualism encourages excessive concern with achievement.
   b. Familism is impacted negatively.
   c. An imbalance is created between individualism and family togetherness.
   d. Child-centeredness has decreased with growth in individualism.

6. Value clarification is a process that helps people to (choose the one correct answer):
   a. Identify their values.
   b. Change their values.
   c. See the difference between their values and family rules.
   d. Question the rights and wrongs about their values.

7. Many ethnic families do not share the same value of individualism that mainstream Americans do (answer *true* or *false*).

8. Several values cluster together, comprising the central configuration of values in the dominant culture. List six values.

Productivity – materialism, individualism, workethic, progress, education

9. Four variables that influence the family's value system are described. List these. *Social class – Rural – urban – Values – family life, generational differences*

ethnicity –

Choose the correct answers to the following questions.

10. Which of the following are sources of value conflicts?
    a. Generational differences
    b. Social class differences
    c. Acculturation differences
    d. Idiosyncratic (personal) differences

11. One of the concepts germane to social class is that when a family and its reference group do not subscribe to the central core values of a society (select all correct answers):
    a. The adjustment to wider society is relatively easy.
    b. The family is able to gain compliance from society.
    c. The more difficult the family adjustment to community life becomes.
    d. The family experiences social stigma.

► family case study—the Gardiners*

After reading the family case study, answer the questions that follow.

The Gardiner family members are Harry, age 37; May, 28; Len, 11; Joanie, 7; and Ann, 3. This African-American family came to the attention of the public health nurse working in a pediatric outpatient clinic when appointments arranged for Len at the diabetes and urology clinics were repeatedly not kept. Although appointments to the diabetes clinic were kept occasionally, no urology visit was made, and the chart showed that the mother at one time had reported continual bedwetting.

Len was originally diagnosed as having juvenile diabetes when he was hospitalized at age 6. After the child was diagnosed and stabilized, the family was

---

* Family case study adapted from Sobel and Robischon (1975).

counseled as to treatment regimen. Subsequent to this time, four hospitalizations had occurred because of diabetic crises.

During the nurse's first visit, Mrs. G. appeared very anxious, explaining that she always anticipates "bad news" about Len. In response to inquiries about Len's missed clinic appointments, Mrs. G. seemed indifferent, stating that they have been too busy and that arranging child care for Ann was a problem. On a later visit other factors, more covert, which contribute to the family's reluctance to keep Len's appointments were noted. The mother's statements clarify these factors: "When they told me what was wrong with Len I worried day and night and wouldn't let anyone play with him or take him any place. I was constantly with him. Then I decided I couldn't worry like that anymore. I know he really isn't sick. No one could play as hard as he does and still be sick!" Mrs. G. seemed unwilling to discuss Len's fainting episodes except to say they were Len's way of getting attention. She also refused to discuss his four diabetic crisis hospitalizations.

Data concerning the health status of other family members were also noted. Mrs. G. was of average weight and neatly dressed. She was quite gregarious as long as she could control the conversation. Her knowledge about nutrition and other aspects of family welfare important to her—shelter, cleanliness, adequate child care arrangements, regular school attendance—were satisfactory. Mrs. G. claims good health, although she has not received any preventive care from a physician, with the exception of prenatal care, and even this was obtained late in the pregnancy.

Mr. G. had been in the Army many years ago and since this time has been under the care of a Veterans Administration Hospital for bouts of depression. Here he regularly receives tranquilizers and occasional counseling. His wife reported that his physical health is average, stating: "He doesn't get sick or go to the doctor, but he sure is tired all of the time."

Joanie, the 7-year-old, was reported to be in good health, attended school regularly, and was doing all right there. Her mother termed her "a good girl." Ann, the preschooler, was active, friendly, and healthy appearing. Mrs. G. complained of her "overactivity." She explained that Ann was constantly into things and interfered with her efforts to keep the house clean and picked up. Ann's health supervision is irregular and her immunizations incomplete. After well-baby care was completed at 1 year, health care has been sought only for acute illnesses.

The family's economic situation has been unstable. Mr. G. works irregularly in a factory, while Mrs. G. works off and on at a car-washing business. To supplement their insufficient earnings, they receive welfare.

Mrs. G's primary expressed concerns had to do with her husband's lack of responsibility for helping with the household and child-care tasks, as well as his overall neglectfulness and his irregular employment. She openly berated her husband in front of him, the nurse, and their children, complaining that he did not bring home enough money for the family to live on and lacks interest in the home, the children, and money matters. Mr. G. sat silently as his wife verbally assaulted him.

There was an impression of little communication or companionship among family members, except in those areas related to the daily activities of living and taking care of the apartment. The children's play was kept at a minimum due to the noise they created. Most communication was in the form of commands, emanating from the mother to the husband and children. Mrs. G.

states she is constantly working to keep the home clean, meals ready, and children cared for. The home was viewed as a place to be kept clean and organized, so that everything was put away; the children were expected to be "seen but not heard"; they were to be home exactly on time; attend school regularly; keep themselves and their surroundings clean; and obey and respect their mother. There were no toys or reading materials visible. The only discernible source of recreation for the entire family was the television set, which was on constantly. Family recreational pursuits were practically unheard of. Life was virtually task oriented, and no enjoyable and fun activities were included.

The family lives in a low-income housing project, for which they are charged a minimum rent. Kitchen equipment, food, and clothing storage facilities are adequate as are their furnishings. Although the outside appearance of the housing project is dirty and visually in a state of disrepair, the inside of their apartment is orderly and well maintained.

Mr. and Mrs. G. dropped out of high school in the ninth and tenth grades, respectively, in order to start working to help out their parents. No further education or skill training has been received since that time. Relatives do not reside near them, nor are they affiliated with any religious or other community groups. The community in which the family lives is part of a large inner-city area that is deteriorating rapidly. Transportation and social, health, and welfare facilities are easily accessible. Shopping for food and other necessities is limited to small neighborhood shops in the area, since they do not own a car. The schools and churches are nearby. The mother feels the neighborhood is crime-ridden (which the nurse confirmed), and hence she has kept the children indoors most of the time.

12. From the limited information contained in the family case study, what are the salient values operating in this family? (Use the assessment process that was suggested in this chapter.)

13. How important are these identified values to the family?

14. Are these values consciously or unconsciously held?

15. Are there any value conflicts evident within the family itself?

16. Given that value conflict between husband and wife is the family nursing diagnosis here, discuss briefly one intervention strategy that could be used here (given spouses are interested in discussing this area).

► chapter 13 study answers

1. a, b, and c.

2. b.

3. b.

4. Four major, recent value changes (any four):
   a. *Individualism.* Greater priority today placed on individual freedom of choice with a concomitant decline in familism.
   b. *Work ethic.* A change from seeing work as an end in itself to a means for obtaining other important aspirations. Decline in belief that hard work will pay off and decline in the intrinsic meaning of work to many individuals.
   c. *Tolerance of diversity.* Studies show that Americans are becoming increasingly tolerant of variation in lifestyles and also of ethnic differences. Weakening of the myth of the "melting pot."
   d. *Equality.* Egalitarianism in families and in society is increasing. Women's liberation is probably the strongest force in bringing about this change, but other oppressed groups have also sought and are receiving a fairer share of the resources and more consideration of their rights. These groups include children, the mentally ill, and other stigmatized groups.
   e. *Consumerism.* There has been an increased exploitation of resources and a rise in material indulgence involving the discarding and replacement of goods rather than saving.
   f. *Health and quality of life.* The increasing numbers of middle-class Americans engaging in lifestyle improvements is evidence of the increased saliency that this value has in society.

5. b, c, and d.

6. a.

7. True.

8. Productivity, materialism, individualism, work ethic, progress, and education.

9. Any four:
   a. Ethnicity, including religious background.
   b. Social class.
   c. Rural versus urban or suburban (geographical location).
   d. Degree of acculturation of dominant cultural values.
   e. Family life cycle stage.
   f. Generational differences.

10. All (a–d).

11. c and d.

12.

American Core Values	Gardiner Family Values
1. Productivity	1. Probably aspired to being successful—at least get by and be self-sufficient—but were not able to succeed. (Note wife's frustration and hostility toward

	husband because of employment problem.)
2. Work ethic	2. Wife appears to be committed to work ethic at home. Husband is not in conformity with this value.
3. Materialism	3. Not present (not realistic for family).
4. Individualism	4. Not evident.
5. Education	5. Not one of the central values for this family. Note lack of educational pursuits by parents and total lack of books at home.
6. Consumption ethic	6. Not present (economically unrealistic).
7. Progress and mastery over environment	7. Progress not implied. Mastery over environment not present. (Again powerless position makes this value unrealistic.)
8. Future orientation	8. Future-time orientation not seen; no planning observed during the time reported. Present oriented.
9. Efficiency, orderliness, and practicality	9. Mrs. G. seemed to place a high value on orderliness. Gives mother a sense of control.
10. Rationality	10. Value not seen.
11. Democracy, equality, and freedom	11. Democratic functioning not observed in home (authoritarian, wife-dominated power structure).
12. Doing orientation	12. Wife appeared to be a very active person at home, but her doing was limited to her mother and housekeeper roles.
13. Health	13. Health was not seen as an important (prime) value. Preventive care not sought. Child-care services utilized due to the obvious necessity of receiving treatment for acute problems. Mother: Denial of health problems noted regarding Len's health problems.
14. Patriarchal authority	14. Not valued (wife-dominated).

13. Practicality, orderliness, cleanliness appear highly valued.

14. Not known.

15. Wife—work oriented; husband—unable to succeed in this area. Value conflict between spouses related to the work ethic. Wife is hard worker and she expects husband to be also, as well as to be the provider for the family, regardless of his emotional problems.

16. Discuss with spouses their beliefs and expectations about husband's working (get each spouses' views). If husband feels that his "bouts of depression" are the basis of problem, encourage him (and perhaps wife) to see doctor to address this area; if husband and wife believe he does not have the job skills necessary to find new job, referral to a vocational rehabilitation or vocational skill center may be appropriate. Discuss with spouses the need for husband to feel he can find and hold down job and how family members can positively encourage these efforts.

The Family Affective Function

Marilyn M. Friedman with Darlene E. McCown

1. State three reasons why the affective function is a vital family function.

2. Explain briefly the three components of need–response patterns.

3. Discuss how mutual support and emotional warmth originate and continue in a family as part of the "spiral phenomenon."

4. Describe the aims of a family in achieving a mutual respect balance.

5. Define concepts of bonding or attachment, response bonds, identification, crescive bonds, need–response patterns, and their significance to the family's fulfillment of the affective function.

6. Discuss the prime task of parents in assisting their children to form a stable, sound identity in the area of separateness and connectedness.

7. Compare and contrast the marital therapeutic role with the affective function of the family.

8. Name two underlying values and/or priorities present in energized families related to the affective function area.

9. Identify several North American Nursing Diagnosis Association (NANDA) nursing diagnoses that could be appropriate when a family's affective function is being inadequately fulfilled.

10. Using the family case situation, complete an assessment of the affective function. Propose a family nursing diagnosis in the area of the affective function. Suggest two family nursing interventions to ameliorate and/or resolve the above affective problem.

11. Describe several interventions that are helpful to families when a family member is dying.

It is generally recognized that the family exists to fulfill basic functions necessary for the survival of the species (societal needs), namely, procreation and child rearing. Additionally, it acts as the necessary mediator between the society and the individual and forms the matrix in which personal needs are met.

Social organizations and institutions such as the school and social services agencies now share in many of the traditional functions of the family. A number of extremely vital functions, however, remain. Of these socialization (see Chap. 15) and affective functions are perhaps the most important. Major functions of the 1990s family include nurturing, partnering, communicating, adapting, respite (Janosek & Green, 1992), and emotional support. *Affect* is a means to achieve family tasks of physical care, reproduction, teaching, personal growth and development, bonding, and providing purpose and meaning (Friedemann, 1993a). Another significant family function also remaining is the health care function, covered in Chapter 16.

▶ IMPORTANCE OF THE AFFECTIVE FUNCTION

The affective function deals with the internal functions of the family—the psychosocial protection and support of its members. The family accomplishes the task of supporting the healthy development and growth of its members by meeting the socioemotional needs of its members, starting with the early years of an individual's life and continuing throughout his or her lifetime. Fulfillment of the affective function is the central basis for both the formation and continuation of the family unit (Satir, 1972).

An individual's self-image and his or her sense of belonging is derived through primary group (family) interactions. Moreover, the family serves as a primary source of love, approval, reward, and support.

In attempting to fulfill the role of meeting its member's socioemotional needs, the family assumes a heavy responsibility, especially in view of the fact that families move frequently and often do not have the social support systems they need. Moreover, today's families are generally smaller in the number of members, and thus there are fewer members to share the tasks of meeting each other's needs for companionship, love, and support.

Loveland-Cherry (1996) points out that affection among family members produces a nurturing emotional climate that positively influences growth and development and a sense of personal competence. Family nurturance is essential for health promotion behaviors and healthy outcomes.

In view then of the increased emphasis on the importance of family relationships, it is not surprising to find a parallel rise in divorce rates. Permissive divorce laws making divorce more accessible to all sectors of society, and a concomitant lessening of social stigma, along with other factors such as gains made by the women's movement, have also facilitated this national trend. Because divorce is an available option in many families today, most families that remain together do so because of the satisfaction that being a family brings rather than out of necessity or because of coercive economic and social pressures.

Because the affective function is vital for both survival and the functioning of the family as a whole and its individual members, assessment and intervention in this area are crucial. Both health counseling and education are critical strategies to employ in helping families shore up their relationships and better meet each other's needs. Consideration of the affective function is particularly vital in working with young families with newborns and infants, where parent–infant relationships are so significant in terms of their long-term impact on the individuals' and family's future.

▶ COMPONENTS OF THE AFFECTIVE FUNCTION

The affective function involves the family's perception of respect for and care of the psychosocial needs of its members. Through fulfillment of this function, the family serves the major psychosocial purposes of building within its members the qualities of humanness, stabilization of personality and behavior, relatability (ability to relate intimately), and self-esteem (Table 14–1).

Maintaining Mutual Nurturance

First and foremost, fulfilling the affective function involves creating and maintaining within the family a system for mutual nurturance. Recall that in Chapter

---

▶ TABLE 14–1

SOCIOEMOTIONAL ATTRIBUTES OF HEALTHY FAMILIES

- A social milieu for the generation and maintenance of affectional bonds within family relationships, where one is first loved and given to, and in turn learns to love and give in return.
- An opportunity to develop a personal and social identity tied to family identity.
- An opportunity for individuals to be themselves. The family provides a home base or haven where its members are permitted to be themselves—to express their true feelings and thoughts (e.g., hostility with less fear of consequences) and to experience security and love without fear of rejection.

13 on family values, one important family value was valuing the family as a haven for warmth, support, love, and acceptance. A prerequisite to achieving mutual nurturance is the basic commitment of a couple to each other and a nurturing, emotionally satisfying marital relationship. This becomes the emotional foundation on which the parents build their supportive structure. The nurturing attitudes and behavior flowing from parents and siblings to younger children will result in a return flow from children to parents as well.

Brown (1978) views this flow as a spiral phenomenon. As each member receives affection and care from others in the family, his or her capacity to give to other members increases, with the result being mutual support and emotional warmth.

The key concepts here are *mutuality* and *reciprocity*. Parents give emotionally to children; this, in turn, is received and fed back to parents and siblings. (The opposite also occurs: rejecting and angry parents breed angry and rejecting responses in their children.) By maintaining the kind of environment in which its members' needs are adequately responded to, the family provides the opportunity for individuals to form and maintain meaningful relationships not only with family members, but with other individuals also.

Development of Close Relationships.

Through the family's fulfilling of the affective function, individuals develop the ability to relate intimately or closely with others. Intimacy is vital in human relationships, because it fulfills the psychological need for emotional closeness with another human being and allows individuals in the relationship to know the full range of each other's uniqueness.

A person usually first experiences an intimate relationship with his or her parents, beginning with early mother–infant bonding. The relationship continues to grow and develop during the years that follow in the family of origin. When achieved, this sense of closeness and trusting gives the person the confidence to reach outside the family confines and establish close and emotionally satisfying relationships with others. As young adults then start their own family, this sense of intimacy and closeness is passed on to the next generation. Conversely, if early bonding and a sense of trust and intimacy does not occur in the family of origin, the individual will not have the confidence and ability to relate intimately with oth-

ers. Unfortunately this inability is usually passed on to the next generation also, unless some intervening factor such as personal experiences and growth at a later stage in life occurs (Byng-Hall, 1995).

We are reminded by Satir (1972) that it is impossible for a family to meet the emotional needs of its members without the presence of functional, clear family communication patterns. Hence communication becomes the vehicle through which the psychological needs of family members are recognized and responded to.*

Mutual Respect Balance

The literature of parent–child guidance presents a well-respected approach to parenting termed the mutual respect balance (Colley, 1978). When operationalized it helps family members to fulfill the affective function. The primary thrust of this approach is that families should maintain an atmosphere in which positive self-regard and the rights of *both* parents and child are highly valued. Thus it is acknowledged that each person in the family has his or her own rights as individuals, as well as developmental needs specific to his or her age group. A mutual respect balance can be achieved when each family member respects the rights, needs, and responsibilities of other members (Colley, 1978).

Maintaining a balance between the rights of individuals in the family means creating an atmosphere in which neither parents nor children are expected to cater to the whims of the other. Parents need to provide sufficient structure and consistent guidelines so that limits are set and understood. Yet enough flexibility must also be built into the family system to allow for freedom and room to grow and individuate. Mutual nurturance is also made possible when a mutual respect balance exists.

Bonding and Identification

The sustaining force behind the perception and satisfaction of the needs of individuals in the family is **bonding** or **attachment** (used interchangeably). Attachment, according to Wright and Leahey (1994,

---

* This statement provides a cogent basis for health care or welfare professionals working with families to direct their efforts toward helping families shore up and improve their interactional patterns.

p. 60) refers to, "a relatively enduring unique emotional tie between two specific persons." Bonding is first initiated in a new family within the marital relationship. This is when a couple discovers common interests, goals, and values and finds that the relationship validates each of them, carries with it certain tangible benefits (prestige, among friends, community privileges, etc.), makes possible the meeting of certain goals that could not be accomplished alone (having children and a home), and provides mutual enjoyment and comfortableness due to their sustained contact with each other (Perry, 1983; Turner, 1970). Bowlby (1977) called the development of this emotional tie "falling in love."

This same kind of bonding or attachment develops later between parents and children and between siblings as they continually and positively relate to each other through the process of identification.

Mother–newborn and infant attachment is crucial, because early parent–infant interactions affect the nature and quality of later attachment relationships, and these relationships influence the child's psychosocial and cognitive development (Ainsworth, 1966). Identification is the critical element in bonding, as well as the heart of family relationships. Turner (1970) explains that in its most uncomplicated definition, **identification** refers to "an attitude in which a person experiences what happens to another person as if it had happened to himself" (p. 66). In other words, when a family member identifies with another member, he or she experiences the joys and sorrows of the other as if these experiences were his or her own.

In order for bonding or attachment to occur in family relationships, positive identification must first be present. As the most pervasive aspect of attachment, it may be based on sympathy or libidinal mechanisms or be solely derived from the internalization of the attitudes of the other whom he or she cares for and depends on. Once established, the long-term consequence of identification and bonding is a change in the individual's self-image toward the characteristics of the other person with whom he or she has identified. Through identification, children attempt to imitate the behavior of their parents (the parents with whom they identify become their role models). As the child's identity is thus enhanced by the learning of behaviors, attitudes, and values of parents, a bond is formed. Through identification

and bonding, parents obtain referent power over their children.

The identification or identity bond depends on positive, giving responses from people in the relationships. Even an infant gives or rewards mother in his or her earliest beginnings of their relationship by feeding, snuggling up, letting the mother comfort him or her, and so forth. Thus, for bonding to be effective there must be support and enhancement of a person's identity through his or her association with another. "Whenever a child shows admiration towards his parent or spontaneously gives affection, the gratification that the parent feels activates a **response bond**" (Turner, 1970, p. 72).

One facet of the response bond is the general sensitivity, caring for, and responsiveness of the other member(s) in the relationship. When one's communication is accepted, and appreciation and feelings supported, this leads to a closeness and a desire to continue sharing together. Bonding may also exist because of special needs that one person meets for the other person. For instance, a dominant, controlling person may bond with a submissive type—with both having their special needs satisfied in the relationship.

Duration of close relationships is also a factor to be considered. Even though the bonding between newlyweds is intense, and the relationship between mother and a newborn child profound, loss of the newly married mate or newborn will generally not be felt as severely as if the relationship had persisted for several years prior to the loss. As family members closely involved with each other continue their relationship, old bonds become intensified and new, stronger bonds emerge; and these stronger bonds unite these individuals together in a unique, sustaining relationship. These attachments are not substitutable—that is, no other person(s) can replace a particular member. Because these enduring bonds are not initially present, and grow through a close, sustained involvement, Turner (1970) terms these bonds **crescive bonds**.

Although crescive bonding sounds like a natural phenomenon, it is not inevitable, and in some situations crescive bonds do not develop. Turner (1970) discusses two factors that inhibit their growth. First, bonds that are situationally based (based on the existence of certain specific needs or circumstances), such as those bonds that meet certain developmental needs that an individual will possibly outgrow, or task-oriented bonds, are far more vulnerable to weakening and eventual breakage. Second, bonding relationships based on contractual agreements, rather than sacred linkages, are also more vulnerable to dissolution, because contracts involve mutual obligations. In this case if one partner fails to live up to his or her part of the contract, the contract can become invalid. Marriages are seen by many in this light. In sacred linkages, the basis for staying together is felt to be God, family, tradition, and/or one's duty. The bond of parent–child is still seen as sacred and immutable. (A case in point: States do not legally permit a parent the right to disown their minor children.)

Assessing the nature of the attachment and quality of the affectional ties between each set of relationships in the family has been suggested by several family therapists and nurses (Minuchin, 1974; Wright & Leahey, 1994). The focus here is on the various affective relationships rather than on the individual members. Later in this chapter, in the assessment questions, the use of an attachment diagram (see Fig. 14–1) is recommended.

Separateness and Connectedness

One of the central, overriding psychological issues involving family life is the way in which families meet their members' psychological needs, and how this affects the individual's identity and self-esteem. During the early years of socialization, families mold and program a child's behavior, thus forming his or her sense of identity. Minuchin (1974) explains further: "Human experiences of identity have two elements—a sense of belonging and a sense of being separate. The laboratory in which these ingredients are mixed and dispensed with is the family, the matrix of identity" (p. 47).

Children's sense of belonging comes from being a part of, or connected to, a family—playing the roles of child and sibling. The development of a sense of separateness and individuation occurs as children participate in roles within the family and in different family events and situations, as well as through involvement in activities outside of the family. As children grow the parents progressively give them more autonomy to develop and to meet their own unique needs and interests (Minuchin, 1974).

Thus in order to perceive and meet the psychological needs of family members, the family must achieve a satisfactory balance of *separateness* or *autonomy* and *connectedness* (Peterson, 1995). Family members are both connected to and separate from one another. Each family handles the issues of separateness and connectedness in a unique fashion, some families placing much more emphasis on one facet than on the other. The balance between autonomy and connectedness is often shaped by a family's cultural background.

Both conditions are basic and constitutive of family life. The young infant begins the separation process at about 6 months. Through the formative years, he or she forms an identity; but individuation and growth continue throughout his or her lifetime. Nonetheless, connectedness is equally basic, taking a variety of forms from physical proximity to intense involvement that excludes other interests (Handel, 1972).

The family needs to provide opportunities for the mastery of this duality. On the one hand, it must help its members want to be together and to develop and maintain cohesiveness or connectedness. On the other hand, it must gradually provide appropriate amounts of freedom and avenues of expression for members to individuate and become separate individuals.

How much of family life is regulated by power considerations is important here. Parental authority—its scope and the manner of its exercise—is one of the forces shaping the patterns encouraging individuality (separateness) and cohesion (connectedness). Parents differ in how extensively they impose their image on their children. When parents expect children to do all the adapting, there is little room for negotiating, and the chances of promoting individuality are hampered.

Also, families vary in how fast they push their children toward separateness and how intensively they encourage connectedness—that is, how soon they expect their children to grow up and to separate from parents. Some parents encourage babyish, dependent behaviors in their children, while others pressure their children to act more adult at an early age. The pace set for their children's growing up is often based on the parents' aims for themselves and their children. For example, if both parents are working and see dependency as a burden and frustrating to their goals, they will push their children at a faster pace to become self-sufficient and independent. As in other dimensions of family life, parental ideas about child growth and development and the acceptability of various behaviors are also influenced by the family's culture and social class background (Handel, 1972; Peterson, 1995).

In assessing separateness and connectedness within a family, Hartman and Laird (1983) look at the characteristics of the family in terms of enmeshment–disengagement (a continuum). Minuchin originally (1974) generated the notions of enmeshment and disengagement in families. He refers to an enmeshed family as one in which individual and subsystem boundaries (like spousal subsystem boundaries) are continually violated by members outside those boundaries. In enmeshed families, family members interpret or speak for each other and are supersensitive to family members' signals for help. Enmeshed families are families that do not allow room for separate opinions or autonomous behavior. Members tend to be too close (overinvolved) and too restrictive of individual freedom and personal identity. Conversely, in disengaged families, there are closed, rigid boundaries between subsystems and individuals, and very little sensitivity to members' calls for assistance. In these types of families relationships are too distant and there is little recognition or meeting of family members' personal needs. Moreover, there is an absence of involvement with each other. Neither extremes on the continuum are healthy.

Minuchin, Rosman, and Baker (1978), in their studies of troubled families, find that certain types of families are generally enmeshed, including psychosomatic families and families with school phobic and schizophrenic children.

Need–Response Patterns

The affective component of family relationships needs to be evaluated in terms of the extent to which family members seem to care for and about each other (Hartman & Laird, 1983). Parad and Caplan (1965) address this concern in their discussion of the assessment of the **need–response patterns** in families. This concept is essentially synonymous with that of the family affective function. Mutual nurturance, respect, bonding, and separateness–connectedness aspects emerge as vital prerequisites or necessary

corequisites to satisfactory need–response patterns in families (Table 14–2).

Three separate and interlocking phases are inherent in a family's affective response to these needs. First, family members must perceive the needs of the other individuals, within the constraints of the family's culture. Next, these needs must be viewed with respect and seen to be worthy of attention (as discussed under mutual respect balance). And lastly, these recognized and respected needs must be satisfied to the extent possible in light of family resources. It is especially propitious if family members each have confidants within the family with whom they can unburden themselves.

This triad of perception, respect, and satisfaction of family members' needs is very much influenced by American sociocultural perspectives—viewing individuals as separate persons who are deserving of recognition and respect as well as a fair share in the family's resources. This tendency to view family members as unique, evolving individuals corresponds with the high value this society places on individualism.

In working with families it was observed that the family's sensitivity to, and thus perception of the individual members's actions and needs, varies greatly. Most families usually fall somewhere between being extremely sensitive (sign of enmeshment), and thus highly responsive to an individual member's input, and being extremely insensitive and unresponsive to individual members' inputs (sign of disengagement).

The extent to which basic psychological or socioemotional needs are met also varies depending on the family's social support system. Some families have a greater, more involved social network, such as an extended family, from which to draw support. In these families the meeting of family members' psy-

---

▶ TABLE 14–2

THE SOCIOEMOTIONAL NEEDS OF FAMILY MEMBERS

1. Love for one's own sake
2. A balance between support and independence with respect to tasks
3. A balance between freedom and control
4. The availability of suitable role models

Adapted from Parad & Caplan (1965).

chosocial needs can be accomplished by individuals who are both inside and outside of the nuclear family. In contrast, families that are truly isolated from social support systems—closed families—have limited outside resources and hence, depend primarily or solely on family members to meet all their psychological needs. Naturally, this latter state imposes a great burden on family relationships, because probably no one person, such as a mate, can meet all of the other person's needs.

A recent study by Barber and Thomas (1986) found that emotional ties varied depending on the gender of the child and parent. The researchers surveyed 527 largely Mormon college students about their relationships with their parents. Fathers were found to be more physically affectionate to daughters, while mothers showed the same amount of physical affection to children of both sexes. Mothers typically had more companionship with daughters, and fathers with sons. Physical affection was found to be positively associated with self-esteem in both sexes. Another study (Wenk et al., 1994) using longitudinal data from 762 children, ages 7 to 11, showed that children's perceptions of emotional and physical parental involvement were equally important to the well-being of both boys and girls. Feeling loved and respected by parents and having time with parents fosters self-esteem and mental health in children.

The Therapeutic Role

In Chapter 12 the therapeutic role of spouses was discussed as one of the emergent roles increasingly expected of mates entering into marital and family life from all social classes, but particularly in the middle class. This role is quite similar to the mates' role in meeting the affective needs of their mates. While the affective function describes the broad mental health function of the family—as a group designed to meet the psychological needs of its members—the therapeutic role describes an important socioemotional role within the marital subsystem. This role has been explained by Nye (1976): "The behavior . . . is therapeutic in assisting the spouse to cope with and, hopefully, dispose of a problem with which he is confronted" (p. 111). When this role is extended to include the rest of the family, children and adults alike, some very important elements of family behavior come to light. Nye (1976) continues: "Listening

and giving the family member an opportunity to verbalize, acting as a 'sounding board' for the ideas or reactions of the other, supplying additional information, concepts, or insights, and taking concrete actions in sharing the solution of the problem are all involved" (p. 115). Some of these behaviors, of course, would not be appropriate (therapeutic) in relating to a young child or infant, but with older children, much of the same therapeutic, assistive relating can occur.

Primarily, the therapeutic role spouses play is problem oriented. It involves listening to the problem, sympathizing, giving reassurance and affection, and offering help in solving the problem. In Nye's (1976) study of spousal roles, he reported that over 60 percent of both husbands and wives indicated that mates have the duty to enact this role, the remainder indicating the desirability of this role in marriage. Moreover, Nye found that 63 percent of wives usually engage in this role. More women than men enacted this role well; they also valued it more highly.

▶ THE AFFECTIVE FUNCTION IN ENERGIZED FAMILIES

It is important to know how healthy, functional, or, as Pratt (1976) calls them, "energized" families achieve their affective function, because this will give us an optimal standard to use for comparative purposes.

> A feature of energized family structure . . . is the tendency to provide autonomy and to be responsive to the particular interests and needs of individual family members. . . . This includes the tendency not only to accept, but to prize individuality and uniqueness, and to tolerate disagreement and deviance. Respect and acceptance are given unconditionally, without continuous comparison of the person to others or to prescribed standards. . . . The family members are encouraged in their various endeavors, especially in seeking new areas of growth and in developing their creativity, imagination, and independent thinking. (pp. 84–85)

The one limitation of this description is that it was based on a study of largely middle-class white families. Obviously, a family's social class and cultural variability must be considered in evaluating what is healthy and less healthy behaviors in a family.

▶ THE FAMILY UNDER STRESS: THE AFFECTIVE FUNCTION

Maintaining a nurturing familial environment is often a formidable task, as many stressors tend to disrupt family homeostasis and make family members less sensitive and loving toward each other. One of the threats to mutual nurturance is the health/illness stressor.

When the psychological needs of family members are not being adequately perceived and addressed due to the stress of illness in a family member, symptoms in the form of distress signals from one or more family members may become apparent. These symptoms of family dysfunction include various emotional responses such as anger, anxiety, and depression; delinquent or acting-out behaviors; and somatic complaints and illness. This dysfunction, in turn, further inhibits clear, functional communication within family relationships, resulting in a downward-spiraling process until some positive step is taken to curtail further disorganization and reverse the tailspin.

Parad and Caplan (1965) do not believe that the temporary periods of low response to members' needs are necessarily harmful to their mental health. However, persistent, long-standing need frustration is deleterious, and even a temporary inattentiveness to a family member's needs may be harmful if the loss occurs when that individual is particularly vulnerable, such as during a critical phase of a child's development.

Family health professionals note that family problems and dysfunctions generally become worse or more apparent during the terminal phase of an illness or during bereavement (Rolland, 1994). When the family is grieving, conflicts in the family often become overt and the affective needs of family members are usually not acknowledged.

The death of a family member is probably the most catastrophic event for a family member or family (Arnette, 1996). The seriousness of this event is demonstrated in the higher mortality rates of spouses up to 2 years after the death of a mate. Bereaved persons are at higher risk for multiple diseases. These are primarily the chronic diseases of middle and late age. The excess risk of mortality due to bereavement is higher among widowed men than women (Kosten et al., 1985). Some studies found increased risk of death in the first 6 months of bereavement (Bowling & Windsor, 1995). A recent study found that middle-aged

people who lost spouses, siblings, and siblings-in-law generally adjusted more poorly than younger or older individuals and were more prone to health problems in the bereavement period (Perkins & Harris, 1990).

With death comes loss. People who are closest to the person who has died are immediately affected by the loss. Eventually, as in an earthquake, the whole system of relationships is shaken (Gelcer, 1986).

Concerning childhood bereavement, it has been well documented that bereaved siblings show a higher level of behavior problems compared to standardized norms for age and sex (Birenbaum et al., 1990; Davies, 1995; Mahon & Page, 1995; McCown & Davies, 1995). Studies report that between one-fourth and one-third of bereaved siblings have serious problems. These problems include behaviors such as sleep problems, poor school performance, and attention seeking. Grief behaviors in children tend to be internalizing behaviors. Some additional research (Worden, Davies, & McCown, 1996) compares the adjustment of children following a parent versus a sibling death. Approximately one-fourth of the children in each group had behavior problems. However, boys scored higher in the parent loss group and girls scored higher in the sibling loss group. Reasons for these differences need further exploration.

Family members' psychological needs for support are much greater during the period when the family member is dying and after the death. If the member's death is unexpected, stress and grief will be more extreme. When death is prolonged over a period of months or even years, stress is continuous and circumstances ambiguous. Family members are often left emotionally depleted in terms of helping themselves or supporting others in the family. Other stressors occur after a death in the family (numerous arrangements that must be made, settling of the estate, medical bills, and family role transitions); it is easy to see that the adult member(s) would have difficulty supporting child members of the family. This is often a time when the family's social support system (both formal and informal) can play an important role in supporting grieving families. Functional families also pull together during this period and try to share their grief and support each other. Elements of this process have been described by McCubbin and McCubbin (1993) in the Resiliency Model of Family Stress, Adjustment, and Adaptation.

The affective need of family members during the time of a major loss is to be able to grieve for the loss.

Constructive grief work depends on the ability of the social support network (family and the family's social network) to be permissive of feelings, positively accepting and supportive. Family members' energies should be directed to the actual loss as experienced collectively and individually. When feelings are shared there needs to be an open stage for discussing, recalling, memory associating, and reliving of past events. Moreover, certain beliefs may need to be confronted, especially when guilt is expressed based on irrational assumptions of a person's responsibility for events that were beyond the control of that person.

Children also need to be able to grieve. Sharing feelings and thoughts with children and communicating with them at their cognitive and emotional levels of maturity are most important. The parents' handling of death with children and adolescents is most significant in terms of helping them with their psychological needs (Shapiro, 1994). Those families who are open to expressing their emotions are more successful in adjusting to the loss of a family member (McClowry et al., 1989). For long-term adjustment, it is also important for children to review the death event at each new developmental phase in order to reintegrate the experience with a more mature level of understanding.

Several articles have been written about the similarity between divorce and death in a family in terms of adjustment to the loss. Increased risk of illness and distress among both the recently divorced and widowed has been found. The impact of certain factors upon adjustment to widowhood and divorce (economic, social support, cause of divorce/death, timing of event, and attachment) makes a difference as to how difficult both divorce and widowhood are (Kitson et al., 1989).

FAMILY AFFECTIVE FUNCTION: APPLYING THE FAMILY NURSING PROCESS

► assessment questions

The following questions have been included to assist the assessor in appraising the family affective function.

Family Need–Response Patterns

1. To what extent do family members perceive the needs of the other individuals in the family? Are the parents and spouses able to describe their children's and mate's needs and concerns? How sensitive are family members in picking up cues regarding other's feelings and needs?

2. Are each member's needs, interests, and differentness respected by the other family members? Does a mutual respect balance exist? Do they show mutual respect toward each other? How sensitive is the family to each individual's actions and concerns?

3. Are the recognized needs of family members being met by the family, and if so, to what extent? What is the process for emotional release (unburdening) in the family?

For questions 1 through 3 it is suggested that a list of the family members be included with their needs identified (as perceived by family members) and the extent to which these needs are being met.

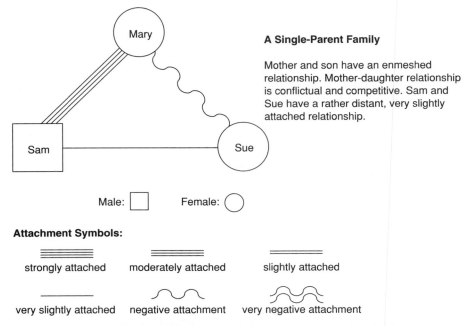

A Single-Parent Family

Mother and son have an enmeshed relationship. Mother-daughter relationship is conflictual and competitive. Sam and Sue have a rather distant, very slightly attached relationship.

Male: ☐   Female: ◯

Attachment Symbols:

strongly attached   moderately attached   slightly attached

very slightly attached   negative attachment   very negative attachment

Figure 14–1. An example of an attachment diagram. Shows a single-parent family. Mother and son have an enmeshed relationship. Mother–daughter relationship is conflictual and competitive. Sam and Sue have rather distant, very slightly attached relationship. *(Adapted from Wright & Leahey, 1994.)*

Mutual Nurturance, Closeness, and Identification

4. To what extent do family members provide mutual nurturance to each other? How supportive of each other are they?

5. Is a sense of closeness and intimacy present among the sets of relationships within the family? How well do family members get along with each other? Do they show affection toward each other?

6. Does mutual identification and bonding or attachment appear to be present? Empathetic statements, concerns about others' feelings, experiences, and hardships are all indications of this being present.

To answer questions 5 and 6, use of an attachment diagram is recommended. Attachment diagrams depict both the strength and quality of the affective relationship or emotional ties between members of the family. The focus is on the relationship and the reciprocal nature of the affectional tie.

The evidence gathered to depict the bonds between family members is largely subjective. Both observational and interview data can be used. Observations about relationships include expression of feelings toward a family member as well as signs of affection or distancing (kissing, hugging, eye contact, smiling, comforting, cuddling, sitting close or far away). Verbal (interview) data include responses to questions about how close member A is to member B. For example: How do A and B get along? What's their relationship like? Which of the siblings is closer to parent A? Also historical information often gives clues as to how close a relationship is. An example is the case of the mother who has constantly cared for the chronically ill child in hospital and home, while the father and older child have rarely been involved in caregiving.

Figure 14–1 illustrates an attachment bond and the symbols used in these diagrams. The present relationships are diagrammed rather then past relationships. Bonds that are very close or very negative (conflictual) are typically maladaptive, although situational crisis sometimes forces very close relationships on a short-term basis and these very close relationships serve a necessary supportive purpose.

Separateness and Connectedness

7. How does the family deal with the issues of separateness and connectedness? How does the family help its members want to be together and maintain cohesiveness (connectedness)? Are opportunities for developing separateness stressed adequately, and are they appropriate for the age and needs of each of the family members?

► FAMILY NURSING DIAGNOSES

In families where the psychological or affective needs of family members are not being met, a myriad of family problems may be manifested. A number of North American Nursing Diagnosis Association (NANDA) diagnoses may be appropriate when there is altered family affective functioning (Table 14–3). In these cases, inability to meet the psychological needs of all family members would be a defining characteristic.

► FAMILY NURSING INTERVENTIONS

Family nursing diagnoses for this area were addressed by using NANDA's classification of germane nursing diagnoses (see Table 14–3). For interventions related to the NANDA diagnoses mentioned previously, the reader is referred to Carpenito (1995) and McFarland and McFarlane (1993). General suggestions for assisting families to better meet the psychosocial needs of their members are briefly explained in the present section.

Interventions Promoting Healthy Need–Response Patterns

The assessment of this area (asking members to tell the nurse about each family member, what his or her psychological needs are, and if family members are responding to these needs) is an education for families in and of itself. Some teaching should preceed this exercise, such as explaining to the family that each person has his or her own individual needs; that many of these needs are based on the person's developmental stage; and that family members need to recognize these and respond to them as well as possible—without interfering with other members' needs. In large families or families that are not psychologically oriented, this may be new information. In fact, there is a misperception by some parents that children should be treated exactly the same, so that no favoritism is involved. With this belief parents often don't see their children's uniqueness. Teaching the family members about individual and family growth and developmental characteristics may be very helpful for sensitizing parents to their children's needs.

Another strategy for helping family members, especially the parents, become more sensitive to individual family members' needs is by asking, "What is Johnnie like?" When parents respond, and the nurse asks further questions about the child's differentness, comments can then be made that interpret a child's behavior so that parents better understand their child. By commenting on a child's behavior, this helps reframe their children's actions in a more positive, informed way. (Example: A mother labels her son's incessant talking as indicating that he is a spoiled brat. The family nurse relabels the behavior, helping the family see the son as anxious and wanting parents' attention.)

► TABLE 14–3

NANDA DIAGNOSES FOR ALTERED FAMILY AFFECTIVE FUNCTIONING

Diagnosis	Example
1. Altered family processes. Definition: The state in which a family that normally functions effectively experiences a dysfunction.	The family is under stress and all the family members' energies are being diverted to handle the stressor, thereby neglecting or overlooking family members' psychosocial needs.
2. Altered parenting. Definition: Occurs when the ability of the nurturing figure(s) to create an environment that promotes the optimal growth and development of another human being is compromised.	A family with marked dominance by the mother (mother is very controlling) and marked passivity by father does not allow oldest adolescent son to individuate or separate from the family, thereby not meeting his psychosocial needs.
3. Potential altered parenting. Definition: Same as above, except that "potential" is added to compromised.	The same as the above family example, except the oldest son is in fifth grade and has not entered puberty. Because of the mother's controlling, overbearing mothering, the potential for a problem occurring when the son reaches adolescence is very great.
4. Dysfunctional grieving. Definition: A maladaptive process that occurs when grief is intensified to the degree that the person is overwhelmed, becomes stuck in one phase of grieving, and demonstrates excessive or prolonged emotional responses to the significant loss.	Dysfunctional grieving is being extended to include the grieving family—which is grieving dysfunctionally. The usual family dysfunction is the *denial* of the death in the family. (Ineffective denial could also be stated.) A family rule is established that it's not all right to talk about the loss, to express feelings about the loss, or to recall memories of the loved one or events where the loved one was present. The memories, feelings, and thoughts are not shared, leading to other problems: psychosomatic illness, depression, pseudomutuality, emotional cutoff, and emotional distancing of family members from each other.
5. Ineffective family coping, compromised. Definition: Involves insufficient, ineffective, or compromised family support, comfort, assistance, or encouragement that may alter the family member's or family's competence in adaptive tasks related to the presenting health challenge (may be short or long term).	Mother has been hospitalized for 1 week due to having surgery. She is the primary nurturer in the family—to both the husband and children. The husband-father has attempted to give the children attention and love, but they (age 2 and 3) are upset and resentful that their mother abandoned them.
6. Ineffective family coping, disabling. Definition: Refers to the behavior of one or more family members that incapacitates the family (or individual members) to adapt therapeutically to the existing health challenge.	Within this family the wife and husband (both are remarried) have two children—a son, age 10 from the husband's previous marriage, and a daughter, age 5, from the mother's previous marriage. The son has been labeled the troublemaker in the family, and is outwardly called this. The daughter is labeled the "sweet one," and comparisons of the children's personality differences are made when the parents get angry at the son.
7. Potential for violence. Altered role performance. Social isolation. Self-esteem, low. Altered growth and development.	These problems could also be present given the situation in which family members' psychosocial needs are not being adequately met.

Source: Adapted from McFarland and McFarlane (1993).

Promoting Mutual Nurturance

To help families maintain or initiate mutual nurturance, communication patterns in the family need to be analyzed. Parents need to feel that they are the ones who must stop circular patterns of angry, rejecting, or dysfunctional messages. For instance, they can do this by not responding to messages that start the dysfunctional pattern going or they can learn not to initiate these interactions themselves and instead communicate so that mutual respect is shown. It is not easy to break repetitive communication patterns. However, if parents understand the dynamics of problematic interactional patterns and are aware of what is happening, they can make definitive steps to change dysfunctional communications. (See Chap.

10 for more elaborate discussion.) Nurses can act as communication role models to families, to help them see that a more healthy mutual respect balance can be achieved in family interactions.

Assisting Families With Closeness–Separateness Issues

Closeness–separateness problems may be due to parents' knowledge deficit, but this is rarely so. These types of problems often have to do with the way the parents themselves were raised and unresolved intergenerational problems. In health settings, overcloseness or enmeshment is a much more common problem than disengagement. This is because there is a tendency in some families for the adult member(s) to become oversolicitous and protective of a family member who has a serious or disabling illness. In some cases, the whole family may be highly resonant (or hypersensitive) to the "identified patient's" needs.

If overcloseness is a long-standing problem in a family and is of the intensity that family members' growth and development is being significantly impeded, then usually family therapy is needed, and a referral should be initiated if the family also believes this is necessary. Minuchin (1974), a noted family therapist, would work to restructure the enmeshed family, while Bowen (1978), another noted family therapist, would work on helping family member(s) become more differentiated.

Assisting Families With Grieving

Several authors have presented guidelines to facilitate grief resolution following a loss or death in the family (Corless, Germino, & Pittman, 1995; McClowry et al., 1989; Kahn, 1990; Shapiro, 1994). In order to help family members who are in anticipatory grief (family member is dying) we need to understand tasks of family members during this difficult time. Rando (1986) describes the tasks of family members:

1. Family members should keep the dying person involved in family decisions as long as possible, so that he or she feels some sense of control and that his or her opinions still matter.

2. The well family members need to individuate from the dying family member. They must come to grips with reality that the loved one will die, and to start contemplating the future without the loved one.

3. Family members need to begin dealing with the reallocation or shifting of roles in the family to establish a new family homeostasis. This shifting of roles is very difficult and family system functioning is often precarious.

4. Family members need to learn to manage the feelings aroused by the terminal illness and death. Sadness, guilt, anger, memories, and reactions to past losses are common emotions that need to be shared and managed.

5. Family members need to face reality in terms of discussion of what needs to be done when death occurs (medical requirements, funeral arrangements, finances, etc.).

6. Family members need to "say goodbye." This should be done by each family member—verbally or nonverbally. This critical area requires support and role modeling from caregivers. Family members need to know when death is imminent.

Turning to the role of the family nurse during this period, a central thrust of her or his care should be to help family members achieve patient–family member comfort. Rando (1986) suggests that to achieve this end family nurses can assist by helping to "maintain the relationship between the dying person and family by encouraging open communication to the extent the family style allows" (p. 75). Another intervention family-focused nurses make is assisting the family to assume new roles (having family conferences is one way to assist family members to adjust and take on additional duties and make practical plans). A third exceptionally important intervention is to facilitate the expression of emotions, and support the family members in their grief. Family members need to know that their feelings are normal and part of the grief process that has to occur. And lastly, assisting the family to understand and absorb pertinent medical communication about the course of illness and treatment is a central role of the family nurse. Holding family conferences to explain illness and treatment concerns and encourage family cohesiveness is very helpful .

► study questions

1. Discuss three reasons why the affective function is so important.

2. The need–response pattern includes not only the perception of family members' needs and the meeting of these needs in the family. What other component is part of this pattern, the component that makes meeting the needs possible?

3. The spiral phenomenon relative to the generation and continuance of emotional support and warmth among family members can be explained as (select the best answer):
   a. Hate begets hate; love begets love.
   b. I'm okay, you're okay principle.
   c. Self-fulfilling prophesy.
   d. Marital role modeling, plus mutual nurturance.

4. The results and goals of achieving a balance in familial mutual respect are (select appropriate answers):
   a. Members of the family do not encroach on the rights of the other individuals in the family.
   b. No family members are expected to cater to the whims of other family members.
   c. Parents treat children as people, not "inferiors" (objects to be manipulated and dominated).
   d. Children do not develop "brat" syndrome, where they seek and receive gratification for their needs, but consider the needs, rights, and responsibilities of parents.

5. Match the four terms and/or concepts in right-hand column with definitions and descriptions in left-hand column.

Definitions/Descriptions

   a. Responsiveness of other member(s) to a family's positive feelings toward them.
   b. Empathy or role making.
   c. Sustaining force behind perception and satisfaction of family members' needs.
   d. Develops in familial relationships where there is continuity and positive interaction.
   e. Grows in intensity with time.
   f. Identification precedes it.
   g. Parents obtain referent power when this is present.
   h. Receiver's reaction to sender's affection and warmth.

Terms/Concepts

   1. Bonding or attachment
   2. Identification
   3. Crescive bonds
   4. A response bond

6. Answer briefly: What is the parental task relative to dealing with connectedness and separateness?

7. The spousal therapeutic role differs from the family affective function in that (select all appropriate answers):
   a. They do not differ; both are synonymous terms.
   b. The spousal therapeutic role deals in a subsystem rather than entire family system.
   c. The therapeutic role is largely problem focused, whereas the affective function covers therapeutic aspects and other supportive and nurturing elements.
   d. The family affective function deals only with being sensitive to family members' feelings, while the therapeutic role suggests more skilled assistance.

8. Pratt describes energized families and how they can achieve their affective function. From her description, list two salient values or priorities that energized families display relative to this area.

> ▶ **family case study**

A family case study is presented with the study questions in Chapter 17. From this family study, answer the following questions concerning the assessment of the family's affective functioning.

9. To what extent do family members perceive and meet the needs of other family members?

10. Does a mutual respect balance exist, where each member shows respect for the other's feelings and needs?

11. To what extent do family members provide mutual nurturance to each other? How supportive of each other are they?

12. Is a sense of closeness and intimacy present among the sets of relationships within the family? How compatible and affectionate are family members toward each other?

13. Does mutual identification and bonding appear to be present?

14. How does the family deal with the issues of separateness and connectedness?

15. Propose one family nursing diagnosis in the area of family affective function.

16. Recommend two family nursing interventions to resolve or ameliorate the above problem.

> ► chapter 14 study answers

1. a. Provides matrix necessary for individuals to grow and develop into healthy, functional, satisfied people.
    b. This function is central to the formation and continuity of the family unit (without this function being met, the basis for continuing as a family would become tenuous).
    c. No other societal system (institution) is sufficiently involved in fulfilling this task.

                                or

    d. Through fulfillment of this function, the family teaches growing individuals how to relate warmly and closely to others.

2. Mutual respect for needs and concerns of family members.

3. a.

4. All (a–d).

5. a. 4.
    b. 2.
    c. 1.
    d. 1, 2, and 3.
    e. 3.
    f. 1.
    g. 1 and 2.
    h. 4.

6. The parental task relative to connectedness and separateness is: (1) to provide opportunities for family and children to be together, (2) to have a sense of belonging and familial cohesiveness, and (3) identification so that the children will want to continue to be together and relate as a family. Concomitantly, the parents must provide opportunities for child to progressively have the freedom and autonomy to individuate, become self-directed, competent, and independent outside the family. The family, via parents, must achieve a satisfactory balance of separateness and connectedness, with both being present and properly emphasized.

7. b and c.

8. Values or priorities (any two):
    a. They are responsive to particular interests and needs of individual family members.
    b. They prize individuality and uniqueness.
    c. They give respect and acceptance to members unconditionally.
    d. Members are encouraged to be independent, creative, and innovative.
    e. Family emphasizes separateness more than most families do.

► family case study

Affective Area:

9. To what extent do family members perceive and meet needs of other family members? This involves an analysis of need–response patterns of family.

Family Member	Perceived Need by Parents	Extent Being Met
John (father)	Did not discuss in the vignette.	From study, no evidence that his socioemotional needs are being met; behavioral evidence is that family is not meeting his needs (avoidance behaviors—staying away and drinking excessively).
Ruby (mother)	No family recognition of her feelings of loss and depression or needs (to be able to be good parent) evidenced.	No data implying that family is meeting her needs; in fact, there is evidence that her emotional needs are not being met (physical illness, depression, and suicidal thoughts). Priscilla, her former confidant, is focused on her own needs and is unable to meet Ruby's relational needs.
Priscilla (age 13)	Parents recognize her needs to take on mother role and to be independent.	Since Ruby feels threatened by Priscilla's successful management of the younger siblings while she was gone, she is not able to positively reinforce her parenting efforts now. Neither parent encourages and/or facilitates Priscilla's separating efforts (becoming less involved with the family and more involved with her peer group).
Cindy (age 10)	None expressed.	Obviously, she likes being industrious and involved in projects and social activities outside of the home, which she is able to do. Family is not meeting this need. Her behavior, especially staying away from the home for long periods of time, may be because of the family's inability to meet her socioemotional needs. Priscilla does serve as Cindy's confidant, which provides a vehicle for meeting some of her emotional needs.

(Continued)

(Continued)

Family Member	Perceived Need by Parents	Extent Being Met
John Jr. (age 6)	Only need expressed was that Ann's leaving might threaten younger children and make them feel that if they misbehave, they may be taken away from family.	No evidence that John's socioemotional needs are being met; in fact, there is behavioral evidence (school phobia, clinging to mother, poor school work) that his needs are not being attended to adequately.
Lisa (age 4)	Parents are aware of her problem with separation anxiety and the threatening effect Ann's loss may have.	Both parents evidently spend more time with Lisa, or are planning to give her more attention. She presently has behavioral manifestations of unmet needs; clingingness, frightened when mother leaves, and enuresis, but seems to be the child that is attended to affectively by the parents.

10. *Mutual respect existent?*

There is no direct evidence concerning whether mutual respect exists, but one can infer that there is substantial insensitivity and thus very limited respect accorded to each other's needs, because there is so little perception or recognition of individual needs in the family.

11. *Mutual nurturance provided?*

Again, seems to be limited. It was twice noted that the family members did not share their feelings with each other in the face of present difficulties (this is a primary means of emotional support). Lisa seems to be comforted and nurtured more by the parents than the other family members are. Priscilla also provides nurturance to Cindy.

12. *Closeness and intimacy present among family members?*

There appear to be only three sets of relationships in the family that show these traits: between Cindy and Priscilla, Lisa and Ruby, and Lisa and John. Also, Priscilla and Ruby used to have closer relationship in past. Affectionate feelings, according to the parents, are and should be expressed only to the two younger children. The degree of compatibility is difficult to evaluate from this vignette. No open conflict is described between the children and parents except for the arguments between Priscilla and Ruby. John and Ruby show signs of incompatibility, handling it by withdrawal (John staying away and drinking, and both of them not discussing important issues). Part of lack of spousal discussion of important issues and feelings, however, may be due to social class and cultural role expectations (i.e., they do not see this as one of the expected roles in marriage).

13. *Mutual identification and bonding?*

    There is evidence that this is present: (1) spouses are staying together (although marital bonds need to be strengthened); (2) Priscilla's emulation of mother's mothering behaviors and role; and (3) separation anxiety of the two younger children when mother leaves.

14. *Issues of separateness and connectedness?*

    The information in this area is limited. However, more emphasis is placed on the togetherness aspects with Priscilla and the other children. Parents do not stress individuality and personal growth (which is more of a middle-class phenomenon and luxury).

15. Altered parenting of son John Jr. and daughter Lisa.

    Defining characteristics: children clinging to mother, show separation anxiety; John Jr.'s school phobia; the mother is anxious and depressed; the father stays away most of the time.

    Related factors: recent hospitalization of the mother; marital strain; children's psychological needs not being recognized or met; poverty; loss of Ann from the family; dysfunctional communication—avoidance of important issues.

16. Teaching: Promoting of open communication and sharing about important issues in family. Hold family conference and discuss what happened to Ann, reasons for her leaving, and that this will not happen to other children. Discuss mother's health problem—asking for members' understanding of both situations and how they feel things are working out now. Role modeling: Family nurse serves as role model to family when above issues are being discussed. Role model open communication, encouraging that each member's opinions, perceptions, and feelings be shared.

The Family Socialization Function

Marilyn M. Friedman

▶ learning objectives

1. Define and identify the tasks of socialization.
2. Explain how the family's involvement in socialization changes during the life cycle of the child-rearing family.
3. Discuss the role that culture plays in socialization patterns, particularly child-rearing practices.
4. Describe the findings of McClelland and associates relative to their study of child-rearing patterns.
5. Explain the role that social class plays in socialization and identify some broad differences in socialization of children between working-class and middle-class parents.
6. Identify several findings from socialization research.
7. Identify several important issues and/or changes in modern society that have directly affected socialization patterns.
8. Correlate the stage of child development with the stage of parent development and parent tasks according to Friedman's model.
9. Explain one's own biases regarding child-rearing practices and socialization patterns.
10. Using a hypothetical family situation:
    a. Assess the family's socialization function.
    b. Identify one family nursing diagnosis in the area of family socialization.
    c. Propose two family nursing interventions aimed at ameliorating or resolving the identified problem.

It is generally accepted that the family is more specialized in its function today than it has ever been. Nevertheless, one vital responsibility has remained a primary focus of the family: the socialization or the rearing of children. The nurse is frequently in a position to influence, support, and assist the socialization process in families. In an attempt to provide the knowledge needed for assessment and inter-ventions, this chapter defines and identifies tasks of socialization, discusses the influence of culture and social class on parenting patterns, reviews some contemporary trends and research about child-rearing, and examines socialization theory. The chapter concludes with nursing practice guidelines (assessment areas, family nursing diagnoses, and intervention).

► SOCIALIZATION: A FAMILY AFFAIR

Defining Socialization

Socialization begins at birth and ends only at death. It is a lifelong process by which individuals continually modify their behavior in response to the socially patterned circumstances they experience. It includes internalizing the appropriate sets of norms and values for the teenager of 14, the bride of 25, the parent of 29, the grandparent of 55, and the retired person of 65.

Socialization embraces all those processes in a specific community or group whereby humans, through their significant lifetime experiences, acquire socially patterned characteristics (Honigman, 1967). Translated into role terminology, the concept of socialization refers to "the process of development or change that a person undergoes as a result of social interaction and the learning of social roles" (Gegas, 1979, p. 365). The roles can be as diverse as a child learning manners, a convict "learning the ropes" in prison, or a student learning to become a nurse.

Most often, socialization proceeds informally and inexplicitly, so that changes made in response to altering cultural and environmental conditions go quite unnoticed. Through socialization, people learn to live with others in groups and come to play appropriate sex- and age-linked roles. This occurs within the larger context or process of development.

Child-rearing practices are subsumed under the rubric of socialization and are the primary focus of attention of this chapter. The terms "socialization," "socialization process," "child rearing," "parental behavior," and "parent–child interaction" are used interchangeably in both this chapter and in the child socialization literature in general (Gegas, 1979).

In the family, socialization refers to the myriad of learning experiences provided there. These experiences are aimed at teaching children how to function and assume adult roles in society. Reiss (1965) points out that the nurturant socialization of children is found universally within the nuclear family structure.

Because this function is now shared with other institutions and is influenced by many extrinsic factors, the family has a reduced, but essential, role in socialization. It is the family, particularly the parents, who transmit their cultural knowledge to the next generation. Parents are responsible for ferrying children from birth through the various developmental challenges and life events, to adulthood. However, contemporary changes in the level of shared responsibility are such that today, outside influences may conflict with and even negate the primary value system of the family. A case in point is the recent immigrant family, where the school system teaches children values and norms that contradict the non-Western values and norms the immigrant parents have and are trying to transmit to their children.

What has not changed is the fact that the family continues to have the primary responsibility of transforming an infant, in a score of years, into a social being capable of full participation in society. The child has to be taught language, the roles he or she is expected to assume at various stages of life, sociocultural norms and expectations of what is right and wrong, and relevant cognitive structures. Additionally, the child must learn appropriate sexual roles and a sense of creativity and initiative.

One aspect of the socialization process of particular relevance for the nurse involves the child's acquisition of health concepts, attitudes, and behaviors. Typically, the mother is the family's primary health educator and leader. She has the responsibility for deciding who is sick, whether or not to initiate treatment, and what kind it should be. She is also responsible for teaching her children basic health habits and attitudes and, as they grow older, how to care for themselves.

Another important and integral task of socialization is the inculcation of controls and values—giving the growing child (and adult) a sense of what is right and wrong and the internal controls needed for self-discipline. The development of morality has been described by Kohlberg (1970) as a developmental process similar to the stages of emotional and cognitive development of Erikson (1959) and Piaget (1971), respectively. By identifying with parental figures and being consistently reinforced both negatively and positively for their behavior, children develop a personal value system and a set of morals that is greatly influenced by the family (Baumrind, 1996).

Socialization involves learning, which entails the use of social control mechanisms such as discipline. The use of discipline as a means of socializing children includes both positive and negative sanctions.

Positive discipline encourages a person to exploit his or her resources for growth and serves as a positive reinforcer of behavior. Different societies and social classes have their own values regulating what sanctions to employ. For example, middle-class mothers in a New England town in the United States preferred incentives like praise to those of rewarding children materially with candy or prizes for being good (Honigman, 1967). Many American parents present themselves as models to their children to illustrate what they want them to be and not to be.

Negative sanctions, on the other hand, imply punishment and involve a great variety of methods. Although we know that punishment often succeeds in eliminating children's undesirable behavior, in itself it lacks direction and does not teach alternative desirable behavior.

Looking at Outcomes of Socialization and Parental Quandaries

One way to measure family success in socialization has been to evaluate the outcomes of the child-rearing process—that is, to measure child-rearing practices and then how successful or well adjusted these same children are or have turned out to be. To do this, comparative standards are used by which we measure a child's progress according to age-related standards; that is, we expect certain socialization skills will be learned at particular ages. This measure, however, is biased and inaccurate.

It is clear and notable that several other intervening variables also make a difference in child outcomes. To start with, parents share the socialization function with other important institutions: the school system, peers, other reference groups, and the wider community. Children themselves vary so greatly in their temperament and behavioral traits (Dadds, 1995; Kileen, 1995) and influence the way parents relate to them. In fact, there is a recent school of thought that suggests that the general family environment is not a very significant determinant of differences in children's outcomes, but instead, genetic influences on children's behavior are more important (Bussell & Reiss, 1993). Regardless of whether environment or heredity is most influential, both factors are indisputably sources of variation in children's behavior.

Often, even in the most dedicated and healthy families, children have trouble adjusting and learning socially approved behaviors. Woodward and associates (1978) state that parents today often feel powerless in the face of institutional interferences: "The growth of social services, health care, and public education has robbed them of their traditional roles as job trainers, teachers, nurses, and nurturers. And their control over their children's lives is threatened by the pervasive, and increasingly authoritative, influence of television, schools and peer groups" (p. 64). Lasch, in *Haven in a Heartless World* (1977), reiterates this same theme. He believes that outside institutions have robbed the family of one of its central functions, child rearing, and thus have immeasurably weakened the family's foundations. He describes the parents' quandary over child rearing and their faltering confidence in their own judgment and ability to parent.

> The family struggles to conform to an ideal of the family imposed from without. The experts agree that parents should neither tyrannize over their children nor burden them with "over-solicitous" attentions. They agree, moreover, that every action is the product of a long causal chain and that moral judgments have no place in child rearing. This proposition, central to the mental health ethic, absolves the child from moral responsibility. . . . It is not surprising that many parents seek to escape the exercise of this responsibility by avoiding confrontations with the child and by retreating from the work of discipline and character formation. (pp. 172–173)

Many parents, frightened by the prospects of perhaps damaging their children due to their own parental mistakes, have turned to "recipe books," "how to" parenting tools, and child counseling, searching for the right technique that will make them if not perfect, at least adequate parents. It is not surprising that by turning to outside counselors, parents may lose even more of their parental authority and confidence in their ability to parent.

Parents' Declining Child-centeredness and Role Overload

Some authors such as Popenoe (1995) and Lasch (1977) suggest that institutional "overseeing" of the training needs of children has resulted from parents' disenchantment with traditional family roles, as well as their waning commitment to child rearing. It is also argued that part of this decline in enthusiasm for raising children stems from the difficulties parents feel in trying to fulfill their primary roles due to increased economic and employment pressures and increased personal needs for their own development and self-expression (Elkind, 1994; Popenoe, 1995).

Most families have two working parents. A substantial number of fathers hold two jobs to make ends meet. Of the more than 15 million women in the labor force, a large number of them are heads of households (U.S. Bureau of the Census, 1988). In today's busy world even affluent and privileged parents feel overburdened and pressured by the simultaneous demands of work, achievement, information overload, parenting, and being a parent. In a recent national survey, 84 percent of parents said they are having a tough time balancing work and family responsibilities (Mehren, 1996). Feminism has made women conscious of many more options in women's lives and so has contributed to the role overload of modern women—given that they are still expected to carry out all their old roles, in addition to any new ones (Woodward, 1990). Experts tell parents to spend "quality time" and "meaningful" time with their children, but even this is difficult to squeeze in between a multiplicity of other priorities.

Elkind (1994), a noted child development educator, laments over the changes that have occurred in the post modern, contemporary family. He notes: "In the modern nuclear family [the family of the 1950s and 1960s] binding sentiments were largely child-centered in the sense that they give preference to the well-being of children and required the self-sacrifice of parents. In the post modern permeable [contemporary] family, however, the sentimental ties have been transformed and are now more likely to be adult centered to the extent that they favor the well-being of parents and adults and require self-sacrifice from the young" (p. 38). Elkind (1994) states that the pendulum has swung in favor of fulfilling adult needs and has led to a "family need imbalance," where children and youth are under greater stress than adults. Elkind asserts, "Children are under substantially greater stress because the world is a more dangerous and complicated place to grow up in, and in part, because their need to be protected, nurtured, and guided has been neglected" (p. 201).

Green (1994) and his co-authors in the influential book, *Bright Futures: Guidelines for Health Supervision of Infants, Children and Adolescents*, reiterate Elkind's concerns about children when they state that children face new and troubling issues today due to major economic, social, and demographic changes affecting families. As part of these pressures, parents spend less time with their children and there is less contact between children and extended family members, increased geographical mobility, a shortage of quality day-care services, diminished neighborhood involvement, and widespread family restructuring of relationships.

Changes in traditional socialization patterns, responsibilities, and time-honored methods are now occurring at a greater rate than ever before. The dilemma of who will teach children important sociocultural traditions, how and where these are to be learned, and at what age and stage, are the questions we have struggled with in the past and will continue to debate into the future.

► SOCIETAL ATTITUDES TOWARD CHILDREN

No matter which society we observe, the attitudes and approaches to the care and rearing of children are congruent with the social, moral, religious, and economic values of that society at a particular period of time. Over time, the place of children in our society has changed. Extraordinary gains have been made in the understanding and care of children. But along with such advances, new social and economic pressures and realities have introduced other attitudes and concerns.

Goodman's observations in 1978 of these events suggest that we are witnessing warnings that something is changing in the most basic relationship in any society: the relationship between its adults and its children, between its present and its future. Goodman commented on the reemergence of a hostile relationship between adults and children, and expressed a concern for the untoward effects of this generational conflict:

> Now, increasingly, parenthood is regarded as a personal, individual decision—a "lifestyle," whatever that may be—made apart from community

interests. Kids are listed not as economic assets, but as financial liabilities. Each year, someone tallies up the cost of raising them as if they were sides of beef. And each year, someone else tallies up their cost to the local town or city and wonders if they are worth it. In many places, the voters are saying "no."(p. E1).

Child development experts mirror Goodman's concern about societal attitudes toward children. Elkind (1994), a child development expert, says that there are times in history when children fare better than others. But there is no question about it: Children are not well cared for in our society today. Child advocacy organizations cite statistics that show the declining lot of children, e.g., increased poverty, infant mortality, delinquency, teen pregnancy, and child abuse (Children's Defense Fund, 1995).

The professional advice given to parents may be a reflection of the child's changing status in a particular time in society. When one examines the shifts in the advice given to parents over the past 60 years, the fluctuating philosophies and anxieties of a highly industrialized and technological society appear evident. Elkind (1994) and Osborne (1995) note these changes in child-rearing advice across the decades.

- 1910s and 1920s: Spank them, deprive them.
- 1930s and 1940s: Ignore them, reason with them.
- 1950s and 1960s: Love them and spank them lovingly.
- 1970s: Use firmness with love.
- 1980s and 1990s: Apply parenting "techniques" advocated by parenting experts.

Elkind (1994), Osborne (1995), and others have observed a shift from an emphasis on the nurturing aspects of parenting pervasive in the previous three decades to an emphasis on using scientifically based "parenting techniques," which are more democratic and encourage mutual communication, but are also more structured and rule oriented.

With continual changes in the advice parents get on how to parent, perhaps the old folk proverb sums up many parents' thoughts today: "Once I had six theories and no children. Now I have six children and no theories."

An examination of the various historic and contemporary attitudes and approaches to children illuminates the obvious; children have always generated an "air of ambivalence" that permeates society and influences its values and beliefs in the care and rearing of its young. Certainly the ambivalence that exists regarding children extends throughout society. The increased use of drugs and alcohol among school-age children and adolescents, along with their myriad of other health and social problems, only increases this feeling of ambivalence. Still, in the middle of conflicting values and beliefs about children and their place in society, an attempt is also being made to adapt to such ambivalence, change, and conflict by emphasizing the importance of the family in child rearing and "revaluing" the parent–child dyad relationships.

▶ SOCIALIZATION IN A CHANGING WORLD

A real need exists to assess the changes that have occurred in the environment, particularly the family and its impact on child rearing. Single-parent families, father as primary caretaker, working mothers, families immigrating to a new country and culture, and a host of other social changes have given rise to many concerns and calls for a dynamic and flexible approach to our traditional notions of socialization.

We do not yet know the long-term effects of these new social relationships and arrangements, although there have been studies which examined child outcomes in different family forms (see Chap. 1). We cannot say with certainty what the impact will be of increased equity in parenting roles, reassignment of traditional male–female parenting practices, fragmentation of the family into single-parent–child units with the possibility of several nuclear configurations, or realignment of traditional cultural values with those of new host cultures. These changes suggest issues that we will inevitably face in caring for today's children and the emerging families of the future.

Changing Socialization Methods

Methods of child rearing have changed drastically over the decades (Table 15–1). In the 1920s, influenced by Watson, a behaviorist, firm, controlled child-rearing practices were in vogue. In the 1960s

▲ TABLE 15-1

CHANGING CHILD-REARING VIEWS AND PRACTICES

From one generation to the next, parents and pediatricians have altered the way they feed, teach, and discipline their children. Some examples across the decades:

1900s–1910s	1920s–1930s	1940s–1950s	1960s–1970s	1980s	1990s
			Breast-feeding		
Nursing popular although many well-to-do women used wetnurses.	Commercially prepared formulas popular as a convenient and progressive way of nourishing infants.		A return to nursing promoted by women's groups and pediatricians as healthier and providing more nurturance.	Nursing overwhelmingly preferred by middle-class white women, less popular with African-Americans and Latinas.	Nursing preferred by middle-class white women, while less popular among Latinas and African-Americans.
			Thumb-sucking		
Attitudes not uniform, although often discouraged.	Prohibited by most parents and physicians.	Allowed along with pacifiers.	Encouraged, along with pacifiers.	Offered, along with pacifiers but neither discouraged nor encouraged.	Offered to children until a certain age, when they are taken away to prevent orthodontic, overbite problems.
			Potty Training		
Enemas and bowel irrigation popular methods of "cleaning" babies.	Begun as early as 2 months of age.	Delayed until 6 to 18 months.		Child determines time to begin, usually between ages 2 and 3.	May be "hurried" because of need for mother to place child in child-care center where children need to be potty trained.
			Discipline		
Children expected to act like small adults.	Strict and early discipline advocated.	Common sense and nurturance urged.	Permissive era of child rearing.	Moderate discipline that is age appropriate.	
			Learning		
Moral training began early.	Nursery schools proliferated as early education became popular.		Early reading advocated along with early training for disadvantaged children.	"Super babies" urged to be treated normally; day care increasingly becomes a national issue.	Providing many avenues for learning and stimulation. Older children are seen as competent and less in need of guidance and protection.

Partially adapted from Elkind (1994), Rock (1988).

and 1970s there was a return to a permissive, more relaxed way of child rearing. In the 1990s more democratic strategies characterized by a combination of rational control, mutual communication, and high levels of affection are in vogue (Bodman & Peterson, 1995). But what child-care experts are saying is that parents are worried, confused, and uncertain. Parents dash to work and hand their children to a variety of relatives, nannies, sitters, nursery and elementary schools, day-care centers, neighbors, and recreational, social, and religious organizations for after-school and weekend activities (Elmer-Dewitt, 1990). They are *not* raising children the way they were raised and they have little idea of how their children will turn out (Elmer-Dewitt, 1990).

Changing Gender Roles in Child Rearing.
Research on gender roles in child rearing demonstrates modest changes in child-care roles of parents, less, however, than one would hope for given the proportion of women who work outside the home. In middle-class families, there has definitely been more father involvement in child-care activities, particularly when children are older (Thompson & Walker, 1991). Mothers, however, are the primary caregivers through the preschool years of children's lives. Regardless of children's ages, mothers are typically more involved in the daily lives of their children. Fathers tend to take a "helping" or "assistive" role in child care.

In working-class families, gender roles in child care usually follow the traditional pattern. Men and women tend to have segregated roles where wives are responsible for home and family, including child care, and husbands are the primary breadwinners (Hughes & Perry-Jenkins, 1996). According to Hughes and Perry-Jenkins (1996), these wives place very little responsibility on their husbands for the child care and support of their children.

Relative to father involvement there appear to be two divergent trends, despite the above research findings. On the one hand, more and more fathers are getting involved either by choice or because of necessity (both working parents, job loss, single fatherhood, etc.). On the other hand, the absence of fathers, seen in the rise in mother-headed families with absolutely no father involvement, is reaching epidemic proportions (Stolberg, 1996b). Father participation (or a father substitute) is critically needed for positive child outcomes (Snarey, 1993).

More Androgynous Socialization.
Discontinuity with prior practices is evident in many aspects of child rearing. But perhaps the one change that has the most profound impact on socialization patterns is that of sex-role behavior and expectations. Masculine and feminine adult roles are changing in families, especially among the middle class, and as they change, so do the socialization experiences of children. Because motherhood has come to occupy a less significant aspect of many women's adult life and because there are so many married women working, socialization practices are changing. There are fewer sex-based differences in socialization patterns (Hoffman, 1977; Scanzoni & Szinovacz, 1980).

Most parents today are being encouraged to socialize their children in a more androgynous fashion, that is, not as identified with a specific gender. Previous values supporting traditional masculine and feminine roles are still alive in working-class families, however, creating a diversity of child-rearing patterns in American society.

There is a question as to whether the push for a "unisex" upbringing may not also cause some problems in later life. Whatever the ultimate adaptive value of unisex childrearing, our children may be getting inappropriate preparation for a sexist adult world that still remains sexist (Johnston & Sarty, 1977).

Pushing the Child to Achieve.
Another change that seems to be widespread because of the preponderance of married women working today is the phenomenon called the "hurried child." Child development experts believe that today's child is being pushed to act like an adult long before he or she is developmentally ready to do so. Many middle-class parents have the tendency to push their children to overachieve, to become "super babies" or "super kids" (Roack, 1988). Children are being pressured to read before kindergarten and are left unsupervised after school. Some hurried children develop into "harried teens," expected not only to achieve in school but to shop, cook, and care for the family as well (Libman, 1988).

Extending Adolescence.
A seemingly conflicting trend with the hurried child is the trend of extended adolescence. Increasing numbers of young adults are taking longer to get their degree, longer to establish a career, longer to leave home and become

Working Mothers

- In 1985 nearly half of the mothers of preschool children (under 6 years of age) were in the labor force, an increase of 75% since 1970.

- Although mothers of older children are more likely to be in the workforce, between 1970 and 1985 the greatest increase in workforce participation has been by mothers of children under 6 years of age.

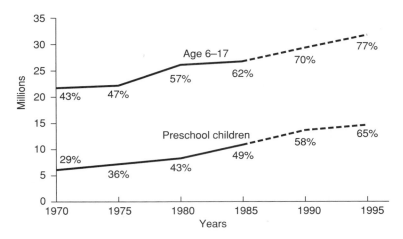

Figure 15–1. Children with mothers in the work force. *(Hofferth & Phillips, 1987.)*

independent, and longer to get married. Many more young adults are living at home after they graduate from school or are cohabitating so as to avoid commitment. With the unprecedented rise in cohabitation 50 percent of all men and women in their 30s lived together before marriage (Woodward, 1990). Premarital sex and part-time employment (they are not related) at minimum wage during high school have also risen sharply. Only about 11 percent of adolescents in school save rather than spend their earnings from part-time employment. These changes reflect a change in values—values adults put in place: consumerism, narcissism, and instant gratification (Woodward, 1990). These values are learned through role modeling and other socialization experiences in and outside of the home.

Redefining Discipline. Some of the most frequently used disciplinary practices of the past are being redefined as "unacceptable," "ill advised," or even detrimental. Physical punishment, from spanking to more severe punitiveness, is being redefined as child abuse by some researchers of child abuse (Gelles, 1990; Steinmetz, 1995). Inasmuch as disciplinary strategies are culturally derived, the cultural context of the family must always be evaluated when assessing families' ways of disciplining children.

The Child Day-care Issue

Day care is the top priority issue for working parents. The proportion of women working who have children continues to rise (Fig. 15–1). Rapid growth in women's participation in the work force means a concomitant growth in child care for preschool through school-age children (after-school programs for those in school). Figure 15–2 shows the growth in day-care programs.

Many of today's working parents are forced to decide who can assist them in terms of day care. Just at the time when mother–child attachments are seen as critical, most mothers are having to deal with the need for day care. Child-care arrangements are one of the major worries and challenges for working parents (Kelleher, 1996). Child care is usually expensive and when it can be afforded, accessibility and quality are often inadequate (Dickinson & Leming, 1995).

Mothers and some social scientists share the concern that day care is ultimately not as good for the child as the mother's care. For instance, Levine (1988) argues that there is compelling evidence that "day-care" children suffer more from diseases and emotional problems (separation anxiety) than children who remain at home with mother, and are poorly socialized when they are sent to day care too soon or for too long. Kagan (1978) disagrees, pointing out that in the studies he reviewed there were no differences in child outcomes between those children staying home with mother and those regularly participating in child care.

Hofferth and Phillips (1987) reported their own evaluation of the research on employment of the mother. They found that employment of the mother has no consistent positive or negative impact on the child. A growing body of research indicates that children of satisfied working mothers tend to do well.

The children demonstrate positive adaptation, self-esteem, and self-aspirations (*Los Angeles Times* Editorial, 1996). These research findings have clearly had a major impact on reassuring working mothers that it is all right to work.

A large number of school-age children go home alone after school, almost 15 percent according to one national survey (Kelleher, 1996). For a great majority of children their "self-care" works out satisfactorily. But for some, it does not. For these children, supervision or after-school programs are needed. After-school hours are a very important and formative part of a child's day.

Legislation Affecting Child Care and Children

The issues surrounding legislation and children are perhaps the least remembered but the most influential in terms of their impact on child rearing. There have been dramatic changes in this century in the laws concerning child care and protection, as well as numerous changes in the concepts of children's rights, parental rights, duties, and responsibilities.

The legal system presents a sometimes contradictory picture of our expectations of parenting. Based on earlier patriarchal patterns of family organization, the father in the past was regarded as the "natural guardian" of the child and was free to punish his child within reasonable boundaries. Loss of parents' rights over the care and discipline of their children could occur only in extreme cases when a "fit person" order was made by the court.

Our laws have evolved considerably from these earlier notions, so much so that the Children's Act of 1975 evidenced a present disenchantment with the natural family as inevitably providing the best care for the child. This change was brought about following the death of a child after being returned to her natural mother. This situation served to strengthen the rights of foster parents, as well as direct the appointment, in appropriate circumstances, of a person to act as guardian of the child or young person in order to safeguard his or her interests.

Legally, children's rights are now widely recognized by the American courts. For instance, in many states children are entitled to the protection of a

Child Care

• In 1985 over one fifth of children under 6 years of age whose mothers worked outside of the home were in day care centers.

• The largest shift in child care arrangements in the last 20 years has been away from relative and sister care toward child care at day care centers.

• Women who work full time tend to use day care centers while women who work part time are more likely to use family care homes.

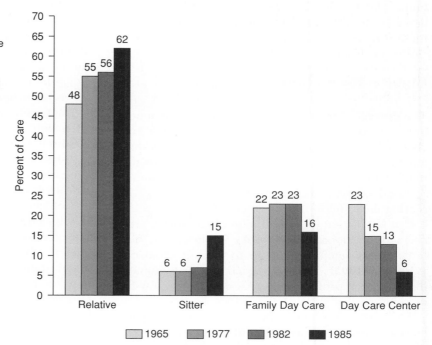

Figure 15–2. Child care arrangements of preschool children, 1965–1985. *(Hofferth & Phillips, 1987.)*

lawyer if they are accused of committing a delinquent act and have to appear in court. Greater civil rights for children make clear to parents that children are no longer considered their property and that outside authorities and agencies have the legal right to question parental actions.

In spite of this recent legislation, children are still inadequately protected in our society. The rise in child abuse is evidence of this. Since 1985 there has been a 40 percent increase in the number of reported cases of child maltreatment (Green, 1994). Baumrind (1994) believes that escalating child maltreatment is symptomatic of societal neglect of the "forgotten half" of our populace.

Another area where we do not adequately protect children is in the area of day care (Belsky, 1995). There are no minimum federal standards to protect the safety and well-being of children in day-care centers (Dickinson & Leming, 1995). And widespread noncompliance with state regulations means that the quality of child care in the United States is frequently poor to minimally adequate (Scarr, 1995).

In 1996, child advocacy groups voiced grave concern about the 1996 welfare reform legislation whereby deep cuts are being made in aid to families with dependent children. Welfare recipients with young children are being forced into the workplace; immigrant families who are not citizens are being denied welfare benefits. The rights of the children in these two types of families are not being protected (Kelleher, 1996).

Making Parenting a Science

The degree of stress and passion parents have about doing a good job raising their children has not changed over the years, but the focus of parent's anxiety has. At a time when 50 percent of all marriages fail, maintaining family life is a high-risk business. Stressed families are searching for guidelines for rearing their children (Brazelton, 1989).

Our fascination with the notion of parenting, proclaimed in a flood of handbooks, implies a new formula for a scientific recipe to raising children (Osborne, 1995). It often appears in this literature that it takes a professional to know the right way to do things.

Today's parents tend to be overwhelmed with parenting issues, as well as with conflicting advice from many sources. Pediatricians and other child-care specialists have become the grandmothers of the 1990s. The tendency for parents to rely on the judgment of others may have been carried to the extreme. "One image that repeatedly struck me," says Beckman, a child development researcher, "was a picture of a mother who hearing her child cry, rushes for the book rather than the baby" (Roack, 1988, p. A24). Another example of this trend is from an article in the *Los Angeles Times* by Dr. Joyce Brothers (1990), a psychologist, on "Testing Parenting Philosophies." Dr. Brothers asks her readers eight questions about "What does being a good parent mean?" Scientific answers are then supplied to correct any faulty information the reader might have; from this it is clear that scientific knowledge becomes the acceptable basis for Brothers' common-sense answers.

▶ THEORIES RELATED TO SOCIALIZATION

Developmental Theories

Erikson's Stage of Generativity.   The most important socialization task for parents is in establishing and guiding the next generation. Erikson's (1963) concept of generativity demonstrates an understanding of the importance of socializing for continuity. In his discussion of generativity versus stagnation, he describes the mature person's need for and dependence on the younger generation. Erikson asserts that when this stage is not fulfilled, regression to an obsessive need for pseudo-intimacy takes place, often with a pervading sense of stagnation and personal impoverishment. Bronfenbrenner (1974) embellishes on the importance of this developmental stage in his comment that we must bring adults back into the lives of children and children back into the lives of adults.

Achieving the motivation for continuity between the generations has become something of a dilemma, because it is difficult to foster the concept of continuity in a time of discontinuity and change. Past traditions, values, and social norms to many parents seem emptied of their utility for the day-to-day functioning of their families. The lack of traditions in families may have subtle, yet important, disruptive effects on the ability of parents to socialize children for continuity.

Stages of Parent Development.

In light of the array of available information on child rearing, the nurse frequently is one of the health care professionals assisting parents to sort out and understand their children's needs and their own responsibilities. In this regard, Friedman (1957), five decades ago, suggested five definitive stages through which parents progress and the appropriate child-rearing task for each period. Each stage reflects the major problems in the child's development with which the parent is grappling. These stages have been observed in a wide variety of sociocultural settings and ethnic groups, as well as in single-parent families, and the basic concept appears to be universal. The five stages of parent development are outlined in Table 15–2.

Theoretical Developments in Socialization Theories and Research

The biggest theoretical breakthrough in the area of child socialization has been the recognition that parent–child relationships are dynamic and interactive (Bodman & Peterson, 1995; Broderick, 1993; Brody, 1994; Rollins & Thomas, 1979). Most research and theoretical discussion up until recently pre-sented a static unidirectional model of parent causation; that is, parents have certain child-rearing techniques, and with these they mold the behavior and attitudes of the child. This one-sided lineal perspective ignored the prior history of interaction between parent and child, as well as the specific immediate antecedent responses of the child to the parents. This "social mold" theory blamed the mother for the child's later problems. Chess (1983), a well-known child development researcher, explains:

> Although the mother's role in child development is significant, development proceeds through a series of interactions with many others, including the father, siblings, teachers and peers. Other factors that influence child development include individual neuro-chemical, genetic and temperamental characteristics of the child. The point, then, that no one factor is overriding makes linear unidimensional models of child development obsolete. (p. 6)

It is crucial that family nurses be aware of the influence that the children's characteristics can have on families and vice versa (Dadds, 1995). Today, using a systems circular causation model, where feedback loops exist, children are viewed as active organisms who contribute significantly to the nature and course of the evolving parent–child relationship. Children are viewed as shaping parents'

► TABLE 15–2

STAGES OF PARENT DEVELOPMENT

Stage of Child Development	Stage of Parent Development	Parental Task
I. Infant	Learning the cues.	To interpret infant needs.
II. Toddler	Learning to accept growth and development.	To accept some control while maintaining necessary limits.
III. Preschooler	Learning to separate.	To allow independent development while modeling necessary standards.
IV. School-ager	Learning to accept rejection without deserting.	To be there when needed without intruding unnecessarily.
V. Teenager	Learning to build a new life—having been thoroughly discredited by one's teenager.	To adjust to changing family roles and relationships during and after the teenager's struggle to establish an identity.

Adapted from Friedman (1957).

behavior and parents as shaping children's behavior. For successful parenting to occur, there needs to be a "goodness of fit" between the child and his or her environment (the expectations and demands of caregivers are consonant with the child's skills and potentials) (Chess, 1983).

▶ CHILD-REARING RESEARCH

It has been years now since Sears and associates (1957) completed one of the most thorough studies of child rearing ever done in the United States. They were particularly interested in how a mother handled a range of developmental problems. Did she cope with these problems by physical punishment, by withdrawing her love, or by depriving her child of privileges? Perhaps more importantly, they began to probe the crucial question in socialization: Did the way the mother treated the child really make a difference in adulthood? What was the impact of whether or not the mother punished, rejected, or smothered her child with love?

Despite all the attention given to these questions over the past years, and the multitude of subsequent child socialization studies, many of these complex questions remain unanswered today, although some empirical generalizations can certainly be made.

There has been an extensive amount of research in the area of parent–child socialization, although the cultural variable was largely ignored in the past and the social class variable was not disentangled from the cultural variable. Earlier research studies based their investigations on social mold conceptualizations, while later research has emphasized bidirectional systemic models (the preceding theories section explains the difference between the two theoretical positions) (Peterson & Rollins, 1987).

Parental Support

Parental support is one of the most robust factors associated with positive child outcomes (Gecas & Seff, 1991). Rollins and Thomas (1979), in an in-depth review and analysis of child-rearing research, which has primarily studied white parents and children, state that there is sufficient empirical evidence to support the following propositions about the effects of parental support.

1. Especially for boys, the greater the supportive behavior of parents toward children, the greater such culturally valued child behaviors as self-esteem, academic achievement, creativity, and conformity.

2. In most instances, a positive relationship is found between parental support and cognitive development in children.

3. The greater the parental support, the greater the moral behavior of children and conformity to adult standards.

4. The greater the parental support, the greater the self-esteem, internal locus of control, and instrumental competence in children.

In summary, parental support was consistently found to have a positive association with all aspects of social competence in children, with the exception of creativity. Here a curvilinear relationship was revealed. Creativity increases in conditions of low to moderate parental support and decreases in moderate to high parental supportive conditions. Creativity also decreases as parental coercion increases.

Parental Control

Different styles of parental control have been found to have opposite socialization consequences (Gecas & Seff, 1991). This was demonstrated in research by Baumrind (1978). Baumrind, based on her research, classifies parental styles of discipline and control into indulgent-permissive, authoritative, and authoritarian. The permissive parental style is characterized by being accepting and nonpunitive in dealing with the child's behaviors. In contrast, the authoritarian style of discipline and control stresses obedience to rules and parents' authority. Control is based on force, threat, or physical punishment. Finally, the authoritative style of discipline and control stresses a rational, issue-oriented, "give-and-take" way of dealing with the child. Control is based on reason and explanation. Authoritarian and indulgent permissive styles are associated with negative or unfavorable socialization outcomes, while authoritative control has positive socialization outcomes. Hence, of the three styles, Baumrind (1978) advocates the third, asserting that it can produce reasonable conformity without loss of autonomy or self-assertiveness.

Epstein and associates (1982, 1993), who studied normal and troubled families over the last 30 years, report additional findings in the area of parental control, which they term "behavior control." They discovered that a flexible behavior control style, where there were reasonable standards and an opportunity for negotiation and change, was the most effective control style. This style is more likely to be present in normally functioning families. In contrast, a chaotic, unpredictable behavior control style was the least effective and found most frequently in dysfunctional families.

Parental Support and Control

The most powerful models explaining effective parenting are those combining parental support and control. Parents have been found to be most effective when they combine a high level of support with authoritative control (Gecas & Seff, 1991).

Parental Affection and Warmth

Several psychologists (McClelland et al., 1978) have argued that parents have very little control over the formation of their child's personality and character and contend that most adult behavior is not determined by specific techniques of child rearing in the first 5 years. They suggest instead that the way parents *feel* about their children matters.

In their study of child rearing, McClelland and colleagues (1978) found that when parents, particularly mothers, "really" love their children, the children were likely to achieve the highest levels of social and moral maturity. The other dimension that was significant for later social adaptation was how strictly the parents controlled their children's expressive behavior. A child was less apt to become socially and morally mature when his parents tolerated no noise, mess, or rough-housing in the home, and when the parents reacted unkindly to the child's aggressiveness toward them, to his or her sex play, or to expressions of dependency needs. Moreover, when parents were concerned with using their power to maintain an adult-centered home,

the child was not as likely to become a mature adult. All in all, it appears that mothers' affection and warmth is a crucial determinant of adult social and moral maturity. Physical punishment by parents was not significantly related to any of the outcomes examined in the study by McClelland and his associates (1978).

Marital Conflict

The presence of interspousal conflict has been found to have a negative effect on parenting and child outcomes. In this area, spouses' ability to handle disagreements constructively and communicate clearly is shown to contribute to children's well-being. The interconnections between marital conflict, troubled parenting, and problems in children tend to persist from toddler through adolescent periods (Gable, Ernic, & Belsky, 1994).

Family Size

One last focus of research has addressed the influence of family size on child-rearing patterns and child outcomes. There is strong research evidence to suggest that small and large families constitute qualitatively different developmental and child-rearing experiences. Children from small families tend to receive more attention than children from large families. Research has linked these differences to intellectual development and school performance (Feiring & Lewis, 1984).

▶ INFLUENCE OF CULTURE ON CHILD REARING

The context in which child rearing and socialization patterns occur was identified by the cultural anthropologist Kardiner (1945). He stated:

1. Techniques which the members of any society employ in the care and rearing of children are culturally patterned and will tend to be similar, although never identical, for various families within the society.
2. Culturally patterned techniques for the care and rearing of children differ from one society to another. (p. vi)

Parents from different ethnic backgrounds use child-rearing techniques that are derived from their unique set of cultural values and role expectations. They draw their parenting practices from the culture(s) with which they identify. Because the process of child rearing is cross-culturally so intricate, social scientists have specialized in studying different age groups and different cultures, with some researchers conducting longitudinal studies. Work in this area has revealed that despite individual variation, children demonstrate patterned behavior that is linked to the culturally patterned behavior of their caretakers.

Cultural factors in socialization are exceedingly difficult to disentangle from environmental, social, and psychological considerations (Julian, McKenry, & McKelvey, 1994). In fact, the relative influence of each is often a matter of conjecture and speculation. Over the years, however, specific cultural responses have been studied and have added to our understanding of the variety of socialization patterns among various ethnic and culturally divergent groups. One serious limitation of research which focuses on parents' child-rearing practices is that the samples are primarily mothers. Research has focused on maternal parenting, not parental parenting. Research about paternal involvement in child rearing is very lacking (Julian, McKenry, & McKelvey, 1994).

Cross-Cultural Comparisons

Caudill's comparative research (1975) of middle-class families in Japan and the United States is one example of comparative studies of infant caregiving. Caudill found that mothers in the two cultures engage in subtly different styles of caretaking that have, however, strikingly different effects. Generally, the American mother seems to encourage her baby to be active and respond vocally, whereas the Japanese mother acts in ways that she believes soothes and quiets her child. By the age of 3 to 4 months, the infants of both cultures seem to have already learned responses appropriate to these different patterns. The striking discovery is that the responses of the infants are in line with certain broad expectations for behavior in the two cultures: in America the expectation that individuals should be physically and verbally assertive, and in Japan that individuals should be physically and verbally restrained.

In middle-class America, the mothers perceive their babies as separate and autonomous beings who are expected to learn to do and think for themselves. The baby is seen as a distinct personality with his or her own needs and desires, which the mother must learn to recognize and care for. She does this by helping her infant learn to express these needs through her emphasis on vocal communication; the baby can thus "tell" her what he or she wants so that the mother can respond appropriately. In contrast, the Japanese mother views her baby much more as an extension of herself; psychologically the boundaries between mother and infant are blurred. As a result of this emphasis on close attachment, the mother is likely to feel that she knows what is best for the baby. There is then no perceived need for the infant to tell the mother what he or she wants. Because of this orientation, the Japanese mother does not place much importance on vocal communication and instead stresses physical contact.

It is not clear in this study what social class the Japanese mothers are from, which is another variable to consider when looking at differences. In cross-class studies of infants in the United States, researchers have often found that middle-class mothers talk more to their infants than mothers in lower socioeconomic groups. Therefore, differences found in this and other cross-cultural studies may possibly be due to differences in social class or the combination of social class and culture.

In looking at the influence of ethnicity in African-American compared to white parents, parental socialization practices of African-American parents mirror those of the wider community. Nevertheless, there is one added dimension to child rearing which is present in African-American families. Because of a history of persistent racial prejudice and discrimination, explicit racial socialization (i.e., teaching of coping skills for survival in a prejudiced society) is clearly a distinctive feature of child rearing (Taylor et al., 1990). A stricter parenting style is believed to be necessary to develop the coping abilities to deal with racism and discrimination. This is buttressed with extensive parental support and open communication.

Lin and Fu (1990) in comparing Euro-Americans' to Chinese-Americans' parenting patterns, discovered that Chinese-Americans exert more parental control and discipline. Chinese-American parents tend to be more achievement oriented and demand more self-control and self-discipline in their children. Parents' demands and control are mixed with devoted sacrifice on the part of the mother, who remains supportive and physically close to the child. This authoritarian child-rearing pattern might seen undesirable from a Western perspective, but to the Chinese culture, this child-rearing pattern is felt to lead to high achievement in their children (Baumrind, 1996).

One interesting cultural difference in childhood training has to do with *modesty*. In the United States in comparison with many other parts of the world, we place an emphasis on modesty. Immediately at birth Benedict (1938) observed that:

> we waste no time in clothing the baby . . . in contrast to many societies where the child runs naked until it is ceremoniously given its skirt or its pubic sheath at adolescence. The child's training fits it precisely for adult convention. (p. 161)

We are rarely aware of how deep and with what precision feelings of modesty are embedded in our culture until we see and feel the response of medical staff and patients dealing with this issue. For example, modesty may be one of the key factors in resistance to cervical examination in cancer detection programs (Alpenfels, 1969).

Many modern parents have never been taught as children how to care for infants and other small children. In contrast, Whiting (1974) notes that in traditional societies where women have important roles in the subsistence economy, children are required to act as nurses to their younger siblings. In all the agricultural societies she studied, mothers designate a child, usually between 7 and 8 years of age, to be their assistant.

Mothers in these same subsistence cultures need to be freed to return to work in the fields, and therefore believe that 7- or 8-year-old children can be trained to be capable caretakers for younger children. In Navajo society children are required to assume child-care responsibilities as soon as they are able, starting with "herding" other children as early as age 3 (Phillips & Lobar, 1990).

These examples indicate the need for a cross-cultural approach to our understanding of families and their child-rearing patterns. Ho (1987), a family therapist, believes that a cross-cultural perspective is crucial in working with families. One unique strength characteristic of all ethnic minorities is the involvement of the extended family in the rearing and guidance of children (Ho, 1987).

Within cultural groups it also needs to be noted that considerable intra-ethnic variation exists. For example, Martinez (1988) conducted a descriptive study of Mexican-American families. She found that mothers' child-rearing patterns varied considerably, with most mothers using authoritarian or authoritative child-rearing techniques.

The role of the father varies widely in child rearing from culture to culture, even though these roles are socially and culturally defined (Lamb, 1987). In traditional Asian, Islamic, and Hispanic families, the father's role in child care and socialization is de-emphasized. He disciplines and controls the children, while the mother provides nurturance and support, as well as takes care of children's day to day needs (Erickson & Gegas, 1991; Ho, 1987). In traditional Native American society, the father is responsible for teaching his children, particularly his sons when they are older, and for acting as a role model. The ultimate power and authority is vested, however, not in the mother or father, but in the community as a whole (Phillips & Lobar, 1990; Mirandé, 1991).

▶ INFLUENCE OF SOCIAL CLASS ON CHILD REARING

Although it is now well accepted that a child's socialization is influenced by the social class position of his or her family, most of us have only a superficial acquaintance with the distinctions that exist between the social classes relative to child-rearing practices. We often develop ethnocentric or stereotyped notions about the differences that exist between the poor and the middle class. It is not uncommon to find that in dealing with families in a health care setting child-rearing patterns that differ from a white middle-class standard are often seen as deviant, dysfunctional, and/or unacceptable. Most practitioners continue to evaluate families in terms of their own middle-class standards. Nurses are often bothered, uncomfortable, or shocked by behavior they perceive as careless, overdependent, aggressive, pretentious, or uninhibited. Class differences in definitions of what is considered to be good or bad child rearing, normal or abnormal, acceptable or deplorable, present possible barriers to the therapeutic relationship between the nurse and the family. "When evaluating lower class behavior we need to keep in mind that behaviors and attitudes considered maladaptive by white, middle class standards may be quite adaptive given the conditions of lower class family life" (Erickson & Gegas, 1991, p. 116).

Research dealing with social class differences in socialization style continues to show that parents from middle- and lower-class social structures, by virtue of experiencing different conditions of life, go about rearing their children with different conceptions of social reality, different aspirations, and different conceptions of what is desirable and needed.

Stemming from several reviews of child-rearing studies that examined the social class differences in parenting (Gegas, 1979; Julian et al., 1994; Peterson & Rollins, 1987), there is a consensus about the relationship between social class and child-rearing behaviors. These major empirical generalizations can be made on the basis of a number of studies:

1. Middle-class parents tend to use an authoritative, democratic parental style while lower-class parents tend to use a more authoritarian, autocratic parental style.

2. One of the most consistent results in the literature is that lower-class families rely more heavily on physical punishment as a means of disciplining and controlling the child, while middle-class parents use more psychological techniques (e.g., use of guilt or shame). Interestingly, earlier studies showed a greater difference between the lower and middle classes than later studies.

3. Findings dealing with social class differences with respect to the nature of the parent–child relationship reveal that in middle-class families a more democratic or equalitarian relationship is likely, while in lower-class families, a more authoritarian or autocratic relationship is likely.

4. Another set of findings focus on the affective dimension of the parent–child relationship—the degree of support, affection, and involvement the parent shows. Social class is found to be positively related to parental affection and involvement, indicating that the higher the social class, the more likely that parental affection and involvement will be greater.

5. There is a strong positive relationship between the parents' emphasis on independence and achievement for their children and social class, i.e., the higher the social class, the greater the parents' emphasis on independence (Bronfenbrenner, 1969).

6. Language (linguistic ability) is more highly developed in the middle-class child. Lower-class parents rely more on the use of commands and imperatives, whereas middle-class parents tend to explain the reasons for a rule or request. Middle-class parents tend to use reasoning and "psychological techniques" and tend to be more verbal in interactions with their children.

Kohn (1969, 1977) points out that child-rearing practices are related to parents' values and to their idea of what behaviors they need to instill in their children so that they will be able to successfully function as adults in the world as they see it. While the middle-class parent values and perceives that independence, achievement, and verbal ability are attributes that their children need to succeed, working- and lower-class parents value and perceive that respect and obedience to authority are behaviors needed to "make it" as adults in communities that are more dangerous and impoverished (Baumrind, 1996). Therefore, middle-class parents encourage and teach creativity, independence, self-control, and ambition more, while working-class parents encourage and teach qualities associated with respect, conformity, and obedience (Kohn, 1977; Peterson & Rollins, 1987).

▶ OTHER VARIABLES INFLUENCING CHILD REARING

Social class and culture are only two variables that influence child-rearing patterns (albeit sociocultural variables appear to explain the most variance in child-rearing practices). We should also consider that parental behavior and socialization techniques are influenced by the amount of stress and strain parents experience, parents' more idiosyncratic ways of coping and parenting, and the resources available to assist, counsel, and support them.

Age of the parents influences child-rearing practices. Teen mothers tend to be more insensitive to their children's needs and more egocentric in comparison with older mothers. A great deal of parents' child-rearing behavior also results from their own socialization experiences as children, and how they were raised by their own parents.

► SOCIALIZATION IN SINGLE-PARENT AND STEPPARENT FAMILIES

Most of the research and literature on child-rearing patterns applies to the two-parent nuclear family (with the wife working at home or outside of the home). The single-parent family and the stepparent family are two other major types of family forms that should also be addressed in terms of child-rearing patterns and outcomes, because family structure is an important factor affecting socialization.

Single-parent Families

Twenty percent of all family units in the United States are single-parent families. Of these 80 percent are mother headed and 20 percent are father headed. In 1991, 15.3 million American children (24.3 percent of all children under 18 years of age) lived with one parent only, an increase of 12.4 percent since 1970 (Fig. 15–3). The growth of single-parent families is due primarily to a high rate of divorce, the increase in births to never-married teenage mothers, and the growth of father-headed families (Bianchi, 1995; U.S. Bureau of the Census, 1993b). There is considerable difference in the proportion of single-parent families among the social classes and ethnic groups (see Chap. 1 for further detail).

Child rearing among single parents is difficult, especially if there are no other adult caregivers available to assist the parent. Single parents struggle against the dual demands of providing financial and emotional support for their children (Weiss, 1994). Poverty and employment of the single parent (usually the mother) add to the difficulty in child rearing (Bowen, Desimone, & McKay, 1995).

Extensive research has been conducted on the effects of the single-parent family on the children—their educational attainment, work, and income. Abundant evidence now exists that demonstrates that children from single-parent families have less success in school, lower earnings, and lower occupational prestige than children reared in intact two-parent families. This has been found even when such factors as income level of the single parent, educational attainment of the single parent, and many other background factors are controlled (Mueller & Cooper, 1986; Nock, 1988;

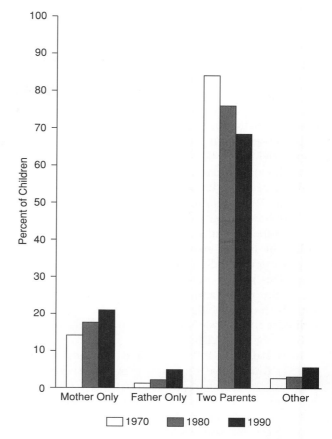

Figure 15–3. Living arrangements of American children under 18 years of age. *(From: U.S. Bureau of the Census, 1988b, 1992.)*

Popenoe, 1995). Children from mother-only families are also more likely to become single parents themselves (McLanahan & Booth, 1989). Moreover, the difficulties mother-only families have are reflected in the finding that single mothers report less satisfaction in their parenting role (Fine et al., 1986).

Stepparent Families

In the stepparent family two of the underlying issues creating role confusion for the stepfather and resultant family disequilibrium are the issues of child rearing and disciplining of children. Each parent draws on his or her own family background when defining child-rearing beliefs, practices, and discipline. Child-rearing practices are quite diverse from family to family, and once set are difficult to change, because they are not objectively based. When parents enter into a relationship in which the stepfather heads the household, but is not really the parent, agreement about child-rearing rules is problematic. Furthermore, the children, through exposure to their natural parents' child-rearing practices, have developed their own behaviors and expectations of what is acceptable or unacceptable for both themselves and their parents.

In the stepparent family the stepfather has no biological rights over the children, and whatever parental rights he may have must be granted to him by his wife. This places the stepfather into a rather untenable position. When conflict arises over the disciplining of a child, the mother feels a natural right to decide the issue. If the stepfather goes ahead and disciplines the child, the mother may either directly become angry, or more often, indirectly strike back by undermining him. This latter course is particularly devastating to the entire family and often exacerbates the conflict, with the mother being torn between the loyalty to her children and to her husband (Furstenberg & Nord, 1985; Visher and Visher, 1993).

In a study of 232 remarried families, Hobart (1987) found that depending on whose children they are, children had different statuses in the family. For instance, first-class children were those born to the remarried couple, second-class children were those from the wife's previous marriage, and third-class children were those from the husband's previous marriage. Parents reported that the most positive relationships were with their shared children. Parent–child relationships varied considerably in the remarried families, and relationship problems were perceived as affecting the spousal relationship.

▶ SOCIALIZATION IN HIGH-RISK FAMILIES

There are a number of situations described in the literature that are likely to produce excessive stress on parents and families. Families under stress are high-risk families. Based on systems theory, we know that a ripple effect occurs when stress is experienced by a member or subsystem. Due to the ripple effect, the whole family system is eventually affected. Parent–child interactions and relationships are always affected to some extent, and when parent–child relationships are affected, so are parenting behaviors (child rearing).

Stressors that create high-risk families may originate in the mother (e.g., the teenage mother), the child (e.g., a child with a chronic or life-threatening illness), or the family environment (e.g., a local disaster).

Examples of high-risk situations are the following. When there is a dysfunctional marital relationship, this negatively affects the parent–child relationship. When mothers are severely disturbed, their parenting abilities are correspondingly diminished (Shapiro, 1983). When parents have seriously ill children, caregiving becomes so demanding that the child's developmental needs are often overlooked and go unmet. The seriously ill child and mother may become so enmeshed in their relationship that other children are neglected (Schor, 1995). Child rearing in both the healthy and ill siblings is thereby impeded. Parents often treat their ill or disabled children differently—as special or vulnerable. This creates particular problems when parents attempt to maintain or return to normal parenting practices.

FAMILY SOCIALIZATION FUNCTION: APPLYING THE FAMILY NURSING PROCESS

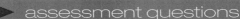

▶ assessment questions

Before discussing the assessment of family socialization patterns, it is important that you, as a family nurse, be very clear about your own biases, attitudes, and expectations that might interfere with assessing family child rearing accurately.

How do you see the way you were raised and the way the families you work with are raising their children? How reasonable are your expectations of parents? For example, is it reasonable to expect a mother of five children never to prop a bottle? In determining the appropriateness of a particular family's child-rearing methods, it is helpful to ask yourself how functional or adaptive the approach is for the particular family being assessed. Another example would be to ask yourself how much of a family's form of child rearing or discipline is culturally derived or influenced.

Related to your expectations about what child rearing should be, are your instructions and advice practical or ideal? How should you adapt your routines and nursing methods to achieve a successful outcome with a particular family?

An important issue for nurses to consider in working with parents and children is the possibility of role confusion. Taylor (1970) reminds us that most adults are protective toward children and that all adults feel some responsibility for children, particularly the very young or the ill. It is therefore difficult for most adults not to interfere when a mother or family seems to be mishandling or abusing a "defenseless" child. This natural response has tremendous survival value for the species but does pose a problem for the family nurse. In one instance, such feelings make it possible to work with families and children who are personally unattractive to the nurse, while on the other hand such feelings make it difficult to remain detached enough to function in a professional capacity.

Because families have diverse sociocultural backgrounds, some families will have child-rearing styles that the nurse has been conditioned, socialized, and taught to recognize as "good" and some as "bad." Most health care specialists who deal with the pediatric client tend to assume that the parents are somehow at fault when a child acts in a "socially unacceptable way" or is sick. This covert attitude is a poor one, making it difficult for the nurse to sustain an objective and effective role. Although the nurse often does things for his or her clients that a mother does for a child, it is tremendously important for the nurse to remember the public and social capacity of the nursing role, and avoid replacing the mother or displacing one's own childhood frustrations on the mother by blaming her for the child's condition. The nurse's ability to support the parents without becoming a surrogate for them is critical for the child, as well as for the self-esteem and potential growth of the parents.

In your assessment of families, the following questions will provide useful data from which to identify potential or actual problems and plan care accordingly.

1. What are the family's child-rearing practices in the following areas?
   a. Behavior control, including discipline, reward, and punishment.
   b. Autonomy and dependency.
   c. Giving and receiving of love.
   d. Training for age-appropriate behavior (social, physical, emotional, language, and intellectual development).

2. How adaptive are the family's child-rearing practices for their particular family form and situation?

3. Who assumes responsibility for the child-care role or socialization function? Is it shared? If so, how is this managed?

4. How are children regarded in the family?

5. What cultural beliefs influence the family's child-rearing patterns?

6. How do social class factors influence child-rearing patterns?

7. Is this a family that is at high risk for child-rearing problems? If so, what factors place the family at risk?

8. Is the home environment adequate for children's needs to play (appropriate to children's developmental stage)? Is there age-appropriate play equipment/toys in the home?

▶ FAMILY NURSING DIAGNOSES

Observing family strengths and problems within the area of a family socialization is very common for family nurses working in schools, pediatrics, community health, family primary care, and mental health, making actual and potential family nursing diagnoses within this area most germane. Family strengths may be covered under "potential" family nursing diagnoses or may be stated as strengths, eliminating the use of family nursing diagnoses. Recalling that the family socialization function covers child rearing, parent–child relationships, and parental behavior, the area is quite broad.

As with the other family dimensions, North American Nursing Diagnosis Association (NANDA) diagnoses were reviewed to identify which diagnoses appear to incorporate actual and potential family socialization problems. Below is a list of the NANDA diagnoses, as described by McFarland and McFarlane (1993), which are appropriate either as the diagnosis or as the outcome or consequence of a problem in this area; in the latter case it could be listed as a defining characteristic.

Nursing Diagnoses

- Altered family processes
- Health-seeking behaviors (health-promotion diagnosis)
- Knowledge deficit
- Parental role conflict
- Altered parenting
- Potential altered parenting

Possible Outcomes of Socialization Problem (Possible Defining Characteristic)

- Altered growth and development
- Altered health maintenance
- Self-care deficit
- Knowledge deficit
- Low self-esteem
- Social isolation
- Impaired social interactions
- Potential for violence
- Noncompliance
- Personal identity disturbance

Two NANDA nursing diagnoses that appear to be directly related to a family socialization problem are Altered Family Processes and Altered Parenting (actual and potential). Altered Family Processes is a more general family nursing diagnosis, but can be used when specific defining characteristics are included. Defining characteristics that McFarland and McFarlane (1993) list are:

- Parents do not demonstrate respect for each other's child-rearing practices.
- Rigidity in function and roles.
- Family does not demonstrate respect for individuality and autonomy of its members.
- Inappropriate or inconsistent family roles.

The other nursing diagnosis, which is more specific to child-rearing problems, is Altered Parenting (actual or potential). The defining characteristics of this diagnosis directly apply to the areas subsumed under family socialization. Table 15–3 is included in

► TABLE 15-3

ALTERED PARENTING (NANDA) NURSING DIAGNOSIS

■ **DEFINING CHARACTERISTICS**

- Lack of parental attachment behaviors.
- Inattention to infant/child needs.
- Inappropriate caretaking behaviors (e.g., feeding, sleep and rest, elimination patterns, clothing, shelter, safety).
- Physical or psychological abuse.
- Abandonment.
- Inappropriate visual, tactile, or auditory stimulation of the child.
- Frequent verbalizations of dissatisfaction or disappointment with the child.
- Frequent identification of negative characteristics of the child.
- Frequent attachment of negative meanings to characteristics or behavior of the child.
- Verbalization of resentment toward child.
- Verbalization of frustration with parenting role or role inadequacy.
- Inappropriate or inconsistent discipline.
- Growth and developmental lag in the child.
- Frequent accidents or illnesses of the child.
- Signs of depression, apathy, disturbed, or bizarre behavior in the child.
- Rejection of caregiver or overcompliance by the child.

■ **RELATED FACTORS**

- Families in which either parent is absent or unable to function because of physical or emotional illness.
- Families in which either parent is unable or unwilling to assume parenting responsibilities.
- Families in which the child is unwanted, displays undesired characteristics, or is physically or emotionally ill.
- Families developmentally lacking parental skills.
- Families lacking external resources, such as contact with or support from own parents or others in the extended family, contact or support from community resources.
- Families in which the parents acknowledge a history of ineffective or abusive relationships with own parents.
- Families in which parents demonstrate a lack of knowledge, cognitive functioning, or role identity as a parent.
- Families in which one or both parents hold unrealistic expectations for self, spouse, or child.
- Families in which the role relationships appear chaotic or inappropriate among the members.
- Families experiencing crises (e.g., financial, emotional, developmental).

Source: McFarland & McFarlane (1993).

this text because this diagnosis is so appropriate here. As previously mentioned, defining characteristics and related factors should accompany the diagnosis.

Identifying parents at risk for child-rearing problems—indicating Potential Altered Parenting—is critical. To name some high-risk groups, they include parents in crisis situations or under stress; teen parents; single parents with limited financial or personal resources or inadequate social support; parents with serious physical or psychological problems; and parents who have premature infants or infants or children with serious or chronic health problems.

► FAMILY NURSING INTERVENTIONS

The Iowa Intervention Project (McCloskey & Bulechek, 1996) have developed listings and descriptions of a broad range of nursing interventions. In most cases, these interventions have been linked to NANDA nursing diagnoses. For instance, altered parenting, the NANDA diagnosis, is linked with 22 interventions (see Table 15–4). The interventions that follow are relevant to health promotional, preventive diagnoses, as well as health restorative types of diagnoses in the area of family socialization. The italicized nursing diagnoses are particularly germane to and/or focused on family socialization diagnoses.

- Child protection, child
- Active listening
- Animal-assisted therapy
- *Anticipatory guidance*
- *Attachment promotion*
- Behavior management (for overactivity/inattention, sexual)
- Behavior modification
- Behavior modification, social skills
- Coping enhancement
- Counseling
- Decision-making support

- *Developmental enhancement*
- Emotional support
- Family integrity promotion
- Family involvement
- Family mobilization
- Family process maintenance
- Family support
- Family therapy
- Infant and newborn care
- Learning facilitation
- Learning readiness enhancement
- *Normalization promotion*

- *Role enhancement*
- *Socialization enhancement*
- Support group
- *Support system enhancement*
- *Teaching (many areas)*

In addition to the broad listing of possible nursing interventions which are relevant in the family socialization area, five intervention areas are discussed more in-depth: supporting parents, making interventions socioculturally appropriate, making interventions appropriate for single-parent and step parent families, teaching and anticipatory guidance, behavior modification, and initiating refer-

---

▶ TABLE 15–4

NURSING INTERVENTIONS SUGGESTED FOR RESOLUTION OF NANDA ALTERED PARENTING NURSING DIAGNOSIS

Parenting, Altered

■ DEFINITION:

The state in which a nurturing figure(s) experiences an inability to create an environment which promotes the optimum growth and development of another human being.

■ SUGGESTED NURSING INTERVENTIONS FOR PROBLEM RESOLUTION:

Abuse protection: child	Family therapy
Anticipatory guidance	Guilt work facilitation
Anxiety reduction	Kangaroo care
Attachment promotion	Mutual goal setting
Caregiver support	Normalization promotion
Coping enhancement	Risk identification: Childbearing family
Counseling	Role enhancement
Developmental enhancement	Security enhancement
Environmental management: Attachment process	Self-esteem enhancement
Family integrity promotion	Support group
Family support	Teaching: Individual

■ ADDITIONAL OPTIONAL INTERVENTIONS:

Behavior management: Overactivity/Inattention	Parent education: Childbearing family
Childbirth preparation	Parent education: Childrearing family
Family integrity promotion: Childbearing family	Parent education: Adolescent
Family involvement	Patient contracting
Family process maintenance	Postpartal care
Health education	Prenatal care
Home maintenance assistance	Respite care
Infant care	Surveillance
Intrapartal care	Teaching: Infant care
Newborn care	

From McCloskey & Bulechek (1996), p. 653. (No part of this work may be altered without prior permission from the publisher.)

rals to parenting programs and early intervention programs.

The Primary Thrust: Supporting Parents

The primary thrust of the nurse's approach in working with families is to reinforce or support parents' natural parenting abilities. This, I believe, is the central intervention strategy for nurses working with parents in child-rearing areas. It is essentially a health-promotion focus. We must assume that all parents want to be good parents. By building up their confidence to deal with their children—who they know best—this approach will prove foundational to all the more specific ways of assisting parents.

Notwithstanding the importance of the above general approach to helping parents, specific parent education strategies are advocated. Advice, counseling, and teaching about parenting is considered to be the responsibility of pediatricians, nurses, teachers, child development specialists, and other professionals. It is not unusual to find "socialization failure" or "inadequate or altered parenting" used as fairly common diagnoses today. Often an attempt is made to involve parents in some type of parenting program in order to assist them in dealing with their children.

Making Interventions Socioculturally Appropriate

In all nursing care, assessments and interventions based on appropriate sociocultural data are important, whether counseling a mother, teaching a child, supervising a medical therapy, or coordinating community resources to resolve identified problems. In each case the nurse should focus on the relevance to the family and not on his or her own values or child-rearing techniques. For example, some families can accept and respond to instructions for improving the diet of their children if the parents are given an explanation that ties in with their own values (e.g., if the children are fed better, they will behave better and the family will be less stressed). In other families, however, having well-nourished children is valued in and of itself, and so a direct teaching approach is used.

Making Interventions Appropriate for Single-parent and Stepparent Families

Child-rearing or parenting problems are generally more problematic in these two common alternative family forms. The stressors on parents are greater than in the two-parent nuclear families, and thus the counseling and educational and referral needs are greater. For guidelines for counseling various family forms, including single-parent and remarried families as well as gay and lesbian couple families, dual-career families, and cohabiting heterosexual couple families, Goldenberg and Goldenberg, two family therapists, have written an excellent book entitled *Counseling Today's Families* (1990). For both health professionals and parents, three American Academy of Pediatrics books are quite instructive. They are: Shelov's *Caring for Your Baby and Young Child* (1991); Shelov's *Caring for Your School Age Child* (1995); and Greydanus's *Caring for Your Adolescent* (1991).

Specific Family Nursing Intervention Strategies

Teaching and Anticipatory Guidance.
Teaching strategies are suggested for helping parents struggling with becoming parents or with rearing a child in the various developmental stages or during a health/illness crisis. This also involves providing anticipatory guidance, supporting, and role modeling. Parents want information about normal developmental behavior of children. They need to understand the importance of modeling the behavior they wish children to adopt and the importance of actively listening and communicating with their children and respecting and supporting them (Schor, 1995). Parents should be referred to some of the books about children and parenting concerns if this is a way they use to gain information.

Behavior Modification.   *Behavior modification* principles are also used in helping parents with child behavior control problems. Because behavior modification is based on the premise that all behavior is learned, this intervention is likewise based on

behavioral learning principles. After gaining a baseline of a child's problematic behavior, so that the frequency of behavior and antecedents to the problem behavior are known, a structured program of reinforcements is implemented. Positive, negative, and neutral reinforcements may be used; although most behaviorists primarily recommend the use of positive reinforcement. This approach can be quite helpful if there are specific child behaviors parents want to eliminate or modify, and the parent can understand the program and have the resources to follow through with the planned, structured approach. Written contracts are developed that detail the planned intervention, so as to guide the parents and health professional (Johnson, 1986; Jones, 1980).

Initiating Referrals to Parenting Programs.

Family nurses also *initiate referrals* to parenting programs. Working closely with the schools, health and other social agencies, family nurses coordinate a variety of resources and a wealth of necessary information to assist families in coping with the complexities of raising children in a changing world of challenging expectations.

Parent education programs are very important resources for parents today. *Both* parents need parenting programs because: (1) education for parenting is typically not provided at home, and very little is included in most educational systems; (2) insufficient and conflicting guidance and many myths are provided in the general media and through parents' social support systems, causing anxiety and confusion; (3) being an effective parent is not easy, and is a vital parental role; (4) parents realize they need help and are seeking help, especially in terms of discipline; and (5) greater father involvement is needed in child rearing (Hammer & Turner, 1985; Osborne, 1995).

Hammer and Turner (1985) and Osborne (1995) have identified different approaches and types of parenting programs popular in communities today. Four of the most popular are described here. The first is Parent Effective Training (PET). This approach/program is based on humanistic psychology and stresses the importance of parent–child communication and parents' listening to and understanding the feelings of children. Gordon's book, *Parent Effectiveness Training* (1970), and the programs that use Gordon's principles

help parents gain the skills needed to be supportive to children.

The second type of program/approach uses *behavior modification* techniques to help parents deal with specific child behavioral problems. Behavioral models of parent education focus on shaping desirable behavior in their children.

The third approach/program to parent education is a life-span, developmental psychology approach. The goal of this type of program is to teach parents about children's development. Parents need to know what to expect of their children and what realistic expectations to have. Most of the very popular parenting books use this approach (i.e., Gesell, Spock, Ilg and Ames, Elkind).

The fourth approach or type of parenting program is based on family systems theory. This approach is a family counseling approach, which focuses on unhealthy relationships/dynamics in the family. It assumes that once these unhealthy interactions/relationships are mended, parents can more successfully parent.

Discipline is undoubtedly one of the prime areas about which parents seek help. Hammer and Turner (1985) and others have developed guidelines to help parents discipline more effectively (see Table 15–5).

By discussing parents' expectations of their role, the family nurse may identify sources of frustration, confusion, and gaps in information. By initiating referrals to parent education programs, conducting parent groups and client education sessions, and providing support and encouragement, parental role transition and confidence can be facilitated.

Initiating Referrals to Early Intervention Programs.

For families at risk with children with special needs and young, high-risk mothers, early intervention has become one of the cornerstones of treatment (Kang, Barnard, & Oshio, 1994; Smith, 1995). Intervention that is interdisciplinary and comprehensive is incorporated in these programs. Regional developmental centers are examples of such services. Family nurses often serve as case managers, coordinating interdisciplinary services, as monitors of the developmental progress of children, as assessors of the home and family environment, and as health educators and counselors to

► TABLE 15–5

GUIDELINES TO PARENTS ON DISCIPLINING CHILDREN

- Parents' goals in disciplining should not be punishment for wrongful actions, but rather punishment to assist children to control their behavior; develop self-discipline, optimal competence, and moral character; accept responsibility for their behavior; and consider the needs and feelings of others.
- Within a responsive and supportive parent–child relationship, prudent use of punishment is a necessary disciplinary strategy.
- Discipline works best when tailored to the individual child and the specific situation.
- Children need consistent discipline from loving parents.
- Failure to discipline can produce serious rebellion and "acting out" behavior during the adolescent period.
- Children want and need structure and limits.
- With young children, when parents decide to use punishment for a given act:
  1. The punishment should immediately follow the act.
  2. The punishment needs to be both deserved and understood.
  3. The punishment needs to be related to the act.
- Parents should remain calm and focus attention on the child's behavior (not the child himself or herself) when disciplining.
- Parents should refrain from venting their own anger at the child's expense.
- Although spanking is acceptable and normative in some cultures, its use should be carefully evaluated, as research has shown negative outcomes relative to children's later behavior. The effectiveness of spanking must be viewed within the cultural context.

From: Baumrind (1996), Dickinson & Leming (1995), Giles-Sims, Straus, & Sugarman (1995), Greydanus (1991), Hammer & Turner (1985), McCubbin & Dahl (1985).

families with respect to children's developmental and health care needs. Counseling here is directed at providing family support; it can also involve helping families obtain food stamps and other community resources and counseling parents about child rear-ing of children with special needs and disabilities (Healy et al., 1985; Kang, Barnard, & Oshio, 1994). Early intervention programs have been shown to reduce child abuse, improve behavior, and improve school performance (Smith, 1995).

► study questions

1. Which of the following is the best definition of socialization?
   a. The act of learning to relate to people.
   b. The training provided to function in a social environment.
   c. The social and psychological development of a child.
   d. Child-rearing practices.

2. The central task involved in socialization of children revolves around teaching them how to function and assume adult roles in a society. Subsumed under this main task are several more specific tasks. Name three of these.

3. American families have retained the primary responsibility for socializing their children during which life cycles of the family (select all appropriate answers):
   a. Stage of marriage.
   b. Childbearing (stage of expansion).
   c. Families with preschool children.
   d. Families with school-age children.
   e. Families with teenage children.

4. Culture plays a dominant role in socialization. Explain briefly.

5. McClelland and associates conducted a study of child-rearing patterns and their outcomes among American families. They found that (select the best answer):
   a. Strict limit setting and clear boundaries produced well-behaved, obedient children.
   b. No one approach to child rearing was superior over another approach.
   c. Parental love and acceptance was the crucial determinant in the child's acquisition of social and moral maturity.
   d. Parents have very little control over the formation of their child's personality and character.

6. Which of the following research findings are true about research in family socialization? (select all correct answers)
   a. The "social mold" theory continues to be the prominent theoretical perspective used.
   b. Parental control and parental support are two major parenting variables found to influence child outcomes.
   c. Androgynous socialization leads to later problems in child adjustment.

7. Social class is another vital variable influencing a family's socialization patterns. Social class makes a difference because (select the best answer):
   a. By virtue of experiencing different life conditions, families from various social classes have varying conceptions of social reality and what is desirable, feasible, and most important.
   b. Social class determines how parents deal with the world and their children.
   c. Being in one social class or another gives a family a limited view of the world and consequently limits its child-rearing techniques to those with which the family is familiar.

8. Research concerning social class differences in child-rearing patterns found that (answer *true* or *false*):
   a. The white-collar family stresses respect and obedience more than the blue-collar family does.
   b. Conformity and individualism are both emphasized more by middle-class families.
   c. Middle-class families rely more on reasoning and talking things over with children, while lower-class families tend to use punishment more as a way of disciplining children.

9. The attitudes and approaches to the care and rearing of children in a society (select all appropriate answers):
   a. Will be congruent with the society's dominant value system.
   b. May or may not be related to the society's dominant value system.
   c. Will be positively associated with the society's dominant value system.
   d. Will be related to the traditions but perhaps not the current values because of cultural lag.

10. Identify several important changes and/or issues affecting child rearing in our society.

11. Match the appropriate stage of parent development and parental tasks in the right-hand column with the child's stage of development in the left-hand column.

   a. Infant   1. To allow independence.
   b. Toddler   2. To accept rejection without deserting the child.
   c. Preschooler   3. Learning to build a new life for parents.
   d. School-ager   4. Learning the meaning of the cues.
   e. Teenager   5. Learning to accept child's growth and development.
                       6. Learning to master anger and frustration.

12. Self-examination of child-rearing biases: What particular beliefs and attitudes do you hold that might limit your effectiveness in working with parents and children in the area of parenting or child rearing?

► family case study

From the following family vignette assess the family's socialization function using the questions provided at the conclusion of the vignette as assessment guidelines.

Mr. and Mrs. Chin, ages 50 and 45, respectively, moved 10 years ago to San Francisco from Hong Kong. The Chins operate a small cleaners, and the family income has always been low despite the long, hard hours of work of both parents. They have four children: Harold, 23, who is at the California School of Technology studying engineering; Lee, 22, who is a registered nurse; John, 17, who is in high school and an excellent student; and Joe, 10, who is attending fifth grade. All the children (including the older ones) are always busy working. John and Joe work extremely hard on their studies, and with school work and home chores there is little time left over for playing or getting into "mischief." The parents have greatly encouraged their children to pursue higher education and academic achievement. Through their accomplishments, the Chins feel the children have brought honor to them.

During the home visit all the children were observed to be respectful of their parents' authority. In the presence of their parents, the two youngest were quiet and did not interject comments or express themselves until directly asked a question, at which time they answered quickly while looking to their mother for approval.

Mrs. Chin states that her husband is strict in child rearing and that if the two younger boys who are still living at home disobey, he administers immediate corporal punishment. Mrs. Chin relates that a misbehaving child in the Chinese community is considered "not trained," meaning that the parents are to blame; thus a child's wrongdoing brings shame and dishonor to the whole family.

When Mrs. Chin was asked how she raised her children, she related that she cuddled and fondled them a lot while they were little. But as soon as they became preschoolers she gradually withdrew her expressions of love and physical hugs and kisses. From school age on, she and her husband have pushed her children to become independent and responsible. Both parents said that they had emotionally removed themselves somewhat from their children lest their children might lose respect for them.

The parent–child relationships appear to be more restrained and formal than in most American families. However, though muted, one was still able to feel the obvious respect and caring they feel for each other.

13. Describe how the family dealt with the following areas of child rearing: discipline, rewards, punishment, moral training, autonomy, initiative, creativity, dependency, giving and receiving of love, and training for age-appropriate behavior (social, physical, emotional, language, and intellectual development).

14. How adaptive are the family's child-rearing practices for their particular situation (social class, culture, environment, etc.)?

15. Who assumes responsibility for the child-care role or socialization function? Is it shared and if so, how?

16. How are children regarded in the family?

17. What cultural beliefs are operating in their child-rearing practices?

18. Based on the brief hypothetical family situation that follows:

    • Identify a family nursing diagnosis in the area of family socialization.
    • Propose two family nursing strategies to ameliorate the problem.

Mrs. Cabrillo is in the pediatrician's office for an infant check-up. She is seen by the pediatric nurse practitioner who, after she has checked the baby, asks Mrs. Cabrillo how she is managing at home with the two children. Mrs. Cabrillo brings up the problem she is having with Mary, who refuses to go to kindergarten.

Family background: Mr. and Mrs. Cabrillo, ages 35 and 25 respectively, have a daughter, Mary, age 5½ years old and a newborn son, John, age 3 months. The daughter started kindergarten 3 months before the baby was born and went to school pretty regularly at that time. Since John has come home, however, she "is a changed little girl." She hits the baby, shouts "no" to her mother when she tries to discipline her or give her commands, refuses to dress herself to go to school, and throws temper tantrums at the breakfast table when her mother says she has to go to school. Mary is so upset and defiant that the mother can't make her go to school, and so she has been staying home with mother.

Mr. Cabrillo (John Sr.) is very impatient about the situation, because, according to his wife, he doesn't understand. "Mary is different with him. She obeys her father, who is very firm with Mary." Mr. Cabrillo works long hours during the weekdays and doesn't get very involved with the children when he is home.

The parents are both from an Italian family—the mother immigrated just before Mary was born and speaks broken English. She has never worked outside the home. John Sr. was raised in the United States and his family lives nearby. Mrs. Cabrillo is fairly socially isolated because she doesn't drive and speaks limited English. Her only friends are her husband's family, who "always take John Senior's side in discussions."

▶ chapter 15 study answers

1. b.

2. Any three:
   a. Language development.
   b. Sociocultural norms and expectations (right and wrong).
   c. Sexual roles.
   d. Individual initiative and creativity.
   e. Acquisition of health concepts, attitudes, and behaviors.

3. b and c.

4. The child-rearing techniques used in a society are culturally patterned, and hence there is a tendency for families within a particular culture to rear their children similarly. These culturally patterned techniques for child rearing differ from culture to culture, as do the ideas and beliefs about the capabilities and needs of children during their stages of growth and development. Moreover, because socialization patterns differ from one culture to the next, so will personality norms and broad expectations for personal behavior.

5. c.

6. a and b.

7. a.

8. a. False.
   b. False.
   c. True.

9. a and c.

10. Several important societal changes/issues affecting child rearing (any three):
    a. Day care for children of working mothers and their feelings of guilt about working and dissatisfaction about the facilities available.
    b. The growing number of single-parent families and how well this type of family can fulfill the socialization function.
    c. The growing number of stepparent families and the complex parenting problems this family form faces.
    d. Methods or approaches for assisting families where child abuse or neglect exists.
    e. The emphasis on "unisex" upbringing and its consequences.
    f. Conflicting information from "experts" on how to raise children.

11. a. 4.
    b. 5.
    c. 1.
    d. 2.
    e. 3.

12. Attitudes or beliefs that limit effectiveness include:
    a. Strong beliefs that orderliness, neatness, obedience, degree of restraint, or assertiveness are desirable and should be important to everyone.
    b. Rigid values and beliefs that hold that there is a "right and proper" way to raise children.
    c. Religious convictions suggesting that certain customs and techniques are "good" and others "bad" or "sinful."
    d. The belief that the mother or parents are solely responsible for their children's behavior (blaming the parents).
    e. The attitude that the family's situation is not relevant, or is less significant, whereas "what is best for the child" should be the focus (excluding consideration of the constraints of the family's environment).

13. *Discipline and punishment.* Father administers punishment; uses physical (corporal) means. Parents consider a child's wrongdoing as a reflection of the parents' failure to train their children adequately, and thus they feel threatened and disgraced by their children's misbehavior. The children certainly feel shame for the "loss of face" they have brought to the family. Hence the punishment is more than corporal, because the child being punished also feels the interpersonal sanctions of rejection, disapproval, and withdrawal of acceptance and love.
    Rewards. Parents did not express how they reward children, except that Mrs. Chin verbally expressed (in front of children?) that her children, by virtue of their achievements, brought great honor to the family. This may indicate a pattern of verbal praise and acceptance.
    Moral training. Family is highly structured and has clear boundaries as to what was right and wrong. This was instilled through careful supervision when the children were young (assumed) and by strict discipline when children were assumed old enough to take on adult behaviors (responsi-

bility, self-sufficiency). When children were young they were given much unconditional love and affection from parents.

Autonomy and dependency. Children were pushed to be autonomous and responsible from school age on; dependency would not be reinforced positively during these same stages of development.

Initiative and creativity. There was no mention of how parents handled the issues of creativity and taking initiative.

Giving and receiving of love. The mother mentioned the extensive expression of affection to children when they were young, but that from preschool age on (gradually) and especially beginning at school age, children were pushed away from parents' affectively. In fact, parents tried to remove themselves to some extent, so that they could maintain the position of respect vis-à-vis their children.

Training for age-appropriate behaviors. Little is mentioned except that social responsibility (home chores) and school achievement (intellectual development) were stressed and promoted in this family.

14. The child-rearing approach is very adaptive for this family. The parents obviously desire their children to have a better life than they have had. Through their socialization patterns they are training children to be self-sufficient, productive, success-oriented, and independent.

15. The mother may have responsibility for the everyday matters, but the father definitely has ultimate responsibility to administer sanctions for misbehavior and thus ultimate responsibility for socialization. The socialization function is seen as a prime responsibility for this family.

16. There is little data from which to draw conclusions about how children are regarded in this family, but one senses that children are highly valued and are central to the aspirations and life goals of the parents.

17. The family is not acculturated to the dominant American culture. The parents are first-generation Chinese-American; they consider themselves part of the Chinese community, and the values and child-rearing practices they describe are congruent with the traditional values of the Chinese. In describing the Chinese child-rearing practices, Sung (1967) verifies that the Chins' socialization patterns are indeed culturally patterned.

> Discipline is strict and punishment immediate in the Chinese household. . . . The Chinese child is taught that when he does wrong, it is not a personal matter between himself and his conscience; he brings disgrace and shame upon his family and loved one. . . . A Chinese baby may be cuddled and fondled, showered with kisses, and rocked to sleep in his mother's arms, but as the child grows older, the mother withdraws her expression of affection. . . . Chinese parents think they can maintain authority if they are careful to keep a certain distance from their children. . . . The father never tries to be a friend to his son, nor the mother a big sister to her daughter. . . . A parent is the authority that demands obedience, and authority must maintain its dignity. (pp. 168–171)

18. *Family nursing diagnosis:* Altered parenting (of Mary by both parents). Defining characteristics: Problem with behavior control (rules and standards change). Mary is allowed to stay home from school when she has a temper tantrum. Mary is disobedient to mother.

    - Daughter is school phobic.
    - Mary hits baby.
    - Mother lacks confidence in parenting Mary.
    - Father is impatient about problem with Mary.

    Related factors

    - Father is relatively uninvolved with Mary's care.
    - Newborn baby in home.
    - Mother is socially isolated (lacks social support) and is unacculturated to American society.
    - Mother from Italian family—where familism is a central value of culture—and her family is not here to assist or support her.

    Three family nursing intervention strategies:

    a. Bring father into child care plan. Both parents together need to sit down with the pediatric nurse practitioner and discuss problems. Father needs to be encouraged to be active in Mary's child care, even though culturally this was not the traditional role of the father.
    b. Set up behavior modification program to eliminate Mary's temper tantrums and refusal to attend school.
    c. Teach parents about sibling rivalry—about its causes and ways to reduce rivalry and sibling's regression. Normalize some of Mary's behavior as being commonly seen as a reaction to introducing a new baby (and competitor) into the home.

The Family Health Care Function

Marilyn M. Friedman and Irene S. Morgan

► learning objectives

1. Recall the various ways in which the family carries out its health care function.

2. Identify three salient factors that influence a family's conceptualization or definition of health and illness, and whether they seek health care.

3. Discuss Baumann's study relative to the three criteria or orientations used to define health and illness, and the group differences found.

4. Explain Koos's central findings in terms of the influence of socioeconomic status on illness recognition.

5. Diagram the Health Belief Model, explaining the several important components of the model and their relationships to each other.

6. Discuss the significance of each of the cognitive-specific cognitions and affect motivation mechanisms found in Pender's Health Promotion Model.

7. Explain the significance of the health belief model for family nursing practice.

8. Summarize Pratt's findings and conclusions concerning how adequately the American family performs its health care function.

9. Enumerate the basic aspects that need to be assessed when completing an appraisal of a family's (a) dietary practices, (b) sleeping and rest practices, (c) physical activity and recreation practices, (d) drug practices, and (e) self-care practices.

10. Identify potential environmental and hygiene practices that could negatively affect family members' health.

11. Describe the basic health promotive and preventive measures recommended for adults and children.

12. Describe how Kleinman's Explanatory Health Model informs our understanding of family beliefs about health, illness, and health care seeking.

13. Discuss four health education areas about which families need information for their own dental self-care.

14. Describe what should be included and recorded in a family health history.

15. List and define four intervention strategies that are used to assist families to modify their lifestyle.

For the family health professional, the health care function is a vital component of family assessment. To place this function in perspective, it is one of the five family functions and entails the provision of physical necessities: food, clothing, shelter, and health care. Shelter (housing and family's neighborhood and community) was discussed previously in Chapter 9 as part of environmental data.

From the perspective of society, the family is the basic system in which health behavior and care are organized, performed, and secured. Families provide health promotion and preventive health care, as well as the major share of sick care for their members. Furthermore, families have the prime responsibility for initiating and coordinating services rendered by health care professionals (Pratt, 1977, 1982).

There has been a pervasive assumption that as the family has become more specialized in its functions, its health care function has been lost—being transferred to the doctor's office and hospital (Adams, 1971). And yet the tremendous role families play in the provision of health care to family members is clearly evident to health care professionals.* With the acknowledgment that major improvements and maintenance in health occur primarily through environmental and personal lifestyle modifications and commitments, the family's central role in assuming responsibility for its members' health is strengthened (Pratt, 1982). Therefore, it is our belief, supported by Pratt (1976) and Forrest (1981), that the provision of health care is indeed a vital and basic family function. We believe that education and counseling for *family self-care* should be a primary goal of family nursing practice.

▶ FAMILY BEHAVIOR RELATED TO HEALTH AND ILLNESS

Health practices and the use of health care services vary tremendously from family to family. Two primary reasons for this diversity in health care practices are family differences in both conceptualizations of what constitutes health and illness and their health beliefs

relative to seeking health care and following through with health care actions.

Conceptualizations of Health and Illness

Conceptualizations of health and illness vary widely from culture to culture, region to region, and family to family. The ubiquity of a disease in a community, and gender, social class, and ethnic differences are additional factors that influence a family's conceptualizations of health and illness.

The Ubiquity of Health Problems

Some health problems endemic to whole communities or groups may be taken as a matter of course rather than defined as illness. Social customs and norms often determine whether particular behaviors are considered sick or healthy (Jahoda, 1958).

A family, neighborhood, community, or society must label a condition or certain behaviors as an illness or disability before that illness or health condition can be considered a health problem to that group. The frequency of a condition often influences whether the condition is labeled an illness or not. For instance, if practically everyone in a community is suffering from malnutrition, the associated fatigue will probably be considered normal. A case in point: in America today we accept colds and dental caries, which occur so frequently, as annoyances that are a part of normal living, and most sufferers of colds or toothaches do not consider themselves ill.

Gender and Social Class Factors

Woods and associates (1988) uncovered some interesting gender and social class findings in their research, which addressed woman's definitions of health. In an attempt to measure the concept of health from a woman's perspective, these researchers interviewed a sample of 528 women living in the Pacific Northwest on the meaning of health. The women, ranging in age from 18 to 45, representing diverse cultures, marital statuses, and educational and socioeconomic levels, reported a rich variety of health definitions. The most frequently reported by the sampled women were: defining health as a clinical notion (e.g., not being ill,

---

* The reader is referred back to Chap. 1, which discusses in depth the role of the family in relation to the entire spectrum of health and illness concerns.

having no aches, pains, or headaches), as a positive affect (e.g., sense of well-being, feeling good), as feeling fit (having stamina and strength, able to be active), as practicing healthy lifestyles (e.g., not smoking, eating a balanced diet), and as being in harmony (e.g., feeling spiritually whole, where life is in balance, feelings of contentment). Women who had more formal education and/or higher incomes reported images of health in which there was a positive sense of "exuberant" well-being. The women who were educationally and/ or economically less advantaged tended to conceptualize health more pragmatically—as the absence of symptoms, the ability to perform their usual roles, and the ability to adapt to the demands of their environment. The study findings suggest that the women from higher social classes probably have more opportunity to develop images or conceptualizations of health that go beyond the limits of clinical symptomatology, role performance, and adaptive notions.

Social Class Differences

People from the same ethnic background and from a similar socioeconomic status often share comparable attitudes, myths, and values concerning their health. This has been particularly documented in poor communities (McLachlan, 1958; Lewis, 1961).

Kane and associates (1976) point out that the interpretation given to "health" by the poor is a natural consequence of the living conditions in which they find themselves. Irelan further explains:

> Their entire orientation is colored by the fact that they live with other poor people; they take on the perspectives of those around them and reinforce each other's beliefs and values. The way they cope with health problems is traceable either to the material situation of poverty itself, to the social structure of poverty, or to the aspects of the life outlook of poverty—the ideals, values, and beliefs to which the poor man adheres. (Irelan, 1972, pp. 56–56)

People have different ways of defining whether they are sick or well. Some people feel they are sick only when they can no longer work or carry on their usual daily activities and roles; others are very attuned to their physiological functioning and recognize even minor symptoms or signs as an indication

of disease and illness; a third orientation to illness is that people are sick when they are not feeling well.

Baumann (1961) demonstrated these differences in an early study she conducted of middle-aged and older chronically ill clinic patients from working-class and lower socioeconomic backgrounds and freshmen medical students in their first 3 years of medical school, who were generally from middle- and upper-middle-class backgrounds and in their early 20s. She compared the two groups according to their definitions of health and illness. Baumann found the three prevailing basic orientations to wellness and illness alluded to above existed in the two groups: (1) a subjective feeling of well-being or ill health (the feeling-state orientation), (2) an absence or presence of general or specific symptoms (symptom orientation), and (3) a state of being able or unable to perform usual activities (a performance orientation). Consistent with American society's productivity value orientation, both groups (representing both age and socioeconomic differences) mentioned an activity orientation in their conceptualization of health and illness. The clinic patients tended to identify subjective feelings as being a significant factor in their definition (supporting Koos's conclusions (1954) that the less educated are less articulate in their thoughts about illness), while the freshmen medical students identified the presence or absence of symptoms as the second criterion in their definition of health and illness.

Koos (1954), in a classic study, demonstrated that socioeconomic position greatly influences an individual's interpretation of symptoms—that is, whether symptoms are perceived as symptoms of illness or not, and when present, whether they constitute indications that medical care should be sought. He found that as one descends the social class ladder, less symptom recognition and perceived need for medical services existed among the study population. Thus the middle-class worker was found to be much more knowledgeable about disease symptoms, while the working-class and lower-class person showed less recognition of symptoms as being signs of ill health and therefore did not view these symptoms as indicating a need for medical attention. Generally, Koos concluded, the poor must reach a stage of being incapacitated before they define themselves as ill.

Social class differences are also quite pronounced relative to a family's overall priorities. In the lower class, health is often found lower on the list of necessities unless a crisis is present. Jobs, food, and shelter are pressing priorities for the poor.

How a family or family members define health and illness has important ramifications for family nursing practice. The family's definition of health needs to be clarified so that we know what goals and priorities are important to the family, as well as what possible areas of health education are present.

As illustrated by the previously mentioned studies of Baumann (1961) and Koos (1954), the more educated a family is, the better the family's knowledge of health usually is. This expectation would have to be validated with a particular client. Also, certain family members, generally the mother, are better informed. Women have consistently been found to have acquired more health education information due to their health role responsibilities in the family.

Cultural Differences

Another major factor influencing family members' conceptualizations and beliefs of health and illness is the family's ethnic background. Arthur Kleinman, an anthropologist and psychiatrist, developed an Explanatory Model of Health and Illness, which describes how cultural factors govern individuals' perception, labeling, explanation, and valuation of symptoms health and illness definitions, prognosis, treatment, and health promotion. Kleinman (1988) and his associates (Kleinman, Eisenberg, & Good, 1978) make an important distinction between disease and illness. *Disease* is the health care professionals' biomedical understanding of the health problem, while *illness* is the patient's personal and unique understanding and definition of what is happening to him or her.

According to Kleinman, cultural factors determine the importance of the various domains of influence. These domains shape people's explanations of health and illness and what they think they should do about health. The three domains of influence that Kleinman identifies are the professional, popular, and folk domains of influence. Within the *professional domain* individuals learn about diseases and treatment from a health professional perspective. Within the *popular domain*, which is the most powerful of the domains of influence, family, relatives, other kith and kin, and the lay community are sources of health and illness information and beliefs. According the Kleinman and associates (Kleinman,

Eisenberg, & Good, 1978), in 70 to 90 percent of all health situations, the popular domain of influence is consulted first. The last domain of influence is called the *folk domain*, whereby nonprofessional healers such as *curanderas/curanderos*, Native American medicine men, or herbalists provide explanations about health events. In unacculturated families, both the second and third domains of culturally derived influences are sources that are transmitted by family and community across generations.

Western societies typically root their explanations of health and illness in natural phenomena (as opposed to supranatural phenomena) and scientific findings; that is, the causes of health problems are thought to be infection, mechanical injury, tumor growth, or stress-induced. In non-Westernized ethnic groups and societies, families hold explanatory belief systems in which health and illness are viewed as resulting from social or supranatural causes or from an imbalance (like hot and cold or *yin* and *yang*) in the body. These explanations are usually holistic explanations—recognizing the interrelationship between the mind and body and between the individual and his or her social environment. The view of treatment of an illness is generally congruent with the beliefs about the cause of the problem (Kleinman, 1980). For example, if the health problem is thought to be caused by disturbed social interactions, social interventions are preferred (Friedman & Ferguson-Marshalleck, 1996). In Native American cultures, "sings" and sand paintings are the therapies used when social interaction and support are needed for problems emanating from interpersonal problems.

Health Beliefs About Health Care Seeking and Health Action

The second major factor identified as influencing health practices is an individual's and a family's health beliefs about seeking care and taking health action. Two related issues are discussed here: (1) the factors that lead to the readiness and intention of an individual to seek health care services and improve his or her lifestyle (i.e., change personal health behaviors); and (2) the variables that influence health promotive and preventive actions themselves (personal health practices and use of health services).

The most comprehensive scheme for looking at disease prevention and illness detection behavior is the Health Belief Model (Beckernovic, 1976), which has been subjected to testing in a wide variety of preventive and curative health areas. Although modified several times since its inception, it is believed to be a useful tool for systematically analyzing personal health behavior, predicting such diverse activities as preventive health actions, medical care utilization, delay in seeking help, and compliance with medical regimens.

The Health Belief Model utilizes Lewin's theories stressing that it is the world of the perceiver that determines what he or she will do, not the physical environment, except as this environment is viewed by the individual. Lewin identifies some aspects of life as having a negative valence (negatively valued), some as having a positive valence (positively valued), and some as having a neutral valence. Individuals seek to avoid the negatively valued aspects, whereas they try to incorporate the positive aspects into their lives.

The original model (Fig. 16–1) deals with explaining preventive health actions—that is, strategies for avoiding the negatively valued regions of illness and disease. In order for an individual to take preventive action to avoid disease he or she would need to believe that (1) he or she was personally susceptible or vulnerable to the disease; (2) the illness was at least moderately severe, so that the consequences of acquiring the disease would significantly disrupt the person's life; (3) taking a particular action would be beneficial in that it would reduce susceptibility to or severity of the disease; and (4) the benefits are outweighed by the barriers, such as costs, pain, time, inconvenience, and embarrassment.

The susceptibility and seriousness of the disease are perceived factors, not dependent on fact but on the person's personal beliefs. Both of these individual perceptions become the "readiness" factors leading to the perceived threat of a disease. In this model there are modifying factors (demographic, sociopsychological, and structural) that are posited to modify perceived susceptibility, severity, perceived benefits versus costs, and cues to action. Cues to action refer to the immediate stimuli needed to trigger recognition in the person's mind of the susceptibility and seriousness of a disease (the threat), and the need for taking action to reduce the threat (Rosenstock, 1974).

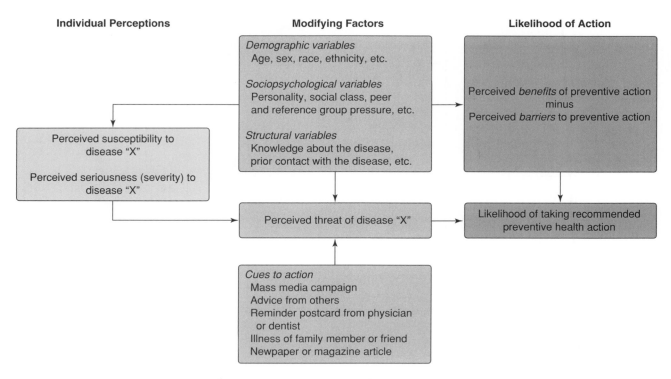

Figure 16–1. Diagram of the (original) Health Belief Model. *(From Rosenstock, 1974, p. 7.)*

In newer, modified health belief models, the readiness factors have been extended to include both the perceived feelings of the susceptibility and seriousness of the health problem (the threat) and positive motivation to maintain, regain, or attain wellness. This motivational factor includes concern about and the salience of health matters in general, willingness to seek and receive medical direction, plans to comply, and existence of positive health practices (Becker, 1974; Rosenstock, 1974).

Pender (1996), extending the Health Belief Model, has proposed a Health Promotion Model that is complementary to the other models of health protection. Health promotion focuses on movement toward a positively valenced state of enhanced health and well-being. The negatively valenced states of illness and disease appear to have minimal motivational significance for health-promoting behavior. Pender suggests that a desire for growth, expression of human potential, and quality of life provides the motivation for health-promotive actions.

Pender's Health Promotion Model (Fig. 16–2), derived from expectancy value and social cognitive theory, has recently been revised (Pender, 1996).

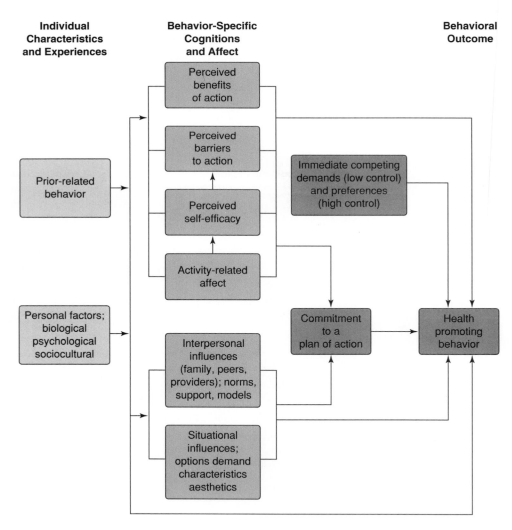

Figure 16–2. Revised Health Promotion Model. *(From Pender, 1996, p. 67.)*

The revised model theorizes about the relationships among individual characteristics and experiences, behavior-specific cognitions and affect, and behavioral outcomes.

In Pender's model individual characteristics and experiences include the effect of prior related behavior and personal biological, psychological, and sociocultural factors. Although personal factors are thought to influence the likelihood of engaging in health-promoting behavior, some personal characteristics cannot be changed, and thus are seldom incorporated into nursing interventions.

The core of the revised Health Promotion Model emphasizes the importance of behavior-specific cognitions and affect as the primary motivators of behavior. These variables could be especially significant for nurses to consider, as they are subject to modification through nursing interventions. The six behavior-specific cognitions and affect considered to be of major motivational significance in encouraging an individual to engage in health-promoting behaviors have been identified within the model as: perceived benefits of action, perceived barriers to action, perceived self-efficacy, activity-related affect, interpersonal influences, and situational influences. Behavior-specific cognitions and affect that are hypothesized to be directly related to health promoting actions include positive perceptions of the anticipated expected outcome, minimal barriers to action, feeling efficacious and skilled, positive feelings about the health behavior, presence of family and peer social support, positive role models, and availability of environmental contexts that are compatible, safe, and interesting (Pender, 1996).

Behavioral outcomes are proposed to be influenced by a person's sense of commitment to a plan of action with identified specific strategies, and the capacity of the person to repress competing demands and preferences. Health-promoting behavior is the action outcome in the model. Pender emphasizes that health-promoting behavior is ultimately directed toward attaining positive health outcomes for the client that should result in a positive health experience throughout that person's lifetime.

In summary, important aspects to remember about the health belief models is that they are rational decision-making models in which the occurrence of personal health behavior is thought to be influenced by factors identified in Becker's Health Belief Model and Pender's Health Promotion Model.

In regard to implications for family health care, these models were introduced to emphasize the significance of the family's belief system. If a family perceives a threat and if avenues are then presented to the family for reducing the threat, such as accessible and effective screening, health services, lifestyle improvements, education, and so on, the family will be more likely to act positively on its behalf. A health practitioner should not use the fear tactic, so as to build up anxiety and thus readiness, without offering an effective and accessible remedial action to handle and reduce the threat.

► HOW WELL FAMILIES PERFORM THE HEALTH CARE FUNCTION

The health care function is not only an essential and basic family function but one that assumes a central focus in healthy, well-functioning families. Pratt (1976, 1982) underscores the significance of effective functioning in this area by stating, "The more numerous and vital the functions the family performs successfully for its members, the stronger the family system" (1976, p. 122). This section focuses on the question of how well families fulfill their health care function.

Pratt (1976) assessed how well the contemporary American family is functioning as a personal health care system among 510 members of families in New Jersey. She examined the families' adequacy of health practices and home care for ill members, use of professional health care services, level of health knowledge, and attitudes about good health. Pratt found the family to be lacking. For instance, there was a serious breakdown between what should take place to promote and maintain family members' health and what usually occurred. Significant indiscretions were present in the family's pattern of nutrition, exercising, rest, smoking, dental hygiene, communication, and self-care practices. Medication problems were commonplace. Care of dependent, sick, or disabled family members was often not possible or was inadequately carried out. And a significant number of families either failed to utilize health care services or used the service improperly, as in the misuse of emergency rooms for primary health care. Preventive health care was spotty, and although the level of health information was improving, it was still not sufficiently high to serve as a sound foundation in most families. Pratt (1976) concluded that "the composite picture is one of fundamental failure in caring for health" (pp. 45–46).

She suggests that the reasons why families are having difficulties providing health care for their members lies with both (1) the structure of the health care system and (2) the family structure. Pratt found that when families had wide associations with organizations, engaged in common activities, and used community resources, they used health care services more appropriately. Also, personal health practices were enhanced when husbands were actively involved in internal family affairs, including matters concerning the health care system. She identified certain basic problems with the structure of the medical care system that made it difficult for families to carry out their health care functions.

1. The health care system is organized predominantly around the interests and needs of health care providers rather than consumers. This is operationalized by the preponderant control physicians have over their clients, hospitals, standard fees charged, and so forth. Professional autonomy is highly valued, resulting in inadequate review and control over the members of professional organizations.

2. Medical care systems are organized bureaucratically, resulting in specialization of functions, rigidity of structure and roles, and depersonalization.

A third reason why families are having difficulties providing health care to their members is the *lack of access to care due to lack of health insurance.*

Race, and level of income and education, contribute to class differences in health care service utilization. Minority populations and those with lower levels of income and education utilize preventive health care services less frequently. Nonwhite populations spend fewer days in the hospital, see a physician less often, and are more likely to be treated in a hospital outpatient department than in a physician's office (U.S. DHHS, 1989). For such groups, poor experiences with the health care system are likely to lead to low rates of service utilization for health examinations and treatments.

One major factor explaining differences in utilization patterns of medical services is the lack of health care insurance coverage. Approximately two-thirds of the U.S. population is covered by employment-related coverage, either individually or through groups sponsored by those other than employers. A total of 74.5 percent of the insured population is privately insured. Ten percent of the population receives coverage from publicly funded programs such as Medicare and Medicaid, according to data obtained from survey findings conducted by the National Center for Health Services Research. An estimated 14.7 percent of the population, or 37 million Americans, remain without private insurance or public coverage to help pay medical needs (Himmelstein & Woolhandler, 1994).

About two-thirds of the uninsured are employed workers and their families. This group represents the largest number of uninsured. Uninsured workers are typically part-time or self-employed, work for small establishments, earn low hourly wages at or near the minimum wage, and work in industries characterized by seasonal or less technical employment such as agriculture, construction, manufacturing, and sales. Individuals who are poor and from minority backgrounds are at highest risk of being uninsured. Nearly 33 percent of Hispanic-Americans, 20 percent of African-Americans, and 10.7 percent of non-Hispanic whites were uninsured in 1990. In addition workers from certain occupations have a high rate of being uninsured. For instance, workers in agriculture, household employment, construction, forestry, and fishing had uninsurance rates greater than 30 percent in 1990. Other population groups that are especially vulnerable for being uninsured and underinsured include children, unmarried young adults, older women, lower middle-income groups, and families without a working adult living at or near the poverty line (Himmelstein & Woolhandler, 1994) (see Fig. 16–3).

Many insured families are underinsured, preventing them from getting comprehensive health care. Furthermore, many poor families who are covered by Medicaid are treated in busy emergency departments and outpatient clinics of public hospitals where care may be fragmented and episodic (Center for Health Economics Research, 1993).

In order for families to become a primary and effective health resource, they must become more

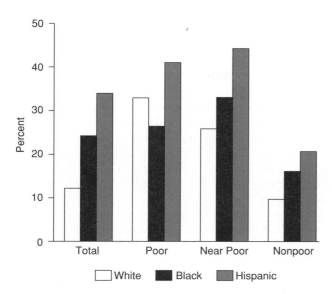

Figure 16–3. Families without health insurance, 1992. *(Source: U.S. Bureau of Census. Current Population Survey, 1992.)*

involved in the health care team and the total therapeutic process (Krozy, 1996). This implies an equalitarian relationship with health care providers in which both parties can openly express and negotiate in term of their particular needs and interests. Pratt (1976) explains: "Families cannot become highly responsible about their health care duties if the professionals exclude them from participating in medical management" (p. 171).

Such a partnership role is needed whether promotive, preventive, curative, or rehabilitative health needs are under consideration. People must be treated as responsible adults, not passive children, if professionals wish them to assume self-responsibility.

Not only must the family be in partnership with health care providers in directing and implementing its own health care, but clients should also be the ultimate decision makers and managers of those health issues affecting their welfare and lives. In order for clients to engage in effective self-care, they must have the knowledge and skills needed to provide good health care. This means that families need access to the primary sources of health information. Thus professionals must be willing to extend their role to include health education directed toward family self-care and family empowerment (Courtney, 1995; Rafael, 1995).

Most families appear to recognize the need to assume strong management of their own health care. However, both professionals and the health care industry—hospitals, pharmaceutical companies, supply companies, and the health insurance industry—discourage it. Data from Pratt's study revealed that families who were most effective in obtaining appropriate medical services and who practiced a wellness lifestyle on their own were the families referred to as "energized" families. These families assertively sought and verified information, made discriminating decisions, and negotiated aggressively with the health care system, rather than passively accepting and complying (Pratt, 1976, 1982).

▶ HEALTH CARE PRACTICES

Promotion of health practices within the family is a basic goal of family nursing. It becomes critical to gain information regarding the family's health practices to assist the family in health promotion and maintenance.

How well is a family performing the necessary health practices to protect and foster healthy growth and development? One often-used indication of the family's level of functioning is the overall level of health of its family members. This is often inferred by gathering information as to the incidence of disease per member in a specific period of time, realizing, of course, that the ages of individuals and their environment play major roles in the genesis and incidence of disease. Large families and families with young children, for example, have a greater incidence of disease per family. Troubled, problematic families are found to have less resistance to disease and thus have higher rates of disease than families that are functioning well.

In addition to looking at the overall health and illness patterns of family members, the presence or the absence of overt health practices are fruitful assessment areas, providing relevant areas for client education. (See Chap. 2 also.) Nine primary areas of health practices will be explored in this section:

1. Lifestyle practices
2. Family dietary practices
3. Family sleep and rest practices
4. Family exercise and recreation

5. Family drug habits
6. Family self-care practices
7. Environmental and hygiene practices
8. Medically based preventive practices
9. Dental health care practices

Family Lifestyle Practices

Hundreds of thousands of Americans die prematurely each year of diseases caused primarily by unhealthy lifestyles. These unnecessary mortalities result from heart disease, cancer, accidents, hypertension, cirrhosis of the liver, suicide, homicide, and diabetes. Recognizing the significance of lifestyle in promoting the health of Americans, the U.S. Department of Health and Human Services published *Healthy People 2000*, a platform for action to help bring the American people toward their full health potential. The report identifies three broad goals: "increase the span of healthy life for Americans, reduce health disparities among Americans, and achieve access to preventive services for all Americans" (U.S. Department of Health and Human Services [U.S. DHHS], 1991, p. 6). To support accomplishment toward these goals, *Healthy People 2000* set forth 300 measurable objectives to be accomplished by the year 2000 in 22 areas of priority for health promotion, health protection, and clinical preventive services. Health promotion strategies are described as

> those related to individual lifestyle—personal choices made in a social context—that can have a powerful influence over one's health prospects. These priorities include physical activity and fitness, nutrition, tobacco, alcohol and other drugs, family planning, mental health and mental disorders, and violent and abusive behavior. Education and community-based programs can address lifestyle in a crosscutting fashion. (U.S. DHHS, 1991, p. 6)

Tobacco use, alcohol use, and poor dietary practices are three major unhealthy lifestyle patterns.

Tobacco Use.   In 1990, approximately 400,000 deaths were due to tobacco use. Cigarette smoking is the leading cause of preventable death in the United States (Manley, 1996). An estimated 61 million Americans were current smokers in 1995. This represents a smoking rate of 29 percent in the adult U.S. population. No significant differences in smoking rates have been found by race or ethnicity. Education level affects smoking rates as demonstrated by a consistent decrease in the smoking rate in groups with a higher level of education. Adult men have somewhat higher rates of smoking than women, but rates of smoking appear to be similar for adolescent boys and girls, aged 12 to 17. Approximately 4.5 million youths, aged 12 to 17, were current smokers in 1995, making the rate of smoking among youths 20 percent. Current smokers are more likely to be heavy drinkers and illicit drug users. An estimated 6.9 million Americans in 1995 were current users of smokeless tobacco (U.S. DHHS, 1996). Tobacco use increases the incidence of heart attacks and strokes, pneumonia and other lung diseases, and even deaths of low birth weight babies whose mothers' smoking habits played a significant role in the stunted development of their unborn infants. Tobacco use accounts for one in three cancer deaths in the United States. The American Cancer Society (1996) estimated that in 1996 approximately 170,000 lives would be lost to cancer because of tobacco use. Health care costs, insurance, and lost economic productivity due to the use of tobacco products cost the United States more than $100 billion annually (American Cancer Society, 1996).

Alcohol Use.   Alcohol, another lifestyle hazard, is used by more Americans than any other drug, including cigarette tobacco. According to national data, approximately 111 million persons age 12 and over were current alcohol users, which was about 52 percent of the total population aged 12 and older (U.S. DHHS, 1996). About 32 million persons engaged in binge drinking, and about 11 million Americans were heavy drinkers. About 10 million current drinkers were under age 21. Alcohol usage rates have not significantly changed since 1994. Euro-Americans continue to have the highest rate of alcohol use at 56 percent. Rates for African-Americans and Hispanic-Americans were 45 and 41 percent respectively. Men were more likely than women to be binge and heavy drinkers. In contrast to the pattern for tobacco use, the higher the level of educational attainment, the more likely the use of alcohol (U.S. DHHS, 1996).

Nearly one-half of all deaths from motor vehicle crashes are alcohol related. It is estimated that 25 percent of all hospitalized persons have alcohol-related problems. The economic cost of alcohol abuse was estimated at $136.3 billion in 1990 (U.S. DHHS, 1990). Excessive alcohol drinking increases the risk of coronary heart disease, hypertension, stroke, chronic liver disease, some forms of cancer of the oral pharynx, neurological diseases, osteoporosis, nutritional deficiencies, and many other disorders. Even moderate drinking carries some risk in circumstances that require neuromotor coordination and judgment (e.g., driving vehicles, working around machinery, and piloting airplanes or boats). Approximately 10 percent of those who consume alcohol in the United States are alcoholics (National Research Council, 1989). Alcohol consumption during pregnancy can damage the fetus, cause low infant birth weight, and lead to fetal alcohol syndrome.

Recreational Drug Use.

Drug abuse involves the regular taking of a deleterious or noxious quantity of any drug, prescribed or illicit, over a period of time. The 1995 National Household Survey on Drug Abuse (U.S. DHHS, 1996), conducted by the Substance Abuse and Mental Health Services Administration, on illicit use of marijuana, cocaine and crack cocaine, heroin, hallucinogens, and inhalants, provides a comprehensive description of substance use and abuse in the United States. Data from the 1995 survey clearly show a continuing increase in the use of marijuana, cocaine, and hallucinogens among adolescents. The survey also demonstrates the aging of the drug-using population. Cohorts who were teenagers and young adults in the 1960s and 1970s are now older, and although most no longer use illicit drugs, many still do. The proportion of drug users that are aged 35 and older has increased from 10 percent of users in 1979 to 27 percent of users in 1995 (U.S. DHHS, 1996). Many of the drug users in this aging cohort have used drugs for many years and have developed severe drug problems. This may partly explain the continuing rise in hospital emergency department episodes, which are more likely to involve heavy users. Reports of increasing heroin and methamphetamine use have been prominent over the past few years, based on data from medical examiners, emergency departments, and drug treatment facilities (Greenblatt, Gfroerer, & Melnick, 1995; National Institute on Drug Abuse, 1996).

Marijuana is by far the most prevalent drug used by illicit drug users; approximately 77 percent of current illicit drug users were marijuana or hashish users in 1995. Between 1994 and 1995 the rate of marijuana use among youths aged 12 to 17 increased from 6 percent to 8.2 percent, continuing a trend that began during 1992–1993 (U.S. DHHS, 1996). In 1995, an estimated 9.8 million Americans were current marijuana or hashish users. This represents 4.7 percent of the population aged 12 and older.

Marijuana has a toxic effect on brain nerve cells. Researchers have found that chronic use of THC, the psychoactive ingredient in marijuana, destroys nerve cells and causes other pathological changes in the brain, possibly placing long-term marijuana users at risk for serious or premature memory disorders as they age. The daily use of one to three marijuana joints also appears to produce approximately the same lung damage and potential cancer risk as smoking five times as many cigarettes. Additionally, marijuana elevates heart rate, increases blood pressure, and is believed to adversely affect reproductive functioning in women.

A second illicit drug that is widely used is cocaine. Most clinicians estimate that approximately 10 percent of those who initially use cocaine "recreationally" will go on to serious, heavy use. It is one of the most powerfully addictive of the abused drugs, and is available in several forms. Cocaine is usually sniffed or "snorted," being absorbed through the mucous membranes of the nose. It can also be injected, or after chemical conversion to a purified form known as "freebase" or "crack," it can be smoked. Compulsive cocaine use may develop even more rapidly if the substance is smoked rather than ingested intranasally.

Cocaine acts as a strong central nervous system stimulant. Specific physical effects include constricted peripheral blood vessels, dilated pupils, and increased temperature, heart rate, and blood pressure. Cocaine's immediate euphoric effects, which include hyperstimulation, reduced fatigue, and increased mental clarity, last approximately 30 to 60 minutes.

Cocaine use ranges from episodic to addictive. Episodic cocaine use may produce nasal congestion and a runny nose. Some consistent users of cocaine report feelings of restlessness, irritability, and anxiety. A possible consequence of chronic cocaine "snorting" is ulceration of the mucous membrane of the nose. Addictive cocaine use can sufficiently damage the nasal septum to cause it to collapse. Continuing high doses of cocaine can also result in physiological seizures followed by cardiac or respiratory arrest, coma, or death. In 1994 and 1995, an estimated 1.5 million Americans were current cocaine users. This represents 0.7 percent of the population aged 12 and older. Rate of cocaine use had declined from 5.7 million in 1985 to 1.4 million in 1992, but has since risen somewhat (U.S. DHHS, 1996).

Estimates of heroin use from the National Household Survey on Drug Abuse (U.S. DHHS, 1996) are considered very conservative due to probable undercoverage of the population of heroin users. Estimates of lifetime heroin prevalence have generally remained at around 2 million since 1979, and no significant changes in the past year have been detected. The estimated number of current heroin users was 117,000 in 1994 and 196,000 in 1995.

Intravenous (IV) drug abusers are at increased risk for AIDS. Since January 1, 1989 data from the National Institute on Drug Abuse indicates that 30 percent of all AIDS cases involve IV drug abuse. Minorities are overrepresented among IV drug users. Among heterosexual IV drug abusers, a disproportionate number (80 percent) of persons with AIDS are African-Americans and Latinos.

Methamphetamine, also known as "crank," "meth," or "speed," once associated with blue-collar workers and biker gangs, now is gaining increased popularity among college students and young professionals. The estimated number of persons who have tried methamphetamine in their lifetime was 4.7 million, 2.2 percent of the population in 1995. In 1994, the estimate had been 3.8 million (U.S. DHHS, 1996). A frightening form of methamphetamine is a newcomer called ice. Produced in rock-like form, ice is smoked. The drug enters the body faster and its effects are longer lasting when compared to cocaine. Also called crystal meth, it is often odorless, colorless, and tasteless.

Hallucinogens such as LSD, PCP, mescaline, and peyote continue to be a significant problem in the United States. Chronic users of these drugs report memory loss, speech difficulties, depression, and weight loss. When given psychomotor tests, PCP users tend to have lost their fine motor skills and short-term memory. Mood disorders occur. The rate of current use of hallucinogens increased from 0.5 percent in 1994 to 0.7 percent in 1995. Among youth aged 12 to 17. The rate increased from 1.1 percent to 1.7 percent (U.S. DHHS, 1996).

During the 1988 to 1989 survey (Turner, 1990) it was found that the use of inhalants, and the nonmedical use of psychotherapeutic drugs such as sedatives, tranquilizers, stimulants, and analgesics, decreased to less than 2 percent of the population, being slightly higher for females than males.

Poor Dietary Practices.   Poor dietary practices leading to obesity is another example of the results of an unhealthy lifestyle. Many Americans are overweight and gain weight as they grow older. Both overweight and adult weight gain are linked to high blood pressure, heart disease, certain types of cancer, arthritis, breathing problems, and other illnesses (U.S. DHHS, 1995). As individuals age, to stay at the same weight, they must balance the amount of energy taken in food (caloric intake) with the amount of energy the body uses (caloric output). Physical activity is an important way to use up food energy. Many Americans spend too much of their day in sedentary activities that require little energy. In addition, many Americans of all ages now spend a lot of leisure time each day engaging in inactive activities, for example, watching television.

The kinds and amounts of food people eat affect their ability to maintain their weight. High-fat foods contain more calories per serving than other foods and increase the likelihood of weight gain. However, even when people less high-fat foods, they can still gain weight from eating too much of foods high in starch, sugar, or protein. Foods from the base of the Food Guide Pyramid (Fig. 16–4) should serve as the foundation for meals. Foods from the grain group, along with vegetables and fruits, are the basis of healthful diets (U.S. DHHS, 1995). Diets high in fat, saturated fat, cholesterol, and salt contribute to Americans' risk for chronic disease. Obesity, high blood pressure, high blood cholesterol, and elevated serum glucose can be modified by a balance of a healthy diet and sufficient physical activity.

In sum, it is clear that many lives can be saved through lifestyles improvement. Personal behavioral changes are needed particularly in the areas of diet, smoking, alcohol, abusive drug consumption, and physical exercise.

Family Dietary Practices

Encouraging all family members to keep a 3-day food diary is very helpful in assessing both the quality of their family's diet and how it meets individual nutritional needs. Such a record, 3 sequential days' intake (2 weekdays plus 1 weekend day), is a stronger indication of a family's eating patterns than is the record of only a single day's intake. A 24-hour food history may not truly represent the family's usual eating patterns (Lacey, 1989). Dietary variations that may occur among individual family members during the day should be included in the journal. Active participation by all family members in completing the food record will enhance the discovery of what family members eat, and where their dietary strengths and deficiencies lie. The 3-day nutrition intake record is an excellent base for assisting families to assess their present nutritional status and begin to develop nutritional goals. The family food diary offered in Figure 16–5 may be used as a guide for data collection.

Assessment of the family's food choices should be a collaborative effort between the family and the nurse. Are a variety of foods consumed from the food guide pyramid each day? Specifically, does the diet contain 6 to 11 servings from foods in the grain group, 3 to 5 servings from the vegetable group, 2 to 4 servings from the fruit group, and moderate amounts of foods (2 to 3 servings) from the dairy group and the meat and beans group. (The food guide pyramid is displayed in Figure 16–4.) Are adequate amounts of dark green or deep yellow fruits or vegetables consumed each day to meet vitamin A requirements? Are vitamin-C-rich fresh fruits and dark green leafy vegetables part of the daily diet? Are low-fat dairy products consumed to meet calcium and vitamin D requirements? Other aspects of the family nutrition analysis should include evaluation for the amount and quality of dietary fat, intake of cholesterol and saturated fat, patterns of complex carbohydrate and fiber intake, consumption of sugar and artificial sweeteners, sodium use, processed food intake, alcohol consumption, coffee and tea intake, and the use of dietary supplements.

In analyzing a 3-day food record, the family nurse should determine individual variances. Are any individual family members underweight or overweight for their height and age group? What does each person eat (types of food and quantity) in relation to the family's dietary practices. By learning about family food practices, preferences, and individual dietary habits,

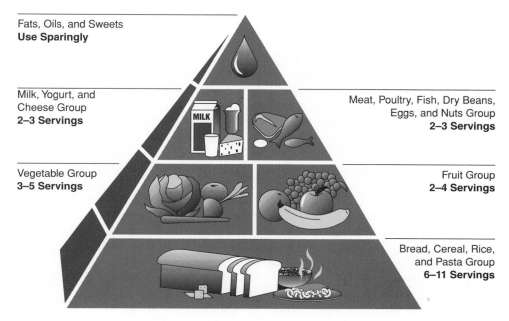

Figure 16–4. The Food Guide Pyramid. *(Source: U.S. Department of Health and Human Services [1995]. Nutrition and Your Health: Dietary Guidelines for Americans, 4th ed. U.S. Department of Agriculture, Home and Garden Bulletin No. 232.)*

	Food Served	Quantity	Comments (Factors such as Place, Activity, Money)
Breakfast			
Snacks (between meals)			
Lunch			
Snacks (between meals)			
Dinner			
Snacks (between meals)			

Figure 16–5. Family dietary diary (record of family dietary intake for 3 days).

the nurse and family will gain a holistic picture of family dietary patterns. For instance, is Johnnie's state of obesity and extensive tooth decay due to his eating excessive amounts of sugars and carbohydrates? If so, is this part of the family's customary diet, along with sedentary activities and poor dental hygiene? Or does the family serve well-balanced meals and Johnnie's sweet intake is at school and/or a reflection of other problems?

Food fads, reduction diets, special dietary beliefs, or culturally based food patterns—such as dietary practices based on a traditional Jewish, Mexican, or Italian pattern, or special food practices based on a philosophical or health commitment such as that held by many vegetarians—need to be appraised. Understanding the family's value system and beliefs underlying their food practices is also important and serves as a suitable foundation for later work with the family on any modification that might be needed.

Because obesity has been repeatedly demonstrated to be one of the key precursors to chronic illness and shortened longevity, assessing the family's caloric intake and comparing this to their actual caloric need becomes germane to practice.

Additional information relevant in assessing family dietary practices includes an awareness of the function of mealtimes for the family and the family's attitude toward food and mealtimes. Does the family eat together (all meals, only dinner, etc.)? Is mealtime (when they are together) a social, pleasurable experience? How are the meals handled when the family does not eat together? When families are more atomistic or individualistic (each family member doing his or her own "thing"), junk foods and a less adequate diet are often found. When family members do not congregate for at least dinner, it makes it difficult for the family to interact and share with each other, because mealtime is often the one opportunity families have to enjoy each other's company and share important and pleasurable experiences, thoughts, and feelings.

Do parents use the giving and withholding of food as reward and punishment? Where this occurs, the child learns to associate food with approval (love) and disapproval (rejection). Pairing food and social needs for love and acceptance is an unhealthy linkage, as counselors who treat the obese will attest.

Shopping, Planning, and Preparation Practices.   What are the shopping arrangements? Where is food purchased? Does the family plan for the week or several days at a time, or do they operate on a meal-to-meal basis, shopping for each meal or one day at a time? (The latter is certainly an inefficient means in terms of time and money.) What kind of budgetary limitations exist in their food shopping? If the need is present, does the family use food stamps? Is food storage and refrigeration adequate? What are usual ways in which food is prepared (fried, boiled, microwaved, eaten cold, variety of means)?

Shopping, Preparation, and Serving Responsibilities.   Who is responsible for each of these tasks? Although we generally assume that the mother-wife is responsible, it is sometimes a role shared with the spouse and/or older children.

Family Sleep and Rest Practices

Sleep is a necessary function for quality living. It is thought to fulfill several physiological needs, such as energy conservation, restoration, and protection against exhaustion (Kick, 1996). A major factor in determining how much sleep family members require is age. Newborns need between 16 and 18 hours of sleep distributed over every 24-hour period. Infants in the first 6 months of life sleep progressively more in the night than in the day, with requirements for 10 to 12 hours of rest nightly and usually two to three daytime naps by the end of the first year. Toddlers will sleep 8 to 12 hours nightly and have one daytime nap. The preschool-age child requires 10 to 12 hours of sleep. The average school-age child requires 9 to 10 hours of rest each night. The need for sleep declines for adolescents to about 7.5 hours daily. Young and middle-age adults require 6 to 8 hours of sleep. Elderly sleep requirements drop to an average of 6.5 hours. An increase in overall health status, improved mental status, and increased longevity has been positively correlated with regular, adequate rest and sleep habits (Baker, 1985).

Every family has patterns for sleeping, even though in some families these patterns may be erratic due to crowding in the family's home, different work or school schedules, illness, or because of caregiving needs as in the family with a new baby. Assessment of the family's sleep should begin with a sleep history. The following assessment questions may be posed:

1. What are the usual sleeping habits of adults and children? Here one wants to know the number of hours of sleep per night. Are these suitable according to individual's age and health status?

2. Are there *regular* sleeping patterns, with regular hours for going to bed and getting up in the morning? Who decides when the children go to sleep?

3. Where do the family members sleep? In separate or shared beds? Are sleeping arrangements crowded or adequate?

4. Do any family members take naps or have any other regular means of resting?

The nurse should assess if any individual family member has trouble sleeping (insomnia) and if so, what specific type of trouble—falling to sleep, or awakening early without being able to resume sleeping. Frequency and severity of the insomnia should be elicited. Often, sleeping difficulties are due to inadequate sleeping arrangements in the home. A simple sleep diary or log individually kept by each family member may provide additional insight into identifying sleep disturbances.

A deficiency in knowledge of family members' sleep requirements, and what makes a good sleep routine, may be found. New parents may be confused about their baby's irregular sleep schedule. Older adults may lack understanding regarding normal sleep requirements and changes that occur with aging. Many families lack a knowledge of the effects that sedatives and other prescribed drugs, over-the-counter drugs, and illicit drugs have on sleep. The nurse should elicit information from the family as to the possible etiologies of any identified sleep pattern disturbances.

Family Exercise and Recreational Activities

Regular exercise promotes general health. Less sedentary or more vigorous activity may help reduce body fat and disease risk. Less than 20 percent of adults in the United States exercise with sufficient frequency and intensity to improve cardiovascular fitness (Jonas, 1996). Among the priorities for health promotion established by the U.S. Public Health Service's *Healthy People 2000* (U.S. DHHS, 1991), physical activity and fitness is listed first. To encourage increased participation in physical activity among Americans, the Centers for Disease Control and Prevention and the American College of Sports Medicine convened an expert panel. The panel's recommendation is that every adult should accumulate 30 minutes a day or more of moderate physical activity on most, preferably all, days of the week (Burns, 1996). The recommendation emphasizes physical activity as opposed to exercise, which some people find difficult to fit into their daily schedules.

The family nurse should assess family physical activity levels. Specific assessment questions suggested are the following:

1. What types of family recreational pursuits (i.e., jogging, bicycling, swimming, dancing,

tennis) are family members engaged in? How often? Who participates?

2. Do common daily activities performed by family members require a moderate level of energy expenditure? Do family members spend at least 30 minutes participating in moderate or heavier physical activity nearly every day?

3. What are the family's beliefs about the relationship of physical activity to health?

Chapter 8 also discusses family recreational activities and the importance of families' engaging in active recreational pursuits as families.

Family's Therapeutic and Recreational Drug Habits

As we know, taking medications is a ubiquitous activity of Americans, with over-the-counter drugs most often used (60 to 70 percent of the time). In a society where pills are regarded as a panacea for everything from sexual problems to headaches, it is no wonder that major community health problems exist in Americans' drug-taking habits.

A significant amount of medication use by families is carried on as an alternative to professional care, because generally the health problems being treated are seen as too trivial to seek medical care for or are conditions that the family can adequately handle. A national survey discovered that one-half of those sampled undertook self-medication for sore throats, coughs, colds, and upset and acid stomachs. Home over-the-counter medication was found to not be limited to gastrointestinal and upper respiratory complaints, but also covered other body system problems, including the central nervous system, urogenital tract, and skin (Roney & Nall, 1966). Home medication is also frequently used as a supplement to professional treatment. Professional treatments are often altered or modified by patients, as seen in the extensive modifications made to diet and insulin regimen by diabetic patients. Prescribed medications, furthermore, are often not taken by patients as directed. One study reported a medication rejection rate of 50 percent (Linnett, 1970).

It is important to assess the family's use of over-the-counter and prescription drugs, particularly for nurses working in primary care and home health care. Nurses should ask about what drugs family members take and for what purpose. By identifying drugs commonly used by the family, the assessor can look for possible side effects or harmful interactive effects. Also, drug usage can tell the nurse something about how the family and/or the family members cope with life events and health problems, as well as how they define health and illness.

Some over-the-counter drugs commonly taken by Americans are potentially harmful, or at best unnecessary. The regular use of laxatives and painkillers are examples. Although most of the fatal medication poisonings are caused by prescribed medications, with barbiturates heading the list, 20 percent are caused by over-the-counter drugs. Of the nonfatal drug poisonings, aspirin is the leading offender, primarily because of its tendency to produce gastrointestinal bleeding.

In homes where young children are present, storage of drugs and other hazardous substances in safe child-proof containers and cupboards is imperative, as the incidence of poisoning among children is very high.

One important factor leading to medication poisonings is the tendency of older families to save and reuse medicines years later. Any nurse who has cared for older patients in their homes will attest to the fact that families will hoard medicines prescribed many years ago. Many of these containers do not even contain the name and dosage of the drug. Such medications undergo change over time and, at best, become ineffective. Often families end up using their old medicines to treat a family member who they perceive to be experiencing the same or similar symptoms as the person for whom the drug was originally prescribed. The possible misdiagnosis by the family presents a further hazard.

In assessing the drug use of older family members, as part of a home health visit, it is suggested that the nurse find a way to tactfully review the kinds and age of the drugs stored in the house. By doing so the nurse will be able to go over with the family both the new and old medications and their usage, which may influence the family to properly dispose of drugs that are old and/or unmarked.

In considering drug habits, assessment not only of the use of medications, but also the consumption of caffeine, alcohol intake, smoking, and recreational drug use is indicated. Smoking and alcohol intake should be assessed in terms of who uses either substance, and how much, when, and under what situations or circumstances. Is the use of tobacco or alcohol by a family member(s) perceived as a problem by that person or other family members? Among drinking members, does the use of alcohol interfere with their capacity to carry out their usual activities? How long has the present use of alcohol continued? What was the pattern of drinking in the past?

The family exercises a profound influence on the onset and continuity of patterns of substance abuse by family members and provides a context for communication of knowledge, skills, and attitudes about substance abuse. Positive social reinforcement (modeling by parents or esteemed family members of substance abuse behavior patterns) may play a major social influence in contributing to youth drug use (Baumrind, 1985). At the other end of the continuum, families may highly discourage substance abuse and openly communicate that illicit drug use is contradictory to family values.

Those family members who do become severely drug dependent most often need specialized treatment to recover. A wide range of treatment is available through public and private entities. Recovery treatment centers that incorporate the family into their plan of care more holistically and effectively treat the substance abuser.

Health care professionals need to be most concerned with helping the teenagers. This is because smoking, drinking, and recreational use of drugs often begin during these years.

Family's Self-care Practices

When assessing a family, especially one in which members are experiencing health problems, a determination is needed of both the family's ability to provide self-care and its motivation and actual competence in handling health matters. For a family to be responsible for its own self-care, it needs to have an understanding of its own health status and/or health problems and the steps needed to improve or maintain its health (Johnson, 1984). Self-care practices involve not only preventive practices, diagnosis, and home treatment of common and minor ambulatory health problems, but also all the procedures and treatments prescribed for the care of illness of a family

member, such as giving medications, using special appliances, changing dressings, and carrying out special exercises and diets.

How adequately is the family able to handle the responsibilities of these therapies? Estimates from the literature report that 75 to 85 percent of all health care is provided by self or family, with self-care being the predominant illness response in the older population (Hickey, 1988). These percentages hold for both populations who have and do not have access to professional health services (Levin et al., 1976). There are no firm data demonstrating that lay-initiated self-care is any less effective than professional care (which is about 35 percent effective), or less dangerous (which involves 20 percent iatrogenic ill effects and 4 to 11 percent complications from nosocomial infections) (Levin, 1977). The authors Elliott-Binns (1973) in Britain and Pederson (1976) in Denmark found that 90 percent of self-care procedures taken prior to professional intervention were appropriate and helpful.

An assessment of the family's self-care abilities, focusing on the family's knowledge, motivation, and motor skill strength or coordination necessary to carry out the physical tasks of care, provides the foundation for evaluating the need for nursing intervention. In identifying the family's strengths, resources, and potentials, the nurse should not overlook the possible stressful effects of caregiving on the family unit. Families that assume the major health care responsibility for members who are frail or suffering severe health problems may experience high levels of physical and emotional strain. Financial burdens may also contribute to a family's level of strain.

Studies have shown that women caregivers tend to exhibit higher levels of stress than males. Adult daughter caregivers especially have been found to experience greater familial conflict and household disruption, particularly when married with dependent children (Bass & Noelker, 1987; Cantor, 1983). Chapter 12 covers the problem of family member caregiving in more depth.

Environmental and Hygiene Practices

Environmental practices consist of habits or patterns that positively or negatively affect the family's or its members' health status. For instance, is the family regularly exposed to smoke, herbicides, asbestos, lead, or other harmful substances? Noise pollution may also be harmful, as well as water pollution and radiation exposure. More and more evidence demonstrates the adverse effects of long-term, low-level exposure to noise and to chemicals in our air, water, and food. A discussion of environmental concerns relative to the home, neighborhood, and community is presented in Chapter 9.

The family's hygiene and cleanliness practices may also be considered as forms of environmental practices. Although cleanliness is not "next to Godliness," there are several general health habits that reduce the possibility of infection and its spread.

1. Washing hands before meals and after toileting.

2. Using separate towels. When an infectious skin condition such as scabies or impetigo is present, sharing towels can be an infection route.

3. Drinking from separate cups and glasses that are clean. In families with several children and an overworked and overwhelmed mother, sharing of baby bottles and cups is commonly seen.

4. Bathing and cleanliness. Although this is certainly needed, community-based nurses have been found to be overly critical of the families they visit in terms of degree of family cleanliness. We need to carefully differentiate between family hygiene practices that are, in fact, deleterious to health and those that are contrary to our own habits and customs but are *not* harmful.

Safety practices could also be included here, but have already been included in Chapter 9 as part of environmental data.

Medically Based Preventive Measures

Although the annual physical examination can detect early-stage disease in the absence of symptoms, there is considerable controversy as to whether such examinations are effective when performed for routine screening of asymptomatic persons. Moreover, there is little scientific evidence that healthy persons experience better outcomes as a result of head-to-toe physical examinations. The U.S. Preventive Services Task Force concluded that health care clinicians should invest most of their time in talking with clients about health behaviors and a healthy lifestyle rather than performing physical examination procedures and tests (Woolf & Lawrence, 1996).

On the other hand, a selective health promotion/disease prevention-oriented physical examination on a regular and periodic basis, and tailored to the client's age, race, and sex are vital and serve several purposes. They provide the necessary information to jointly establish with the client a health maintenance plan. The preventive health assessment identifies risk factors particular to an individual; for example, an adult who smokes and whose father died of heart disease should be counseled about heart risk factors, because a person with that health profile has twice the risk of incurring heart disease as an individual who does not smoke and has no family history of disease.

Major risk factors are related to heredity, sex, race, and age. For instance, individuals whose families have had heart disease at early ages or diabetes have an increased likelihood of inheriting a predisposition toward those diseases. Thanks to their sex hormones, premenopausal women are less likely to have myocardial infarctions than men of the same age group. African-Americans have more than twice the chance of developing hypertension than whites. And generally, the older one gets, the greater the chance of developing a chronic illness.

This does not imply, however, that the above risk factors are inevitable harbingers of future events. In fact, susceptibility to some diseases can actually be reduced if an attempt is made to attenuate risk factors by improving one's lifestyle and seeking routine, preventive health care.

What should be included in the annual health assessment of the well adult? Again, opinion varies. The minimum should probably be a general history (review of the systems and any present complaints), blood pressure, vital signs, weight, and urinalysis; for women, a pap smear and breast and pelvic examinations are indicated; for men older than 30 to 35 years of age, an electrocardiogram, heart auscultation, rectal examination, and lipid panel (serum cholesterol and triglycerides) should be performed. Middle-aged men should also have a protoscopy or sigmoidoscopy of the rectum done for detection of cancerous polyps, and African-Americans should be tested for sickle-cell anemia.

What are the family's feelings about having a "physical" when they are well? Past practices of the family may be a gauge to their feelings; nevertheless, a lack of periodic well-care may also be a function of inaccessibility to, ignorance about, and/or the costs of such services. In order to ascertain the reasons behind not receiving health examinations, more direct questions may be warranted.

Vision and Hearing Examinations.
Health assessments should be supplemented by vision and hearing examinations. This is particularly important, because glaucoma and hearing loss can be detected and can usually be treated effectively or prevented.

Children should have periodic vision and hearing examinations done as part of their well-baby and preschool care. During the school years children are periodically given Snellen tests, a rough screen for common vision problems. Because hearing difficulties can lead to serious behavioral and learning problems in school, children should be routinely given an audiometric test during the early school years. Primary care practitioners should also complete rough screening for hearing during well-child care visits (Green, 1994).

Adults who wear glasses need an eye examination annually, unless visual changes are noted sooner. For others, every other year is adequate. The eye examination should include tonometry testing for detection of glaucoma, which is recommended on a yearly basis for all adults over 40 years of age.

If families do not know of an eye specialist to call, it is helpful to review with the family the difference in training and focus of an optician, optometrist, and ophthalmologist. If while eliciting a family medical history, the nurse finds a history of glaucoma in the family, he or she should stress an annual eye examination even more vigorously, as there is now overwhelming evidence of a higher incidence of glaucoma among siblings and offspring of patients with the disease than among the rest of the population (Perkins, 1973).

Although asymptomatic adults may not need annual audiometric testing, if hearing difficulties are noted or an individual is at high risk, testing is indicated. Progressive hearing loss can occur from exposure to certain types of noise. If a client is exposed to a high level of noise at work or home, the nurse should inquire into his or her use of ear protectors and hearing examinations. Hearing loss can also occur with age, due to vascular insufficiency of the cochlea. Smokers have greater hearing loss than nonsmokers, as smoking reduces the blood supply by vasospasm induced by nicotine, by atherosclerotic narrowing of the vessels, and by formation of thrombi in the vessels (Diekelmann, 1977).

Immunization Status.
The most important and specific measure against preventive disease is that of immunization (Green, 1994). At least 75 to 80 percent of susceptible children must be immunized to effectively protect a community from preventable communicable diseases (Garner, 1978). Hence promotion of immunization services is a vital and integral part of family health care.

In 1985, through legislative regulation of immunization requirements for school attendance and provision of free immunizations for those who were in need, a 96 percent overall immunization level was achieved in the school-aged population (U.S. DHHS, 1985). Unfortunately, however, the level of immunized children has dropped. We must refocus our attention on immunizing preschool and infant populations, as the immunization levels in 1994 were reported to be as low as 58 percent (Wong, 1995).

For infants and children, the need for being adequately protected against tetanus, diphtheria, pertussis (whooping cough), hepatitis B virus, *Haemophilus influenzae*, polio, measles (rubeola), mumps, and rubella (German measles) is crucial (American Academy of Pediatrics, 1995). Smallpox vaccinations are no longer advised, as the risk of untoward reactions to the vaccine are now greater than the risk of contracting the disease. Flu vaccines and tuberculin skin tests are also recommended for certain age groups and under certain situations. (The conditions and age of the person and the community incidence and exposure risk are important variables here.) Booster shots of diphtheria and tetanus are recommended for adults every 7 to 10 years, because both of these diseases are serious and endemic in the United States today.

When completing an assessment of the immunization status of family members, the types of immunizations received, dates, and any adverse reactions to immunization should be recorded.

Dental Health Care Practices

Dental health practices are essential in maintaining good teeth throughout an individual's life span. The prevalence of dental ill health is widespread, especially among the poor of our country.

Dental health care includes both preventive care and curative health practices. In order to maintain high-level dental health, a combination of personal habits or practices, as well as preventive care by a dentist and/or dental hygienist, should be carried out. The four basic elements for dental health maintenance are:

1. Regular preventive dental services, including dental examination, x-rays, cleaning, education, and for children topical fluoride treatments when indicated. The American Academy of Pediatrics (1995) recommends children have dental check-ups, cleaning, and fluoride treatments twice a year.

2. Use of fluoridated water, or if unavailable, prescription for daily oral fluoride liquid or tablets for children.

3. Regular brushing and flossing of teeth after meals.

4. Reduced amounts of certain types of fermentable carbohydrates in the diet. All fermentable carbohydrates have the potential of contributing to the development of dental caries by supplying the raw materials necessary for bacteria in the mouth to produce tooth-decaying acid. Fermentable carbohydrates include sugars, such as found in fruits, honey, and sweets; and cooked starches such as found in bread and potatoes (Loe, 1988).

A survey conducted by the National Institute of Dental Research (NIDR) found that an estimated one-half of the nation's school children aged 5 to 17 have no tooth decay at all. This represents a 36 percent reduction in caries from NIDR studies conducted at the beginning of the 1980s (Loe, 1988). Dental experts suggest factors that have contributed toward the improvement in children's dental health include the widespread use of fluoride, the increased application of sealants, improvement in personal oral hygiene, the receipt of regular professional dental care, and the rise in awareness of the effects of eating habits on the teeth (Loe, 1988).

Fluoride, which can be found in the drinking water supply in some communities, or which is prescribed by dentists as an oral supplement, is recognized as the most effective agent available to protect teeth from decay. Less helpful but still effective are the various means of applying fluoride topically, including the application of fluoride solutions by many dentists, or the self-administration of fluoride rinses or gels by the patient (American Dental Association, 1988). With a combination of fluoride treatment and sealants the incidence of dental caries can be reduced by 90 percent (American Academy of Pediatrics, 1995).

Dental caries result from the interaction of several processes, primarily the amount and type of carbohydrates in the diet, the amount of plaque buildup, and resistance of the teeth. Consumption of foods and beverages high in sugar content contribute toward harmful bacteria producing acid for at least 20 minutes after eating. Snacking should be kept to a minimum and confined to foods that do not promote decay—nuts, popcorn, raw fruits, vegetables, and sugar-free drinks. Professional dental care and practicing good daily oral hygiene (brushing and flossing) can control harmful bacteria by removing plaque. Learning how to brush and floss teeth properly to remove plaque is one of the best investments a person can make in preserving his or her own dental health. It is especially important to remove plaque thoroughly from the teeth before bedtime. During sleep less saliva is secreted, and therefore, bacterial acids are diluted less at night (Kandzari & Howard, 1981).

For American adults, periodontal disease continues to be a major dental problem and is the chief cause of tooth loss. Gum disease is thought to affect at least three out of four adults and may strike 95 percent of the population at some time (Kandzari & Howard, 1981; Loe, 1988). Gum disease can be slowed down or prevented by careful attention to brushing, flossing, and regular professional dental care.

The family nurse, in teaching families about dental health and hygiene, may wish to check the mouths of some of the children or adults for plaque buildup or bring some disclosing solution that they can use to detect plaque themselves. Dental health education should stress that teeth should be brushed at least twice a day after meals, and the sooner the better, to prevent sugars from remaining in the mouth. The object of brushing is to remove plaque and food particles from the teeth, which is done by effective friction of the toothbrush (a soft-bristled one) against the surface of the teeth. The importance of using dental floss once a day to supplement brushing should also be advised, because some surfaces of the teeth and teeth–gum junctions are inaccessible by brushing alone (American Academy of Pediatrics, 1995).

Families (both children and adults) need thorough demonstrations of an effective method for brushing teeth. Due to limited dexterity, children may need some help brushing their teeth until they are between ages 7 and 10. Newer methods of brushing teeth are much more effective than the older vertical (from gum line or down) method taught in the past. Regular, after-meal brushing and flossing teeth is considered essential in the prevention of dental caries, gum disease, and periodontal disease.

Treatment of dental problems has not been mentioned except in passing, but is also of vital import. Although prevention has been stressed, early detection and treatment of dental and gum problems will certainly keep more serious problems from developing. Malposition problems—over- and underbites, causing unequal exertion of pressure on teeth—are targets for early detection in children. Orthodontia may be needed to correct these problems, which if untreated could later cause periodontal disease and speech problems, as well as result in cosmetic ill effects (American Academy of Pediatrics, 1995).

▶ FAMILY HEALTH HISTORY

This area is significant for several reasons. First, family histories will often identify familial risk factors. Second, the family's experience with certain diseases might possibly have resulted in fears, myths, or misconceptions about these illnesses. Family nurses should be sensitive to these possibilities and may want to explore family members' beliefs in this area further. Third, through eliciting a family medical history, the family nurse will learn more about both families of orientation and marriage and thus gain a better understanding of the family's past and present.

The family medical history includes an identification of past and present environmentally and genetically related diseases of the family of orientation—going back to maternal and paternal grandparents and including aunts and uncles and their children. Besides ascertaining the general health status of all these individuals, family-centered nurses should specifically inquire about the presence of the following diseases, because individuals often forget to mention important familial diseases:

1. Environmentally related diseases (to which family members might be or have been exposed).
   a. Psychosocial problems: mental illness and obesity.
   b. Infectious diseases: typhoid fever, tuberculosis, venereal disease, hepatitis, diarrheas (dysenteries), and skin diseases (scabies, lice, impetigo).
2. Genetically linked diseases: epilepsy, diabetes, cystic fibrosis, mental retardation, sickle-cell anemia, kidney disease, hypertension, heart disease, cancer, leukemia, vision and hearing defects, hemophilia, and allergies, including asthma.

Including family history information on the family genogram (see Fig. 8–2) is a useful way of recording this information. The family genogram should include the age of members, whether the individual is living or deceased, the cause of death, level of general health, and presence of chronic disease.

Family Health Records

Families often change health practitioners and are seen at several agencies or by different specialists for different diseases. With passing years, memories fade as to what happened when, underscoring the need for families to keep records of the year-by-year medical events of each family member.

Educating families about the importance of maintaining family medical records is an important health education area for assisting families to become responsible for their health care. The data the family maintains will aid the family when new practitioners are visited and may also obviate the need for redundant expensive and time-consuming laboratory and diagnostic tests. Moreover, information given in the record may assist a family to obtain faster and more accurate diagnoses.

When there are young children in the family or adult members, especially older adults, who have several illnesses and are seeing more than one practitioner concurrently, it is especially critical to have medical record information. For children, immunization records are important to maintain; for adults, diagnostic and laboratory tests, diagnoses, medications taken, and any adverse reactions to them should be carefully recorded.

The following broad areas of health information need to be included:

- Family medical history (see previous section).
- Maternity record.
- Children's heights and weights.
- Adults' weight records.

- Childhood diseases (of children).
- Accident records.
- Major surgeries, illnesses, and hospitalizations.
- Immunization records.
- Allergies.
- Corrective devices (glasses, hearing aids, dental plates, and special shoes are examples).
- Blood groups and Rh factors.
- Blood pressure; and other laboratory tests performed.

FAMILY HEALTH CARE FUNCTION: APPLYING THE FAMILY NURSING PROCESS

▶ assessment questions

The following areas and questions are germane to assessing the family's health care function.

1. *Family's health beliefs, values, and behaviors.* What value does the family assign health? Health promotion? Prevention? Is there consistency between family health values as stated and their health actions? What health-promoting activities does the family engage in regularly? Are these behaviors characteristic of all family members, or are patterns of health-promoting behavior highly variable among family members? What are the family's health goals?

2. *Family's definition of health–illness and its level of knowledge.* How does the family define health and illness for each family member? What clues provide this impression, and who decides? Can the family observe and report significant symptoms and changes? What are the family members' source of health information and advice? How is health information and advice transmitted to family members?

3. *Family's perceived health status and illness susceptibility.* How does the family assess its present health status? What present health problems are identified by the family? To what serious health problems do family members perceive themselves vulnerable? What are the family's perceptions of how much control over health they have by taking appropriate health actions?

4. *Family dietary practices.* Does the family know food sources from the food guide pyramid? Is the family diet adequate? (A 3-day food history record

of family eating patterns is recommended.) Who is responsible for the planning, shopping, and preparation of meals? How are the foods prepared? How many meals are consumed per day? Are there budgeting limitations? Food stamps usage? What is the adequacy of storage and refrigeration? Does mealtime serve a particular function for the family? What is the family's attitude toward food and mealtimes? What are the family's snack habits?

5. *Sleep and rest habits.* What are the usual sleeping habits of family members? Are family members meeting sleep requirements that are appropriate for their age and health status? Are regular hours established for sleeping? Do family members take regular naps or have other means of resting during the day? Who decides when children go to sleep? Where do family members sleep?

6. *Physical activity and recreation.* Are family members aware that active recreation and regular aerobic exercise are necessary for good health? What types of recreational and physical activities do family members engage in regularly? Are these activity patterns representative of all family members or only certain members? Do usual daily work activities allow for physical activity?

7. *Family drug habits.* What is the family's use of alcohol, tobacco, coffee, cola, or tea? (Caffeine and theobromine are stimulants.) Do family members take drugs for recreational purposes? How long has (have) family member(s) been using alcohol or other recreational drugs? Is the use of tobacco, alcohol, or prescribed/illicit drugs by family members perceived as a problem? Does the use of alcohol or other drugs interfere with the capacity to carry out usual activities? Do family members regularly use over-the-counter or prescription drugs? Does the family save drugs over a long period of time and reuse? Are drugs properly labeled and in a safe place away from young children?

8. *Family's role in self-care practices.* What does the family do to improve its health status? What does the family do to prevent illness/disease? Who is (are) the health leader(s) in the family? Who makes the health decisions in the family? What does the family do to care for health problems and illnesses in the home? How competent is the family in self-care relative to recognition of signs and symptoms, diagnosis, and home treatment of common, simple health problems? What are the family's values, attitudes, and beliefs regarding home care?

9. *Environmental and hygiene practices.* These questions are already covered under family environmental data.

10. *Medically based preventive measures.* What are the family's history and feelings about having physicals when well? When were the last eye and hearing examinations? What is the immunization status of family members?

11. *Dental health practices.* Do family members use fluoridated water, or is a daily fluoride supplement prescribed for the children? What are the family's oral

hygiene habits in regard to brushing and flossing after meals? What are the family's patterns of simple sugar and starch intake? Do family members receive regular preventive professional dental care including education, periodic x-rays, cleaning, repair, and for children topical or oral fluoride?

12. *Family health history.* What is the overall health of family members of origin and marriage (grandparents, parents, aunts, uncles, cousins, siblings, and offspring) over three generations? Is there in the past or present a history of genetic or familial diseases—diabetes, heart disease, high blood pressure, stroke, cancer, gout, kidney disease, thyroid disease, asthma and other allergic states, blood diseases, or any other familial diseases. Is there a family history of emotional problems or suicide? Are there any present or past environmentally related family diseases?

13. *Health services received.* From what health care practitioner(s) and/or health care agency(ies) do the family members receive care? Does this provider(s) or agency(ies) see all members of the family and take care of all their health needs?

14. *Feelings and perceptions regarding health services.* What are the family's feelings about the kinds of health services available to it in the community? What are the family's feelings and perceptions regarding the health services it receives? Is the family comfortable, satisfied, and confident with the care received from its health care providers? Does the family have any past experience with family health nursing services? What are the family's attitudes and expectations of the role of the nurse?

15. *Emergency health services.* Does the agency or physician the family receives care from have an emergency service? Are medical services by current health care providers available if an emergency occurs? If emergency services are not available, does the family know where the closest available (according to their eligibility) emergency services are for both the children and adults in the family? Does the family know how to call for an ambulance and for paramedic services? Does the family have an emergency health plan?

16. *Source of payment.* How does the family pay for services it receives? Does the family have a private health insurance plan, Medicare, or Medicaid, or must the family pay for services fully or partially? Does the family receive any free services (or know about those for which it is eligible)? What effect does the cost of health care have on the family's utilization of health services? If the family has health insurance (private, Medicare, and/or Medicaid), is the family informed about what services are covered, such as preventive services, special medical equipment, home visits, and so forth?

17. *Logistics of receiving care.* How far away are health care facilities from the family's home? What modes of transportation does the family use to get to them? If the family must depend on public transportation, what problems exist in regards to hours of service and travel time to health care facilities?

► FAMILY NURSING DIAGNOSES AND PLANNING

In terms of the types of family nursing diagnoses that are often found in the area of the family's health care function, the number of possibilities are large. Certainly family nursing diagnoses that lead to health-promotional or educational strategies are appropriate here, because knowledge deficits of family members are commonly observed. These knowledge deficits are seen in the various areas discussed in this chapter, such as dietary practices, rest and sleep patterns, physical activity and recreation practices, drug and alcohol use, lifestyle practices, and use of health care services.

North American Nursing Diagnosis Association (McFarland & McFarlane, 1993) individual and family nursing diagnoses that are behaviorally oriented and deal with the family health care function are:

Potential Health Problems (Health Promotion and Disease Prevention Focused)	**Actual Health Problems**
Risk for caregiver role strain	Caregiver role strain
Potential for more than requirements, nutrition	Altered nutrition: Less or more than body requirements
Knowledge deficit	Knowledge deficit
Health-seeking behaviors	Altered health maintenance
	Noncompliance
	Self-care deficits

Family health promotion nursing diagnoses may be subsumed under *health-seeking behaviors*. Carpenito (1989) explains that health-seeking behaviors in the family context pertains to a state in which a family or family members who are in stable health "actively seek ways to alter personal health habits and/or the environment in order to move toward a higher level of wellness" (p. 408).

The family nursing diagnosis *altered health maintenance* identifies health care practice areas where the family or family members demonstrate actual or potential inadequate health practices. Carpenito (1989), in extending this diagnosis to the family, states that it pertains to a state in which a family or family members "experience or is [are] at risk of experiencing a disruption in health because of an unhealthy lifestyle or lack of knowledge to manage a condition" (p. 382). Specific examples of problems that could be found under this broad diagnosis are ineffective or inadequate dental care practices, dietary practices, preventive health care practices, and family planning.

Family nurses are challenged to assist the family unit in identifying areas of health risk, in establishing relevant health goals, and in planning for lifestyle changes that will continue as an ongoing family commitment. For health-promotion planning to be effective, it must be compatible with the family's cultural beliefs and practices. Awareness of the family's cultural interpretation of health, illness, and health care is essential prior to embarking on specific goal-oriented interventions. In addition, family goals should be recorded and prioritized. Major sources of stress, along with any recent or current family developmental or situational transitions, also require consideration prior to intervention. Collaboration of the entire family in expressing concerns, setting health goals, and planning for lifestyle modifications should increase the effectiveness of the nursing interventions.

► FAMILY NURSING INTERVENTIONS: GUIDELINES FOR LIFESTYLE MODIFICATION

Working with families to plan lifestyle modifications so that health goals can be met is an important role for the family nurse. Pender (1996) describes useful approaches that may be considered in initiating and supporting family behavior alterations. Specific strategies that nurses may apply in initiating family lifestyle changes include self-confrontation, cognitive restructuring, modeling, operant conditioning, and stimulus control.

Self-Confrontation

The first technique, *self-confrontation*, is based on the assumption that clients make changes when they recognize incompatibilities within their own beliefs, values, and behaviors, or between their own behaviors and those of individuals they hold in esteem and wish to emulate. Once this comparison occurs and contradiction is experienced, the client is more likely to change values, attitudes, and behaviors to achieve greater consistency with the self-concept. The nurse, in reviewing family lifestyle, can provide feedback to families by suggesting areas of inconsistencies between family beliefs or values and current behavior patterns. Contradictions that are of most concern to the family should be the focus for intervention. An example of using this strategy can be found in a family that highly values good nutrition as an essential ingredient in maintaining health, and believes its diet is well balanced. Yet family members admit to regularly consuming "fast foods" for lunch during the week. A family that is confronted with this inconsistency between its beliefs and actual dietary patterns hopefully will be more motivated to change its behavior.

Cognitive Restructuring

The *cognitive restructuring* method of behavior adjustment, which was originally described by Ellis and Grieger (1977), is also known by the term "rational-emotive therapy." The premise behind this approach is that the manner in which the family perceives and evaluates a specific situation determines its emotional reaction to the situation. Irrational or illogical self-statements may be generated by unsatisfactory past experiences, with the client skeptical of achieving behavior changes.

Goldfried and Sobocinski (1975) have outlined specific steps for applying cognitive restructuring strategies to improve clients' emotional outlook and foster feelings of success. The nurse utilizing this approach should counsel family members to recognize the irrationality or the constraining nature of certain beliefs (Wright, Watson, & Bell, 1997). An example is where all of a family's members are overweight and firmly convinced that "none of us will ever be thin; we have always been heavy." Cognitive restructuring as an intervention promotes the acquisition of rational positive self-statements and contributes to clients feeling an increased sense of personal control.

Modeling

Modeling is a common strategy used in behavior therapy. It is based on the premise that a person will learn through observation of role models, beginning with early childhood and continuing through to adulthood (Bandura, 1977). Modeling is especially helpful when clients are uncertain as to which behavior(s) is (are) necessary in order to achieve a specific goal. Clients should identify with their models in order for this technique to be effective, with family members and nurse working together to select suitable models. The family nurse is in a powerful position to positively influence family health by being a role model of healthful living. He or she does this by demonstrating skills that the family seeks to learn by providing needed health education, and by expressing encouragement to promote desired family behavior. The technique of modeling may also be used in community organized health promotion classes, and in mutual self-help groups such as Weight Watchers or Alcoholics Anonymous. Self-help groups function by offering a setting for role modeling and mutual support (Roth, 1996b).

Operant Conditioning

Operant conditioning, based on the principle that behavior is determined by its consequences, can be an effective behavior modification strategy. Desirable behavior is reinforced (not as "consequences") to increase the probability that the behavior will be repeated. Positive reinforcers, or rewards, are more effective motivators of behavior change than negative reinforcers or punishments. Nurses applying this intervention strategy should work with families to choose behavior to be changed. Schedules should be developed of how to gradually move toward selected targeted health-generating behavior, and reinforcement contingencies should be set up. In order to attain family goals, a nurse–family contract with designated rewards for desired behavior may be entered into, so as to provide responsibility guidelines for all family members. Contracting can be enjoyable for the entire family, with family members serving as an important source of motivation for each other. Pender (1996) suggests that operant conditioning works best if the behavior to be reinforced is countable, so that reinforcement may be used correctly.

Stimulus Control

In *stimulus control,* attention is directed toward changing the antecedents rather than the consequences of behavior as in operant conditions (Pender, 1996). This method of behavior control suggests that by changing events that precede undesirable behavior it is possible to decrease or eliminate such action, and increase target behavior. Stimulus control concentrates on arranging environmental cues to promote only the desired behavior. Both the original Health Belief Model and Pender's Health Promotion Model agree that cues are important factors in promoting health behavior change. Nurses should work with families to accomplish stimulus control by accurately identifying under what conditions desirable behavior occurs more frequently, and under what circumstances undesirable behavior is prompted. Nurses should offer instruction on how to develop sensitivity to appropriate cues, and counsel families on ways to facilitate opportunities for encountering those that are appropriate. Behavioral cues may be taken from a variety of sources. Examples of possible sources include contact with health care professionals, significant others, the communication media, or visual stimuli from the environment such as viewing others participating in the target activity. In addition to environmental cues, nurses can further influence desired action by encouraging families to develop a positive set of internal cues such as "feeling good" or an increased sense of self-esteem. External cues, such as having a family member or friend invite you to an aerobic exercise class, can be combined with internal cues, such as remembering feeling more energetic after exercise sessions. Multiple cues potentiate each other.

In summary, nurses and other health care professionals can assist families to attain a healthier lifestyle. Specific lifestyle modification strategies have been suggested as possible nursing interventions to support families to increase their health-promoting activities and attain their family health goals. Perhaps one of the most lasting contributions to a family's health may be the interventions the family nurse undertakes to assist a family to attain and maintain a healthy lifestyle.

► study questions

1. Which of the following are major ways that the family carries out its health care functions? (Select all appropriate answers.)
   a. Family provides preventive health care to its members at home.
   b. Family provides the major share of sick care to its members.
   c. Family pays for most health services received (directly or indirectly).
   d. Family has prime responsibility for initiating and coordinating health services.
   e. Family decides when and where to hospitalize its members.

2. List three primary factors that influence a family's conceptualizations of health and illness and whether they seek health care services.

3. Name the three basic orientations used to define health and illness (according to Baumann). Keeping in mind the two groups studied, correlate the orientation(s) each group identified more frequently.

4. Describe what Koos' central research findings were.

5. Fill in the missing components in this representation of the health belief model (original model).

Health belief model (original):

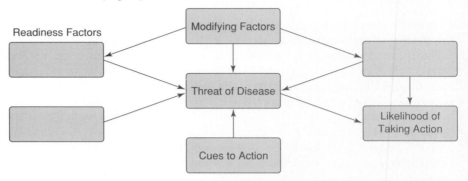

6. Recall in Pender's model the behavior-specific cognition and affect variables suggested as influencing the likelihood of engaging in health-promoting behaviors. What other modifying factors are thought to contribute in activating health-promotion behaviors?

7. Pratt found that on the whole most American families were not adequately performing their vital health care function. On what basis did she conclude this? What are three basic reasons for this inadequacy?

8. Kleinman's Explanatory Model of Health and Illness is significant because (select best answer):
   a. It explains what kind of health beliefs a family is likely to have.
   b. It brings out the importance of culture in forming health explanations.
   c. It discusses the important role that popular and folk domains of influence have.

9. List four assessment areas to cover when appraising a family's dietary practices.

10. The following is a list of several areas that should be assessed under family's sleep and rest practices: number of hours usually slept each night by family members, who takes regular naps during day or what other rest techniques do family members use, and where family members sleep. What important area(s) has (have) been omitted?

11. Formulate three basic questions to ask a family in relation to its physical activity practices.

12. Which of the following substances constitute drugs that need to be assessed by the family completing a family health assessment? (Select all appropriate answers.)
    a. Coffee, tea, cola, and cocoa.
    b. Alcohol use.
    c. Over-the-counter medicines.
    d. Tobacco use.
    e. Recreational drugs such as marijuana and cocaine.

13. An appraisal of self-care practices involves an assessment of:
    a. Preventive and diagnostic practices.
    b. Home treatment practices, including home care of sick or disabled members.
    c. Determination of the family's ability to provide self-care.
    d. (fill in) _____.

14. Which of the following family nursing intervention strategies would be appropriate in assisting a family with school-aged children to change the children's dental health practices in the area of brushing and flossing teeth? (Select all correct answers.)
    a. Cognitive restructuring.
    b. Modeling.
    c. Operant conditioning.
    d. Stimulus control.
    e. Self-confrontation.

15. Safety was a major area covered under environmental practices. Identify two general areas of health advice related to family safety.

16. Name four salient general health education areas for families to learn about concerning dental health.

17. Which of the following measures are generally recommended for plaque control? (Select all appropriate answers.)
    a. After-meal toothbrushing.
    b. Reduction in dietary sucrose.
    c. Daily flossing of teeth.
    d. Use of an antiseptic mouthwash twice a day.

18. A family medical history consists basically of two parts. First, information would be elicited about each family member (going back to maternal and paternal grandparents) and his or her present and past health status. What would be the second area of assessment?

► chapter 16 study answers

1. All but e. Physicians and health insurance companies have practically total control over when and where to hospitalize their patients.

2. a. Socioeconomic status (also can identify level of knowledge, which is correlated with the educational status and socioeconomic status).

b. Gender differences.
c. Ubiquity of health problem in community (certain prevalent symptoms or problems are accepted as being part of living and thus viewed as inevitable, unavoidable, and "normal").
d. Cultural differences.

3.

Orientations	Groups That Mentioned Orientation More Frequently
a. Feeling-state orientation.	Chronically ill clinic patients (lower socioeconomic group).
b. Performance orientation.	Both groups.
c. Symptom orientation.	Medical student group (younger, presumably well, and of middle- and upper-middle-class background).

4. Koos' study found that as one descends the socioeconomic scale, a lack of recognition of and indifference to symptoms of illness increase. Also when individuals failed to recognize behaviors as indicative of possible disease, they failed to see that medical care was indicated.

5. See the diagram of the (original) Health Belief Model below:

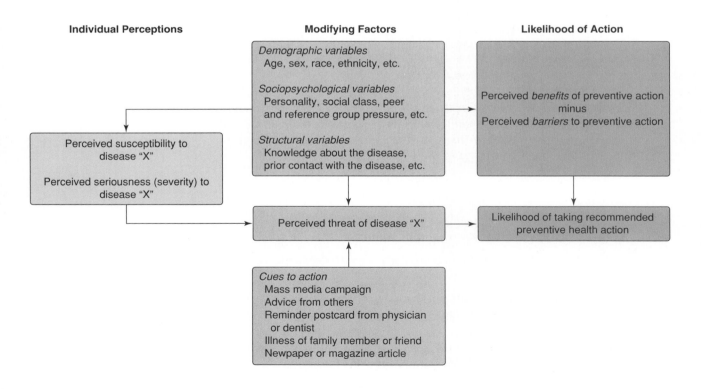

6. Six behavior-specific cognitions and affect factors are identified in the model as the primary motivational mechanisms for engaging in health promoting behavior. They are: (1) perceived benefits of action, (2) perceived barriers to action, (3) perceived self-efficacy, (4) activity-related affect, (5) interpersonal influences, such as family and peers, and (6) situational influences. Individual characteristics and experiences (including the effect of prior related behavior and personal biological, psychological, and sociocultural factors) are thought to contribute to activating the above six behavior-specific cognitions and to direct impact on health promotion behaviors. Additionally, the likelihood of a person engaging in health-promoting behaviors is conceptualized as being influenced by a person's sense of commitment to a plan of action with specific strategies and the ability of the person to subdue competing demands and preferences.

7. Pratt concluded that American families were generally inadequate in carrying out their health care function based on the following observations:

   • Many homes not suitable for maintaining health and controlling infectious disease and accidents (crowdedness, safety hazards, pollution, lack of infectious disease control).

   • Widespread unhealthful personal and family health practices.

   • Medication misuse widespread.

   • Dependent and/or disabled family members not cared for or inadequately cared for.

   • Insufficient or inappropriate use of health services found frequently.

   • Level of health knowledge inadequate.

   • Family's self-care practices not satisfactory.

   Reasons for this inadequacy:

   1. Basic structure of the health care system (health care provider dominated; bureaucratic structure).

   2. Family structure itself (family needs to be more widely involved with community and husband-fathers need to be actively involved).

   3. Lack of access due to lack of health insurance.

8. c.

9. Any four of the following:
   a. Nutritional history (the 3-day family food record).
   b. Observe for variations among family members in terms of quality and quantity of diet. Does visual inspection indicate normal limits for height and weight?
   c. Identify any special family food preferences (culturally, philosophically, or trend-based dietary food patterns).
   d. Psychosocial aspects of mealtimes and eating (food used as a reward or punishment)?
   e. Shopping, planning, food preparation characteristics.

10. a. Are the number of sleeping hours appropriate for the age of each of the family members?
    b. Are there regular times established for children to go to bed and get up?
    c. Do any members of the family have sleeping problems? If so, what kinds of problems?

11. a. What types of family recreation involving physical activity does your family engage in?
    b. How frequently do you as a family engage in physical activity? Does everyone in the family participate?
    c. What effect do you think physical activity has on your family's health?

12. All (a–e).

13. Caregiving needs and the potential for caregiver strain.

14. All intervention strategies could be effectively utilized in this situation.

15. a. Always follow the manufacturer's warning on cleaning solutions, powders, or chemically treated materials.
    b. Store toxic, abrasive, or caustic substances properly and out of the reach of young children.
    c. Do not save and re-use old prescribed medicines.

16. Any four of the following:
    a. Importance of fluoride for increasing resistance of tooth to decay.
    b. Importance of brushing and flossing teeth (and use of an effective method of brushing).
    c. Role of carbohydrates (starches and sugars) in producing dental caries.
    d. Importance of regular dental examinations and cleaning of teeth.
    e. Early treatment of dental caries and treatment of major orthodontic problems.

17. a, b, and c.

18. Asking about specific diseases (both genetically based and environmentally related diseases) that family members or their parents or grandparents might have had.

17

Family Stress and Coping Processes: Family Adaptation

Marilyn M. Friedman with Elra Kolbrun Svavarsdottir and Marilyn McCubbin

▶ learning objectives

1. Describe the importance of family coping strategies and processes.

2. Present evidence of changes in family life that require coping strategies and processes.

3. Define and differentiate the meanings of these terms and concepts: stressor, stress, crisis, individual coping, family coping and adaptation.

4. Explain what coping tasks are appropriate for each of the three time phases of stress.

5. Trace the sequence of events that occur during a family crisis.

6. Identify three major variables involved in the development of crisis or successful resolution of the problem (noncrisis), according to Hill's family stress theory.

7. Discuss in what way the Resiliency Model is an extension of Hill's family stress theory.

8. Identify six categories of family stressors and strains as described in the Resiliency Model.

9. Explain two family strengths depicted in the Resiliency Model that can help to explain family adaptation to stressful life situations.

10. Discuss helpful and harmful coping strategies as described by Burr and associates.

11. Briefly describe four functional coping strategies used by families and four dysfunctional adaptive strategies used by families.

12. Differentiate whether specific adaptive strategies are functional, dysfunctional, or both (could be either healthy or unhealthy).

13. Identify the two basic purposes of social support systems.

14. Utilizing a family case example:
    a. Assess the family in terms of family coping processes and strategies.
    b. Identify one family nursing diagnosis in the area of family coping.
    c. Propose two family nursing interventions appropriate for resolving or ameliorating the problem.

Families constantly face the need to modify their perceptions and lives. The stimulus for this change comes from within and without. The normal, continually evolving developmental needs of all the family members, in addition to the presence of unexpected situations involving family members, make up the inner demands for change. The external stimuli for change come from the changing society as it interacts with the family during the family's life cycle. General systems theory and family developmental theory both stress the inevitability and ubiquity of family change. Family stress theory focuses on family responses to stressful life situations and what facilitates successful adaptation. Continual demands force the family to adapt in order for the family to survive, continue, and grow. Family coping processes and strategies are essential for making this possible. A family's perceptions and handling of its problems through use of various resources and coping strategies are crucial to the family's success in dealing with the demands placed on it.

Most important, moreover, family coping processes and strategies serve as vital processes or mechanisms through which the family functions are made possible. Without effective family coping, the affective, socialization, economic, and health care functions cannot be adequately achieved. Hence family coping processes and strategies constitute the underlying processes that enable the family to enact its necessary family functions.

Assessing family resources, coping strategies and processes provides the foundation for assisting families in their adaptation and in their attainment of a higher level of wellness. Achieving a higher level of wellness is the goal or the raison d'être of family nursing practice. Strengthening and encouraging adequate adaptive responses and capacities, as well as reducing the actual and potential stressors from within and outside the family, are part of this broad and encompassing goal. Whether the family is essentially healthy or dysfunctional or somewhere in between (in their location on the health–illness continuum), the family health nurse is still dealing with the same issue: assisting families to help themselves achieve a higher level of functioning or wellness within the context of their particular aims, aspirations, and abilities.

▶ THE GENERAL STATE OF FAMILY HEALTH TODAY: HOW WELL FAMILIES ARE COPING

Families in the United States have great strengths but face considerable challenges today (see Chap. 1). One of the main strengths of U.S. families is their durability (Fine, 1992). Despite all the technological changes that have occurred in society, families are still the basic institution where individuals are socialized and nurtured. Other strengths of American families are their ethnic and structural diversity (i.e., the array of family forms such as nuclear, intergenerational, single-parent, stepparent, cohabiting, and gay and lesbian). Nonnuclear family structures have reached a greater level of acceptance today than before, although many of these families and their members still face discrimination in school, workplace, and community settings. U.S. families also can be characterized by their resilience (Fine, 1992). Despite all the economic, social, and political pressures, most families can be considered to be functioning quite satisfactorily. The majority of adults in the United States are employed, are in relatively good health, have meaningful social relationships, have at least a high school education, and are not involved in criminal activity (Fine, 1992). These individual achievements can certainly be influenced by how well families are performing their functions in society.

The National Survey of Families and Households (Bumpass & Sweet, 1991) in a random national sample of 13,017 U.S. individuals aged 19 and over, examined family experiences of these individuals during childhood and when they left the parental home: cohabitation and/or marriage, fertility history, having first- and later-born children, any marital disruptions, as well as their education and employment histories. Deliberate oversampling was carried out of single-parent families, stepfamilies, minority families, cohabitors, and recently married persons to focus on these groups which are often underrepresented in other surveys. The main changes in family patterns were found to be in the early stages of the life course. About half of all children in this sample and in the United States experience living in a one-parent household sometime during their childhood due to higher divorce rates and increases in nonmarital childbearing. The experience of living in a one-parent household was found to be more common in African-American and Hispanic-American families and for those not completing high school.

Changes in marital behavior and fertility also were found (Bumpass & Sweet, 1991). Marriage rates have declined for all ages, especially in the early 20s age group; but at the same time a remarkable increase was found in cohabitation. Fertility declined, especially in the early childbearing years. Marital disruption increased by 50 percent in the first 10 years of marriage, with almost half of all recent marriages involving at least one previously married partner. Adult children who returned to the parental home after leaving did so mainly because of marital disruption or financial difficulties. Poverty in working poor and mother-headed families has increased significantly recently to a 30-year high. Children have been hit the hardest, with nearly one-fourth of all children living in poverty (Leeds, 1996).

These structural and situational changes in American family life—increased cohabiting, more single-parent and stepfamilies, higher divorce rates—as well as downsizing of both small businesses and major corporations (resulting in decreased employment opportunities, need for dual earners for financial survival), and a growing elderly population—all create both new opportunities for growth and increased stress and demands for coping to fulfill family functions.

Families cope with and adapt to stressful life situations on a daily basis. In addition, over the life course, families also need to cope with situational (unexpected) stressors such as unemployment; acute or chronic illness in child, adult, or elderly members; abusive behavior; alcohol or drug abuse; adolescent pregnancy; and/or accidental death or injury. Health care professionals such as nurses are in contact with families in hospitals, clinics, and in communities for either a short or a long period of time. This chapter can serve as a conceptual framework for guiding family nursing assessment and interventions in families who face a variety of different stressful family life situations.

▶ BASIC CONCEPTS AND DEFINITIONS RELATED TO STRESS AND COPING

All of the concepts and terms defined below, with the exception of family coping, are well established and their meanings fairly well agreed on. In defining family coping, definitions of coping as applied to the individual have been adapted to the family.

Stressors refer to the initiating or the precipitating agents that activate the stress process (Burr, Day, & Bahr, 1993; Chrisman & Fowler, 1980). The precipitating agents that activate stress in the family are life events or occurrences of sufficient magnitude to bring about change in the family system (Hill, 1949). Family stressors can be interpersonal (inside or outside of the family), environmental, economic, or sociocultural events or experiences. Perceptions color the nature and gravity of possible family stressors, because families react not only to the presence of actual stressors, but also to events as they perceive or interpret them. The family's perceptions are of paramount importance. It is significant to note that families that are crisis prone consistently tend to perceive events in a distorted, subjective manner. Events that healthy families would look at objectively and/or positively as a challenge are viewed by crisis-prone families as threatening and overwhelming. In these cases extensive stress is experienced which in turn taxes family adaptive capacities.

Stress is the response or state of tension produced by the stressor(s) or by the actual/perceived demand(s) that remains unmanaged (Antonovsky, 1979; Burr, 1973). It is the tension or strain within a person or social system (individual, family, etc.) and is a reaction to a pressure-producing situation (Burgess, 1978). Because stress or tension in a family is so difficult to measure, researchers and practitioners alike often assess the accumulation (pile-up) or magnitude of stressors in a family's life to get an estimate of the amount of stress the family is experiencing (Olson et al., 1983). McCubbin and Patterson (1983a) define the concept of pile-up of family life stressors as the sum of developmental (expected) and situational (unexpected) events as well as intrafamily strains (tensions in relationships among family members).

A **family crisis** has been defined as a continuous condition of disruptiveness, disorganization, or incapacitation in the family system (Burr, 1973; McCubbin & McCubbin, 1993). A crisis results because the family's current resources and adaptive strategies are not effective in handling the stressor(s) (see Fig. 17–1). Hence, a family crisis refers to a disruptive state or period in a family's life when an extremely stressful event or series of events significantly taxes the family's resources and coping abilities, with no resolution of the problem in sight. The family's usually effective problem-solving skills become useless or diminished during this psychosocial emergency (Kus, 1985).

There are two types of situations that can put families into a crisis: developmental and situational. Developmental or maturational events are those stemming from families' experience in the process of the psychosocial growth of members (e.g., becoming a parent; child maturing as adolescent; retirement). They are inherent within the stages of the normal life cycle of both the family and its members. Situational events are not common or normally expected, such as the death of a child or serious illness of one of the family members. Depending on the family's resources, coping abilities, and perceptions of these events, developmental and situational events can become crises for the family.

Individual coping strategies are viewed as positive or negative strategies of adaptation. Coping consists of problem-solving efforts by an individual faced with demands highly relevant to his or her welfare, but taxing the person's resources (Lazarus, Averill, & Opton, 1974). Pearlin and Schooler (1978) add the notion of presumed effectiveness of coping responses when they define coping as any response (behavioral or perceptual-cognitive) to external life strains that serves to prevent, avoid, or control emotional distress. Simply stated, coping efforts or behaviors are positive or negative, problem-specific, active strategies geared toward resolving a problem. Coping is a term that is limited to actual behaviors or cognitions people employ, not to resources they potentially could use.

Family coping denotes a family group level of analysis (or an interactional level of analysis). Family coping is defined by McCubbin (1979) as an active process where the family utilizes all existing family resources and develops new behaviors and resources that will strengthen the family unit and reduce the impact of stressful life events. By shifting from the individual level to a family level of coping, coping becomes much more complex. Because of the difficulty in assessing family coping efforts, most family coping studies describe a combination of individual and family coping responses made by family members and the family. Family coping responses or behaviors are the specific actions or cognitions family members employ (McCubbin et al., 1981), while coping patterns and strategies are similar responses that cluster into homogeneous sets. Family and individual coping strategies develop and change over time, in response to the demands or stressors being experienced (Menaghan, 1983).

Adaptation is a process of managing the demands of the stressors through the use of resources, coping, and problem-solving strategies. The outcome is an altered state of functioning that may be positive or negative, resulting in the increase or decrease of a family's state of wellness (Burgess, 1978). For example, seeking help from community agencies may be a very positive move when outside assistance is needed to help a child with learning problems, but the same adaptive strategy may be negative if it becomes the predominant way a family solves its problems. This is because the family does not learn to utilize its own inner resources.

Family adaptation is functionally defined by McCubbin and McCubbin (1993), as a "process in which families engage in direct responses to the extensive demands of a stressor, and realize that systemic changes are needed within the family unit, to restore functional stability and improve family satisfaction and well-being" (p. 57). According to McCubbin and McCubbin (1993), adaptation involves the process of restructuring family patterns of functioning. In a concept analysis by Clawson (1996) that focused on family adaptation to chronic illness of a child family member, family adaptation was defined as an ongoing family system process identified by the use of multiple coping strategies to achieve adaptive tasks in a chronic illness situation. Both of these definitions emphasize that family adaptation is a process that takes place over time when family members are adapting to stressful life situations such as caring for a child with chronic illness. However, these definitions differ in that the McCubbins' definition emphasizes the need for families to make systemic changes in family functioning while Clawson stresses the need for families to utilize their coping strategies in response to a specific situational stressor, in this case a child member with a chronic illness.

▶ TIME PHASES OF STRESS AND COPING STRATEGIES

Nurses need to be aware of the time phases of stress, as well as the coping strategies family members and the family unit might use during each of the three time periods.

Antestress Period

In the period before actually confronting the stressor (such as the hospitalization of a child), anticipation is sometimes possible; there can be an awareness of impending danger or the perceived threat of the situation. If families or helping persons can identify a future stressor, anticipatory guidance as well as preventive coping strategies to weaken or reduce the impact of the stressor may be sought or provided.

Actual Stress Period

Adaptive strategies during the period of stress usually differ in intensity and kind from those utilized prior to the onset of the stressor and stress. There may be very basic survival, defensive strategies used during this period if the stress in the family is extreme. With tremendous energy expended in dealing with a stressor(s) and stress, many family functions (some which may be crucial to family health) are often temporarily set aside or are inadequately performed until the family has the resources to deal with them again. An example of the latter situation is when families totally organize their family life around the care of a member with a chronic illness. In these situations they become very dysfunctional over time as the developmental needs of the healthy members are unmet and the developmental course of family life is distorted (Reiss, Steinglass, & Howe, 1993). The most helpful coping responses during stressful periods are often intrafamilial (to be discussed later), and the seeking of spiritual support (Friedman, 1985; Pravikoff, 1985).

Poststress Period

The coping strategies employed following the initial acute stress period, termed the posttrauma phase, consist of strategies to return the family to a homeostatic, balanced state. To promote family wellness during this phase, the family needs to pull together, mutually express feelings, and solve its problems (Burgess, 1978) or seek out and utilize familial supports for resolving the stressful situation. Four possible poststress outcomes have been cited: (1) family functioning at a higher level than before; (2) family functioning at the same prestress level; (3) family functioning at a lower level than before; or (4) family dissolution (i.e., separation, divorce, abandonment) (Mederer & Hill, 1983). When a family ends up functioning at a lower level of wellness or in a state of family dissolution, family members often need professional assistance to help them increase their repertoire of effective coping strategies (Reiss, Steinglass, & Howe, 1993).

▶ FAMILY STRESS THEORY

One of the primary tasks of a family nurse is detecting when a family is in crisis (although in actuality families range from functioning well to poorly rather than falling neatly into crisis or noncrisis categories). In assessing a family in trouble, it is important to determine (1) whether or not the family's problem is being adequately managed by the family members; (2) if a crisis state exists; or (3) whether the existing problem is part of a chronic inability to solve problems. Nursing intervention varies substantially in each of these cases. Moreover, in working with a family that is not presently having problems but has had a history of being crisis prone, a family nurse would want to be attuned to this tendency so that early problem recognition and assistance can take place.

Two family stress theories, one emphasizing the precrisis stage (the ABCX Model) and one emphasizing postcrisis (the Resiliency Model), are discussed next as useful guides for the nurse working with families managing stressful situations. One of the differences between these two models is that in the ABCX Model (Hill, 1949) a crisis situation is viewed as a negative outcome for the family, but in the Resiliency Model (McCubbin & McCubbin,

1993), crisis is viewed as an indication that the family must make some fundamental changes in how it usually functions in order to adapt to stressor events (McCubbin & McCubbin, 1993).

Hill's Family Stress Theory

Hill's (1949) classic family stress theory is the most eloquent, parsimonious model that describes the factors producing crisis or noncrisis in families. Based on research Hill conducted on war-induced separation and reunion, he developed a family stress theory called the ABCX Model in which he identified a major set of variables and their relationships that led to family crisis. He also theoretically described a postcrisis "roller coaster" adjustment process which families went through. These two parts of his theoretical framework have remained virtually unchanged for the last 40 years. Moreover, this theory has been the basis for many research studies in the family stress and coping area, and has been foundational to the work of Caplan (1964) and other clinicians in generating practice theory and principles in crisis intervention.

This ABCX framework has two parts. The first is a proposition dealing with the determinants of family crisis: "A (the event and related hardships) interacting with B (the family's crisis meeting resources) interacting with C (the definition that the family makes of the event) produces X (the crisis)" (Hill, 1965, p. 36). The second part is a more process-oriented statement regarding the course of adjustment following a crisis. Hill (1965) explains that the course of family adjustment following a crisis involves (1) a period of disorganization, (2) an angle of recovery, and (3) reorganization and a new level of family functioning.

Figure 17–1 presents a visual representation of an adaptation of Hill's model. To elaborate further on Hill's model, this model explains what precipitates a crisis in one family and not in another. As seen in Figure 17–1, there are three basic factors involved.

The first is the actual presence of stressors or stressor-events (factor A). The second basic factor influencing the outcome–crisis or noncrisis in dealing with a stressor is the family's resources and use of coping mechanisms (factor B). Major stressors initially force stereotypic defenses. Later, coping efforts emerge. If the family does not make use of its resources and coping mechanisms from its repertoire of possible responses, the result is the same as if the family did not possess the coping resources. However, the intervention is easier in this case because it is less difficult to assist families to utilize past coping patterns than to help families learn new ways of responding.

Third and most important of the three contributing factors is the family's perception and interpretation of the stressors or stressor-events (factor C). Lazarus and co-workers (1974) emphasize that it is the person's or group's cognitive appraisal of the stressor that influences what coping efforts are made as well as the final outcome. Recall that families that consistently perceive and define events and their situation as threatening and dangerous rather than challenging will most likely be crisis prone. Functional families are able to see events as understandable and manageable.

Antonovsky (1994) posits two views of individual and family health: (1) the pathogenesis and (2) the salutogenesis way of thinking. Antonovsky's (1979, 1994) emphasis is on the salutogenesis way, which directs one to think and study health fundamentally differently than the pathogenesis way of thinking. Nurses often use a pathogenesis model in assessing for disease symptoms in an individual or family. In contrast, salutogenesis explains what facilitates successful coping with stressful life situations and what moves individuals and families toward health (Antonovsky, 1994). In Antonovsky's (1979, 1987) Salutogenic Model of Health, the main concept is sense of coherence (SOC). SOC is believed to shape an individual's core of specific coping and to encompass one's sense of comprehensibility (where internal and external stimuli are seen as predictable and structured); manageability (the belief that available resources are meeting the demands/stressors), and meaningfulness (the belief that stressors/demands are

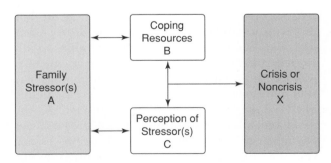

Figure 17–1. Hill's Family Stress Theory (1949). *(Adapted from McCubbin & Patterson, 1983b.)*

worth investing in) in stressful life situations. The SOC concept has been widely studied in individuals, and those with strong SOC been found to experience a higher sense of well-being (Carmel et al., 1991; Larsson & Setterlind, 1990; Petrie & Azariah, 1990; Ryland & Greenfeld, 1990), less dysfunction (Langius & Björnvell, 1993), and less life stress (Flannery, Perry, Penk, & Flannery, 1994). Family sense of coherence, while less studied, also has been found to have a positive influence on adaptation to life-threatening and disabling illness (Anderson, 1994; Antonovsky & Sourani, 1988).

Returning to Hill's Family Stress Theory, factor X deals with crisis or noncrisis. Hill (1965) discusses this factor in terms of crisis-proneness in families. Crisis-proneness describes how families handle the B and C factors of the theory. When families are crisis-prone, they tend to experience stressor events (A) with greater frequency and greater severity and define these (C) more frequently as crises. These types of families are more vulnerable to stressor events also because of the meager resources and coping abilities (B) they possess. In addition, they typically fail to learn from past crises, leading them to see new stressor events as threatening and crisis provoking.

The X factor tends to be seen by Hill as an "either/or" outcome, although gradations of crisis or noncrisis certainly exist. The disorganizing effects of crisis in the family are seen in family relations and role performance of family members. Hill (1965) observed that sexual behavior of the marital couple was a most sensitive index of the presence of crisis (Hill, 1965).

Subsequent to Hill's seminal theory building, other family stress models have been built on Hill's original work. The most recent family stress model emphasizes the factors that influence the family's postcrisis response.

The Resiliency Model of Family Stress, Adjustment, and Adaptation

The Resiliency Model of Family Stress, Adjustment, and Adaptation (McCubbin & McCubbin, 1993) is a theoretical framework that also emphasizes family adjustment and adaptation when families experience stressful life situations. The Resiliency Model builds on the earlier work of Hill's ABCX stress model (Hill, 1949, 1958) as well as later family stress models (McCubbin & McCubbin, 1987, 1989; McCubbin & Patterson, 1983a). The main emphasis of this model is on the resiliency of families or their ability to recover from adverse events and what strengths and capabilities influence this process.

The Resiliency Model is based on four fundamental assumptions about family life:

> (a) Families face hardships and changes as a natural and predictable aspect of family life over the life cycle; (b) families develop basic strengths and capabilities designed to foster the growth and development of family members and the family unit and to protect the family from major disruptions in the face of family transitions and changes; (c) families develop basic and unique strengths and capabilities designed to protect the family from unexpected or normative stressors and strains and to foster the family's adaptation following a family crisis or major transition and change; and (d) families benefit from and contribute to the network of relationships and resources in the community, particularly during periods of family stress and crises. (McCubbin & McCubbin, 1991, p. 3)

In the Resiliency Model (Fig. 17–2), families' responses to stressful life events and transitions occur in two phases: (1) the adjustment phase, and (2) the adaptation phase.

The Adjustment Phase of the Resiliency Model. The adjustment phase of the model depicts family response to events that do not present major hardships and require only minor changes in how the family unit is currently functioning *or* the *initial* response of the family to a more major event. Situations that may require only adjustment by the family could be family vacations, a family member's brief acute illness with complete recovery, or a family member receiving a ticket for a minor traffic violation. Families who experience such stressors will adjust to the stressor by calling upon the families' established ways of functioning with only minor changes being made; the family's definition of the stressor (family appraisal), the family's existing resources, family problem-solving and coping abilities. However, if minor changes in family functioning are not adequate to manage these events, then the family moves into a crisis situation and the adaptation phase of the model.

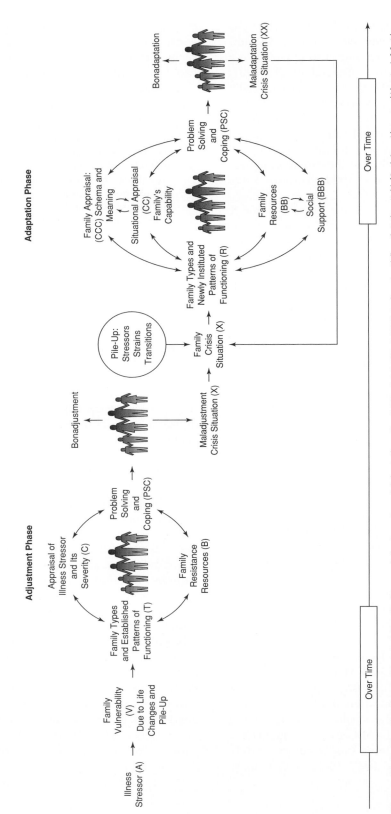

Figure 17-2. The Resiliency Model of Family Stress, Adjustment, and Adaptation. *(From McCubbin, M. & McCubbin, H. [1993]. Families coping with illness: The Resiliency Model of Family Stress, Adjustment, and Adaptation. In C. Danielson, B. Hamel-Bissell, & P. Winstead-Fry, Families, health and illness [pp. 21–63]. St. Louis: Mosby.)*

The Adaptation Phase of the Resiliency Model.

In this model, the crisis situation is not necessarily viewed as pathological or detrimental to the family, but rather indicates that the family needs to make fundamental structural or systemic changes in functioning in order to adapt to the situation. In other words, old ways of functioning are no longer adequate and new solutions must be found. Both developmental and situational stressors can create a crisis and require adaptation by the family.

Crises in the family call upon the family unit to make some systemic family changes to restore stability to family member and family unit functioning (McCubbin & McCubbin, 1993). Family crisis is conceptualized in the model as a "continuous condition of disruptiveness, disorganization, or incapacitation in the family social system" (Burr, 1973, cited in McCubbin & McCubbin, 1993, p. 31). Therefore, since families in crisis need to make major changes in functioning in order to adapt to stressful life situations, family crisis is viewed as a necessary precondition in order for the family to adapt to stressors or demands that family members are experiencing (see Figure 17–3) (McCubbin & McCubbin, 1993).

In the adaptation phase of the model (see Fig. 17–2), response to a crisis situation is determined by the pile-up of demands, stressors, transitions, and strains, as well as the strengths and capabilities of the family unit. These include newly established patterns of functioning; the family's appraisal of how the demands are being met and the family's world view; resources within individual family members, the family unit, and the community; and the family's existing and newly developed problem-solving and coping responses. Each of the major variables in the model are subsequently described.

Pile-up of Demands.

Families are often dealing with more than one stressor at a time. In the Resiliency Model, six categories of stresses and strains are identified: (1) The stressor event and associated hardships (e.g., when families of children with chronic asthma need to stabilize the family environment in the home by keeping the air clean and dust free, not having pets, and asking family members to give up smoking); (2) normative transitions (e.g., birth of children, children entering school, adolescent stage, retirement); (3) preexisting family strains (e.g., difficulty getting along with an ex-spouse); (4)

situational demands (e.g., work hours increase or extensive requirements for work-related travel with frequent absences from family); (5) consequences of the family efforts to cope (e.g., one member quiting his or her job to care for a member with chronic illness, which decreases family income; or the use of drugs and alcohol as a coping strategy); and (6) intra-family and social ambiguity—lack of clear guidelines from both within and outside the family as to how to manage this situation, such as what to do about infertility or having miscarriages (McCubbin & McCubbin, 1993).

Newly Instituted Patterns of Functioning.

The importance of the family establishing new patterns of functioning in a crisis is emphasized in the Resiliency Model. Instead of looking at just one aspect of family functioning at a time, two aspects of functioning are considered simultaneously to construct a "family type." Family types are defined as the set of family attributes that explain how the family functions as a unit (McCubbin & McCubbin, 1993). Although there may be many family types or combinations, three family types will be briefly described.

The **regenerative family** type is characterized as possessing family hardiness and family coherence. Family hardiness refers to the internal strengths and durability of the family unit and is comprised of the family members' ability to work together and have a commitment to solve problems; an ability to see stressors and change as challenges rather than enormous obstacles that family members cannot surmount; and the feeling that the family has some influence in how things turn out and that they can achieve some degree of mastery or control over the situation. Family coherence refers to the family's sense of comprehensibility, manageability, and meaningfulness, as noted earlier from Anotonovsky's model (1979, 1994). The **rhythmic family** type focuses on family time and routines (e.g., mealtime and bedtime routines); and the valuing of these times and routines as an integral part of daily family life. These routines provide some predictability for the family during times of stress and crisis. The **resilient family** type highlights family flexibility (the ability to change) and family bonding (emotional closeness between family members). Families who are high on both hardiness and coherence, time and routines and the valuing of these, and flexibility

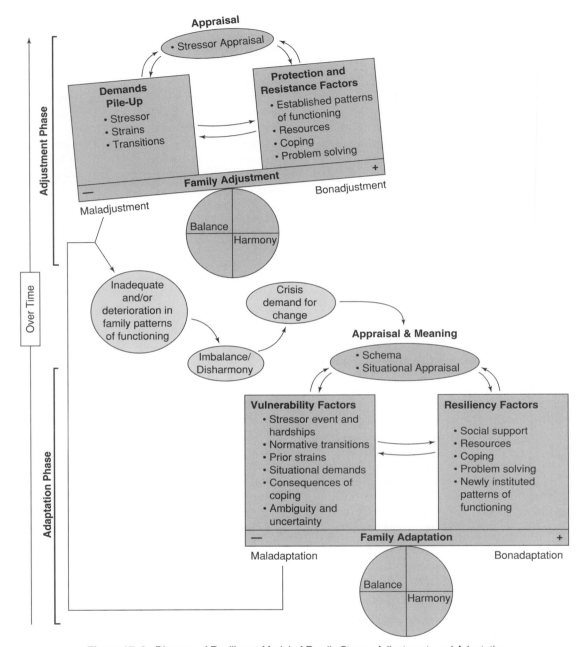

Figure 17–3. Diagram of Resiliency Model of Family Stress, Adjustment, and Adaptation.

and bonding have been found to be better able to adapt to stressful situations (McCubbin, Thompson et al., 1988).

Resources.

Resources are those attributes and supports that are available for use by the family in crisis situations. McCubbin and McCubbin (1993) emphasize three different sources and levels of resources: the individual, the family unit, and the community. Resources of individual family members may include: (1) intelligence, (2) knowledge and skills, (3) personality traits (e.g., optimism), (4) physical health, and (5) emotional health such as self-esteem or sense of mastery. Family unit resources may include organization, decision-making skills, and conflict-resolution abilities. Community resources include both personal support (e.g., relatives, friends) and institutional support (e.g., health care services) that are available outside the family.

Social Support.

Social support is a community support that can be a vital help to families in crisis. Social support will be described more fully later in this chapter but in the Resiliency Model, social support is defined as "information exchanged at the interpersonal level that provides: (a) emotional support (individuals in the family believe that they are loved and cared for); (b) esteem support (family members believe that they are respected and valued); and (c) network support (family members believe that they belong to a network of communication where mutual support and understanding is emphasized)" (Cobb, 1976, cited in McCubbin & McCubbin, 1993, p. 48). In addition McCubbin and McCubbin (1993) also emphasize (d) appraisal support (information that allows family members to assess how well they are doing), and (e) altruistic support (information received as goodwill from others for giving of oneself). Community resources can be a valuable source of social support if the family is willing to access and use this source of support.

Family Appraisal in Adaptation Phase.

In the adjustment phase, the family appraisal encompasses only the family's definition of the stressor (the first level of family appraisal). Two additional levels of appraisal are introduced in the adaptation phase of the model. The family's situational appraisal (the second level) is viewed as the family's shared assessment of the stressor, the hardships created by the stressor, and how well the family is managing these demands (McCubbin & McCubbin, 1993). This second level of appraisal may bring about changes in how a family is coping and functioning. Family schema or world view is the third level of family appraisal. This level of appraisal refers to the families' view of shared values, goals, and expectations that is constructed over time. This level of appraisal is influenced by the family of origin of the adult family members, the cultural and religious background of the family, and societal norms and values. The family world view is usually quite sta-

ble, but can be altered by the occurrence of catastrophic events such as the premature death of a young father in an accident or the birth of a child with Down syndrome.

Problem Solving and Coping.

In the Resiliency Model, coping behavior is defined as the effort and resources families use to manage a stressor (McCubbin & McCubbin, 1993). Thus, resources are what the family possesses and coping is what the family does. Four strategies of coping are identified in the model: (1) action to reduce the demands (e.g., putting a disabled family member in a nursing home), (2) action to obtain additional resources (e.g., finding home nursing care for disabled member), (3) managing tensions and relieving stress (physical exercise, doing enjoyable activities together as a family), and (4) reappraising the situation using reframing strategies (e.g., being thankful for the good things, believing you are doing all that is possible). Reappraisal will be discussed more fully later in the chapter.

The role of parental and family coping has been examined in many studies. For example, in a study on parental coping in a sample of 71 families with an infant 1 year old or younger who was newly diagnosed with congenital heart disease (Svavarsdottir & McCubbin, 1996), the mothers of more severely ill infants reported more helpful coping behaviors related to understanding the health care situation than did fathers. Fathers with higher caregiving demands and higher family system demands (pile-up) found coping behaviors related to maintaining the family unit, maintaining their own psychological stability and use of social support, and understanding the health care situation more helpful than fathers who reported lower caregiving and family system demands. These results demonstrate that coping plays a role in managing both child caregiving demands and the pile-up of family demands in chronic illness of a child.

Problem-solving communication also influences how families adapt. In the Resiliency Model, two types of family communication are identified: (1) incendiary or a conflict-escalating type of communication, which increases stress and tension (e.g., yelling, screaming, blaming tactics); and (2) affirming or a stress-reducing type of communication, which has a calming, supportive, and soothing effect on family members' interaction. Telling members they are doing a good job, conveying warmth and appreciation, and listening to concerns are examples of this type of communication. Families that have lower levels of incendiary and higher levels of affirming communication have been found to adapt better (McCubbin & McCubbin, 1991).

Family Adaptation.

In the Resiliency Model, family adaptation is depicted as occurring at two levels: individual to family and family to community (McCubbin & McCubbin, 1993). At the first level, family adaptation occurs after the family has accepted changes in its functioning in order for the family to work together as a unit. At this level, families are able to carry out their functions—affective, socialization, health care—effectively without compromising the physical health and emotional well-being of family members. At the second level, family adaptation occurs through daily transactions and interactions between the family and the community. Families adapting to stress will need to adapt at both the individual-to-family and the family-to-community levels of functioning because change at one level influences family functioning at the other level (McCubbin & McCubbin, 1993). If the family is not able to make these changes or a new stressor challenges the family's existing level of adaptation, the family can move back into a crisis situation (see Fig. 17–2).

▶ IMPACT OF STRESSORS

Families are daily bombarded with tension-producing stimuli, some of which are only mildly irritating and hardly noticed, such as traffic noise and poor housing, and some of which are potentially or actually devastating to families, such as marital disruption or the loss of a child (McCubbin & Patterson, 1991; Pearlin & Turner, 1987). As depicted in the Resiliency Model (McCubbin & McCubbin, 1993), families are seldom dealing with a single stressor at a time but are often exposed to both normative and situational stressors simultaneously.

For over 50 years researchers have realized the great quantitative and qualitative differences that stressors have on individuals. As early as 1949, researchers systematically studied the quality and quantity of life changes and their impact on the health of individuals (Holmes & Rahe, 1967). From these studies, weights were assigned to a variety of life events (both positive and negative life changes) that were associated with poor health outcomes (Nickolls, 1975). From these early studies, later researchers developed family-based tools that assessed life changes in families. One such widely used tool is the Family Inventory of Life Events and Changes (FILE) (McCubbin, Patterson, & Wilson, 1983).

The FILE (McCubbin, Patterson, & Wilson, 1983) is an instrument that can be used to assess the pile-up or accumulation of family stressors in a family. It has 71 items, grouped into nine subscales: (1) intrafamily strains or difficulties in family relationships, such as strains between parents and children or between ex-spouses; (2) marital strains; (3) pregnancy and childbearing strains; (4) financial and business strains; (5) work–family transitions and strains; (6) illness and family "care" strains; (7) losses (deaths in nuclear and extended family); (8) transitions "in and out" (children being launched or returning home after leaving); and (9) family legal violations. The FILE questionnaire has been validated in many research studies. Families with a higher accumulation of life events (i.e., higher scores on the FILE) have been found to have lower family functioning and poorer health of family members (McCubbin & Patterson, 1991).

On the FILE each life event is weighted as to how stressful it is (Table 17–1). The seven most stressful life events in the *total* FILE scale are: (1) a child member died; (2) a parent or spouse died; (3) spouse or parent was separated or divorced; (4) the presence of physical or sexual abuse or violence in the home; (5) a member became physically disabled or chronically ill; (6) spouse or parent has an affair; and (7) a member went to jail or juvenile detention. Table 17–1 illustrates the three most stressful items under each of the nine subscales of the FILE.

Family life strains and stressors stem from multiple factors, suggesting how difficult it is to assess families. We have tended to think that in order to eliminate a problem one would need to find a way to eliminate or treat a particular causative factor, rather than view the situation more broadly. By assessing the balance between the stressors (their duration and strength)

THE MOST STRESSFUL LIFE EVENTS (WEIGHTED SCORES) BY SUBSCALE IN THE FAMILY INVENTORY OF LIFE EVENTS AND CHANGES SCALE (FILE)

Family Life Changes	Value
■ LOSSES	
A child member died	99
A parent/spouse died	98
Married son or daughter was separated or divorced	58
■ MARITAL STRAINS	
Spouse/parent was separated or divorced	79
Spouse/parent has an "affair"	68
Increased difficulty with sexual relationship between husband and wife	58
■ FAMILY LEGAL VIOLATIONS	
Physical or sexual abuse or violence in the home	75
A member went to jail or juvenile detention	68
A member ran away from home	61
■ ILLNESS AND FAMILY "CARE" STRAINS	
A member became physically disabled or chronically ill	73
Increased difficulty in managing a chronically ill or disabled member	58
Increased responsibility to provide direct care/financial help to husband's/wife's parents	47
■ INTRAFAMILY STRAINS	
A member appears to depend on alcohol or drugs	66
A member appears to have emotional problems	58
Increased difficulty in managing teenage child(ren)	55
■ PREGNANCY AND CHILDBEARING STRAINS	
A unmarried member became pregnant	65
A member gave birth to or adopted a child	50
A member had an abortion	50
■ WORK–FAMILY TRANSITIONS AND STRAINS	
A member lost or quit a job	55
A member stopped working for extended period	51
A member retired from work	48
■ FINANCE AND BUSINESS STRAINS	
Went on welfare	55
A member started a new business	50
Change in agriculture or stock markets which hurt family income	43
■ TRANSITIONS "IN AND OUT"	
Young adult member left home	43
A member was married	42
A member moved back home or a new person moved into the household	42

Source: McCubbin, Patterson, & Wilson (1983).

and the nature and strength of supportive or protective elements, both intrafamilial and extrafamilial, one can either attempt to eliminate or reduce the potency of stressors or to build up and strengthen the family's resources (assets).

Given an assessment of the duration and strength of the family's stressors or current life stressor and other risk factors on the one hand, and their psychosocial, physical, and environmental strengths and capabilities on the other, it should be easier to anticipate which families are at risk; it may then be possible to reduce or eliminate certain stressors, or conversely to strengthen or add certain assets or resources to modify the balancing of forces in favor of the family's greater health. Furthermore, many of the most stressful life events that cannot be changed may have their impact weakened by preparing the family for the event (anticipatory counseling) or providing reality, present-oriented, short-term counseling such as crisis intervention during the time when the overwhelming stressors are being experienced (Nickolls, 1975).

► FAMILY COPING PROCESSES

The picture of family adaptation to stress emerging from research and theoretical efforts up to about the mid-1970s was that the family was merely a reactor to stress, a "defensive" manager of resources with much tendency towards dysfunction. Fortunately this trend is changing. Many subsequent investigations have shifted away from the dysfunctional emphasis to a more positive and broadened interest in the wide array of resources and coping strategies families utilize. Thus, the healing properties of families and their ability to "bounce back" after adversity has received greater emphasis. With this focus, families tend to be seen as resilient social change agents, innovative and surprisingly effective under stressful conditions (Burr, Day, & Bahr, 1993; Burr et al., 1994; McCubbin & McCubbin, 1993; McCubbin, Olson, & Larsen, 1991).

Family Coping Strategies

Coping strategies have been defined as behaviors or processes families use when adapting to stress (McCubbin & Dahl, 1985). One inclusive framework of coping strategies for families under stress includes: (1) cognitive strategies (e.g., gaining of useful knowledge, being accepting of the situation and others), (2) communication strategies (e.g., being open and honest, listening to each other), (3) emotional strategies (e.g., expressing feelings and affection, dealing with negative feelings), (4) relationship strategies (e.g., increasing togetherness, increasing cooperation and trust), (5) spiritual strategies (e.g., becoming more involved in religious activities; having faith in God), (6) environment/community strategies (e.g., seeking help from others), and (7) individual developmental strategies (e.g., increasing self-sufficiency and independence, developing hobbies) (Burr et al., 1994).

In a recent study of 46 families, the extent to which 80 different coping strategies were helpful or harmful in managing various types of stressors (bankruptcy, displacement of the homemaker, infertility, a troubled teen, child with chronic illness, or institutionalized handicapped child) was evaluated by Burr and associates (1994). In-depth interviews and observations were made of these families who had actually experienced the above kinds of situational stressors. In compiling the results from the total sample, the two most helpful coping strategies were identified as spiritual and communication type strategies (see previous examples). Coping involving individual development, emotional strategies, and relationship strategies were noted to be the next most helpful. The two least helpful coping strategies were community support and cognitive strategies.

Family and individual coping efforts and behaviors are conceptualized as being problem or situation specific. Different circumstances and different problems demand different solutions; that is, different coping responses need to be employed. Burr and associates' study (1994) confirmed that coping strategies were stressor specific. For example, the cognitive strategy of accepting the situation was helpful for 90 percent of displaced homemakers, but perceived as more harmful by 39 percent of couples managing infertility problems. They concluded that if displaced homemakers accepted their situation, they could then go on to seek more education, find employment, and build new relationships. In contrast, accepting the situation for infertile couples meant they were giving up on having a biological child and this was not helpful for them (Burr et al., 1994).

The Process of Family Coping

Family stress scholars have suggested that using a variety of coping strategies to cope with stress is more important than using one or two particular coping strategies all the time (Burr, Day, & Bahr, 1993; Burr et al., 1994; McCubbin, Olson, & Larsen, 1991). It is assumed that the following coping strategies are usually functional—although perhaps the exclusive/predominant or inappropriate use of a particular coping strategy could produce dysfunctional family outcomes. Burr and associates (1994) found the most harmful coping behaviors to be: keeping feelings inside (suppressing emotions), taking out feelings on others (in relationships), keeping others from knowing how bad the situation was (lack of communication), and denying, avoiding, or running away from the problem. Without being specific as to the particular situational and family context as noted above, the real functionality of any behavioral pattern cannot be determined. However, families do have certain coping styles or propensities, which also influence the particular types of coping efforts the family brings to bear on a problem.

Another way to view family coping is to look at whether the coping strategies come from within the family or rely on supports and resources outside the family. Family coping strategies are classified as internal or external to the family system (see Table 17–2). A description of these specific coping strategies follows.

Internal Family Coping Strategies

Under internal family coping strategies, seven general types of intrafamilial coping strategies are discussed: family group-reliance, the use of humor, greater sharing together, controlling the meaning of the problem by reframing/passive appraisal, joint problem solving, role flexibility, and normalizing.

Family Group-Reliance.   Certain families when under stress cope by becoming more reliant on their own resources. Families accomplish this by creating greater structure and organization in the home and family. Established family time and routines such as those involving mealtime, bedtime, house-

▶ TABLE 17-2

EXAMPLES OF INTERNAL AND EXTERNAL COPING STRATEGIES: THE F-COPES SCALE

Strategies

- **INTERNAL COPING STRATEGIES**

Confidence in Family Problem Solving

Knowing that we have the strength within our own family to solve problems.

Facing the problems "head-on" and trying to get solutions right away.

Knowing we have the power to solve major problems.

Reframing Family Problems

Accepting stressful events as a fact of life.

Accepting that difficulties occur unexpectedly.

Defining the family problem in a more positive way so that we do not become too discouraged.

Family Passivity

Knowing luck plays a big part in how well we are able to solve family problems.

Feeling that no matter what we do to prepare, we will have difficulty handling problems.

Believing if we wait long enough, the problem will go away.

- **EXTERNAL FAMILY COPING STRATEGIES**

Church/Religious Resources

Seeking advice from a minister.

Participating in church activities.

Having faith in God.

Extended Family

Sharing our difficulties with relatives.

Asking relatives how they feel about problems we face.

Seeking advice from relatives.

Friends

Seeking encouragement and support from friends.

Sharing concerns with close friends.

Seeking information and advice from persons in other families who have faced the same or similar problems.

Neighbors

Asking neighbors for favors and assistance.

Sharing problems with neighbors.

Community Resources

Seeking professional counseling.

Seeking information from the family doctor.

Source: McCubbin, Olson, & Larsen (1991).

hold chores, visits with extended family, and the valuing of these routines can be a source of strength and predictability when the family is under stress (McCubbin & McCubbin, 1991). When families establish greater structure, it is an attempt to have greater control over the subsystems and is comparable to the "tighter" regulation of troops in the military under combat conditions. This usually involves tighter scheduling of members' time, more tasks per family member, a more close-knit organization, and a more rigid, prescribed routine. With the closing of family boundaries comes a call for greater family organization and discipline of members, coupled with the expectation that members will be more self-disciplined and conforming. Families utilizing greater control, if successful, also achieve greater integration and cohesiveness.

This type of family coping usually stems from the influence of the traditional Protestant ethic, which values and sees self-control and self-sufficiency as particularly necessary during hardship periods. Concomitant with structuring is a need for some families to be "strong" and to learn to conceal feelings and master tension within themselves. However, "strong" families sometimes have weak bonds. A case in point is a study by Reiss and associates (1986). The researchers observed that members with a chronic illness in "strong" families who rigidly adhered to the medical regimen for their end-stage renal disease died sooner than family members with a chronic illness who took a day off from their strict treatment regimen to spend time with the family, have a meal together, and socialize (Reiss et al., 1986). Thus, rigidity and control can be helpful in managing stress, but if carried to extreme, appear to be detrimental to both individual and family functioning.

Burgess (1978) points out that this particular coping strategy, involving self-discipline among family members, may be very necessary *initially* in stressful situations such as when parents are confronted with a serious accident at home. They must maintain composure and the capacity to problem solve, because they then are responsible for their own lives and those of their children. And, in fact, Pearlin and Schooler (1978) found that self-reliance was an efficacious coping response in the area of enacting one's marital and parental roles. Time management is one particular coping response that follows within this broader coping strategy.

Nonetheless, this strategy also can be dysfunctional if in certain circumstances outside help is needed but not sought. For example, a family caregiver for a member with Alzheimer's who does not seek outside help when the member's condition deteriorates to needing total physical care may seriously impair his or her own physical and mental well-being. Also if family group-reliance becomes a habitual, pervasive mode of adaptation, the needed flexibility is lost.

Use of Humor.

A sense of humor is an important family asset that can contribute to improving the family's attitude toward its problems and health care. Wooten (1996) emphasizes that humor and laughter can be viewed as self-care tools to cope with stress whereby the ability to laugh can give one the feeling of power over the situation. Humor and laughter can therefore support a positive and hopeful attitude instead of feelings of helplessness or depression in a stressful situation. According to Wooten (1996) "laughter provides an opportunity for the release of uncomfortable emotions that, if held inside, may create biochemical changes that are harmful to the body" (p. 54). Humor and laughter are also generally known to provide a way for individuals and groups to relieve anxiety and tension. However, even though humor is identified here as functional, if it is used repeatedly to mask direct emotional expression and cover up and shun problems, its use is obviously dysfunctional.

Greater Sharing Together (Maintaining Family Cohesion).

One way of bringing the family closer together and maintaining and managing stress levels and the necessary family morale is by sharing of feelings and thoughts, and engaging in joint family experiences or activities. Greater sharing together produces higher family cohesion, a family attribute that has received wide attention for being a central family attribute (Olson, 1993). Olson (1993) views family cohesion as "the emotional bonding that family members have toward one another" (p. 105). Extreme families are either very high or very low on cohesion. When families are very high on cohesion, the family is said to be enmeshed and there is little individual independence or autonomy. When the family is disengaged or is very low on cohesion, family members are not close to one another and have little commitment to the family unit. Families that have moderate levels of cohesion tend to be more functional and better able to adapt to stress (Olson, 1993). The level of cohesion that is functional for the family also is influenced by cultural background;

higher levels of cohesion in certain cultural groups are both desirable and functional.

The most crucial relationship requiring cohesiveness or sharing together in the family system may be between the spouses or adult partners, particularly in middle-class families. A confiding relationship, especially between mates, in which individuals can talk intimately about themselves and their concerns has been shown to be critical for good psychological health in times of stress. The sharing of concerns and feelings is also very advantageous in reducing the family tension level. High family cohesiveness is especially helpful when a family has been traumatized, because family members are in much greater need of support (Figley, 1989).

A family's involvement in family rituals that have meaning and value to the family is another way in which the family shares together. Rituals in families are repeated social processes or patterns of interaction that preserve the family identity and give family members a shared definition of the world (Hartman & Laird, 1983). An excellent cultural example of a family ritual is the traditional Jewish custom of sitting shivah for a 7-day period after a funeral in which relatives and close friends visit with the bereaved family and share their thoughts and feelings, providing mutual emotional support and nurturance.

Leisure-time family activities are especially important coping resources to rejuvenate a family's cohesiveness, morale, and satisfaction (McCubbin & McCubbin, 1991; Olson, 1993). Like so many sayings, the adage, "A family that plays together, stays together" contains much truth. This coping strategy is ultimately aimed at building greater integration, cohesiveness, and resiliency in the family.

Controlling the Meaning of the Problem by Reframing and Passive Appraisal.

One of the primary means Pearlin and Schooler (1978) found to be effective in coping was by use of the mental mechanism—controlling the meaning of the problem, which ameliorates or cognitively neutralizes threatening stimuli that are experienced in life. As mentioned earlier, the interpretation given to events can make the difference between overresponding to a situation (wherein the family experiences great stress), reacting in a realistic way (wherein the situation is seen objectively, appraised accurately), and underreacting (wherein an element of denial may be present and less stress is elicited). Two ways to control the meaning of the problem are presented here; reframing and passive appraisal.

In the family mental health literature, *cognitive reframing* is encouraged most often as a way for controlling the meaning of a stressor. The terms "optimistic beliefs" and "positive appraisal" (Burr, Day, & Bahr, 1993; Folkman et al., 1986) are also used synonymously. Families that use this coping strategy tend to see the positive facets of life's stress-producing events, as exemplified by the making of positive comparisons ("count your blessings"; "it could have been worse"); selectively ignoring the negative aspects ("I've learned a lot from this negative experience"); and making the stressful events or experiences less important in terms of the family's hierarchy of values (Chesler & Barbarin, 1987; Pearlin & Schooler, 1978). Redefining and reframing the situation was found to be especially helpful for families that had a child with a chronic illness (Burr et al., 1994).

Reframing is an individual or family perceptual way of coping and is often influenced by family beliefs. Families have shared perceptions or shared subjective realities, and the reframing process will be influenced by these perceptions. Rolland (1994) emphasizes that individual and family beliefs function as a cognitive map that guide family actions and decisions. Beliefs can, in that way, be in harmony with the families' world view, family paradigms, and family values. According to Rolland (1994) families develop paradigms or belief systems about how the world operates. These beliefs shape how families experience and interpret their environment and are an important factor in the family's process of reframing and redefining its situation. The role of religion and spirituality also plays an important role in forming beliefs. Families will note in stressful situations that they believe that "God would not give us anything we couldn't manage" or that "God will help us through this situation."

A second way families control the meaning of a stressor(s) is by *passive appraisal*, sometimes referred to as a passive acceptance. Here families use a collective cognitive coping strategy of viewing the stressor or stressful demand as something that will take care of itself over time and about which there is nothing or little that can be done. As Boss (1988) points out,

passive appraisal can be an effective stress-reducing strategy in the short run in cases where nothing can be done. By passively accepting the situation, a family may more easily tolerate the inevitable or immutable. However, if this strategy is used consistently and over time, its use then inhibits active problem solving and change in families.

Joint Problem Solving.   Joint problem solving among family members is a family coping strategy that has been extensively studied via laboratory research methods by a group of family researchers (Klein, 1983; Reiss, 1981; Strauss, 1968) and in the natural setting (Chesler & Barbarin, 1987; Epstein et al., 1993; Figley, 1989). Focusing on the routine and expectable disruptions in family life, researchers have looked at the differences in families' use of joint problem solving. Joint problem solving can be described as a situation where a family jointly is able to discuss a problem at hand, search for a solution governed by logic, and reach a consensus on what to do based upon a fully shared set of cues, perceptions, and suggestions from the various family members. Effective family problem solving involves seven specific steps: (1) identifying the problem, (2) communicating about the problem, (3) coming up with possible solutions, (4) deciding on one of the solutions, (5) carrying out the action, (6) monitoring or making sure that the action was carried out, and (7) evaluating the entire problem-solving process. By incorporating these problem-solving strategies into family life, families are believed to function more effectively (Epstein et al., 1993). Reiss (1981) calls families that use effective problem-solving processes environment-sensitive families. These types of families see the nature of problems as being "out there" and do not try to make the problem an internal one.

Figley (1989) identified "solution-oriented problem-solving" as being a type of functional coping. Families coping with trauma usually only "get stuck" briefly on who is to blame for the current problems the family is experiencing. The families then move to mobilize their resources to resolve the stress-producing situation (Burr, Day, & Bahr, 1993; Figley, 1989).

Role Flexibility.   Because of the rapid and pervasive changes in our society and hence in family life, role flexibility, especially among mates, constitutes a powerful type of coping strategy. Olson (1993) has emphasized role flexibility as one of the major dimensions of family adaptation. The spouse or adult partner subsystem's ability to role share and change roles when needed is very important. In research on levels of functioning of grieving families, Davies and colleagues (1986) corroborated the importance of role flexibility as a functional coping strategy. They found that the degree to which family roles were flexible or rigid differentiated levels of functioning in their sample of grieving families, with flexible roles associated with better functioning.

Normalizing.

Another functional family coping strategy is the tendency for families to normalize things as much as possible when they are coping with a long-term stressor that tends to disrupt family life and household activities. Multiple authors have used the term "normalizing" to conceptualize how families manage a member's disability (Knafl & Deatrick, 1986). Davis (1963) was the first researcher to use the term "normalization" to describe a family's response to illness or disability. He found that families with children who had polio normalized their situation by minimizing abnormalities in the child's appearance, participating in usual activities, and maintaining ongoing social ties. Normalization is a management process often used by families of children with chronic health conditions. Normalization is an ongoing process that involves acknowledging the chronic condition but defining family life as normal, defining the social effects of having a child with a chronic condition as minimal, and engaging in behaviors that show others that the family is normal (Knafl & Deatrick, 1986; Shepard & Mahon, 1996).

Gender Differences in Coping

It is important to note that men and women have been found to use different coping strategies. Out of the 80 coping strategies examined by Burr and associates (1994) men and woman differed significantly in the use of ten coping strategies. Women found it more useful to share concerns or difficulties with friends, openly express positive and negative feelings and emotions, and spend time on self-development and hobbies. On the other hand, men tended to use more withdrawal strategies such as trying to keep feelings inside, trying to keep others from knowing how bad things were, and using alcohol more. Thus, tensions can arise in a family when the man wants to withdraw and keep distant from a stressful situation while the woman wants to cope by talking about the situation and expressing her feelings. Research on coping among dual-career men and women across the family life cycle (Schnittger & Bird, 1990) also revealed gender differences in coping. In this study women, when compared to men, coped significantly more often by delegating, using social support, using cognitive reframing, and limiting their avocational activities such as recreation and hobbies.

External Family Coping Strategies

Although internal coping strategies are crucial, most authors writing in this area today also emphasize the necessity for families under stress to bring in or receive greater external information, tangible goods, services, and support. External family coping strategies of seeking information, maintaining active linkages with the broader community, using social support systems, and seeking spiritual support will be discussed more in-depth in this section. Most of the discussion in this section describes nuclear family support systems, because social support from the extended family is considered a type of external family coping strategy.

Seeking Information.

Families that are more cognitively based respond to stress by seeking knowledge and information concerning the stressor or potential stressor. This acts to increase feelings of having some control over the situation and to reduce fear of the unknown; it also helps the family to appraise the stressor (its meaning) more accurately.

Parents who actively cope with parenting by seeking out new information and other resources demonstrate positive results and feelings of coping well with parenting responsibilities (Pearlin & Schooler, 1978). Provision of information is often one of the major ways nurses and other health care professionals intervene with families. Many studies have born this out. For example, providing information related to self-care and early recognition of children's asthma symptoms resulted in significant reduction in emergency room visits for intervention groups (Alexander et al., 1988; Fitzpatrick, Coughlin, & Chamberline, 1992); and programs focusing on informing families about asthma medication observed improvement in the child's asthma management after the intervention (Barnett et al., 1992; Hunter & Bryant, 1994).

Maintaining Active Linkages With the Community.

This category differs from coping by using social support systems in that it is a continuing, long-term, and general family coping effort, not one geared to alleviate any one specific stressor. In this case, family members are active participants (as active members or in leadership positions) in clubs, organizations, and community groups. Recall that one of the assumptions in the Resiliency Model (McCubbin & McCubbin, 1993) is that families contribute to and benefit from an active network of community supports and services. The rationale for the importance of this linkage as a coping effort is grounded in systems theory, which states that any social system must have a movement of information and activity across its boundaries if it is to perform its functions (Whitchurch & Constantine, 1993). Because the family alone cannot serve all its member and group needs without enrichment from other sources, the initiation and promotion of growth-producing relationships within the neighborhood, town, and wider society is essential (Pratt, 1976). If, however, the family's boundaries are continually open and do not sufficiently allow for family integration and control over input, this strategy would then be dysfunctional.

Using Social Support Systems.

Seeking and using social support systems within the family's social network is the major external family coping strategy. In addition to extended families and the whole network of professional services, experts, and organizations, there exists a great reservoir of potential help: kin, friends, neighbors, employers, fellow employees, classmates, teachers, and groups with which a family shares common interests, goals, lifestyles, recreational involvements or social identity. Subcultural and reference groups are examples of these types of groups. The family's social networks serve as a third "set of players" for the family wrestling with making suitable arrangements in matters of education, child care, health and welfare services, and so forth (Howell, 1975).

In addition to the discussion in this chapter about seeking family social supports as a type of external family coping strategy, a section within Chapter 8 discusses the concept of social support, social support research findings, and how to assess family social support, using interview questions, the genogram, and the ecomap.

According to Caplan (1974) there are three general sources of social support. These consist of spontaneous, informal networks; organized supports not directed by professional health care workers; and organized efforts by health care professionals. Of these, the informal social network (defined above as the social network) is viewed as the group providing the greatest amount of help in times of need.

The duration and permanency of support systems vary. Some family support systems are long-term, composed of continuous sets of individuals and groups that assist the family in more general life issues such as developmental tasks and situational crisis (e.g., a loss of family member). Other support systems may be crisis oriented, dealing with specific issues and are short-term in duration (Hogue, 1977) such as a group of families who all have a member in the intensive care unit at the same time.

A family copes with its problems within a social network; needless to say, it is impossible to survive in isolation from outer resources. Accessing support can be difficult in some circumstances. For instance, if a member is critically ill, the family may have a strong need for a support person but it may not always be able to request such a support, because of the critical nature of the health problem or its treatment (Hupcey & Morse, 1995).

Purpose of Social Support Systems.

Social networks of support systems have two primary coping purposes: nurturance and emotional support, and direct assistance to family members (Hogue, 1977; MacElveen, 1978). In these types of relationships the nurturing persons or groups care for, support, and emotionally meet some of the psychosocial needs of the family members. Support systems also are concerned with the morale and welfare of the family as a group, and will work to sustain or improve the group's morale and positive motivation.

Extended families or close friends encourage members to communicate freely about their personal difficulties. When the family then shares its problems with this support system, it is offered individualized advice and guidance in keeping with the family's traditions and values. The superiority of extended family and close friends over professionals who do not know the family, in terms of giving help and advice, is often expressed by clients (Friedman, 1985). After all, who knows the family better than these supportive individuals? Can health care professionals have the same keen sense of uniqueness of a particular family that close friends and family have? And who has the greater and more lasting interest in the family's welfare and happiness? The answers to these questions speak for the vital nature of informal social networks. The family's informal social network also can provide feedback to the family about its expectations, perceptions, and priorities; this, in turn, can improve the family's communication with outside community supports (Wade, Howell, & Wells, 1994).

The second primary purpose support systems achieve is that of task-oriented assistance that extended family, friends, and neighbors often provide. An important element of this assistance is not only telling family members how to find sources of care and assistance in the community, but also giving direct assistance. In our society, usually only close relatives will provide extensive long-term help. Assistance from extended family also takes on the form of direct help, including continuing and intermittent financial aid, shopping, care of children, physical care of old people, performing household tasks, and practical assistance in times of crisis (Caplan, 1974). In coping with caregiving for an elderly family member, most families have been found to cope well with caregiving demands and use institutions or formal services only as their last resort (Neundorfer, 1991). However, a significant proportion of family caregivers do experience depression, anxiety, and/or other negative health outcomes as a result of their caregiving. The use of outside community supports can often alleviate some of these burdens associated with long-term caregiving.

The absence of such assistive relationships can generate a sense of vulnerability, especially where use of these assistive relationships, e.g., the extended family, is an important culturally derived way of coping. For instance, Friedman (1985) found that the absence of extended family support in Latino as compared to Anglo families that had a child with cancer was much more disruptive. Another case in point, where absence of social support made a difference, was in a study by Murata (1995). Murata studied family stress, social support, and sons' behavior problems in 21 low-income inner-city African-American mother-headed families. In her sample, higher family stress, greater behavioral problems of sons, and higher levels of depression were all positively associated with the mothers' perceptions of having lower levels of social support.

Inadequate Use of Social Networks.   There is both concern and evidence that many people do not seek needed external help (Pearlin & Schooler, 1978). Several factors inhibit families, especially those in the middle class, from fully utilizing these resources. First, the belief exists that professional services are often best, but because they are very costly and often beyond the family's means, no outside help is sought. Second, while the family is thought of as a place where individuals can let down their defenses and receive and give support and care, some believe that in facing the outside world the family should exhibit independence and self-sufficiency. Despite the fact that family members often yearn to be interdependent, to be supportive of others outside of the family, and to receive support in return, a feeling persists that asking for help or support is a sign of weakness and fallibility. Thus, when a family "fails" to handle its own problems, it "should" be prepared to turn to paid professionals to resolve the problem (Howell, 1975).

In the case of family "failure"—that is, where the family is unable to succeed solely through its own means—professional services are available. The services available to the lower-income family or to those who cannot pay full fees, however, are often inadequate or inaccessible (Wilson et al., 1995). Unfortunately, professionals, rather than encourage self-care and self-control, often rob families of their control over their own problems and, ironically because of their lack of real understanding and knowledge of the family, may very well provide unsatisfactory solutions (Hogue, 1977).

In contrast to closed families who inadequately utilize informal social support, it has been suggested that open families are able to define their boundaries more loosely and flexibly, according to the needs of members and the group and according to outside demands and requests for help from the social network. Because such boundaries allow for a greater exchange of energy, matter, and information, these families are better able to use the family's informal social network.

A family's use of its social network as a resource for assistance will alter the use of professional services in a more appropriate direction, namely, for those specialized or complex needs that cannot be met by the family's social support system or self-care resources.

Mutual Aid or Self-help Groups.   Even though the extended family and other informal social networks usually serve as primary sources of support for many individuals and families, self-help groups are another very important source of social support in communities (Pender, 1996). Many family members find that they need to share and seek help from others who have the same concerns and need to share. And their usual support system does not adequately provide for these needs, some of which are more specialized in nature. Hence, participating in a self-help group provides a supportive and/or assistive system that is sufficiently sharing to mediate communication, guide action, and make personal experiences more bearable (Miller & Katz, 1992; Vickers, 1971).

Individuals and families join mutual aid groups as a coping strategy to meet a wide variety of special needs. Hence self-help groups include a broad gamut of organizations, established with varied purposes and processes. For instance some self-care groups, such as PFLAG (parents and friends of lesbians and gays) provide education, support, and understanding for this often marginalized group; parents of murdered children band together to share their grief and rage; Vietnam veterans' groups are alternative caregiving systems; some groups, such as ostomy clubs, are adjuncts to the health care professional's services; some are an expression of democratic, political ideals, such as the National Organization for Women (NOW); and some are vehicles for promoting individual change, such as Parents Anonymous and Alcoholics Anonymous. These self-help groups maintain either face-to-face, telephone, newsletter, and/or computer support networks among members.

There is a tremendous growth in urban areas of recovery-oriented self-help groups for family members with addictions (the addicted person and his or her "codependents"). This rapid growth is evidence of the extent to which addictions (alcohol, drugs, eating, gambling) are a problem today, as well as the tendency for families to use self-help groups for coping with these growing problems. More recently support/education groups also have been formed for prevention of such problems. The DARE (drug awareness resistance education) program to prevent drug use in children and adolescents is one example.

Seeking Spiritual Support.   Although most people would think of seeking and relying on spiritual support as being an individual coping response, several studies have reported that family members find it a family way of coping too (Burr, Day, & Bahr, 1993; Chesler & Barbarin, 1987; Friedman, 1985; McCubbin, Olson, & Larsen, 1991; Olson et al., 1983). In fact, belief in God and prayer were identified by family members as being either the most important way the family coped with a trying health-related stressor or a very important and frequently employed method in two studies (Friedman, 1985; Pravikoff, 1985). In Pravikoff's study of 28 family members of post-myocardial infarction patients, the sample was composed of older WASP (White, Anglo-Saxon, Protestants) who were middle-class. In Friedman's study (1985) of 55 families with a child with cancer, the families were one-half Anglo and one-half Latino. Latinos, in comparison to Anglos, relied much more heavily on religion as their most important way of handling their child's cancer. Ethnic differences in family coping with respect to the helpfulness of spiritual supports were quite evident. Olson and associates (1983), in surveying 1200 white middle- and upper-middle-class Lutherans, also found that for coping with everyday life problems, use of religious supports was ranked as very helpful. Spiritual supports have helped families tolerate chronic, long-term strains and contribute to maintaining the family unit. Olson and associates (1983) found that the use of this strategy varies in the family's life cycle stage. For instance, families in their study reported that they used spiritual supports less during the early stages of family life, but used spiritual supports more thereafter.

▶ DYSFUNCTIONAL FAMILY ADAPTIVE STRATEGIES AND PROCESSES

Whereas functional families experiencing stress tend to act in a direction that reduces stress, dysfunctional families tend to use habitual defensive strategies that tend not to dissipate the stress or eliminate or attenuate the stressor (Epstein et al., 1993; White, 1974). Dysfunctional adaptive strategies do temporarily reduce stress, but the stress returns because the underlying stressors are not dealt with. Stress-reduction strategies can be functional or dysfunctional. The difference here is that dysfunctional strategies have deleterious effects on family members.

In the McMaster model of family functioning (Epstein et al., 1993) (also see Chap. 1), the dimensions of problem solving, communication, roles, affective responsiveness, affective involvement, and behavior control are emphasized as having the most impact on the emotional and physical health of family members. Families that are dealing ineffectively with functioning on any of these dimensions are believed to contribute to a clinical presentation of dysfunction, but families that are functioning effectively in all dimensions are believed to have optimal physical and emotional health (Epstein et al., 1993).

Families use various specific dysfunctional strategies in attempting to cope with their problems. In most cases these strategies are selected unconsciously, often as responses that their families of origin used in attempting to adapt.

As might be expected, the literature dealing with dysfunctional adaptive patterns is much more voluminous than the literature dealing with healthy ways of solving familial problems, this literature having been generated primarily by family and other psychotherapists interested in family interaction and process among their troubled clients.

Because no all-encompassing typology or classification of family dysfunctional adaptive strategies exists in the literature, the classification in Table 17–3 was generated to describe major types of family dysfunctional adaptive strategies. It should be noted that each of these dysfunctional family adaptive strategies is used to reduce family stress or tension.

▶ TABLE 17–3

TYPOLOGY OF DYSFUNCTIONAL FAMILY ADAPTIVE STRATEGIES

■ **DENIAL OF PROBLEMS AND OVERT EXPLOITATION OF ONE OR MORE FAMILY MEMBERS**
  • Nonphysical, but active overt emotional exploitation, scapegoating, use of threat.

■ **DENIAL OF FAMILY PROBLEMS; ADAPTIVE MECHANISM IMPAIRS THE FAMILY'S ABILITY TO MEET AFFECTIVE FUNCTION**
  • Denial seen in family belief system: Family myth.
  • Denial seen through communication patterns: Triangling.
  • Denial maintained through establishment of emotional distancing: Pseudomutuality.
  • Authoritarianism: Submission to marked domination.

■ **FAMILY DISSOLUTION AND ADDICTIONS**
  • Loss or abandonment by family member.
  • Drug and/or alcohol abuse.

■ **FAMILY VIOLENCE**
  • Spouse abuse.
  • Child abuse.
  • Sibling abuse.
  • Elder abuse.
  • Parent abuse.
  • Gay/Lesbian abuse.

Denial and Overt Exploitation of Family Members

There are several overt exploitative ways that families reduce tension for the family as a group, at the emotional expense of one or more individual members.

Under this broad category of denial and exploitation, two family dysfunctional patterns are briefly discussed: scapegoating and the use of threat.

Scapegoating.   Scapegoating is a dysfunctional adaptive mechanism because although it reduces the tension level of the family system and makes the continuance of family homeostasis possible, it does this at the expense of the emotional health of one of its members—the scapegoat or "the identified patient" (Fischer & Wampler, 1994; McCreery, 1981). The scapegoat's function is to effect a total clearance of the emotional ills that beset the family. This pattern is fairly common in troubled families and can be recognized when a family has achieved unity and cohesiveness while at the same time negatively labeling and stigmatizing one of members. The identified patient or scapegoat is "selected" to be the focus of the family's difficulties, thus hiding the real problems within the family (e.g., the marital relationship).

How is the scapegoat selected? First, the person must not be someone who has great significance for family survival; thus, children are by far the most common choices for being scapegoats. Children are in a relatively powerless position, cannot separate from family, are pliant to behavioral changes, and can adopt the roles parents assign to them. Usually the first child is more vulnerable, because in a faulty marriage further strained by the advent of a child, the stressful marital difficulties are quickly displaced onto the first available and "appropriate" object— the first child. A particular child may also be selected because of his or her age or sex, intelligence, health status, developmental stage, resemblance to another family member with negative attributes, or simple availability. Also, a family member who has already been negatively labeled is particularly vulnerable to scapegoating (Klose, 1995; Roberts, 1975).

How does the scapegoating process start and continue? The scapegoating process often starts when families are faced with some unresolved tension that hinders their natural development. For example, when couples are experiencing marital stress they may be having deep-seated fears about the marital relationship but at the same time need to deny that the problem exists (Bell & Vogel, 1968; Hardwick, 1991). The family's problem is perceived to be insoluble and beyond its resources and coping abilities. Because of this, the situation is felt to be a threat or danger to the family's survival and the life goals of its members. Concomitantly, the tension and stress levels rise and throw the family into a state of disequilibrium.

As a result of increased stress level and precarious family stability, the family attempts to reduce tension through the exploitation of one or more of its members. Scapegoating reduces family tensions, because tensions, hostilities, and guilt can be directed toward (or displaced onto) the identified problem member. Furthermore, the scapegoat begins taking on the assigned roles, which started as negative labeling and later became internalized, i.e., into the role of being the scapegoat.

When scapegoating has become an established family adaptive mechanism, family homeostasis is achieved. There is open acknowledgment and labeling of the identified patient or scapegoat. Psychic economy results as group tensions are attenuated by the displacement of anxieties, guilt, and hostility onto an object acceptable to the value system of the family.

Later, when the problem has been further walled off, the individual is reclassified in the family structure as a "problem member" different from all other family members. Although the scapegoat is the victim of hostile projections, because the family is an interactive system, the scapegoat concomitantly works to maintain his or her position as a scapegoat. The parents, to avoid criticism of their treatment of their scapegoated child, define themselves as being victimized by the "problem child" (Hajal, 1990; Vogel & Bell, 1960). Eventually the outside world verifies this differentness by also labeling and stigmatizing the scapegoat. Such labeling maintains the family system's dysfunctionality.

Why would the scapegoat maintain his or her unpleasant role? The answer lies in the self-fulfilling prophesy: a person does what is expected and responds to the reinforcement he or she receives to maintain a certain role. Reinforcement consists of secondary rewards of extra attention, even if negative, and exemption from responsibility.

If the scapegoat leaves the family, is removed by the community, or does not enact the proper role (because of psychiatric treatment), the family will face another homeostatic crisis. At that time the scapegoat may step back into the former role or a new scapegoat may be selected.

In summary, the scapegoating mechanism can be viewed as functional for the family, in that the scapegoat produces family equilibrium on a short-term basis; but it is dysfunctional in the long run for the emotional health of the exploited member and, for that matter, the health of all family members.

Use of Threat.   Threat is another dysfunctional coping strategy used as a means of keeping the family together at the expense of the emotional health of its members. Therefore, threat can be viewed as a recurrent family dynamic in some troubled families (Gagne, 1992; Smoyak, 1969). This technique is employed by the family to produce and maintain connectedness and discourage members' efforts to individuate and achieve separateness. The purpose of doing so is to ensure the survival of the family.

Gagne (1992) and Smoyak (1969) describe the control technique involved in using threat. The initial basis for needing this means of ensuring family survival is that the family system views its surrounding environment as hostile and threatening. The family feels the only way it can survive is to stick together as a closed family system. Family preservation then becomes emphasized over the individual needs of its members, and the family value of connectedness becomes elevated to a place of high importance to maintain the family. Minuchin (1974) and Olson (1993) refer to these families as "enmeshed;" Bowen calls them "undifferentiated" families (Miller & Winstead-Fry, 1982).

When one or more family members acts in an autonomous, individualistic fashion, the other family members become threatened by the separating individual's impending breach with the family, and thus take action to bring him or her back into the fold. They may do this by themselves threatening to leave the family system, including threats of suicide or self-destructive acts; by threatening social ostracism, and forbidding reentry into the family; by threatening an aggressive act against the separating individual; or by threatening emotional rejection—withdrawal of affection and support. These maneuvers, if successful, result in the "deviant" family member retreating from his or her separatist efforts and again conforming to the value of connectedness. Furthermore, once reintegrated, this individual may then take part in sanctioning another member who attempts to individuate.

Forcing deviating members back into the family so that all members espouse connectedness restores the family's equilibrium. However, individuals from such families have severe adjustment problems when they leave the family environment, because they have not learned autonomy, self-directedness, and how to relate effectively with the outside world.

Denial of Family Problems

Denial is a defense mechanism used by family members and the family as a whole. On a short-term basis, family denial is often functional, as it allows the family to "buy time" to protect itself while gradually accepting painful event. But in the long run, denial is dysfunctional for a family. There are several denial adaptive mechanisms discussed in this section: family myth, triangling, and pseudomutuality.

The Family Myth.   Through the family's belief system, myths can be created about the family that obscure reality and deny some of the real issues and problems within the group, these problems being perceived as either too painful to be brought out in the open or as unnecessary to discuss because doing so will only make things worse (Byng-Hall, 1988). A family myth refers to a belief that is generated in response to the unfulfilled wishes and expectations of the family, instead of being based on a rational and objective appraisal of the situation (Battiste, 1975). The concept of family myth has been clarified as being "a series of fairly well integrated beliefs shared by all family members, concerning each other and their mutual position in the family life, beliefs that go unchallenged by everyone involved, in spite of the reality distortions they may conspicuously imply" (Ferreira, 1963, p. 457).

As wish-fulfillment fantasies, family myths are established early in the family life cycle to serve as a defense against the limitations that the reality of family life imposes. Family myths thus tend to suspend reality. The more myths a family has, the less realistically that family can judge a situation and the fewer the alternatives it has to draw from. For instance, if a myth exists that the mother needs to be protected and helped, then during times of the father's absence, the family's role flexibility is diminished because the mother's ability to function in an instrumental role is stifled by the family myth.

Myths are inner images of the family group, not only the facade that the family holds out to outsiders. Examples of these family myths are: "We all like to do things together"; "We stay married only because of the children"; "Father is the strong one"; "We're a happy family" (Battiste, 1975). Battiste further explains when to suspect that family myths are operating: "When these inner images a family has of itself seem to not ring true to the outside observer, but when the family clings tenaciously to them, one is probably on the track of a family myth" (p. 101).

As previously mentioned, most family myths begin in the early days of the family, when relationships are being formed and cemented. Family myth formulas for togetherness are sought to promote closeness and set limits on possible untoward interpersonal reactions. Circular, repetitive communication patterns, as well as roles, power, and value characteristics develop based on a myth, which in turn, preserves the family unit (Battiste, 1975; Pillari, 1992).

Occasionally, during a time of family crisis, a family myth will be used as a balancing mechanism. As a means of achieving homeostasis, the myth is called into play when a family experiences stress that threatens to disrupt family functioning. Thus, the family myth functions as a defensive mechanism in that it prevents the family from destroying itself by maintaining, and sometimes even increasing, the level of family organization through the establishment of patterns set up as part of the family myth—a myth such as, "When in times of distress, we all help each other" (Peters, 1974).

On the surface, one might say that this "coping" strategy is functional—after all, it provides satisfaction for the family, automatic agreement, a common frame of reference, and stabilizing reassuring rituals. However, it is a dysfunctional adaptive mechanism because it narrows the vision of reality and the choices or alternatives available. Members react to family issues in a stereotypical, nonindividualized way and become limited in their repertoire of responses used to deal with significant issues and life problems. Thus the growth of the family and its members is stifled because, in the presence of family myths, they will not acquire the feelings of confidence and growth that come from meeting life's problems head-on and confronting life's disappointments with a broad range of possible solutions (Battiste, 1975; Price, 1990).

Triangling.   Another way of reducing stress either on a short-term or long-term basis within the family is through the use of triangling. This concept was developed by Bowen (1976), a noted family therapist, and applies to the reduction of tension in a dyadic relationship by adding a third member, who then absorbs and diffuses the ongoing tension in the dyadic relationship (Hallen, 1978). In other words, bringing in a third member relieves the emotionality between the original two by shifting the tension to the new dyadic member and making one of the initial partners into an "outsider." The balance of forces within triangles is fluid and may shift either fre-

quently or over long periods of time. In periods of very high stress, a system will triangle in more outsiders, again reducing the stress within the family (Miller & Winstead-Fry, 1982).

For instance, a husband and wife may be involved in an unsatisfactory, argument-laden relationship that results in neither of their needs being met. Triangling in a third person, one of the couple's children, reduces the marital relationship strain. Both mates begin to focus on the child, although one mate usually develops a dyadic relationship with the child and the other mate becomes the third person—the outsider. This process forces the child to take sides: for one parent and against the other. The parent who forms the close relationship with the child tries to fulfill his or her emotional needs through the parent–child relationship, putting new unrealistic demands on this relationship, so that often the newly formed dyad also becomes strained. As a result, the outside parent may again be triangled in, resulting in a shift back to the marital dyad. "If a triangled person remains in this position for a period of time, it is quite possible he/she will develop some physical or emotional problem as an outlet for his/her anxiety" (Francis & Munjas, 1976, p. 38).

Triangling is included here as a dysfunctional coping strategy because it is a commonly used way in which to reduce interpersonal tension within the family without treating the underlying ills of the situation (Juni, 1995). Although triangling can be looked on as a phenomenon occurring to some extent in all emotionally laden interactions, and especially in dyadic ones under stress, the pervasive use of this stress-reducing mechanism over a long period of time may be considered to be dysfunctional because it does nothing to alleviate the stressor and is injurious to long-term emotional needs of family members.

Pseudomutuality.   Pseudomutuality may be classified as a long-term dysfunctional adaptive strategy because it maintains family homeostasis at the expenses of meeting the family's affective function—that is, recognizing and responding to the socioemotional needs of its members (Schreiber, 1992). The real problem, the inability to foster and maintain intimate, close affective relationships, is covered up by a facade of solidarity and cohesiveness among family members.

Pseudomutuality has been defined as "a type of relatedness in which there is a preoccupation of family members with a fitting together into formal roles at the expense of individual identity" (Wynne et al., 1958, p. 205). As with the use of threat, individual separateness or divergence is forbidden. Individual differentness or divergence is perceived as leading to disruption of the relationship and must therefore be avoided. The use of threat is sometimes used in families displaying pseudomutuality.

These families may desire closeness and intimacy but are afraid of it and are unable to reach one another on a feeling level. Affective communications are almost nil. Each family member strives for relatedness, but feels that other members block his or her efforts at closeness.

To the outside world these families usually present a picture of family solidarity, because their face-saving needs are great. However, they are able to approach this desire only through much formalized or ritualized action, such as giving gifts, celebrating birthdays, holidays, and so forth.

Pseudomutuality is a long-term adaptive strategy used by families. It presents "a stifling structure that constricts autonomy . . . consists of ambiguity, meaninglessness, and emptiness. . . . Individuality poses a great threat, especially with family members who have poor ego structures to begin with" (Silver, 1975, p. 111).

Authoritarianism.
Submission to marked domination is included in this section as a long-term dysfunctional adaptive strategy, because through the submission of family members to a dominant, ruling figure, usually the husband/father, family equilibrium is achieved—but again, at the emotional expense of the subordinates and less obviously, the dominator. Peace and balance may be accomplished on either a short- or long-term basis, but when it is reluctant and forced, anger rages beneath the surface—to be either repressed, with conformity and dependence the outcome, or expressed as depression, somatization, or through acting-out behaviors of defiance, antisocial acts, destructiveness, and so on.

Authoritarianism refers to the tendency to give up one's independence due to feelings of powerlessness and dependency and to fuse self with somebody or something outside one's self in order to acquire the power or strength felt lacking. In an authoritarian family, people renounce their own personal integrity and become part of an unhealthy, submissive–dominance symbiosis. The submissive family members are very dependent on the dominant individual. Life as a whole is felt by the submissive members to be something overwhelming, all-powerful, and uncontrollable. There may also be a defiant family member in these types of families who reacts to the domination with resistance. Interestingly enough, the dominating family member is also dependent on his or her subordinates, because the need for power and control is paramount. Along with having absolute power over the other family members and making them into instruments to be used and exploited, the dominator holds the feeling, "I rule you because I know what's best for you" and "I have done so much for you, now I expect something in return."

As with all the other dysfunctional adaptive strategies, all members in these families suffer. This authoritarian symbiosis curtails efforts of family members to individuate, grow, and become self-directed and independently proficient in life. Moreover, they learn only two ways of relating to people—either as the ruler or the ruled and with this background they perpetuate these roles in all their other relationships and transmit these interpersonal patterns to the next generation. The types of families that fit into this category are those families that do not negotiate on issues, and where the dominant one seeks no input from others before decisions are made.

Many families are mildly husband-dominated and function very effectively. It is only when this dominance pattern becomes exaggerated that it becomes a dysfunctional way to adapt to life's stressors.

Cultural patterns must be taken into account when examining whether authoritarianism is an adaptive strategy the family is using. For instance, both Hispanic and Asian families are traditionally patriarchal. However, even in these families marked domination is not salubrious and does not follow the social mores of these cultures.

These dysfunctional adaptive strategies—scapegoating, use of threat, denial of family problems, perpetuation of family myths, triangulating, pseudomutuality, and authoritarianism can lead to dysfunctional family adaptation. The family may dissolve through abandonment, separation, or divorce or exhibit psychosomatic illness or patterns of family violence or addiction. Nurses in family health care settings often encounter families in these situations.

Family Dissolution and Addictions

To reduce tension or stress in the family, the family members may physically or psychosocially separate from each other. This includes loss of a family member through abandonment, separation, or divorce, and psychosocial loss of family member through the member's involvement in an addiction (alcohol, drugs). Only the addicted family is discussed here.

The Addicted Family.
Addictions of family members are being understood today as family system problems rather than as individual problems. Alcohol and drug use have been found to have an intergenerational pattern. Abusive drinking in young adults has been found to be influenced by dysfunction in the family of origin (Fischer & Wampler, 1994). Steinglass and associates (1987) explained how alcoholism is a family systems problem when they examined the family system of the alcoholic. In *The Alcoholic Family*, they clearly demonstrated the role that alcohol plays in reducing tension in the family and maintaining homeostasis (albeit, short-lived). Their research charts the developmental course of alcoholism in the family and explains the role that other family members play as co-dependents or enablers of the alcoholic. The 10-year study upon which *The Alcoholic Family* was based challenges many of the commonly held notions about alcoholism and proposes a family systems approach for treating alcoholism.

The role of drugs in families is similar to that of alcohol—only the substance is changed (it should be noted that many individuals are addicted to more than one drug or to drugs and alcohol). Certainly the recent growth in drug use, particularly among teenagers aged 12 to 17 years (Savage, 1996), and addictions has had a tremendous influence on the health care system and treatment modes. In addition to professionally led recovery programs, self-help groups following the 12-step program, originally developed to assist alcoholics, are mushrooming nationwide. Many strands of psychosocial and practice theories converge in the current thinking about addiction and its treatment, including family systems theory, chemical dependency theory, child abuse theory, and group therapy theories.

Concerns for family members is evidenced in the literature and in the growth of self-help groups for the "adult children of the alcoholic." Adult children of alcoholics have been profoundly affected by growing up in an alcoholic family, as growing up in these types of families places specific and constant strains on all the family members. Easley and Epstein (1991) found adult children coping with alcoholic parents who use passive appraisal of the problem, attempt to avoid the problem, and blame themselves, are more likely to have poorer adult functioning. In addition, Steinglass and co-workers (1987) showed the tension stress level in alcoholic families is like the ocean tides—always changing, with continual ups and downs and maneuvers to keep the system afloat. Researchers have found that binge drinking by the member with alcohol dependency is more stressful for the family than a member who has steady drinking habits. In the case of binge drinking, the family never knows exactly when the member will decide to engage in heavy drinking (i.e., go on a "binge") so that family members are in a constant state of tension as to whether the member's behavior will disrupt family plans, embarass them in public places, or require intervention (i.e., taking away car keys). Families of steady drinkers, on the other hand, know that this individual is a continuous abuser of alcohol so there is less uncertainty and unpredictability in that person's behavior and they grow accustomed to the addicted member not performing family roles and responsibilities (Jacob, 1992).

Family Violence

Extreme uses of threat, scapegoating, and authoritarianism can result in family violence. Family violence is recognized as one of our major public health problems today (Straus & Gelles, 1990; Wallace, 1996). The professional literature about child abuse and spouse abuse has mushroomed, and there is concomitant rapid growth of research in this area.

One of the main problems in examining family violence data and studies is that the terms "abuse" and "violence" are not conceptually equivalent terms; nor are they consistently defined in the literature. Straus and associates' (1980) definition of wife and child abuse refers to only those acts of violence that have a high probability of causing injury to the victim. Wallace (1996) defines family violence as "any act or omission by persons who are cohabitating that results in serious injury (physical or emotional harm) to other members of the family" (p. 3).

Family or domestic violence is not confined to any one social class. Most domestic violence is directly related to social stress in families (Wallace, 1996). The violent family is often one that is socially isolated (Gelles & Maynard, 1987).

Those individuals who experienced a violent and abusive childhood are more likely to become abusers. The National Center on Child Abuse and Neglect estimates that 30 percent of individuals who were physically or sexually abused or extremely neglected as children become abusive parents themselves.

Although the basic mechanism of violence (use of physical force by one family member against another) is the same, there are actually six types of family violence, depending on who the abuser and victim are: spouse/marital partner abuse, child abuse (physical and sexual), violence between siblings, elder abuse, parent abuse, and violence in gay and lesbian relationships. The first two types are more numerous and widely acknowledged than the latter four.

Spouse Abuse.

Although the use of physical force by one mate against the other (largely husbands against wives) has recently been recognized by the mass media and professionals as a significant social problem (Gelles, 1980; Straus & Gelles, 1990), it has been a commonly used tactic for the handling of frustration and stressors throughout our country's history and, as such, has been societally sanctioned in the past. Even though women are generally victims of spousal abuse, they can also be the perpetrators. Some studies have found that men as victims of spousal abuse are more common than people thought (Wallace, 1996). However, the abuse that women suffer is more common and more severe than the abuse men experience in spousal relationships (Wallace, 1996). Spousal abuse is defined by Wallace (1996) as "any intentional act or series of acts (physical, emotional, or sexual) that cause injury to the spouse" (p. 164). Straus and Gelles (1990) estimate that over 16 percent or one in six couples in America experience couple abuse.

In a study based on a subsample of the National Survey of Family and Households, (n = 4088), the results indicated considerable underreporting of marital violence (Szinovacz & Egley, 1995).

Wallace (1996) believes that spousal abuse has multiple sources in society. For example, social stress, power differences in the marriage (see Chap. 11), women's dependency on their husband, alcohol abuse among husbands, pregnancy, and the marriage license (license being viewed as ownership and rights of control by any means) have all been found to be factors indicating a higher probability of spousal abuse (Wallace, 1996). Further, many studies have found that abusers have low self-esteem, abuse alcohol, and have experienced violence in the family of origin. Nevertheless, Lackey and Williams (1995) found married men (n = 424) who had developed strong attachments to their partner, friends, or relatives to be less likely to be violent to their female partner even though they had experienced violence in their family of origin.

Women who are beaten by their husbands often stay in the marriage with the hope that the husband will change, although statistics indicate this almost never happens. Also many battered women lack alternatives (alternate places to live, financial resources). Many of these women remain very passive and are unwilling to run away because they often have come from families where violence was customary, and thus see their predicament as part of "normal" married life. Moreover, some women say that they want to keep the family together and have very traditional values about family life. In fact, many wives are unaware that it is illegal for their husband to beat them up. Moreover, many batterers are "supermacho" types who will not let their wives go out alone, and follow and harass them if they try to run away, leaving the wives with the idea that they will never be able to become free (Benedek, 1978; Wallace, 1996).

Despite the vast numbers of wives who remain in marriages where spousal violence is present, increasing number of wives and their children are leaving their home. In response to this trend, shelters for battered women are now found in many communities across the nation. Nurses need to know about these community resources, as well as hot lines and professional and peer group counseling services for battered women in order to make appropriate referrals.

Child Abuse. Public awareness of child abuse did not come about until the 1960s when the diagnosis "battered child syndrome" was coined. Family violence as an academic topic of research remained virtually hidden until the early 1970s. Hence, the whole area of family violence and the important underlying family dynamics are relatively new for family health professionals.

The number of cases of child abuse appear to be rising rapidly (see Figure 17–4); however, some of this rise is due to improved record keeping. Some family violence researchers believe that the incidence of child abuse has probably not changed dramatically from previous eras, but that the increase is due to greater public and professional awareness of child abuse, and less public tolerance for it, as well as a better recording system (Straus et al., 1980; Straus & Gelles, 1990). Nevertheless, complete statistics of this ubiquitous problem are impossible to gather. If accurate and complete data were available, however, child abuse could turn out to be a more frequent cause of death than such diseases as leukemia, cystic fibrosis,

and muscular dystrophy, and could even rank with automobile fatalities.

Child abuse can be physical, emotional, or sexual, or a combination of any two or all three. Physical abuse in children has been defined as "any act that results in a nonaccidental physical injury by a person who has care, custody, or control of a child." (Wallace, 1996, p. 29)

Child abuse has been found to occur in all social classes, races, and among both men and women. Generally, children who are 5 years old or younger and older teenagers are at greater risk for experiencing abuse by their caretakers. Parental behaviors that are associated with physical abuse in children include life stress, loneliness, depression, anxiety, negative parenting attitudes and practices, poor conflict resolution in the marital relationship, and excessive alcohol use (Milner & Murphy, 1995; Straus & Gelles, 1990). Even though all children are at risk for being physically abused, children who are difficult to manage or control may be at higher risk (Straus & Gelles, 1990; Wallace, 1996).

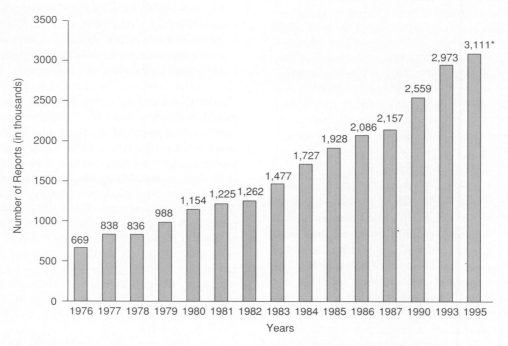

Figure 17–4. National Estimates of Child Abuse and Neglect Reports, 1976–1995. *3,111,000 cases of reported child maltreatment translates into 46 out of 1000 children in the United States reported for child maltreatment in 1995. (From Children's Defense Fund [1995], National Committee to Prevent Child Abuse [1995], and the United States Department of Health and Human Services [1989].)

Children who have been sexually abused often react to abuse by changing their behavior. Feelings of guilt, shame, fear, and anger are often shown. These changed behaviors often manifest themselves in school; abused children may also experience sleep disturbances, have eating disorders, or show regressive or depressed behavior (Wallace, 1996). Briggs, Hubbs-Tait, Culp, and Blankemeyer (1995) studied 134 college students (67 males and 67 females) who had either been sexually abused, had a mother who was dying from cancer, or were normal. Students who had been sexually abused experienced more psychosocial problems than the other two groups.

Several underlying frameworks have been used to explain child abuse in our society: (1) the psychopathological model, where the characteristics of the abuser are viewed as the primary cause of child abuse; (2) the interactional model, where child abuse is seen as the result of a dysfunction in the family itself; and (3) the environmental–sociological model, where child abuse is viewed as a result of the social stresses in society (Wallace, 1996). The first and third frameworks are supported by the findings of the following 1990 report. According to the U.S. House Ways and Means Committee (Harris, 1991), adult drug use has been implicated as a predominant contributor to child abuse: in child-protective service agencies in 22 states and the District of Columbia the most salient characteristic of the adult abuser was his or her use of drugs.

Sibling Abuse.   Most of the discussion about family violence and physical child abuse can be applied to the discussion of sibling abuse. Sibling abuse has been defined as "any form of physical, mental, or sexual abuse inflicted by one child in a family unit on another" (Wallace, 1996, p. 101). Often, sibling abuse occurs when the older or more powerful sibling has control over another sibling (the victim). In addition, sibling abuse has been found to be higher in families where child abuse and or spousal abuse occurs (Straus & Gelles, 1990). The types of sibling abuse that have been reported are: physical abuse (e.g., striking, kicking, punching); emotional abuse (e.g., name-calling, ridicule, degradation, exacerbating a fear, and destroying personal possessions); and sexual abuse (Wallace, 1996).

Elder Abuse.   Elder abuse and neglect, according to a watershed 1985 report by a congressional subcommittee (Larsen, 1989) is a problem that is increasing nationally. In an extensive review of family violence literature, Steinmetz (1987) reported that elder abuse is an area of research that has been virtually ignored until recently. Most of the published articles represent personal observations and/or expert opinion.

Wallace (1996) defines elder abuse as "conduct that results in the physical, psychological, or material neglect, harm, or injury to an elder" (p. 221). One study of elder abuse, conducted by Steinmetz (1987), described circumstances under which elderly abuse occurred. Ninety-one percent of her sample were 70 years or older and 85 percent had experienced diminished physical functioning. All elders shared a home with one of their children. The abusive techniques used by the caregiving children "ranged from screaming and yelling (30%); threatening to send elders to nursing home (8.5%); withholding food or medication (17%); . . . to physically restraining elder (7.5%) and slapping, hitting and shaking (2.5%). Overall, 12% of the caregivers had used physically abusive acts or the threat of physical violence in an attempt to maintain control" (p. 738).

Families caring for an elderly parent that are experiencing high levels of stress are much more likely to be involved in elder abuse. Also, caregivers who perceive caregiving tasks to be stressful are more apt to engage in elder abuse (Pagelow, 1984; Steinmetz 1987).

Parent Abuse.   Another form of abuse is that in which children are old enough to now perpetrate violence against their parents. The children at one point were recipients of violence, and through role modeling learned that the use of violence was a feasible and acceptable mode of expressing anger. In studies that examined this phenomenon, the children were adolescents. In the first national study published (Straus et al., 1980) of 2143 intact families with adolescent children (10 to 17 years old), 9 percent of the parents reported experiencing at least one attack by one of their children and 3 percent said they had experienced severe violence. In both single- and two-parent families, mothers were more likely to be the victims and sons the perpetrators (Steinmetz, 1987).

In data from another nationwide study of parent abuse (Agnew & Huguley, 1989), abusing adolescents were more likely to have friends who also assaulted their parents and approved of delinquency, including violence. These white adolescents who were weakly attached to their parents believed that the probability of official sanction for parental assault was low.

Gay and Lesbian Abuse.

Gay and lesbian family violence is believed by some researchers to be at the same rate as among heterosexual couples or around 25 to 35 percent (Wallace, 1996). However, this form of violence has not been widely studied. Gay and lesbian families share emotions and financial responsibility in their relationship that can lead to conflict situations. Generally, both lesbian and gay abusers use similar types of violence on their victims as heterosexual couples, such as rape, threats, economic control, psychological or emotional abuse (e.g., humiliation, mind manipulation, isolation, and lying), homophobic control, breaking household items, assaults with weapons, biting, and scratching (Wallace, 1996).

▶ SUMMARY

In summary, many changes have taken place in American family life over the last decade. For example, the divorce rate has increased and more children are now experiencing a one-parent household than before (Bumpass & Sweet, 1991). Remarriage is common with stepfamily structures and relationships are becoming more and more complex. Poverty and rising crime rates afflict families living in both urban and rural environments. Some families have to adapt to unexpected life events such as unemployment, hospitalization, chronic illnesses, or drug and alcohol abuse.

How families cope with these stressful life events differs. Some families adapt very well to stressors and strains by changing patterns of functioning, using resources and helpful coping strategies to manage the stress. These families go on to fulfill family functions and have satisfactory relationships within the family and with the community. Other families utilize harmful or dysfunctional coping strategies that may only temporarily reduce the stress. Outcomes for these families sometimes result in family violence and abuse, child neglect, or drug/alcohol abuse. Health care professionals such as nurses, who are in contact with families both in institutional and community settings, are in a key position to assess both family stresses and family strengths and intervene with these families to bring about more optimal family adaptation. Hence assessment questions, possible family nursing diagnoses, and general intervention guidelines are briefly presented next.

FAMILY STRESS, COPING, AND ADAPTATION: APPLYING THE NURSING PROCESS

▶ assessment questions

The following questions have been included to assist the nurse or professional in appraising family stressors and family coping processes and strategies.

Stressors and Strengths

1. What stressors (both long- and short-term) are being experienced by the family? Refer to the Family Inventory of Life Events Scale (FILE) for examples of significant stressors. Consider environmental and socioeconomic stressors. What is the family's definition of its situation? Is it possible to estimate the duration and strength of the family stressors?

2. What strengths counterbalance the stressors? Is the family able to handle the usual stresses and strains of daily family life?

3. Is the family able to act based on a realistic and objective appraisal of a stressful situation or event?

Coping Strategies

4. How does the family react to stressful situations? What coping strategies are being used? What coping strategies has the family employed to deal with what types of problems? Do family members differ in their ways of coping with their present problem? If so, how?

5. Does the family use the following internal coping strategies?
    *   Family group-reliance.
    *   A sense of humor.
    *   Sharing of feelings, thoughts, and activities (maintaining cohesiveness).
    *   Controlling the meaning of the problem/reframing.
    *   Joint problem solving. What are the problem-solving abilities of various family members? Are they able to articulate their needs and concerns? Can they proceed through the steps of the problem-solving process? (Epstein et al., 1993)
    *   Role flexability
    *   Normalizing

6. Does the family use any of the following external coping strategies?
    *   Seeking information.
    *   Maintaining linkages with the community (general external involvement).
    *   Seeking and using social support.

        Informal support systems (friends, family, neighbors, employers, employees, organizations and groups—e.g., self-care or mutual aid groups and other groups with which family members have common interests or goals).

        Formal support systems (professional services, both in health and health-related areas).
    *   Seeking spiritual supports.

7. Assessment of family coping may also be done by using a coping instrument such as the Family Crisis Oriented Personal Evaluation Scale or F-COPES by McCubbin, Olson, and Larson (1991). This instrument assesses a family's use of internal and external family coping (see Table 17–2).

8. What dysfunctional adaptive strategies has the family used or is the family using? Are there signs of any of the dysfunctionalities listed below? If so, record their presence and how extensively they are used.
    *   Scapegoating.
    *   Use of threat.
    *   Family myth.
    *   Triangling.

- Pseudomutuality.
- Authoritarianism.
- Alcohol and/or drug abuse.
- Family violence (spouse, child, sibling, elder, or gay and lesbian).
- Child neglect.

▶ FAMILY NURSING DIAGNOSES

According to the North American Nursing Diagnosis Association (NANDA) classification of nursing diagnoses, there are four nursing diagnoses that specifically cover the focus of family coping processes and strategies. These are:

1. Family coping: Potential for growth
2. Ineffective family coping: Compromised
3. Ineffective family coping: Disabling
4. Potential for violence (McFarland & McFarlane, 1989)

Other less specific diagnoses—such as knowledge deficit, social isolation, altered health management, and alteration in family processes—could also be used, but they would have to be specified in the defining characteristics and related factors to be sufficiently problem-focused.

The diagnosis of *family coping: potential for growth*, is family-systems based and is appropriate for situations where the family nurse's goals are to assist families in coping effectively with the family demands/stressors. Families may be successfully adapting at this time, but are anticipating certain future health stressors and in need of information to promote health and prevent problems in the future.

The diagnosis of *ineffective family coping: compromised*, is appropriate to use when the family assessment data show that the family is employing adaptive strategies that are ineffective for resolving present stressors. Because of the use of ineffective adaptive strategies, its functioning or adaptation is compromised.

The diagnosis of *ineffective family coping: disabling*, is used "when the behavior of one or more family members incapacitates the family (or individual members) to therapeutically adapt to the existing health challenge" (McFarland and McFarlane, 1989, p. 943). Although the generation and description of this diagnosis was guided by family systems theory, the above definition is ambiguous in terms of how family coping is used. Family coping in this text refers to the coping behaviors or responses made by a subsystem, such as parent–child or spousal subsystem, or the family as a whole—indicating an interactional level. Hence, the use of this diagnosis for family coping diagnoses should not include individual coping or adaptive responses; the outcome "disabling" would then refer to the family outcome(s).

Although *ineffective family coping: disabling* can be long- or short term, the family is having greater difficulties adapting when this diagnosis is used than when the previous diagnosis is used. Family health and growth are adversely affected here (McFarland & McFarlane, 1989).

In reviewing the diagnosis of *potential for violence*, the diagnosis, defining characteristics, and suggested interventions are focused on the potentially violent individual. Using a family-centered approach, each of these areas needs to be broadened to incorporate the family system and the family members at risk.

▶ GENERAL FAMILY NURSING INTERVENTIONS

Because of the breadth of coverage in this chapter, only general family nursing interventions are outlined here. Please refer to Chapter 18 for elaboration of the interventions identified in this section. Interventions are based on family assessment data pertaining to family stressors and coping (as outlined in the assessment section), as well as on the family nursing diagnoses.

Assisting Families at Risk to Cope

Several guidelines are recommended:

- Encourage all family members to be involved, especially fathers.
- Support (reinforce) effective coping strategies that families and family members are using to either reduce family tension, control the meaning of stressor(s), or eliminate stressor(s).
- For families that need to learn additional coping strategies, literature resources are provided

that elaborate on stress management, cognitive reframing, lifestyle alteration, and use of self-help groups (see Table 17–4). Chapter 16 also covers lifestyle modifications.

For families that are employing ineffective family coping strategies, the family nurse should differentiate between whether the family is chronically dysfunctional (in that case referral for more long-term therapy is indicated) or in acute crisis but functioning within normal limits until the onset of the stressor(s). In this case, family crisis intervention principles and an empowerment perspective are suggested as guides to family interventions.

Family Crisis Intervention Principles. Family crisis intervention extends crisis intervention theory by incorporating a family focus. Very briefly, family crisis intervention is a short-term practice model for families experiencing crisis or stress to help them cope with present stressor(s) and future stressor(s). It involves: (1) defining the precipitating stressor event and hazardous life events, (2) assessing the family's interpretation of the event(s), (3) assessing the family's resources and methods for coping with stressors, and (4) assessing the family's state of functioning. Based on this model, a supportive yet focused problem-solving approach is used to assist the family to mobilize resources (its own and community resources) to resolve the present crisis, and to learn how to prevent and cope with future stressful experiences (Kus, 1985).

Empowering Families. Boss (1988) and Figley (1989, 1995), family researchers and clinicians, describe an approach involved with empowering families. Their suggestions extend and enrich the family crisis intervention model. Boss (1988) points out that for families that have been traumatized or victimized, learned helplessness is a common family reaction. If helplessness can be learned, she reasons, then helpless can be unlearned. Empowerment comes when family members regain their self-esteem and self-confidence and take pride in the family as a team, regaining control over what happens to the family collectively and individually, making sense out of what happened by finding some meaning to the problem(s), and sharing with other family members while actively attempting to prevent the problem or event from reoccurring. Reassuring families that their reactions to traumatic situations are common and predictable, thereby "normalizing"

their situation, is an effective supportive technique (Figley, 1989).

Figley (1989) implies that empowering families is as much a philosophical attitude toward working with traumatized families as it is engaging in certain specified activities. When he views and treats troubled families, his approach is tempered by his genuine respect for the natural resourcefulness of families. In the following passage, he explains this perspective:

> I try to empower the family by creating the kind of intervention context that results in the resolution of the traumatizing experience but, just as importantly, that results in the family's giving themselves most of the credit for the accomplishment. Moreover, this approach makes the family feel more confident to face any future traumatic experience equipped with the necessary information, skills, and problem-solving methods. (p. 42)

Protecting Family Members Who Are at Risk for Violence

This goal may be accomplished by:

1. Recognizing and reporting child abuse.
2. Supporting and referring abused spouses, elders, siblings, parents, gays and lesbians, the abuser, and the family unit.
3. Coordinating care to families and family members, working collaboratively with other health and welfare workers (Gilliss et al., 1989).

Referring Families That Exhibit More Complex Family Coping Problems and Dysfunction

When family stress and coping problems of families are beyond the services the family nurse can provide, referral and follow-up of ongoing family counseling or therapy is often indicated. Referral to a counselor who uses a family systems approach is also suggested.

Educating Families about Effective Coping to Promote and Maintain Family Health

Use of teaching strategies to provide family health education in the content areas listed in Table 17–4 is a major intervention.

▶ TABLE 17–4

LITERATURE RESOURCES ABOUT STRESS MANAGEMENT, COGNITIVE REFRAMING, LIFESTYLE ALTERATION, AND USE OF SELF-HELP GROUPS

■ STRESS-MANAGEMENT STRATEGIES

Buckwalter, K. C., Hartsock, J. & Gaffney, J. (1989). Music therapy. In G. M. Bulechek & J. C. McCloskey (Eds.). *Nursing interventions: Treatments for nursing diagnoses* (pp. 58–74). Philadelphia, PA: W. B. Saunders.

Mealy, A. R., Richardson, H., & Dimico, G. (1996). Family stress management. In P. Bomar (Ed.), *Nurses and family health promotion* (2nd ed.). Philadelphia: Saunders.

Pender, N. J. (1996) *Health promotion in nursing practice* (3rd ed.). Stamford, CT: Appleton & Lange.

Scandrett-Hibdon, S. & Uecker, S. (1992). Relaxation training. In G. M. Bulechek & J. C. McCloskey (Eds.). *Nursing interventions: Essential Nursing Treatments* (2nd ed.) (pp. 434–461). Philadelphia, PA: Saunders.

Steiger, N. J., & Lipson, J. G. (1985). *Self-care nursing: Theory and practice*. Bowie, MD: Brady.

■ COGNITIVE REFRAMING OR REAPPRAISAL

Minuchin, S. & Fishman, H. C. (1981). *Family therapy techniques*. Cambridge, MA: Harvard University Press.

Scandrett-Hibdon, S. (1992). Cognitive reappraisal. In G. M. Bulechek & McCloskey, J. C. (Eds.), *Nursing interventions: Essential nursing treatments* (pp. 462–471) Philadelphia, PA: Saunders.

Wright, M., Watson, W. L. & Bell, J. M. (1997). *Beliefs: The heart of healing*. New York: Basic Books.

■ LIFESTYLE ALTERATION

Bomar, P. (Ed.). (1996). *Nurses and family health promotion* (2nd ed.). Philadelphia, PA: Saunders (Chapters on family recreation and exercise and family nutrition and weight control.)

Bulechek, G. M. & McCloskey, J. C. (Eds.). (1992). *Nursing interventions: Essential nursing treatments*. (2nd ed.). Philadelphia, PA: Saunders. (Chapters on exercise, patient contracting, smoking cessation, and weight management.)

Pender, N. J. (1996). *Health promotion in nursing practice* (3rd ed.). Norwalk, CT: Appleton & Lange (Chapters on lifestyle modification, stress management, exercise and nutrition.)

■ USE OF SELF-HELP GROUPS

Danielson, C. B., Hamel-Bissell, B. & Winstead-Fry, P. (1993). *Families, Health, and Illness*. (Chapter on social support and mutual support groups, pp. 213–230). St. Louis, MO: C. V. Mosby.

Kinney, C. K., Mannetter, R., & Carpenter, M. A. (1992). Support groups. In G. M. Bulechek & J. C. McCloskey (Eds.), *Nursing interventions: Essential nursing treatments* (2nd ed.) (pp. 326–339). Philadelphia: W. B. Saunders.

Pender, N. J. (1996). *Health promotion in nursing practice*. (3rd ed.). Stamford, CT: Appleton & Lange.

Steiger, N. J. & Lipson, J. G. (1985). *Self-care nursing: Theory and practice*. (2nd ed.) Bowie, MD: Brady.

▶ study questions

1. Family coping is vitally important because (select the best answer):
   a. It is the mechanism through which family functions are made possible.
   b. It provides opportunities for family members to learn.
   c. It leads to problem solving and mastery over family issues and stresses.
   d. It either eliminates stressors or leads to stress-reduction activities.

2. Changes in family life in North America come from within and outside the family. Major recent changes in families include (select all correct answers):
   a. Families are becoming more isolated from kin.
   b. There is greater diversity of family forms.
   c. Marriage rates have declined, especially in early 20s age group.
   d. Divorce rates are dropping dramatically.
   e. Poverty has increased significantly among working poor families.

3. Match the definitions in the right-hand column with the concepts and terms in the left-hand column.

Concepts/Terms	Definitions
a. Crisis	1. Part of salutogenic model of health.
b. Sense of coherence	2. Active, effective adaptive efforts.
c. Defense mechanism	3. The precipitating or initiating events or agents that generate stress.
d. Stressors	4. The general process of adjustment to change.
e. Stress	5. The strain, disequilibrium produced by threat or actual existence of stressors.
f. Adaptation	6. Habitual, stereotypic responses to threat or actual presence of stressors.
g. Coping	7. In the presence of the stress and stressors, the family's failure in use of effective adaptive strategies.

4. McCubbin and McCubbin (1993) have identified six categories of stresses and strains; name four of these.

Are the following statements true or false?

5. In the antestress period, anticipatory guidance would be contraindicated.

6. Defensive tactics are often necessary adaptive responses during the actual stress period.

7. During the poststress period, coping tactics consist of strategies to return the family to a homeostatic state.

8. McCubbin, Patterson, and Wilson (1983) developed the Family Inventory of Life Events and Changes Scale (FILE) to (select the best answer):
   a. Identify positive correlation between stressors and stress.
   b. Assess pile-up of life events and strains experienced by families.
   c. Identify cause-and-effect relationships between number of life change events and presence of illness.
   d. Assess correlation between stress and wellness.

9. In the Resiliency Model (McCubbin & McCubbin, 1993) an indicator of family adaptation is (select the best answer):
   a. Family is experiencing no stress.
   b. Family has not gone into crisis.
   c. There is a "fit" between the family and the community.
   d. Family members do not have a chronic illness.

10. Burr, Klein, and associates (1994) identified both helpful and harmful coping strategies and found the most helpful coping strategies to be (select all correct answers):
    a. Keeping others from knowing how bad the situation was.
    b. Spiritual support.
    c. Increased family communication.
    d. Community support.
    e. Cognitive strategies.

11. Which of the following are two primary variables involved in whether crisis develops or not?
    a. Compliance with environment.
    b. Perception of event or change.
    c. Coping resources.
    d. Choice to grow or stagnate.
    e. Open or closed communications.

12. Select four functional family coping strategies (two internal coping resources and two external coping strategies) and describe each of these briefly.

13. Select four dysfunctional family adaptive strategies and describe each of these briefly.

Choose the correct answers to the following questions.

14. The two prime purposes of social support systems are to:
    a. Provide direct assistance.
    b. Become a family advocate.
    c. Replace professional services.
    d. Provide emotional support.

15. Indicate which of the following are functional (F) or dysfunctional (D) or which could be either (E), depending on the situation.
    a. Family group-reliance.
    b. Scapegoating.

   c. Pseudomutuality.
   d. Sense of humor.
   e. Increased linkage with community.
   f. Spouse violence.
   g. Child neglect.
   h. Triangling.
   i. Social support systems.
   j. Seeking of information.
   k. Role flexibility.
   l. Controlling the meaning of the problem by reframing.

16. Effective coping responses by families usually occur when (select all correct answers):
   a. The family has adequate inner and outside resources to draw from.
   b. The crisis-provoking event is interpreted in an objective, realistic manner.
   c. Family bonds and unity exist.
   d. The family has the capacity to shift course and modify roles within the family.

17. The purpose(s) for families utilizing threat as a control mechanism is (are) to:
   a. Maintain authoritarian structure within the family.
   b. Maintain or reinstate connectedness within the family.
   c. Insure the survival of the family group.
   d. Decrease family members' attempts to behave in an autonomous, individualistic manner.

18. In tracing the usual sequence of events that occurs when a family experiences a crisis or after the family is faced with a stressful event with which it cannot effectively cope, what consequences then follow?

► family case study*

Read the following family study, then assess the family in the areas of affective functioning and family coping functioning.

Mrs. Ruby Nichols, a 34-year-old obese woman, came to the mental health clinic because, she said, "I just don't know what to do." She was crying hysterically and unable to respond to further questioning. After remaining with her for an hour, the nurse was able to elicit that her 5-year-old foster daughter was being removed from her home per court order. Welfare funds, her only support for herself, her unemployed husband, and their five children, were being

*Adapted from Black (1974).

terminated in a week, leaving her unable to pay the bills or buy enough food for her family. Although Mrs. Nichols was still tearful and depressed, she was able to be driven home by a community worker.

The following day the nurse made a visit to the Nichols' home. Mrs. Nichols related the following history.

Ruby and John Nichols had been married 15 years. Four children were born of the marriage: Priscilla, 13; Cindy, 10; John Jr., 6; and Lisa, 4. They also had a foster daughter, Ann, age 5. The couple had known each other a year before their marriage in their home town of Smithfield, Louisiana. John was an unskilled laborer, but had always managed to be employed. Ruby had attended business school prior to the marriage and was employed as a book-keeper until the first child was born. She described her early marriage as fine except for moving so many times, caused by John's "meddling mother." The family would move to get away from his mother, but she would always manage to locate them and appear on the scene. "We were a healthy, happy family and everything was fine as long as John's mother stayed away." Ruby related that this source of conflict between herself and John was resolved each time by a move on their part. However, she and John never really discussed their mother-in-law problems according to Ruby. Following each new move, Ruby would join clubs and organizations to make new friends and John's work provided a similar opportunity for him. John also spent several evenings a week in the local bar, "shooting the bull" with the boys from work.

The last move was 6 months ago. After 2 months John lost his job and was unable to find another. This resulted in the family going on welfare, which Ruby and John felt ashamed of, as they had always prided themselves on paying their own bills. Shortly after this, John's mother found the family and moved into town. When she came to visit, a bitter argument ensued regarding John's mother and since then John had been staying away from home and drinking a lot. Moreover, 3 months ago Ruby had abdominal surgery which was followed by complications and a prolonged hospitalization period. During her absence from home, the role of mother was assumed by Priscilla, who managed well with the help from the next door neighbor, Mrs. Law.

Ruby was released from the hospital 3 weeks ago as sufficiently recovered to stay at home. When she got home she perceived that the children had functioned "very well" in her absence; in fact, she felt that they did not need her and even seemed to resent her. John remained away most of the time and was minimally involved in family life during her hospitalization, as well as presently.

A week ago she learned of the court's decision to remove Ann from the home and the termination of welfare funds. Ruby felt herself becoming less and less able to manage and admitted to depression and suicidal thoughts. However, her concern for her children prevented her from doing anything self-destructive. The next-door-neighbor, Mrs. Law, realizing the gravity of the family's situation, told Ruby to go to the mental health clinic for help.

Subsequent visits to the family revealed that the children were having problems and that Ruby had difficulties relating to their problematic behaviors. It was observed that the children and parents did not discuss these problems or their concerns with each other, and that there was no movement toward sharing their feelings about Ann's leaving, the mother-in-law's disruptive influence, or Ruby's health problems.

Priscilla, age 13, seemed to resent Ruby's return, because it meant the loss of her mothering role. She and her mother have engaged in frequent arguments over the discipline of the younger children, what they should wear, and how they should act. The arguments usually ended with Priscilla leaving the house for long periods of time without telling Ruby where she was. This caused Ruby to worry. Priscilla was not interested in school, her main interest being to grow up as quickly as possible and emulate her mother. She also wanted desperately to be independent and make her own decisions in life. Ruby had "weaned" Priscilla early in terms of her being self-sufficient at home: from age 6 on, Priscilla was caring for her younger siblings and helping her mother out in the home.

Cindy, age 10, seemed unaffected by the situation. She was quite involved with her school activities and Campfire Girls and spent much time in these activities and at her friends' homes. Priscilla and Cindy evidently have a closer sibling relationship than the other siblings do. Cindy tells "all her secrets" to Priscilla when she is upset, worried, or needs someone to talk to.

John Jr., a first grader, was refusing to go to school. Every morning it was now a struggle to get him off to school. He would cry and hang on to his mother. His teacher reported poor school work and lack of attentiveness when he was present.

Lisa, age 4, displayed similar clinging behaviors to those of John Jr. She seemed frightened when mother left the home and was wetting the bed again after having no problems in this area for 2 years. Both John Jr. and Lisa frequently questioned their mother about the recent absence of Ann. They asked if Ann went away because she was "bad."

On the third contact between the family (the parents) and the nurse at the mental health clinic, the nurse asked the parents to describe each child, what he or she was like, and what personal needs or problems they were trying to assist their children with at that time. It was noted that specific information on each child was difficult to obtain. For instance, these general statements were made: "Oh, he (she) is just the average 6-year-old (or whatever age applied)," or "Priscilla's just like all other teenagers, wanting her way all the time," or "I treat all my children the same, regardless." They were able to recognize, though, Priscilla's need to care for her younger siblings and to be independent, but were not open to her staying away from the family very much, or developing a set of friends outside the family with whom she might have frequent social contact.

The mother also recognized that Lisa was very attached to and dependent on her, and needed reassurance that mother would be back when she left home. Additionally, both parents thought Ann's leaving was threatening to the younger children, who might think this might happen to them if they misbehaved. Ruby was trying to spend more time with Lisa to help her with her fears over the mother's separation and Ann's leaving. John showed interest in "comforting" and being involved with Lisa also, since Lisa always responded "in such a cute, loving way to her daddy," according to the mother.

Both parents are able to show affection and warmth to the younger children (John Jr. and Lisa), but do not feel that it is appropriate to be so "physical" when they get older. It was noted that the parents were not physically affectionate to each other and seemed emotionally distant during the interviews. Ruby says that they have never shared their personal concerns with each other much. "It takes another woman to understand my feelings. I used to confide in Priscilla a lot, but since she is upset with me, I haven't been able to talk with her."

19. What short- and long-term stressors are impinging on the family? What strengths counterbalance these stressors?

20. Is the family able to act based on a realistic and objective appraisal of the situation?

21. How does the family react to stressful situations? Both functional and dysfunctional strategies should be described.

► chapter 17 study answers

1. a.

2. b, c, and e.

3. a. = 7.   e. = 5.
    b. = 1.   f. = 4.
    c. = 6.   g. = 2.
    d. = 3.

4. Any four of the following categories:
    a. Stressor events and associated hardships.
    b. Normative transitions.
    c. Pre-existing family strains.
    d. Situational demands.
    e. Consequences of family efforts to cope.
    f. Intrafamily and social ambiguity.

5. False.

6. True.

7. True.

8. b.

9. c.

10. b and c.

11. b and c.

12. Internal Coping Strategies (two):
    a. *Role flexibility.* Ability of family members to adapt by shifting roles as needed.
    b. *Family group-reliance.* The tighter structure and control over subsystems, greater degree of family organization and cohesiveness.

c. *Use of humor.* Improves attitude toward problems and gives some respite and lightness to a stressful situation.

d. *Greater sharing together.* Increasing family efforts to converse about feelings and thoughts, participate in family activities.

e. *Normalizing.* When confronted with a long-term stressor, parents normalize family life to minimize family disruption from stressor.

f. *Controlling the meaning of the problem.* Interpreting or defining a change or event realistically, objectively (where cognitive mastery is involved). Reframing the situation more positively.

g. *Joint problem solving.* The family is able to jointly discuss a problem, search for a solution, and reach a consensus.

External Coping Strategies (two)

a. *Seeking information.* Pertinent information sought to deal with issue/problem at hand.

b. *Maintaining active linkages with broader community.* This is a more general lifestyle characterization, where family members have open boundaries and continually participate and involve themselves in community organizations and activities.

c. *Seeking and using social support systems.* Social support systems function to provide support and assistance either more generally or on an as-needed basis. These social support systems are composed of friends, extended family, employers, employees, neighbors, groups (including mutual aid groups), organizations, and professional persons and agencies.

d. *Seeking spiritual supports.* This type of support includes engaging in prayer, rituals, belief in God and attending church/temple together as a family.

13. Dysfunctional family adaptive strategies (any four):

a. *Spouse violence.* In response to pent-up frustrations in marital relationship and hostility of marital partners, one spouse attacks the other.

b. *Child abuse.* Physical violence, usually by one or both parents, against one or more of their children.

c. *Scapegoating.* Selecting one or more family members to be the identified family problem. Negatively labeling and imposing unhealthy exploitative role on to the scapegoat.

d. *Use of threat.* By use of threat or ostracism, expulsion or self-destructive acts, family keeps all its members in conformity. "Separateness" actions by individuals are thus curtailed.

e. *Triangling.* Introduction of a third member into a stressful dyadic relationship when stress level reaches point where stress reduction is sought. This is exploitative of third member and does not confront the problem in the relationship.

f. *The family myth.* Beliefs developed in family about itself which have themes of wish-fulfillment. These tend to hide real problems and limit family's alternatives and problem-solving resources.

g. *Pseudomutuality.* Maintaining pseudo or false closeness. Family members have difficulty in expressing affection and closeness. As a result, they build up all sorts of customs and rituals that structure family members' responses and establish a facade of closeness and solidarity.

h. *Authoritarianism.* This is a long-term adaptive response to deal with feelings of powerlessness and dependency. One member becomes the dominator and the others the subordinates. All "lose" in this type of family structure, because there is no opportunity provided to learn the value of negotiation, discussion, and how to relate effectively with others and yet be autonomous.

14. a and d.

15. a. E.   g. D.
    b. D.   h. E.
    c. D.   i. F.
    d. E.   j. F.
    e. E.   k. F.
    f. D.   l. F.

16. all (a–d).

17. b, c, and d.

18. Family functioning continues to decline until either the family seeks or receives assistance and begins to deal effectively with the stressor, or the family reaches a low point in family functioning and then stabilizes at this new, lower level of family function.

> ► family case study

19. Short-term stressors impinging on the family:
    Husband's unemployment.
    Being on welfare and then the threat of termination.
    Ann's loss (removal from the home).
    Ruby's recent ill-health, hospitalization, and convalescence.
    Ruby's depression and suicidal thoughts.
    Long-term stressors impinging on the family.
    The perceived interference of John's mother.
    Emotional distance and lack of communication in family and especially within marital relationship.
    Continual geographical movement, from one community to the next, so that no stable and sufficient social network is established.
    Husband's minimal participation in family life and his excessive and frequent drinking bouts.
    Family strengths:
    Presence of social support system, although small: receiving help from mental health clinic, Mrs. Law, neighbor.
    Ruby's caring for and commitment to children.

Parents' staying together and father's interest in Lisa and his potential of greater participation in family life.

Parents' motivation to find employment, be financially self-sufficient.

Priscilla's interest in and ability for child care.

20. The parents' ability to act based on objective and realistic appraisal of a situation is limited. In terms of the interference of John's mother, they perceived events as problems over which they had no control. They see the problem being John's mother's behavior, rather than a situation in which they need to communicate with each other and John's mother in order to define problems and identify a mutually satisfactory way of handling situation. Data do not reveal their perception of why Ann was removed or why welfare was terminated. Ruby personally distorts the parenting situation, feeling that her children did well without her and did not wish her back.

21. 1. Functional adaptive strategies:

No evidence for the use of some of the internal coping strategies related to family's inner resources such as greater family reliance on themselves, increased sharing of feelings and thoughts, shared activities, and controlling the meaning of the stressors.

Family (Ruby and then family) did seek a key support system when problems reached crisis proportions—the mental health clinic. The neighbor, Mrs. Law, has assisted family. But the family, because of its continual moving, has not developed an adequate social support system.

2. Dysfunctional adaptive strategies:

Use of spousal withdrawal—both spouses do not communicate openly with each other; husband withdraws from family physically and through his drinking.

Use of denial as to the family's real problems. They have seen their major family problem as John's "meddling mother." Use of family myth around this source of conflict was apparent. The family myth, more specifically, has been that "we are a happy family as long as John's mother stays away."

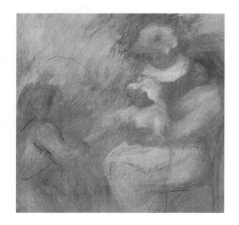

four

GENERAL FAMILY NURSING INTERVENTIONS

Part IV contains only one chapter, a chapter that was added in the third edition and expanded upon in the fourth edition. Chapter 18 focuses on the major family nursing interventions that cut across the many possible family nursing diagnoses. It should be referred to when the reader needs more information about one of the six major family interventions: teaching, counseling, contracting, case management, collaboration, and consultation.

18

Family Nursing Interventions

Marilyn M. Friedman

► learning objectives

---

1. Explain how active family participation can be accomplished during the intervention phase of the family nursing process.
2. Relative to the family nursing interventions of teaching, counseling, contracting, case management, and collaboration:
   a. Define and/or explain what the particular intervention strategy entails.
   b. Describe with what types of family nursing diagnoses the intervention strategy would be helpful.
   c. Discuss the limitations of using the intervention strategy.
3. Identify major variables that affect the efficacy of client teaching.
4. Compare the teaching–learning process with the nursing process.
5. Describe the different levels of family involvement in teaching versus counseling.
6. Describe the family nurse's role relative to consultation, client advocacy, and coordination.
7. Identify several family nursing interventions appropriate to use in two family case examples.

Family nursing intervention builds upon family assessment, family nursing diagnosis or statements of family strength(s), and planning, where goals are formulated, alternative intervention strategies and resources identified, and priorities set. It is not routine, random, or standardized, but tailor-made to the particular family with whom the family nurse is working.

In working with families, a wide array of interventions are dynamically and flexibly used. It is clear, however, that descriptions of family nursing interventions in the literature are sadly lacking (Bell, 1995; Gilliss & Davis, 1993; Robinson, 1994; Robinson & Wright, 1995). The literature on research and clinically based family nursing interventions is so sparse that Janice Bell, editor of *Journal of Family Nursing*, twice put out the call for descriptions of studies documenting the effectiveness of family nursing interventions. Her last plea makes this poignant request:

> Determined, persistent journal editor seeks specific descriptions of nursing practice with families: rich clinical exemplars, case studies, process research, outcome research, questions and answers about the effectiveness of family nursing interventions. (p. 355)

This is not to say that extensive literature is not available on both general and specific types of nursing interventions, but the vast majority of it is individually focused, not family oriented. And the literature that is family oriented is primarily informed by a traditional, nonsystemic (nonsystems) theoretical, lineally focused frame of reference (Robinson, 1994). What we have tried to do in this text is present systemic models of practice (including assessment and intervention). This frame of reference is referred to by Robinson (1994) as nontraditional, containing systemic, subjectively focused and circular notions. More traditional orientations (i.e., objective, lineal, advocating the primacy of the individual) to working with families are also described; the preponderance of literature about nursing interventions of families favors this latter, traditional approach. In the traditional frame of reference underlying family nursing interventions, it is assumed that if the nurse intervenes (the treatment), the client will likely respond in a certain way (the outcome), whereas in the nontraditional orientation, nurses can create a context for change, but families are free to find their own solutions (Robinson, 1994).

In addition to the presence of two differing orientations or philosophical paradigms in the family nursing intervention literature (the objective, lineal, traditional paradigm/frame of reference and the subjective, systemic, circular, nontraditional paradigm/frame), beginning efforts are being made to identify family nursing interventions. Craft and Willadsen's (1992) research using a Delphi process involving 130 nurses expert in family nursing identified nine categories of family nursing interventions (see Table 3–5 for a listing of these). The Nursing Interventions Classification (NIC) Project being carried out by faculty at the University of Iowa (McCloskey & Bulechek, 1996) is further evidence of the work being done to identify family nursing interventions (their interventions are primarily individual-oriented, but some significant family nursing interventions are also identified). Both of these efforts are laudable. Nevertheless, as Bell (1995) reminds us, "further work is needed to articulate specifically what the nurse does when he or she intervenes with families" (p. 356).

One of the reasons why family nursing interventions have been so difficult to identify is suggested by

Beavers and Hampson (1990). They maintain that family assessment and intervention are inseparable elements in clinical practice. Moreover, they assert that for some families assessment (the questions that the clinician asks and resultant feedback) constitutes intervention. They mention that the families who typically make positive changes based on the assessment process and associated feedback are more competent families who are able to constructively use information provided in the assessment process.

In this text there are several locations where family nursing interventions are described. The first detailed discussion is under the intervention section of Chapter 3. A definition of family nursing interventions is presented there, as well as more general principles of family nursing intervention. In addition, Wright and colleagues' Calgary Family Intervention Model (CFIM) is elaborated upon (Wright & Leahey, 1994) in Chapter 3.

The second area of the text where family nursing interventions are found is in the concluding sections of the chapters within Part II (Chaps. 8–17) and Chapter 6. More specific family nursing interventions are described within these chapters, interventions which are most germane to the particular foci of each of the respective chapters. These more focused family nursing interventions and the chapters in which they are located are as follows:

Family Nursing Intervention	Chapter Location
Calgary Family Intervention Model (CFIM)	3 and 10
Sociocultural interventions	8
Financial interventions	8
Social support and social networking, including use of self-help groups	8
Interventions to promote family recreation and leisure-time activities	9
Environmental health promotion	9
Environmental modification strategies	9
Interventions to assist the homeless	9
Conflict management techniques	10
Referral to parenting programs	10 and 15
The empowerment model (family power area)	11

Lastly, more general family nursing intervention strategies are included in this chapter. These are interventions that cut across the wide array of family nursing content areas and are applicable to a broad range of family situations. In addition, with respect to these general family nursing interventions, various theoretical perspectives may be used and different family nursing diagnoses can provide the underlying need. Six major family nursing intervention strategies are explored in this chapter: teaching, counseling, contracting, case management, collaboration, and consultation.

▶ DEFINING FAMILY NURSING INTERVENTIONS

The more traditionally oriented definition of nursing intervention (according to the two contrasting orientations described above) is provided by the NIC Project faculty (Bulechek & McCloskey, 1996) as: "Any treatment, based upon clinical judgment and knowledge, that a nurse performs to enhance patient/client outcomes. Nursing interventions include both direct and indirect care; both nurse-initiated, physician-initiated, and other provider-initiated treatments" (p. xvii). This definition is a good foundation, but needs to be further specified to be more applicable to families. Craft and Willadsen (1992), conceptualizing of the family system as client, developed the following definition of nursing interventions for families:

> Nursing interventions for families are nursing treatments that assist families and their members to promote, attain, or maintain optimal health and functioning or to experience a peaceful death. Currently, the domain of family treatment seems to fit nursing as opposed to medical diagnosis and treatment. It is unusual for a physician to write an order for "family support" or "caregiver support." These interventions are the responsibility of nursing and are nurse initiated. (p. 520)

Wright and Bell (1994) propose a process-oriented, systemic definition of family nursing interventions. They refer to these as: "action(s) or response(s) of the nurse, which include the nurse's overt therapeutic actions, that occur in the context of a nurse–client relationship to affect individual, family or community functioning for which nurses are accountable" (p. 3).

▶ FAMILY AS ACTIVE PARTICIPANT AND PARTNER

In keeping with the premise that families have the right and responsibility to make their own health decisions, families and nurses need to form a partnership to promote health and address families' health concerns. This partnership between health professionals and families is at the core of all good health care systems (Green, 1994). Active family participation is an essential approach to incorporate into each of the subsequent family nursing intervention strategies. Family involvement in the implementation phase often means to engage the family in mutual problem solving, as well as to create a context for change through therapeutic conversations in which family strengths are drawn forth. Family members are then freed to decide what makes sense to them and what they should do on their own behalf (Robinson, 1994; Wright & Leahey, 1994).

Inclusion of as many family members as possible in planned educational and counseling/supportive sessions is very helpful (Doherty & Campbell, 1988; Rolland, 1994). It allows family members to express themselves and support each other. It also stimulates much-needed group discussion and feedback and assures that all attending members obtain the needed information. One family member may ask novel questions, which then exposes the rest of the participating members to the discussion that follows.

In families with a chronically ill child it often happens that only the mother is involved in managing the child's illness. This most common constraining arrangement leads to the father and healthy siblings feeling "left out" (Drotar et al., 1984; Rolland, 1994), and it progressively distances them from the mother–sick child dyad. It also keeps them from having first-hand information about the health problem and treatment and from having opportunities to share concerns and support each other.

In caring for a sick family member in the hospital or home, especially if the illness is life threatening, the family members often feel helpless, powerless, and stressed. Wright and Leahey (1994) provide several intervention suggestions aimed at involving the family and reducing its stress. These include teaching caregiving techniques and how to touch and hold the patient without disrupting treatments, as well as encouraging family members to take on particular caregiving roles. Involvements such as these provide the family with a sense of competency (Power & Dell Orto, 1988).

▶ TEACHING

Including the family in patient education is vitally important. Educating the patient without the family will frequently result in poor self-care and poor recovery outcomes (Rankin & Stallings, 1996). Teaching or health education is one of the major family nursing intervention approaches. It may cover many areas of content and focus, including health promotion and disease prevention, illness/disability concerns and impact, and family dynamics. Teaching strategies are processes that facilitate learning. The aims of learning are to support healthy behaviors or to change unhealthy behaviors, albeit alterations of behavior are not always immediate or observable. Four specific goals of family health teaching are presented in Table 18–1.

Watson (1985) stresses that education provides information to clients, thereby assisting them to cope more effectively with life changes and stressful events. Gaining meaningful information helps family members feel a greater sense of control and less stress. It also enables them to more clearly define their own options and more successfully problem solve.

▶ TABLE 18–1

GOALS OF FAMILY HEALTH TEACHING

1. To provide information so that clients are able to make informed decisions with regard to health and illness.
2. To assist clients to participate effectively in their care.
3. To assist clients to adapt to the realities of an illness and its treatment, trajectory, and prognosis.
4. To assist clients to experience the satisfaction of seeing their own efforts contribute toward improvement of health.

Adapted partially from Steiger & Lipson (1985).

In the era of managed care and the emphasis on self-care and self-responsibility, the need for client education is greater than ever before. Hence, health teaching needs to be geared toward assisting patients and families to engage in self- and family care and self/family responsibility. Adults and children, as early as possible, need to feel that they have the capacity to care for themselves and their family members, and the right to sufficient information so that they can make their own informed decisions. If this philosophy is established early in family–nurse relationships, then the traditional hierarchical model, with superordinate–subordinate positions, is no longer appropriate. As health educators, we need to play the role of facilitator and resource person to clients who will decide which options are best for them.

Teaching interventions today increasingly involve teaching skills to family caregivers. With the advent of Diagnostic Related Groups (DRGs), managed care, and other cost-saving policies, growing numbers of hospitalized patients are being discharged early. Both inpatient nurses and home health nurses are assuming much greater responsibility in teaching family caregivers how to care for their recovering family member in the hospital and home.

Teaching–Learning Process

The teaching–learning process is similar to the nursing process in that both contain the same basic steps: assessment, problem statement (in teaching these are called "learning needs"), goals, implementation, and evaluation.

Assessment of Need.
When formally teaching, assessment of the family members' readiness to learn is part of the assessment and is crucial to ascertain before proceeding further. Two types of readiness need to be considered: emotional and experiential readiness of learners. **Emotional readiness** involves the motivation to learn, while **experiential readiness** includes adequacy of background knowledge, mastery of specific skills, and knowledge, attitudes, and values related to learning (Steiger & Lipson, 1985). Readiness is more complex and difficult to assess in a family, because readiness varies among family members. Adults, in particular, learn best when they are ready and willing to learn (Knowles, 1973). Watson (1985)

contends that more emphasis should be placed on the client's learning process. Part of assessing readiness factors in family members should involve discovering family members' perceptions and informational and skill needs.

Problem Identification.
Generally speaking, learning needs of families regarding health and illness matters are extensive, especially when a family member has a serious and complex health problem. Knowledge deficits about family health promotion and all that this entails should, however, not be overlooked as a central focus for teaching also.

Among the North American Nursing Diagnosis Association (NANDA) diagnoses that are relevant with respect to teaching interventions, knowledge deficit is one of the most germane diagnoses for family nursing. It is a very general diagnosis, and so must be further specified in the defining characteristics and contributing factors. Although the NANDA diagnosis is individually oriented it can easily be extended to include the family.

Planning.
The establishment of goals or objectives is the first part of the planning process. There are three domains relative to learning objectives: cognitive, affective, and psychomotor (Bloom, 1956). Planning also involves identifying what measures will be used to estimate how well the objectives have been met. Short-term and long-term realistic, client-centered goals are usually indicated. The simple imparting of information cannot be considered teaching, particularly if there is no evidence that the client has learned or met the objectives of the teaching. Needless to say, for learning to occur, it is crucial that the health educator and client share similar objectives.

Determining the particular teaching strategies to be employed is also part of planning.

Implementation of Teaching Plan.
Working with the whole family or sets of relationships within the family makes the actual teaching more complex. First of all, there maybe two different generations to teach and they have different emotional and experiential readiness levels. Teaching a whole family demands that a more flexible, interactive teaching modality be used. Many times role modeling is used, especially when teaching families how to communicate more clearly and openly with each other.

Teaching in family nursing means much more than the formal, structured imparting of information. It entails informal teaching—that which goes on in spontaneous client–nurse interactions. It includes modeling, demonstrating, and experiential strategies, which help the family learn new competencies or gain a more positive definition of their situation (called "reframing"). It involves "coaching" family members through an illness or medical regimen or procedure, or how to negotiate with the health care system (Benner, 1984). And lastly, it acknowledges and incorporates clients' interpretations of their health or illness and/or that of their family members. Some of these interpretations are socioculturally based. Family-oriented health educators should also utilize principles of teaching–learning in their implementation strategies. See Table 18–2 for principles of teaching–learning.

Documentation and Evaluation. Documenting the client's response to teaching and the extent to which the objective(s) have been met—as perceived jointly by nurse and family—completes the teaching–learning process. Within nursing today, increased emphasis is on client outcome evaluations (Sparks, 1995).

As with the nursing process, if the goals or objectives are not fully met, then analysis of what barriers to learning existed is in order. With barriers identified, modification of the teaching–learning plan typically follows (Steiger & Lipson, 1985).

▶ TABLE 18–2

PRINCIPLES OF TEACHING—LEARNING

- Start where the learner is.
- Proceed from simple to complex.
- Proceed from the familiar to the unfamiliar.
- Use terminology that is appropriate for the learner.
- Set both short-term and long-term goals.
- Apply knowledge to enhance learning.
- Provide positive reinforcement to enhance learning.
- Incorporate the "four Cs" into teaching (display confidence, act competent, communicate clearly, and demonstrate caring).
- Use teaching materials that are suitable for the literacy skills of the learner.

Source: Partially adapted from Doak, Doak, & Root (1996), Rankin & Stallings (1996), Sparks (1995).

Types of Learning

Learning involves acquiring new thoughts and ideas (cognitive learning), attitudes (affective learning), and behaviors (psychomotor skill acquisition) (Bloom, 1956). Recognition is needed of the three kinds of learning when planning teaching interventions because all three types of learning are important (Lester, 1986). Moreover, the three types of learning are interdependent. For example, sufficient knowledge (cognitive learning) is foundational to the other two types of learning. When our attitudes about food and nutrition positively change, then behavioral changes often follow. Acquiring self-care skills can also lead to more positive attitudes about self-care.

Some educators draw on the sage words of Confucius to illustrate why and how to teach psychomotor skills. He said, "I read and I forget, I see and I remember, I do and I understand."

Variables Affecting Teaching Effectiveness/Learning

There are numerous factors that can positively or negatively influence the efficacy of the teaching intervention. Client and contextual variables that affect teaching effectiveness are listed in Table 18–3.

Informal Teaching: Provision of Information

Where sharing of information occurs in spontaneous encounters between nurse and family members, or information is communicated to family members in an unstructured manner, informal teaching is involved. Doherty and Campbell (1988) detail the skills that health care professionals need when providing ongoing medical information and advice to families. The skills are:

- Regularly and clearly communicating health findings and treatment options to family members.
- Attentively listening to family members' questions and concerns.
- Advising families how to handle the health and rehabilitation needs of the patient. (p. 132)

► TABLE 18–3

VARIABLES AFFECTING TEACHING EFFECTIVENESS

■ **CLIENT FACTORS**
   • Motivation of family members. Motivation is the critical force or drive that activates persons to change.
   • Ages of family members.
   • Members' psychological state (e.g., anxiety, depression level).
   • Family members' perception of health problem(s).

■ **COMMUNICATION FACTORS**
   Communication involves the exchange of information between the sender and the receiver. Barriers to communication include those due to:
   • Lack of comprehension of subject matter.
   • Cultural and language barriers.
   • Socioeconomic barriers.
   • Inability to communicate clearly with teacher and each other.

■ **SITUATIONAL FACTORS**
   • The environment in which the teaching–learning takes place.
   • The timing of the teaching.
   • The teaching modalities used.

The breadth or depth of health information provided may vary depending on the family members with whom one speaks. Accuracy of information is paramount, however, and who provides what information should be coordinated when teaching efforts are interdisciplinary.

Providing Information to Families With Critically Ill Members.

Clinical practice and family research indicate that in health care settings families desire more information than they obtain from health professionals (Wright, Watson, & Bell, 1997). This need for information is heightened when family members are hospitalized and critically ill (Wright & Leahey, 1994). Families want to be regularly informed about their loved one's condition, treatments, and progress. One important informal teaching strategy suggested for the hospital nurse is to make regular telephone contact with the family (Bozett & Gibbons, 1983). This strategy has benefits for both the nurse, who now controls the dissemination of information and no longer sees the family as being disruptive and bothersome, and the family,

which feels that it does not have to be constantly at the hospital. Family members will be less anxious because of the supportive information that is regularly provided in the telephone calls.

Role Modeling

In addition to informal teaching strategies, role modeling is a powerful modality for teaching family members how to modify their behaviors. Bandura, a social learning theorist, points out how central role modeling is in learning. He contends that "learning through observing complex behaviors and then modeling such patterns is the source by which the most important learning of the social world takes place" (Jacob & Tennenbaum, 1988, p. 9). This approach is particularly important for pediatric family-centered nurses who serve as important role models when teaching parents; for primary care and community based nurses when they teach positive health behaviors; and for family mental health nurses when they teach family members how to communicate and interact more functionally. "Practice what you preach" is the well-used adage here. "There is nothing less motivating than a health care provider who encourages the client to stop smoking or lose weight yet is overweight and smells of tobacco" (Steiger & Lipson, 1985, p. 15).

Anticipatory Guidance

Anticipatory guidance is an important facet of health teaching. It provides the family with information on what to expect with respect to a future event, a potential problem/issue, or a child's next developmental phase. Discussing probable events, feelings, and situations with the family provides for clarification of ideas, reduction of anxiety, and future role change adaptability. Anticipation of and preparation for a coming event, a subsequent developmental phase, or a probable trajectory or prognosis of an illness will make the event less traumatic for the family and allow family members to better handle the situation (Green, 1994).

An example of the benefits of anticipatory guidance is the success that Lamaze classes enjoy. When labor begins, both parents trained in the Lamaze technique are fully prepared and usually go through the labor and delivery with excitement and positive feelings. A positive birthing experience gives parents positive feedback about their ability to handle future parenting challenges.

In conclusion, teaching interventions are one of the most essential types of family nursing interventions. Family health professionals need to keep in mind, however, that knowledge in and of itself does not necessarily lead to needed changes in behavior. As Health Belief Models describe (Rosenstock, 1974; Pender, 1996), changes in health behaviors are due to multiple factors with knowledge alone not being sufficient. A meta-analysis (a synthesis of multiple studies) of patient teaching research demonstrated that presentation of knowledge alone is not the most effective option. Approaches that combine information with emotional support to relieve anxiety were reported to be superior to the provision of information alone (Mumford et al., 1982).

▶ COUNSELING

Until recently, counseling has been thought by most nurses to be appropriate only for those in psychiatric–mental health nursing. It is now widely accepted, however, that there are levels of sophistication and complexity in counseling and that basic family counseling (called family interviewing by Wright and Leahey, 1984) is a core family nursing intervention. Family therapy and family systems nursing, advanced forms of family counseling, are viewed by this author as well as by the American Nurses Association Council of Psychiatric–Mental Health Nurses (1994) as requiring advanced practice nursing education.

Although not called counseling, nursing has long been concerned with nursing's therapeutic interpersonal process (Peplau, 1952). Patterson and Zderad (1976), in their description of humanistic nursing, assert that the crux of nursing is the existence of an authentic dialogue between nurse and patient and that the goal of this dialogue is growth promotion and nurturance of the human potential. Counseling and supportive intervention strategies are congruent with these ideas about nursing's role and goals.

Defining Counseling

Although there are numerous approaches in counseling, all connote an interpersonal intervention

process. Banks (1992) offers the following broad definition of counseling:

> Counseling is an interactive helping process between a counselor and a client characterized by the core elements of acceptance, empathy, genuineness, and congruency. This relationship consists of a series of interactions over time in which the counselor, through a variety of active and passive techniques, focuses on the needs, problems, or feelings of the client which have interfered with the client's usual adaptive behavior. (p. 281)

The core elements of counseling, then, are empathy, or the experiencing or sensing of another's feelings and behaviors; acceptance or positive regard for the client; and congruency or genuineness, being unpretentious and honest in the client–nurse relationship (Rogers, 1951; Truax & Carkhuff, 1967). Underlying these attributes is a respect for others, free of authoritarian judgments and coercive pressure (Banks, 1992), as well as a caring for and about the family.

Counseling is a process that seeks to help families and their members address, resolve, and effectively cope with their problems, and to utilize their competencies and other resources more fully. Encouraging family members to express and share their concerns, perceptions, and feelings with other family members is an essential part of this process. Assisting family members to positively reframe or cognitively restructure their thoughts and perceptions about events—in order to bring about healthier behavior—is also a major intervention approach (Goldenberg & Goldenberg, 1996; Minuchin & Fishman, 1981). Working with individual family members, family subsystems, whole families, and groups of families are ways to provide family counseling services (Greiner & Demi, 1995).

Family counseling strategies are very broad, covering a wide array of more specific techniques and foci. These strategies also range in complexity from very basic supportive counseling interventions to family therapy or family systems nursing where advanced practice preparation is needed. At a basic level of counseling, it is difficult to distinguish when teaching ends and when counseling begins. It is also difficult to identify the conceptual differences between teaching and counseling. Doherty (1995) addresses these two issues by suggesting that teaching and family therapy (an advanced form of family counseling) are part of a continuum, where educational approaches are the focus at one end of the continuum and therapeutic approaches are the focus at the other end of the continuum. To demonstrate his idea about this issue, he devised *Levels of Family Involvement,* guidelines for family professionals working with families. Table 18–4 outlines these five levels of family involvement, which start with very minimal involvement (i.e., level I, patient teaching) to an intensive level of involvement (i.e., level V, family therapy). Family nurses—without advanced family nursing practice preparation—should be able to work with families at levels I through IV.

Level V, or the advanced level of family involvement, involves family therapy or as Wright and her colleagues term it, family systems nursing. This level of involvement or practice is well described in Wright and Leahey's (1994) *Nurses and Families: A Guide to Family Assessment and Intervention* (2nd ed.) and in a chapter on family therapy by Watson in Bulechek and McCloskey, *Nursing Interventions: Essential Nursing Treatments* (1992). Systemic belief therapy, a more focused family therapy or advanced family systems nursing approach, is also outlined in the article by Wright and colleagues, "The Influence on the

Beliefs of Nurses: A Clinical Example of a Post-Myocardial Infarction Couple" (1995) and elaborated on in Wright, Watson, and Bell's recent book, *Beliefs: The Heart of Healing in Families and Illness* (1997). This advanced nursing practice counseling model has been successfully developed and used in working with families experiencing various serious health problems. Convinced that a family's problem is their constraining beliefs about their problem, Wright and colleagues focus on the assessment of and intervention in family members' beliefs about their illness (Wright et al., 1995).

As with teaching, counseling interventions can be used in addressing many different types of family nursing diagnoses and problems. Of the NANDA diagnoses relevant for family nursing (see Table 3–2), counseling could be an appropriate type of intervention for all these diagnoses. A nice example of the use of family counseling interventions is presented by Follen, Johnson, and Kronenwetter (1994). They describe the family counseling approaches they used in the critical care setting: interventive questioning, empowering family members to translate the meaning of their experience, facilitating patient–family dis-

---

► TABLE 18–4

THE TEACHING–COUNSELING CONTINUUM AS SEEN IN HEALTH PROVIDERS' LEVEL OF FAMILY INVOLVEMENT

Level of Family Involvement	Description of Involvement	Teaching or Counseling
I	Minimal emphasis on family. Individually oriented education/teaching.	Patient teaching.
II	Collaborative educational activities with members; providing information and advice.	Family teaching.
III	Adds to level II involvement by the eliciting of feelings and experiences of family members.	Combination of supportive teaching and educationally focused counseling.
IV	Brief focused family assessment and interventions. Particularly suited for work with families with health promotion and health problems, as well as families in high-risk situations. Basic family assessment and interventions included here.	Basic family counseling.
V	Family therapy aimed at treating serious psychological and family problems. Advanced skills needed to deal with treatment of intense personal and family distress, conflict, and resistance to needed change.	Advanced family counseling (family therapy).

Source: Partially adapted from Doherty (1995), Doherty & Campbell (1988).

cussion about patients' preferences for care and about care outcomes, and redefining the context of relationships.

Family Counseling of Families in Crisis

Family counseling is often used to help a family deal with a crisis (Hartman & Laird, 1983). The most widely used model of working with families in crisis is the family crisis intervention model (Ell & Northen, 1990). Kus (1992) defines the crisis intervention model that may be used with individual or family clients:

> Crisis intervention is the systematic application of problem-solving techniques, based on crisis theory, designed to help the client in crisis move through the crisis process as swiftly and painlessly as possible and thereby achieve at least the same level of psychological comfort [or family functioning in the case of families] as experienced before the crisis. (p. 181)

The major goals of family crisis intervention are to decrease the immediate negative effects of stress felt by family members and the family as a whole, as well as to mobilize their coping capabilities in adaptive ways (Ell & Northen, 1990). Reframing family members' view of their problem(s) is often used to assist them to search for alternative behavioral, cognitive, and affective responses to their problem (Hartman & Laird, 1983; Minuchin & Fishman, 1981).

The family nurse's functions using this model are to initially and quickly provide access to needed services and then, after the initial stress level is reduced and immediate problems are addressed, to assist the family in problem solving and coping, with the aim being to have the family and its members return to their previous state of family functioning or hopefully to a higher level of functioning. Helping families develop their own methods for coming up with solutions to their problems is congruent with a self-care approach and represents an empowering counseling intervention.

Barriers to Counseling Effectiveness

The barriers to counseling effectiveness are similar to those associated with teaching. Socioeconomic and cultural differences between nurse and family can pose a particularly troublesome barrier if the nurse is not competent in modifying his or her approach to be socioculturally appropriate (Pedersen et al., 1996). Family client motivational problems are also critical barriers to successfully assisting families.

Four additional limitations often curtail what nursing can do in counseling families. First, if the organization for which the family nurse works is not supportive of family nursing counseling interventions (Wright & Leahey, 1994), and hence does not allocate time for this type of intervention or reward the nurse for counseling families, this serves as a major barrier. Second, if the families themselves do not see nurses fulfilling this role, they may be resistant to counseling, unless the nurse can clarify his or her role and gain the participation of the family. A third basic limitation to counseling by family nurses is the reality of today's cost-containment practice mileau. With time and efficiency highly valued to keep costs contained, family counseling activities are often neglected or not feasible. A fourth barrier to counseling effectiveness is the nurses' preparation. If the family has complex problems, advanced nursing preparation is often necessary to adequately address these more difficult family needs.

The Decision to Counsel Families

The decision as to whether to counsel a family is ultimately based upon several primary factors. The first of these is the family's level of functioning, which then implies the extensiveness of the family's problems—or the reverse, the family's strengths or competencies. The family nurse's competence to counsel a particular family is a second consideration. And a third consideration is the work context. Within the present work environment, is it feasible to counsel the family as needed? If counseling is indicated, and it is possible within the work environment and mutually agreed upon, then what areas to focus on, who to see, and how long to work with the family are key considerations (Wright & Leahey, 1994).

▶ CONTRACTING

An effective means by which a family-centered nurse can realistically assist individuals and families to make behavioral changes is through the use of contracts. Contracting is also an excellent way to involve a family in a collaborative process.

Client contracting has been used in nursing since the 1970s and has been particularly efficacious when working with certain types of families such as families with substance abuse, pain control, or compliance problems, as well as families with marital and child behavioral problems (Goldenberg & Goldenberg, 1996; Jensen, 1985).

A contract is a working agreement made between two or more parties, such as between a family and a nurse or between parents and a child. To be timely and relevant, contracts are continuously renegotiable and cover the following areas: goals, length of the contract, client responsibilities (commitments), and health care team members' responsibilities, steps toward meeting the goals, and rewards for meeting goals (Sloan & Schommer, 1975; Steiger & Lipson, 1985). A contract may be written (Table 18–5) or verbal. One of the advantages of making a contract is that at the end of the contract period, progress is evaluated and either a new contract made or the relationship terminated (Boehm, 1992; Wright & Leahey, 1994).

Usually the contract is written, straightforward, simple to construct, and noncoercive (Goldenberg & Goldenberg, 1996). It also clarifies expectations for the parties involved (Boehm, 1992). The philosophy underlying the use of contracts is that of client involvement and the encouragement of self-care and self-responsibility. The contract draws clients in as the chief partners in their own health care. In fact, effective use of contracts is dependent on family involvement. For contracts involving family health problems, it is essential that the contract be made with the responsible and appropriate family members. Otherwise, family system problems cannot be properly addressed.

▶ TABLE 18–5

BASIC COMPONENTS OF WRITTEN CLIENT CONTRACTS

- Purpose or goals of the contract: short term and/or long term.
- Implementation: activities taken to reach goals and by whom.
- Priorities in terms of goals or activities.
- Reward when goals are met.
- Time parameters: when activities are to be accomplished.
- Reevaluation date to determine progress.
- Cosigners and date.

Nursing Diagnoses and Contracting

According to Jensen (1985), client contracting is particularly appropriate for clients with the following types of nursing diagnoses: noncompliance, knowledge deficit, ineffective coping, alterations in parenting, and self-care deficit diagnoses. Contracting has also been useful in addressing parenting problems or problems created by parent–child differences (Goldenberg & Goldenberg, 1996). Loveland-Cherry (1988, 1996) encourages family-centered nurses to also use contracting with family health-promotion diagnoses.

Limitations to the Use of Contracting

In client contracting, first and foremost the clients must be actively involved in the development, goal setting, and implementation. Because of this requirement, certain types of clients are automatically not appropriate candidates. Families in which the adult members are very dependent, disturbed, cognitively impaired, retarded, or not responsible, are poor candidates because of their inability to help develop and carry out their part of the agreement. Very young children within the family, unless the parent(s) is involved, are also not able to develop or carry through on their commitment.

It is also pointed out in the literature that client contracting takes time and effort. Moreover, in contracting the nurse may feel some loss of control, because the majority of the responsibility for implementation shifts to the family client.

In summary, two essential components of this intervention according to the literature (Boehm, 1992) are identified as (1) active client input into goal setting; and (2) when the goal has been met, the provision of positive reinforcement.

▶ CASE MANAGEMENT

Although nursing case management of the family as client is not directly discussed in the nursing literature, recently nursing case management of the individual client has received extensive attention and interest (ANA Task Force on Case Management, 1988; Cary, 1996; Smith, 1988; Zander, 1988). Case management has a long history of being part of public health nurses' role; more recently its prominence in the acute care setting has emerged (Cary, 1996).

The growth in managed care has been a prime force behind the emergence of case management (Cary, 1996). Managed care's emphasis on controlling costs and improving efficiency of care, while maintaining quality of care and client satisfaction, has definitely shaped the way case managers are functioning (Jones, 1994; MacPhee & Hoffenberg, 1996).

Defining Case Management

Case management is seen as a system, a clinical decision-making process, a technology, a role, and a service (Bower, 1992). Many definitions of case management appear in the literature. Nevertheless, there is a consensus that the process involves five essential steps: client assessment; planning; linking (referring, coordinating, and advocacy); monitoring; and evaluating (ANA Task Force on Case Management, 1988; Joint Commission for Accreditation of Community Mental Health Service Programs, 1976; Weil et al., 1985). As a process of determining, integrating, and monitoring complex client needs, it seeks to balance quality of care outcomes with efficient use of existing resources (Bower, 1992). Specific characteristics of case management identified in the literature include (1) its emphasis on active client participation; (2) its holistic orientation; (3) its self-care, self-deterministic orientation; and (4) the coordination and efficient use of a wide range of human services (Bower, 1992; White, 1986).

As can be seen from the preceding definition, the case management process and the process used in nursing practice (the nursing process) appear very similar. The crucial difference lies in the breadth and scope of the client assessment (the case management assessment is more comprehensive relative to assessment of psychosocial, environmental, and health-related variables) and the planning and resource identification with clients and members of the service network. This entails greater service coordination (Martin & Scheet, 1992; Weil et al., 1985).

Zander (1995), a nursing expert on case management in the acute care setting, states that case management builds on nurses' existing professional roles by adding three new dimensions to their job: (1) authority—the heightened authority to coordinate

client services; (2) accountability—for favorable financial and clinical outcomes; and (3) time—a greater time commitment. Many parents and families require sequencing or organizing multidisciplinary services across settings—hospital, clinics, home, hospice. Managing these transitions is a crucial role for family-oriented case managers.

Client Advocacy

A major component of case management is client advocacy (Smith, 1993). An advocate is one who speaks for and on behalf of some other person or group. It is also someone who vindicates or espouses a cause by argument, a defender or intercessor, such as the position of defense attorney assumes. Kosik's (1972) definition relative to client advocacy by nurses extends the above definitions, incorporating a deeper commitment to the client. She explains:

> For me, patient advocacy is seeing that the patient knows what to expect and what is his right to have, and then displaying the willingness and courage to see that our system does not prevent his getting it. The goals of patient advocacy are, first, making a person more independent because he knows the what, why, and how of the system and, second, changing the system to make it more sensitive and relevant by revealing injustices and inadequacies, thereby making complacent continuation of the status quo impossible. The nurse may have to make waves. She may have to see that workers and agencies do their jobs and expose the indifference and inhumanity of care givers. (p. 694)

The role of being a client advocate involves informing clients and then supporting them in whatever decision they make (Bramlett, Gueldener, & Sowell, 1990; Kohnke, 1982). Although a goal of client advocacy is client independence, the advocate may have to accept and perhaps even foster dependency temporarily, for many people, especially the poor, have never had their dependency needs met. And thus we need to start there and assist the person or family to grow.

Although there are multiple ways of defining what advocacy means, in all cases there is a basis in ethical principles—using the principle(s) of self-determination (autonomy), justice (fairness and equality), beneficence (doing good), and nonmaleficence (doing no harm) to guide each of varied definitions of advocacy. Some nurses see advocacy as the philosophical foundations of nursing (Curtin, 1979; Gadow, 1980).

Community-based family nurses are in a strong position to act as advocates. They are in the community working with families that are often poor and feeling powerless and hopeless. Not only *is* there a greater need for these nurses to assume this role because of client needs, but unless the advocacy role is assumed, the rendering of other essential services may not be obtainable. Nurses in hospitals also have an important opportunity to act as family advocates—making sure that families and their members receive needed services and that the services they are receiving are appropriate and of good quality.

Thus the family nurse can be a client advocate in at least four ways: (1) by assisting clients to obtain services they need and are entitled to, (2) by trying to make health care systems more responsive to client needs, (3) by advocating for the inclusion of more socioculturally appropriate services, and (4) by advocating for more responsive social policy (Canino & Spurlock, 1994). Family advocacy can range from calling the welfare department before referring a family, in an effort to pave the way for them, to testifying in court on behalf of a client, calling a meeting with representatives from several agencies to coordinate and improve services to the community, or acting as a political activist working in the political and legislative policy areas to create needed changes in health and human services for families.

Clark (1984) points out that "advocacy necessitates involvement and commitment. The effective community health nurse cannot be content with the attitude, 'I'd like to help you, but my hands are tied.' Advocacy is not a popular concept" (p. 53), because it often means standing up to other health care and social service professionals and health care agencies for the rights of families. Advocacy also means assisting families to learn how to speak up for themselves—to be their own best advocates.

Rafael (1995) examines the various meanings of advocacy and how advocacy and empowerment have similar, yet different features. She concludes that existential or human advocacy (where the client is viewed as subject rather than object, and the nurse as a caring, valuing person) and empowerment are synchronous.

Coordination

One of the most widely accepted roles of the client advocate is the coordinator (Leddy & Pepper, 1985). Because the essence of case management is also coordination, the notions of advocacy and coordination substantially overlap. In fact, case management is often referred to as service coordination (particularly in the social work field), designed to provide multiple services to clients with complex needs within a single locus of control (Seltzer et al., 1989).

The family nurse in community and home health, as well as in primary care, is often a key person in the provision of comprehensive, continuous family health care. In addition to the particular functions the nurse is implementing, he or she supports other team members and interprets the nursing objectives and service, as well as coordinating health services with the various other agencies from which the family is receiving assistance.

Without coordination the client may receive a duplication of some services from different agencies or, even more distressing, a gap in essential areas of need. An illustration of this problem from home health care follows. A rehabilitation clinic patient once remarked to various members of the health care team that she was having difficulty getting out of the bathtub and had no shower facilities to use. Each time she mentioned this to the team members they noted her response, but no one made any suggestions of what to do. A social worker, sanitarian, homemaker-home health aide, and visiting nurse were all visiting the family concurrently. In this type of situation it was the nurse's responsibility to make sure that collaboration was taking place and coordinated efforts being achieved. With a greater number of more acutely and seriously ill patients discharged early from hospital to home and followed by multiservice home health agencies, the nurse's role as case manager or coordinator of services is being expanded. Hospice home care programs are examples of interdisciplinary programs where the nurse plays a vital coordination function.

Discharge Planning.   Promoting continuity of care for hospitalized and long-term, chronically ill clients and their families is a particularly significant need. Discharge planning from one level of care to another within a hospital or from the hospital to home or another health care facility is one example of continuity of care (Kelly, McClelland, & Day, 1992). Effective discharge planning is a central component of case management/coordination. It is essential to the individual patient and family that an appropriate plan and transition be made. From a health care agency's fiscal perspective, it is also critically important to have effective discharge planning to expedite the earliest possible appropriate discharge. Because discharge planning addresses health care access, quality, and cost, this component of case management is receiving wide attention (Kelly et al., 1992).

In this role, the nurse must make continuing efforts to improve referral systems between the various health care and social service agencies in the community, and must be willing to share information with referring agencies, given the client's approval. Referral is a two-way street, and communication must flow in both directions for the system to be functional.

In summary, family-oriented nurses often function across settings as a bridge between the family and various services by acquainting families with available community resources, effecting continuity of care, and coordinating and monitoring the services clients are receiving.

In the case management role nurses must often balance the caring behaviors of being an advocate and a coordinator with the resource control or gatekeeper role they also assume (Seuntjens, 1995). Kane (1988) believes this is possible ethically as long as a case management program is designed to serve a defined population with finite resources. Here the case manager advocates on behalf of the individual, family, and the defined population she or he serves.

Case Management: For Whom?

Great optimism is expressed about how implementation of case management by nurses improves care. For both acute and community settings, among patients for whom complex and serious health and social problems exist, case management is looked upon as a cost-effective, comprehensive practice strategy.

Case management first appeared in connection with workmen's compensation and physical rehabili-

tation in the 1940s (Jellinek, 1988) and later, in the 1970s in the social welfare literature (Grau, 1984). Although public health nursing had been using the term "case management" for many years to describe its services, it was not until the middle and late 1980s that the broad field of nursing rediscovered case management.

The client populations for which case-management strategies have been targeted are the frail elderly (Kemper, 1988; Steinberg & Carter, 1983); the physically disabled/rehabilitation client (Kemp, 1981; Roessler & Bolton, 1978); the chronic mentally ill (Goering et al., 1988); the developmentally disabled; the abused/neglected child (Weil et al., 1985); the AIDS client and clients with other complex chronic and life-threatening illnesses (Fisher, 1987; Martin, 1987), and acute care patients (Fisher, 1987; Newman, Lamb, & Michaels, 1991; Zander, 1988).

Inasmuch as the real thrust of case management is the initiation of linkages between client and needed resources and coordination and advocacy activities, a case management approach should be appropriate for any type of nursing diagnosis. Nonetheless, a case-management strategy and process is a particularly useful type of intervention for use with family clients diagnosed with serious, long-term, or complex needs. Using NANDA nursing diagnoses, the following family-centered nursing diagnoses appear most germane: ineffective family coping, particularly those related to domestic abuse and child abuse or neglect; alterations in family processes; grieving; health maintenance alterations; impaired health maintenance; alterations in parenting; and potential for violence.

Case Management in Various Nursing Specialties

Within the community health context, particularly the home health context, nurses are generally viewed as case managers (Cary, 1996; Dickinson et al., 1988; Martin & Scheet, 1992; MacPhee & Hoffenberg, 1996; Wahlstedt & Blaser, 1986). For example, Dickinson and associates (1988) maintain that case management is a primary role of community health and home care nurses, explaining that they help establish and coordinate the many health care, social, fiscal, and environmental services needed for clients and their families. Moreover, case management is viewed as a major nursing intervention in primary care (Seuntjens, 1995), in acute care (Zander, 1995), in mental health (Pearson, 1995), and in school nursing (Kub & Steel, 1995).

Limitations and Barriers to Nursing Case Management

There are three primary limitations or barriers to using a case management approach in family nursing. The first of these is the reimbursement policies that exist in health care. Nurses, except for those in specialized positions where case management is identified as one of their functions, are not paid for providing case management to individuals, let alone to families. Completing a more comprehensive assessment, actively involving the family, and linking, coordinating, and monitoring services takes time. Adequate funding must be available for case management services to be effectively provided.

Second, nurses are often not sufficiently educated to function as case managers using the broadened definition of case management described above. "Few basic nursing education programs today, regardless of their level of preparation, provide nurses with the knowledge and skills to function efficiently as case managers" (ANA Task Force on Case Management, 1988, p. 8). Nursing programs typically do not emphasize the assessment of social, economic, and environmental areas, or the initiating linkages and coordinating services to families. For instance, referral for assistance with financial problems resulting from health care expenditures involves the family health professional being knowledgeable about available services and programs, agency referral procedures, and how best to refer the family.

Special programs that teach case management skills to nurses have been recently developed and implemented. These programs have been evaluated as increasing nurses' documentation of case management services to clients, particularly nurses' patient counseling, education, and health promotion interventions (Connors, 1988; Winder, 1988). Because case management is being seen in nursing schools as an advanced nursing practice role, the number of masters-level nursing case management programs is growing.

A third limitation—which is related to the first two barriers—is that some health care agencies do not see nurses as operating as case managers (in these cases social workers are generally seen in this role), or the agencies do not see this broadened responsibility as being within their scope of provided services. In spite of social workers being better educated in some aspects of case management, when clients have complex health problems, nursing case managers often are more appropriate. The consequences of a complex and life-threatening disease demands a case manager who is well educated in both health and psychosocial/environmental areas.

▶ COLLABORATION

Another intervention of growing importance to family nursing is collaboration. It is vital to the provision of comprehensive health care to families. As members of a health care team, nurses collaborate and plan comprehensive family-centered care with other team members, as well as with their family clients.

Defining Collaboration

Collaboration, according to Lamb and Napadano (1984), is "a process of shared planning and action over time with joint responsibility for the outcomes and the ability to work together for common goals using problem-solving techniques" (p. 26). Collaboration is a synergistic alliance, in which the outcomes are different and better than any of the collaborators could generate on their own (Kyle, 1995). The end result should be the enhancement of client care and greater professional satisfaction (King, Parrinelo, & Baggs, 1996). The positive impact of collaboration is being increasingly recognized and advocated by nursing and other professional organizations, as well as by accreditation agencies (Lee & Cohen, 1995).

Collaboration can be considered both as a separate family nurse intervention strategy and as an important strategy used in case management. In the various ANA standards of practice, one standard of practice focuses specifically on the nurse's involvement in collaboration. Collaboration in most of the ANA standards of practice includes the client (individual and family) as part of the collaborative process also.

Ability to communicate clearly and negotiate effectively are interpersonal skills necessary for successful collaboration. "Collaboration involves the mutual give and take of cooperativeness and an active participation of all parties . . ." (Kyle, 1995, p. 174).

Collaboration implies a professional, collegial relationship—in which there is mutual respect, egalitarianism and joint decision making (Clark, 1984). An authoritarian type of relationship, where the leadership and direction flow from the physician to nurse to nurse's aide to patient, cannot be considered a team or collaborative relationship. With a hierarchal model (where one person is in charge), communication is not open, direct, or truly two way, and team members' contributions and effective functioning are seriously stifled.

Collaboration: With Whom?

The composition of the health team (or health and welfare team) may vary depending on an agency's available resources, the health care professionals' practices, and a family's needs. Doherty (1988), a family therapist, identifies the therapeutic triangle composed of family, family professional, and medical team as being the treatment context within which collaborative health care should take place when families have chronically ill family members.

In a home health agency the team is commonly composed of a community health nurse, a licensed vocational nurse, a homemaker-home health aide, a social worker, and a physical therapist. The occupational therapist and nutritionist are also often members, or act as consultants to the team. The family physician acts only partially and indirectly as a team member, because he or she is not present, is often difficult to reach, and is typically involved in the medical aspects of care only. Many independent health goals need to be formulated by the home health team based on medical information, physician's orders, and client assessments of patient and family. The patient and family themselves are also central members of the team. In dealing with chronic illness and long-term care, effective collaboration is essential to address the many-faceted interdependent needs of clients (Marosy, 1994).

In primary health care, the health care team usually involves the physician, nurse practitioner, and clinical nurse. A social worker, nurse's aide/voca-tional nurse, clinical psychologist, and other physician specialists may also be members of the team. Because nurse practitioners often work very closely with physician colleagues, the ability to collaborate effectively is vital to delivering care.

In the official public health agency, the team may be broader or smaller in size depending on the family's particular health, welfare, and educational needs. The community health nurse working in an official health care agency may be a member of a community-based team working with a young, child-rearing family where the school nurse, teacher, probation officer, caseworker, and psychologist are a part of the team. School nurses routinely function as collaborative members of teams that assess and plan educational programs for the learning and physically disabled student.

In an acute care setting, physician, nurse, social worker, patient, and family usually make up the team. Family professionals (nurse, social worker, and/or psychologist) need to maintain access and collaboration with the patient's physician, as the disease process and its treatment are affected by the family context.

Kindig (1975) points out that the structure of each health care system and the mix of people working on a health care team depend on the needs of the patient population and on available resources. For the team to function effectively, all members must have a common understanding of their respective roles and responsibilities, as well as clients' needs and the goals of treatment plan. Moreover, when a health care team continually works together, there is a great need for members to work out the process by which decisions are made, communications channeled, and procedures adopted. If a team runs smoothly, this frees more energy for client care, as less energy will be needed for team maintenance and coping with members' interpersonal concerns.

Costs and Barriers to Collaboration

Doherty (1988), speaking about collaboration in primary and secondary care settings, reminds us of one of the major costs of collaboration:

> Collaborating, however, takes effort and accommodation. . . . Physicians must give up some of their unilateral power and psychosocial profes-

sionals must give up some of their righteous superiority on the interpersonal dimensions of patient
care. (p. 209)

The need for an interdisciplinary process, whereby
the efforts and skills of different professionals are
coordinated, is clear when one adopts a family systems
perspective and focuses on ways in which the family
both affects and is affected by the health or illness of
its members (Glenn, 1987). Moreover, in research
studies, collaboration has been shown to be both therapeutically and cost effective (American Nurses
Association, 1992; Koerner & Armstrong, 1984). But
as we all are aware, the organization of health care services, especially since cost-containment measures
have tightened, is characterized as a biomedical
model. Specialist care and fragmentation of services
are the norm (Glenn, 1987). Some integrated health
care systems are still in place, but the biopsychosocial
model, because of economic, political, and social conditions, is presently on the decline. As a result, reimbursement barriers exist, as previously discussed, as
well as health care delivery barriers.

Glenn (1987), a family physician and advocate of
collaborative health care, writes about another common cost or barrier to collaboration. He addresses the
problem of power conflicts between health care professionals. "The main conflicts that emerge involve
turf and money, authority and power" (p. 160). The
problem of physician dominance and nurse deference
is widely cited as a collaborative barrier (Kyle, 1995).
Crucial to successful collaboration is trust and mutual
respect among the collaborators (Kyle, 1995).

The most basic issues underlying collaborative
health care are economic, however, Who is paying
for what and to whom? The way health care dollars
are divided is an intrinsic factor that determines
health care professionals' roles. Psychosocial aspects
of health care receive low priority in terms of reimbursement; and insurance companies generally do
not reimburse health agencies for nurses providing
family psychosocial care.

In conclusion, collaboration is an increasingly
exciting, promising, and vital role in the nursing of
families because it facilitates a holistic approach and
the achievement of shared goals. For the family
nurse, collaborative health practice can be energiz-
ing, rewarding and both therapeutically and cost
effective (Daka-Mulwanda et al., 1995).

▶ CONSULTATION

Consultation is included as a general family nursing
intervention because family nurses often serve as consultants to other nurses and other professionals and
paraprofessionals when individual and family client
information and assistance are needed. Most of the
literature indicates that consultation requires both
expert clinical practice skills and knowledge and
advanced nursing practice preparation (American
Nurses Association, 1992; Fraley, 1992; Kearney &
Yurick, 1996).

Consultation is defined by Caplan (1970) as "a
process of interaction between two professional
persons—the consultant, who is a specialist, and the
consultee, who invokes the consultant's help"
(p. 19). The consultant's role is often to provide
problem-solving assistance with clinical issues. In
the consultation process the consultee is free to
accept or reject the consultant's recommendations
and remains directly responsible for implementing
action and outcomes of care.

In nursing, consultation may take the form of
deliberating together about a particular case or
client and giving suggestions/information about
clients with particular health problems. Or it may
entail interviewing a family and providing another
assessment of the family and its needs. Lewis and
Levy (1982) classify the consultation process into two
types. The first type in the above description is an
example of indirect consultation, where a case-
centered meeting is held and the family is not interviewed by the consultant. The second type of consultation is the latter example, where family members
are directly interviewed by the consultant and a second opinion is given. This particular model is used
extensively in medicine and substantially in psychiatric nursing where psychiatric clinical nurse specialists act as consultants to hospital nurses when
patients are experiencing psychological and behavioral problems (Kearney & Yurick, 1996).

Family-oriented nurses who function as clinical
nurse specialists, school nurses, family counselors,
community health nurses, and occupational health
nurses include consultation as one important component of their practice. Many family nurses develop
special areas of expertise—such as family and child
abuse, family crisis intervention, genetic counseling,

family health promotion and diabetes education programs, and parenting—and provide assistance to other professionals in these special areas.

▶ FAMILY EMPOWERING INTERVENTIONS

Empowerment is a popular "buzz word" in many helping professions today, particularly nursing. The literature on empowerment has grown exponentially in the last decade. Rodwell analyzes the various meanings of empowerment in a recent (1996) concept analysis article. She identifies four defining attributes of empowerment:

1. It consists of a helping process.
2. It involves a partnership that values self and others.
3. It is characterized by mutual decision making.
4. It includes freedom to make choices and accept responsibility.

From Rodwell's (1996) literature review and analytical process, she generates the following inclusive definition of empowerment. "In a helping partnership, it is a process of enabling people to choose to take control over and make decisions about their lives. It is also a process which values all those involved" (p. 309).

An empowerment philosophy underlies all the interventions described in this chapter. They are designed to increase families' knowledge, skills, and capacity for effective action on their own behalf for

the ultimate goal is to assist families to become their own best advocates and resource. Table 18–6 identifies key family empowering interventions.

▶ TABLE 18–6

FAMILY EMPOWERING INTERVENTIONS

- Encouraging active family and family member participation.
- Acting on and carefully listening to family members' concerns and starting where they want.
- Recognizing families as equal partners or team members in the health care system.
- Expanding families' visions of what options and possibilities exist.
- Encouraging family self-help.
- Enabling clients to exercise their autonomy and self-determination in deciding which options to chose.
- Appreciating that families and nurses each have their own specialized expertise in maintaining health and managing health problems.
- Recognizing that both families and nurses bring strengths and resources into their relationship.
- Discovering and affirming the strengths and resources of families, which becomes a foundation for trust.
- Advocating on behalf of families at the client, health care system, and health policy levels.
- Helping families develop more social supportiveness within their own families through the development of family relations skills.
- Giving families the credit for positive changes and accomplishments that occur.

Sources: Figley (1989), Leahey & Harper-Jaques (1996), Malinski (1987), Zerwekh (1992).

▶ study questions

1. Ways to actively involve families during the implementation phase include (check the appropriate choices):
   a. Asking them questions about how they have solved similar problems in the past.
   b. Advising them to follow prescribed recommendations.
   c. Encouraging them to discuss the various options available to them to meet their needs.
   d. Bringing all the family members together to discuss what might be done and who could do it.
   e. Recognizing that clients often lack the competency to make their own health decisions and, hence, need advice on what decisions to make.

2. Match the specific family interventions (from the left-hand column) with
    the descriptions of the interventions (in the right-hand column). More
    than one answer is correct for each intervention.

    ____ Teaching   a. Role modeling.
    ____ Case management   b. Involves intra-agency and/or
                                         extraagency linkages.
    ____ Coordination   c. A working agreement between two
                                         or more parties.
    ____ Advocacy   d. Processes that facilitate learning.
    ____ Collaboration   e. An interpersonal, interventive
                                         process.
    ____ Consultation   f. Assist families to use their own
                                         problem-solving skills and strengths.
    ____ Contracting   g. Giving professional advice to
                                         another helping person.
    ____ Counseling   h. Speaking for or on behalf of a client.
                                     i. Working closely with another
                                         professional to provide health
                                         services.

3. Match the types of limitations/barriers in the right-hand column with the
    interventions in the left-hand column. More than one limitation/barrier
    can be associated with each of the interventions.

    ____ Case management   a. Decreased client motivation to
                                         change health behaviors.
    ____ Teaching   b. Cultural and language barriers
                                         between involved parties.
    ____ Collaboration   c. Families do not see nurses fulfilling
                                         this interventive role.
    ____ Contracting   d. Organization for which nurse works
                                         is not supportive of nursing
                                         intervention.
    ____ Counseling   e. Setting for sustained or sufficient
                                         interaction inadequate.
                                     f. Working relationships are often
                                         hierarchical or stratified.
                                     g. Families are leaderless, chaotic, or
                                         very dependent.
                                     h. Inhibiting economic factors (lack of
                                         reimbursement, payment for
                                         intervention).

Fill in the spaces in the following questions (4–7).

4. Identify three NANDA nursing diagnoses for which teaching would be an
    appropriate intervention.

a. _____
b. _____
c. _____

5. Identify three NANDA family nursing diagnoses for which counseling would be an appropriate intervention.
   a. _____
   b. _____
   c. _____

6. For what types of families would basic supportive family counseling versus family therapy be more appropriate?

_____

7. For what type of health problems would family case management be most indicated?

_____

Are the following statements (8–18) true or false?

8. The steps in the nursing process and the teaching–learning process are the same.

9. In the assessment phase of the teaching–learning process, the sole focus is assessing the learner's readiness to learn.

10. Learning needs are analogous to assessment in the nursing process.

11. Determining the particular teaching strategies to be employed is part of the implementation phase.

12. Contracts can be unwritten or written.

13. Contracts are legal agreements between two sets of individuals.

14. Contracts encourage self-responsibility and self-care.

15. Using contracts greatly aids in the evaluation process.

16. A contract must contain time limitations.

17. A contract is made by the nurse and signed by the patient.

18. A contract spells out goals to be achieved and the respective responsibilities of the involved parties.

19. There are many factors that serve to promote or inhibit learning in families. Identify several important inhibiting factors.

20. The nurse is working with a family referred by a physician. Sammy, the 8-month-old son, was recently diagnosed as having leukemia. When the nurse arrives at the home, she discovers that the mother has little knowledge of leukemia, a limited income, and no transportation to medical services. The mother is overprotective and terribly solicitous in her care of her infant son. Identify three appropriate family nursing interventions.

21. The visiting nurse has made her first home visit to an elderly couple. The husband, Mr. Paul, age 80, has severe emphysema and has just been discharged from a local general hospital. The wife is also 80 and has assumed the caretaker role. In completing a nursing assessment, one of the observations the visiting nurse made is that Mr. Paul is seeing three doctors (a pulmonary specialist, an internist for his "heart condition," and a general practitioner who is a lifelong friend and sees Mr. Paul for immediate problems or "anything else"). The family's bathroom is filled with prescriptions—new, old, same drugs with different doses, and several drugs that have similar actions—prescribed by the different physicians. The patient, being quite concerned regarding his health, is complying by taking all of these. The wife is confused and finds caring for her bedridden husband alone a real burden. She complains of a continual backache and fatigue. Propose four family nursing interventions.

▶ chapter 18 study answers

1. a, c, and d.

2. Teaching—a, d, and e.
   Case management—b, f, and h.
   Coordination—b and c.
   Advocacy—h.
   Collaboration—b, c, e, and i.
   Consultation—e and g.
   Contracting—c.
   Counseling—a, d, e, and f.

3. Case management—b, c, and h.
   Teaching—a, b, e, and h.
   Collaboration—b, f, and h.
   Contracting—a, b, g, and h.
   Counseling—a, b, c, e, g, and h.

4. With virtually all NANDA diagnoses, educative interventions could be relevant if clients are able to understand and learn. Examples (there are many correct answers): (a) knowledge deficit, (b) altered role performance, and (c) health maintenance alteration.

5. a. Ineffective family coping.
   b. Alterations in family processes.
   c. Alterations in parenting. Many more would be appropriate also.

6. Supportive counseling: Families with health problems/concerns who do not have complex and intense problems. With more complex problems, family therapy level of counseling is indicated.

7. Families with serious, complex, and/or long-term health needs. Targeted populations include families with frail elderly, AIDS clients, child abuse, chronically mentally ill, developmental disabled, and physically disabled/rehabilitation patients.

8. True.

9. False.

10. False.

11. False.

12. True.

13. False.

14. True.

15. True.

16. True.

17. False.

18. True.

19. Examples are (a) decreased motivation (denial of learning needs); (b) lack of open communication and/or insufficient exchange of information; (c) environment is poor for teaching–learning to take place (space, noise problems, interruptions); (d) sociocultural differences; and (e) teaching not geared to literacy level of family.

20. Teaching, case management (initiating referral), and counseling.

21. Teaching, counseling, case management (service coordination), and collaboration.

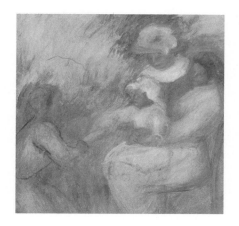

five

CULTURAL DIVERSITY AMONG FAMILIES

In the last section of this book, a description of families from America's three largest minorities or ethnic groups is presented, in order to show the significance of cultural variation in family life. After a brief overview of each of the ethnic groups, the Friedman Family Assessment Model (discussed in Chaps. 6 and 8–17 and appendices A and B) is used as a framework for describing the family groups. Chapter 8 provides the foundational sociocultural content for these chapters.

The Hispanic-American Family

Marilyn M. Friedman

> ▶ learning objectives

1. Identify what peoples constitute Hispanic-Americans and their respective percentages of all Hispanic-Americans.

2. Explain the criticism that is made about early writings of social scientists with respect to the Hispanic-American family.

3. Discuss why the Latino family has not integrated into the mainstream of American society to the extent that other ethnic groups have.

4. Interpret the meaning of two major family values within the Hispanic-American family: familism and the ethic of reciprocity among kin.

5. Describe briefly how the traditional role and power structure of the Latino family is changing.

6. Describe two general socialization patterns among Latino families.

7. Compare American core values with traditional Hispanic-American values.

8. Identify the most important structural change occurring in Hispanic-American families today.

9. Recognize the functions and primary role of these folk healers: *yerbero, curandero, santeria, espiritualisto*, and *brujo*.

10. Recall several common Latino folk illnesses.

11. Identify two central culturally derived family coping patterns of Latinos and a practice implication emanating from knowledge of culturally derived family coping patterns.

12. Explain three health care practice implications based on Hispanic-American culturally patterned beliefs and practices.

Family nurses are increasingly aware of the need for a transcultural and pluralistic perspective in working with diverse ethnic, religious, and cultural groups in American society (Friedman, 1990). There is both a demographic imperative and a practice imperative for having a good understanding of the Hispanic-American family.* The sheer numerical growth of this group in the United States, and the fact that Hispanic-American family members tend to have more frequent and serious health problems, provide additional rationale for becoming

---

* The terms Latino and Hispanic-American are used interchangeably throughout this chapter.

knowledgeable about the Latino family and its family life patterns.

▶ DEMOGRAPHIC PATTERNS OF HISPANIC-AMERICANS

Hispanic-Americans are those people of Spanish origin who classify themselves on census documents in one of the specific Spanish/Hispanic categories—Mexican, Puerto Rican, Cuban, and South or Central American. Recent census projections report that the Hispanic-American population is rapidly increasing and will after the turn of the century become the largest ethnic minority group in the United States (Vega, 1990). Mexican-Americans are the largest ethnic group within the larger Hispanic or Spanish-speaking population within the United States (62 percent or six out of ten Hispanics are Mexican-American). Puerto Ricans constitute 11 percent of Hispanic-Americans, while Cubans make up 4.7 percent, and South and Central Americans 14 percent of Hispanic-Americans (Garcia, 1993).

According to data from the Immigration and Naturalization Service, more than at any time since World War I the United States population increase is driven by immigration, both legal and illegal. Immigrants—7 to 9 million over the 1980 to 1990 decade—are largely from Mexico and Central America, as well as from Asia, South America, and the Caribbean (Barringer, 1990).

The rapid and large growth in the Hispanic-American population is confirmed by U.S. Bureau of the Census data (1983; Rosenblatt, 1996), which estimate that in 1960 there were 3.1 million Hispanic-Americans; in 1970, 9.1 million; in 1980, 14.6 million; and in 1996, 26.5 million. Whereas the white population in the United States increased 9.4 percent from 1970 to 1980, people of Spanish origin increased 61 percent during this same period.

Latinos are more concentrated in some regions of the United States—primarily in the Southwestern United States. The number of Latinos in California has increased fivefold, now constituting 25 percent of California's population. Latinos are a relatively young population with more children than Anglo families. Many are recent immigrants (Hayes-Battista, 1990; Ortiz, 1995).

What specific factors are involved in the tremendous increase in the Hispanic population? The rate of nat-

ural increase (births over deaths) among Hispanics is 1.8 percent, one-third higher than for African-Americans. The fertility rate of Latinos is over 50 percent greater than that of whites (Hayes-Battista, 1990). Certain Hispanic subgroups are growing much faster than others. Since 1980, immigration from Central America has risen sharply because of devastating social upheaval in those countries of origin. Hispanic immigration (legal and illegal) is running at the astonishing rate of an estimated one million people per year. Extrapolating from these figures, Hispanics will outnumber African-Americans around the turn of the century (see Figure 19–1).

Whereas African-Americans are united by race and a common historic experience of slavery, Hispanic-Americans are united by three powerful forces: their language (Spanish, except for Brazilians who speak Portuguese), their strong adherence to Roman Catholicism, and their common values and beliefs rooted in a history of conquest and colonization (Garcia-Preto, 1996). Nevertheless, there are also many factors that divide them into diverse groups.

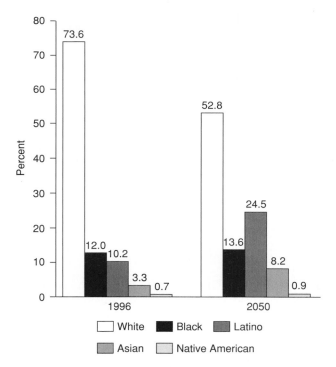

Figure 19–1. Dramatic changes expected in ethnic portrait in United States, 1996–2050. *(Source: Rosenblatt [1996]. Based on 1996 U.S. Census Figures and Projections.)*

The focus of research on the Hispanic-American family has been overwhelmingly on the Mexican-American family, which is more homogeneous than the larger Hispanic-American grouping. In spite of Mexican-Americans being more homogeneous, this subgroup of Hispanic-Americans evidences great intra-ethnic variation also. People of Mexican heritage vary by country of origin (United States or Mexico) and self-identification. In addition, socioeconomic, generational, regional, and idiosyncratic factors account for further intragroup diversity (Falicov, 1982).

Mexican-Americans are a blend of both Indian and Spanish cultures and races. Most Mexican-Americans are *mestizos*, of mixed Caucasian and Indian blood lines (Kuipers, 1995). Generally speaking, first-generation individuals speak Spanish and identify themselves as "Mexicano," whereas second- and third-generation people of Mexican descent speak English and Spanish and usually identify themselves as Mexican or Chicano (Keefe et al., 1978).

▶ THE HISPANIC-AMERICAN INTERFACE WITH AMERICAN SOCIETY

The major waves of Latino immigrants came to the United States after World War II. The pattern and timing of the migration usually has corresponded with economic depression and/or political turmoil in the immigrants' native land (Garcia-Preto, 1996). The Hispanic-American historical interface with the United States has varied by subgroups. The Mexican experience is described first.

The Mexican-American Experience

The pattern of labor utilization of Mexicans and Mexican-Americans provides a significant path for understanding the growth and obstacles to the Mexican-American subculture's assimilation into the American cultural mainstream. Historically Mexican immigration has been closely tied to Southwestern labor needs (Gonzalez, 1991). Until recently, job-starved Mexican nationals worked competitively and at lower wage scales than Mexican-Americans either by crossing the border daily or coming over as *braceros*. The bracero program, now defunct, permitted Mexican workers to work under contract to the

United States when the supply of field workers in this country was evaluated as insufficient (McLemore & Romo, 1985; Queen & Haberstein, 1974).

According to Queen and Haberstein (1974), Mexican-Americans, because of their proximity to Mexico, the fluidity of the border, and the exploitation of the Anglo-dominated agricultural system, have never been able to participate in the usual social processes used by European immigrants to become integrated into and socially mobile within the mainstream of American society.

Mexican-Americans have been, and continue to be, isolated from wider society by religion, language, culture, and social class. Language has served a vital role in maintaining the culture: the Mexican-American family, more than other immigrant families, has continued to speak its native language—Spanish—in the home and community. Social class has also served to isolate Mexican-Americans who are poor from the mainstream of the American middle-class society.

Furthermore, Anglos' oppressive and discriminatory practices and stereotypical view of the Latino culture have created further problems of social integration. Adding to this situation is the view that some Mexican-Americans hold, that the *gringo* is someone from a world alien and hostile to their own way of life (Castro, 1978; Garcia-Preto, 1996).

Compounding the problem of incompatibility between the larger society and the Mexican-American culture is the social and political ferment being generated by the drastic increases in the population of Spanish-speaking immigrants, mostly Mexican and Central American, in many of the areas in the Southwest. The passage of two anti-immigration propositions in California (Proposition 187 and Proposition 209) are evidence of the politicization of the immigration influx (Falicov, 1996). The vast influx of Latinos, particularly illegal immigrants, is a prime source of conflict, dissension, and lack of acceptance, because of the social, economic, political, law enforcement, educational, and health impact this rapid population influx is having (Davis et al., 1988).

The Central American Experience

Immigration from Central America (Guatemala, El Salvador, and Nicaragua primarily) has been recent and dramatic. With civil war, poor socioeconomic conditions, and violation of human rights rampant in the three above-mentioned countries from the 1970s on, record numbers of refugees and illegal immigrants have come to the United States. Political refugees from these countries have not been recognized by the U.S. government; hence, until recently, when amnesty regulations took place, many Central Americans were forced to remain hidden (Conover, 1993).

The Puerto Rican Experience

Puerto Rican families began migrating to the United States in great numbers after World War II. Most came for economic reasons and settled in the Northeast, particularly in New York City. Their pattern of immigration has been a back-and-forth one—going back to the island and then returning for jobs and economic stability. However, migrating here has not been easy for them; one-third of all Puerto Ricans on the mainland are unemployed and poor (Garcia-Preto, 1996).

The Cuban Experience

Cubans arrived in the United States in large numbers in the 1960s, after Fidel Castro won the revolution of 1959 and established a harsh communistic society. The United States at that time opened its doors to Cubans fleeing Castro's government. A second wave of Cubans came in the 1980s, escaping Cuba in boats. Most Cubans live in four states: Florida (concentrated in Miami or "Little Havana"), New Jersey, New York, and California (Garcia-Preto, 1996).

Family–Society Interface Affects Family Life

The type and quality of the interchanges between the family and the external social system significantly affects internal family activities and integration. A major way this occurs is through children's school participation and the father's employment experiences. For instance, the lower- or working-class Mexican-American head of the household has often been unemployed or underemployed in menial positions that constantly erode his self-esteem. He has often had very little access to resources that could change his situation, and has had few effective means

of making institutions in society respond to his needs. This damaging, limiting process invariably diminishes the internal functioning and role relationships within his family. It has an adverse effect on family leadership and the integration and solidarity of families and their members.

Socioeconomic Considerations

Although most Latinos have come across the border in search of jobs, higher wages, and better working conditions, many experience discrimination in employment, housing, and education. Skin color, language difficulties, and Spanish surnames have all contributed to the continued isolation, discrimination, and exploitation Latinos have experienced (Falicov, 1996; Kuipers, 1995).

The impact of social class stratification has received sparse attention in the literature about the Hispanic-American family, and yet must be taken into account. Social class stratification of Hispanic-Americans reflects their disadvantaged social class status. For instance, the proportion of Mexican families in the various social classes does not conform to the American social class distribution of families. Instead, social class distribution is more restricted, reflecting limited social mobility. According to Vega and co-workers (1983), there are four classes in Mexican-American society: the underclass, the low income, the working class, and the middle class.

The underclass is composed of new immigrants who are still in the transition process, while the low-income families are still poor, but have stable unskilled, low-paying employment and residential stability (Vega et al., 1983). This is probably the largest group of Hispanic-American families today (Fulwood, 1996).

The other large Latino social class group in most urban areas is the urban working class. Working-class parents have achieved stable employment in skilled or semi-skilled occupations and are not economically marginal like the under- and lower-class Latinos.

The middle class is similar to the Anglo-American middle class in that it is a nuclear unit and predominately English speaking. Education is highly stressed and a significant proportion of men are in the skilled trades or in business (Vega et al., 1983).

Two indicators of Hispanic-American families' precarious status are income and education. In 1995, it was estimated that the median Hispanic family income was about 50 to 63 percent of the median U.S. family income (Fulwood, 1996; Ortiz, 1995). Educationally, the Latino is also at a disadvantage when compared to the Anglo; 44 percent of all Hispanic adults reported having a high school education, while 79 percent of Anglos had a high school education in 1990 (U.S. Bureau of the Census, 1993). A recent Rand Corporation study of high school students found that only 74 percent of all Latino immigrants between the ages of 15 and 17 were in high school, as compared to 95 percent of natives and other immigrant groups. Many of these young immigrants do not simply "drop out," but have never entered the U.S. school system (Woo & Lee, 1996).

A significant factor that lowers the Hispanic's economic status is family size. Hispanics tend to have larger families and more children than non-Hispanics. Hence the ratio of dependence, or the number of persons who rely on the income of the family head, is considerably larger for Hispanics than for non-Hispanics. With larger families and a reduced salary, 30.3 percent of all Hispanic families have incomes below the poverty level (Fig. 19–2). Latinos are twice as likely to be poor, when compared to the white U.S. population (Fulwood, 1996; Mirandé, 1991). In fact, in 1996, when the general U.S. population showed a small rise in income and a reduced proportion of families living below the poverty level, Latinos were the only ethnic group to show a decline in income: 5.1 percent from 1995 to 1996. Cuban families are the exception when discussing the socioeconomic status of Hispanic-American families. They currently earn 17 percent more in income than other Latino subgroups. Their success is explained by their migration pattern. The large Cuban migration of the 1960s primarily included white, educated professionals who had the resources to improve their status here. In addition, being white, they faced no color barrier (Bernal & Shapiro, 1996).

The Issue of Acculturation

Sociologists have assumed in the past that Hispanic-Americans would become acculturated (make the transition from traditional values and behaviors to

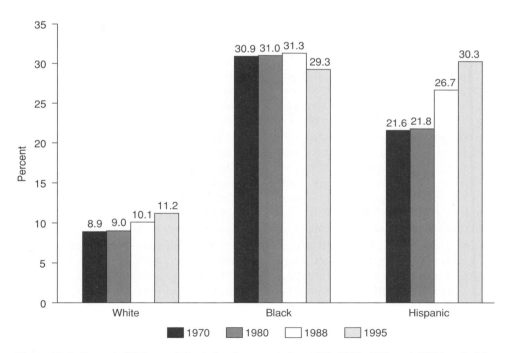

Figure 19–2. Percent of U.S. population below the poverty line, 1970, 1980, 1988, and 1995 by ethnicity. *There were 36.4 million or 13 percent of persons in the United States below the poverty level in 1995. (From: U.S. Bureau of the Census, 1980, 1990, and 1995, cited in Fulwood, 1996.)*

modern, Western values and modes of behavior) and that length of time living in the U.S. was positively associated with modernization, implying that the longer an individual or family is exposed to a dominant culture, the more adoption of the host culture occurs. Although such a formulation has some explanatory value, it fails to delineate which aspects of ethnicity and culture persist over time or the demographic and sociopsychological factors that are likely to affect the acculturation process.

Because of the above shortcomings and the implication inherent within the acculturation notion that the "American" family is the ideal and the "un-American" family less desirable, there is a tendency to move away from acculturation as the sole and central framework for explaining the changes in Hispanic-American families. Also, in spite of intergenerational differences, Hispanic-American families exhibit a wide range of differences in the extent to which they are acculturated to Anglo society.

Increasing attention is now being devoted to the study of ethnic identity among Latinos by more objective empirical methods. There is growing recognition that families can be both "modern and ethnic" at the same time (Baca-Zinn, 1981). Latinos retain a strong sense of ethnic identity, regardless of the number of generations in the United States (Vega, 1995).

There has been tremendous criticism of published Hispanic-American family literature in the early social science literature. Much of the criticized literature is based on opinion and personal observation (Jaramillo & Zapata, 1987). Researchers in their writings failed to recognize and account for the many societal processes (work situation, educational institutions, socioeconomic constraints) affecting the Latino family. Oversimplifications and inaccuracies were inherent in the broad generalizations made about Latino families (Vega, 1995). In addition, most studies were limited to the lower-class Mexican-American family, and social scientists tended to paint pictures of "black and white" stereotypes of family life and family roles—many times in a pejorative, ethnocentric manner. Current family science is "more concerned with understanding the accommodations, vulnerabilities and resilience of the Latino family . . ." (Vega, 1995, p. 5).

Although acculturation has been the primary process used to describe differences between Mexican-American families, we know that this is an uneven process and that some cultural patterns seem to be retained regardless of length of residency in the United States. The pace of acculturation is more rapid among children than parents. The acculturation process unfortunately may also involve adjusting to minority status, diminished life opportunity, and dangerous environments (Vega & Amaro, 1994).

Cultural adaptation varies by socioeconomic status, number of generations in the United States, and ability to speak English (Sorofman, 1986; Vega, 1995). Also, families in urban California areas tend to be more acculturated than are families living in more rural areas, such as in Texas (Dickinson & Leming, 1995).

The findings of one study (Keefe et al., 1978) clearly show that even though Mexican-Americans undergo acculturation as evidenced by a decrease in cultural awareness and/or ethnic loyalty, some things do not change. In particular, the importance of the extended family does not wane. In fact, the extended family appears to grow in structure and function when studied across several generations.

▶ THE NORMATIVE FAMILY FORM

Due to the deep commitment to family, more Hispanic-American persons live in traditional nuclear families (two parents with children) than white or African-American persons. According to 1990 Los Angeles County, California data, 47.1 percent of Latinos lived in nuclear families while 24.6 percent of whites and 21.8 percent of African-Americans lived in nuclear two-parent families (Hayes-Battista, 1990). The idealized Latino family is the extended family, although the extended family living under one roof is not common. Nevertheless, relatives other than nuclear family members often live in the same household (Miller, 1986).

Children traditionally do not separate from their families of origin psychologically or socially. As children grow up and marry, their families become extensions of the original unit, even though they probably do not live within the same household. The mother's and father's kin are generally of equal importance, with special recognition given to the mother's sisters. Both sets of grandparents are revered. First cousins are especially important secondary kin and are some-what like sisters and brothers (Keefe, 1984; Queen & Haberstein, 1974).

The Latino family is typically described as a large and cohesive kin group including both lineal and col-lateral relatives. Strong and extensive linkages beyond the nuclear family are present, with all rela-tives having reciprocal rights and duties. In other words, the extended family system, as a concrete man-ifestation of a familistic orientation, refers to that net-work of relatives including primary kin (siblings, children, and parents) and secondary kin (aunts, uncles, cousins, nieces, nephews, grandparents).

New immigrants, especially those who are undocu-mented, tend to live in multiple family arrange-ments. Single immigrant men tend to live together in the same household to conserve money and other resources (Chavez, 1986).

Godparents (*compadrazgo*) may hold an important place in the family, although the presence and/or role of godparents in Mexican-American families today is more limited (Ramirez & Arce, 1981). *Compadrazgo* refers to the ritual kinship pattern whereby a special linkage is established between two families or two persons by the baptismal ritual. *Compadres* provide coparenthood in time of need but also generate social and interpersonal cohesion, and godparents and godchildren are expected to visit each other and cultivate a close relationship (Kuipers, 1995; Queen & Haberstein, 1974).

Recently the number of teenage Latina mothers has risen sharply. From 1983 to 1993 there was a 45 percent increase in the number of Latina teenage pregnancies. Some of these girls remain home with their parents, some marry, and some establish female-headed families of their own. Reasons given for the sharp rise are: a taboo against discussing sex in the family; a religious prohibition against abor-tions; inaccessibility of family planning services; and girls' perceptions of the women's role as being to stay home and have and raise children (Roan, 1995).

Puerto Rican families have a much greater propor-tion of families headed by women than other Hispanic-American groups. Thirty-nine percent of all Puerto Rican families in 1990 were identified as female-headed, versus less than 20 percent of Mexican and Cuban families being female-headed (Ortiz, 1995).

▶ ENVIRONMENTAL ISSUES

Assessment of the Hispanic-American family's envi-ronment is often crucial. This includes the physical as well as the social environment. If the family is an immigrant family, are they suffering from the loss of their traditional social support network, which was left behind in their country of origin? Are language and lack of familiarity with U.S. institutions interfer-ing with their access to health and other community services?

With immigrant families, asking the question, "What is your country of origin?" and listening to the family members' stories of immigration helps to build an understanding about the country and cul-ture the family left behind and their reasons for leav-ing (Garcia-Preto, 1996).

Many new immigrants are preoccupied with the tasks of basic survival—adjusting to a new social envi-ronment, new jobs, new neighborhoods, new friends, and new social networks. For some, this process can take years, or even a lifetime.

Immigrants may have witnessed the terror and vio-lence that recently has dominated the Central American region. Hence, when working with refugee Hispanic families, assessing the degree to which fam-ily members' past trauma is affecting their current health and adjustment is a primary assessment con-sideration (Hernandez, 1996).

▶ FAMILY STRUCTURAL CHARACTERISTICS

The descriptions of the Latino family that follow are culled primarily from fairly recent sources. Even then, the nurse should particularly keep in mind the possible bias of social class. The nurse also needs to keep in mind that cultural norms tend to refer to what ought to be, and that these cultural prescrip-tions sometimes do not coincide with how things "really" are in families. Because recent research has clarified the wide variation of behavior in Hispanic-American families and has dispelled some of our stereotypes of these families, many of the traditional classic descriptions of family life and roles are deleted.

Family Values

Cultures "hang together" on the basis of commonly shared value orientations. For traditional Hispanic-Americans, orienting values are present and pervasive, although their actual adherence to these values in family life varies. "An appreciation of their existence and potential impact on family life provides an invaluable perspective for understanding cultural behaviors and expectations" (Vega et al., 1983, p. 199).

Familism.

The major theme dominating both the classic and modern portrayal of the Latino family is the deep importance of the family to all its members. The set of norms or values related to the importance of the family is referred to as familism. Here "the needs of the family collectivity supercede the needs of each individual family member" (Grebler et al., 1970, p. 369). Heller (1976) states that familism, the opposite of individualism, denotes a set of rights and obligations pertaining to members of a kin network. Interdependencies are seen as both healthy and necessary. When strong familistic attitudes prevail, role obligations are seen as mandatory (Casas & Vasquez, 1996; Diaz-Guerrero, 1975).

Mexican-American family values reinforce the system of mutual obligations, support, and reciprocity. Vega and associates (1983) explain that other values must also be mutually acknowledged in order for mutual support and reciprocity to occur.

> These [values] are mediated by certain values which have received broad attention in the literature: *orgullo* (pride and self-reliance), *dignidad* (dignity), *confianza* (trust and intimacy), and *respecto* (respect). (p. 199)

Table 19–1 compares American and traditional Latino values in some of the major areas of family and personal life. Although clear differences are identified here, again it needs to be stressed that in both American and traditional Hispanic-American families heterogeneity abounds and intra-ethnic variation is, indeed, great.

Traditional Latino values, with the exception of familism and a religious orientation, are more prominently found among the unacculturated and the poor. Moreover, social class status is a prime determinant of the viability of traditionalism (Moore, 1970).

Martinez (1976) asserts that the poor Latino family shares many values with other poor families and that these values are actually not so different from those of the middle class. The main difference is that many of the values are ideals or "what should be," rather than what "is." Poor families' realistic assessment of their possibilities has been called fatalism, "contentment with their lot," and lack of concern. All imply pathology, differentness, and wrongness. It is this sort of stereotyping that leads people in positions of dominance and control to expect stereotyped behavior and to act accordingly (Martinez, 1976).

Value Conflicts.

One of the serious problems that occurs as the Hispanic-American family interfaces with the larger society is that value conflicts arise. Hispanic-American children's socialization experiences (in school and in the *barrio*) often provoke value conflicts between the generations. Many of the primary values of the Hispanic-American are incongruent with American core values. This naturally poses significant adaptation problems for Latino families and individuals (Hernandez, 1996). For instance, when Latino children start school, they soon learn that they and their families are "out of synch" with the wider society.

Vega and co-workers (1983) point out that in low-income areas where Mexican-American families live in *barrios*, the *barrio* also is a powerful socializer.

> The *barrio* has an independent culture and tradition that is neither Mexican alone nor middle class Anglo-American. . . . Often immigrant parents perceive these manifestations as harmless idiosyncracies. However, they may also represent a fundamental affront to values, customs, and decency. (p. 205)

Expectations and sanctions for not conforming to values and social roles within the family are probably more rigidly defined and controlled among Latinos than Anglos, but nonconformity outside the home is typically not rigidly controlled, as parents perceive limitations on their ability to control the external environment.

Family Roles and Power

The early classic literature about Latino cultures takes cognizance of male dominance in the home.

▶ TABLE 19–1

AMERICAN AND TRADITIONAL HISPANIC-AMERICAN VALUE DIFFERENCES

Area/Issue	American Central Value Orientation	Traditional Hispanic-American Value Orientation
Family	Americans see themselves as individuals first and as members of families second.	Latinos see themselves as members of families first and as individuals second.
Self versus kin obligations	American culture stresses individuality and independence from family after a certain age. Self-reliance, autonomy, and achievement are emphasized.	Latinos believe in ethic of reciprocity within family and kinship group and inter-dependency.
Respect and authority structures	Americans value democratic ideals and egalitarianism (to a much greater extent). The elderly do not receive great respect. The authority of the masculine role is gradually diminishing as a result of the societal trend toward egalitarianism.	Greater value on male leadership and respect toward the elderly and toward authority figures.
Progress versus tradition	Americans value progress and change.	Hispanic-Americans show more reverence and respect for tradition.
Work	Work and productivity are central, often prominent values of the Anglo culture. Work often becomes a value in itself (more true in the past than today).	Work is seen as a necessity in order to live. Other life experiences—social and emotional experiences—are valued more than work.
Materialism	Materialism is a central American value. Possession of material goods is seen as a sign of success and becomes an end in itself. The cynosures of society are the businessman and financier.	Material objects are viewed as necessities and not as ends in themselves. Social status and prestige are more likely to be derived from an ability to experience things directly and/or through social and family relationships rather than through past successes and accumulation of wealth. Hispanic-Americans generally have great reverence for philosophers, poets, musicians, and artists.
Time	"Time is money." Punctuality is equated with goodness and being responsible.	Time is a gift to be enjoyed. More flexible attitude towards time. "Wasting time" is not understood. Punctuality is not an important moral value.
Present versus future time orientation	Making plans for the future (planning) is highly valued as a means of getting ahead. Future-oriented.	Enjoyment of the present. Less concern for always living for the future. More present-oriented.
Interpersonal relationships	Americans value openness and directness in communications. (Americans are viewed as being blunt and succinct by Hispanic-Americans.) Use of kidding to get messages across more indirectly is acceptable. In interpersonal conflict situations, Americans value "leveling," open dissent, and criticizing each other. Value rational expression of thoughts and not emotional expression as much.	Latinos value diplomacy, smooth and pleasant social relationships, and tactfulness, and show concern and respect for others' feelings and dignity. Their manner of expression is more elaborate and indirect. They value agreement, respect, and courtesy, and are very sensitive to criticism regardless of manner presented. They value being expressive and showing feelings toward other persons.

(Continued)

▶ TABLE 19-1   *(Continued)*

AMERICAN AND TRADITIONAL HISPANIC-AMERICAN VALUE DIFFERENCES

Area/Issue	American Central Value Orientation	Traditional Hispanic-American Value Orientation
Environmental responses	Americans are less sensitive to the environment and its various forms of stimulation.	Hispanic-Americans value greater sensory stimulation within their environments, using a fuller range of senses to experience their environment (vivid colors, expressive music and art, spicy foods).
Relationship to environment	Americans see themselves as mastering the environment.	Latinos place more value on living in harmony with the environment.
Education	Education highly valued as means to success and way to be productive. Correlated with work and productivity values.	Education is valued but has often been inaccessible, with schools being culturally incongruent with traditional Hispanic-American values. Also, many Latinos are not in tune with success and scientific, individualistic values associated with American education.
Religion	Most Americans are more secular today.	Religion is more highly valued. Over 95% of Hispanics are Roman Catholic. Acceptance of God's will is widespread way of coping.

Adapted from Andrews (1995), Falicov (1996), Garcia-Preto (1996), Marin & Marin (1991), Murillo (1971).

Here, the father is described as unquestionably the head of the family, as well as being "hard, unyielding and strong," exemplifying the traits of *machismo* (Castro, 1978). Family members must show respect for him or he will become angry and may give vent to his wrath by physically striking out. Paz (1973), a noted Mexican author, and Ingoldsby (1995b) have described the *macho* or masculine role as incorporating the following elements of arbitrary power: superiority, fearlessness, aggressiveness, insensitivity, hypersexuality, and invulnerability. Along with the Latino male's authoritarian role, he is characterized as providing for his family in the best possible manner he can, priding himself on being the sole provider and being economically self-sufficient.

In this same literature the ideal mother is seen as a soft, nurturing, and self-sacrificing woman, with her traditional and positive role of being in the home, with responsibility to her husband and to her children. In fact, her status and roles are usually defined solely by her marriage and her children.

There has been much criticism over this stereotyping of Hispanic-American family roles, both of the conclusions reached and of the theoretical models underlying these past studies (Mirandé, 1991). The focus of recent studies is toward understanding gender roles as flexible and responsive to environmental conditions (Vega, 1995). Empirical studies show that patterns of absolute male dominance in conjugal decision making have never been the behavioral norm among Mexicans either in the United States or Mexico (Cromwell & Ruiz, 1979; Grebler et al., 1970; Hawkes & Taylor, 1975). Although the family structure is described as male dominant, the evidence generally suggests the presence of a more egalitarian structure and process, especially when the wife works or the family is not poor (Hernandez, 1996; Ybarra, 1982). Moreover, the influence and predominance of *machismo* and the presence of female submissiveness and lack of power are equally controversial generalizations being challenged in Latino family literature as studies refute the existence of these stereotypes. Latino scholars on the family argue that there is much diversity within the Latino family and that many of its present adaptations are due to discrimination and socioeconomic barriers.

Several authors have noted the influence that immigration, urbanization, social mobility, and acculturation have on the Hispanic-American family. The

Latino family is being subjected to many of the same societal changes that the Anglo family is facing. The most noteworthy and profound change, as noted in recent studies, revolves around the declining primary authority of the male and the greater egalitarianism of spousal roles (Hernandez, 1996). The husband's pervasive power has given rise to the wife's feeling a sense of injustice, particularly as she is exposed to American mores and values. Latino women's participation in the workforce has increased rapidly and almost equals that of American women generally (Falicov, 1996). Working educated Latino women espouse new aspirations for independence and professional status (Wilkinson, 1987). Large families and the difficulties of finding employment with good wages also compromise the husband-father's ability to provide adequately for the family, which tends to diminish the base for his authority.

Many women, especially the younger ones, are challenging women's traditional roles (Baxter, 1996). In the urban areas, the *chicanitas* (adolescent girls) are venturing outside their homes to join social clubs and gangs. Young Latino women express a need for greater equality in the family and society. Given the increasing occupational opportunities for women and the wish for a higher standard of living, more and more Hispanic-American women are working (Falicov, 1996). As a result, traditional male–female roles are changing, particularly among the younger and middle-class couples, and the women of these groups are finding a greater flexibility and choice of options (Mirandé, 1977). As with the Anglo families, when women take advantage of educational opportunities and find employment outside the home, their self-image and role expectations considerably change. Education and labor force participation of Latino women are beginning to effect revolutionary changes in the Hispanic-American family (Wilkinson, 1987). Given women's emancipation, generational conflicts, and the decline of the male's patriarchal authority, the Latino family is facing substantial transition and occasion for stress.

Family Communication Patterns

Strong affective communication patterns are characteristic of many Latino families. There is much warmth and affection shown between mother and children when children are young. In traditional families, respect is shown by children to parents and elders, and females to males of the family.

The Spanish language, being more emotionally expressive and elaborate than English, shapes the cognitive structure of its speakers. Interpersonal relationships are noted for their tones of respect and hierarchical relationships. As seen in the summary of values in Table 19–1, Hispanic-Americans value courtesy, respect, maintaining one's dignity, diplomacy, tactfulness, expressiveness of feelings (emotionality), and agreement (Falicov, 1996). Kidding and open confrontation are not generally sanctioned, because the need to show respect and to "save face" are important.

▶ FAMILY FUNCTIONAL CHARACTERISTICS

Socialization Patterns

Differences in child rearing and disciplining are notable among Hispanic-American families of diverse social classes. Although parental desires for their children may not vary, the ability to realize aspirations does, and hence socialization experiences are clearly varied between social classes (Vega et al., 1983). Nevertheless, despite social class differences, children are at the center of family life (Wilkinson, 1987). Also, sex role distinctions through child-rearing practices appear to be reinforced in most Latino families. A male is taught how to think and behave like a man, and a female like a woman (Mirandé, 1985).

Traditionally, the raising of children has been the mother's job, while the father's role has been to work and to form associations with his *compadres* (godparents). However, as with American families generally, this rigid demarcation of roles is rapidly declining. Much more sharing of the child care role is occurring among Chicano couples (Mirandé, 1979).

Hispanic-American babies are wanted, cherished, and pampered. They are regarded as *angelitos*, untouched by evil and sin. Parents and older siblings respond to young children in very indulgent, affectionate ways (Queen & Haberstein, 1974). There is a longer state of interdependence between mother and child than in Anglo families (Falicov, 1996).

In more recent studies of child-rearing patterns among Latinos, some researchers have discovered substantial diversity, ranging from permissive, to authoritarian, to authoritative parenting styles. More acculturated mothers tend to use authoritative parenting (Martinez, 1993).

Socialization strains are common among immigrant Hispanic families. Researchers have found that children acculturate at a faster rate than adults in the family—a difference that leads to profound intergenerational conflicts. These conflicts are then aggravated by parental attempts to gain control over their children and children rejecting parental efforts (Hernandez, 1996; Vega, 1990).

The Health Care Function

Among Hispanic-Americans the structure and values of the family are important influencing factors relative to understanding an individual's health attitudes and practices. One can also better understand the shorter longevity and the higher mortality and morbidity rates of Latinos versus the general American population when the high percentage of this group living at or below the poverty level is taken into account (Angel, 1985). The health of family members is affected by their living conditions, the community resources, and the social environment.

Health care needs are diverse and depend largely on the specific vulnerabilities and risks associated with social class, environmental, occupational, and lifestyle patterns. Major health problems and poor access to health care are concentrated among the poor, the least assimilated, the illegal migrant, and the migrant worker (Angel, 1985; Zambrana, Dorrington, & Hayes-Bautista, 1995).

Health Care Beliefs and Practices.   Early studies of health care behavior of Hispanic-Americans emphasized the widespread use of folk medicine (Madsen, 1964; Saunders, 1954). Saunders (1954) asserted that Mexican-Americans considered health care as encompassing both scientific and folk cures. Research on Mexican-Americans in the Southwest shows that folk medicine and beliefs still persist in rural and urban areas among the lower class (Farge, 1975; Keefe, 1981).

Use of folk healing in the urban areas appears to have declined considerably, except among recent, poor immigrant families. In Keefe's (1981) large study of Mexican-Americans in three Southern California communities, there was little indication that *curanderismo* (Mexican traditional folk medical care system) was used. Only 7 percent of the respondents in Keefe's second survey consulted a *curandero* in the last year and one-half of those did so only for a minor medical problem. *Curanderismo* was adhered to most frequently among recent Mexican immigrants who came to the United States after the age of 15, were Spanish-speaking, identified themselves as "Mexicano," and were in the lowest socioeconomic stratum. The respondents who had used *curanderos* believed that folk healers were superior for curing folk illnesses, for curing minor ailments not serious enough to require a doctor's care, and for treating illnesses that physicians could not cure (Keefe, 1981).

Regardless of the degree to which folk medicine is relied upon, there is no empirical evidence indicating that folk medicine and scientific medicine are mutually exclusive systems (Farge, 1975; Kay, 1978; Keefe, 1981; Nall & Speilberg, 1978). Urban Mexican-Americans appear to readily accept modern health care, sometimes supplementing folk medicine with modern medical care or vice versa. Usually there is little incompatibility perceived between the indigenous and the scientific forms of health care.

When both systems of health care are used in health settings (folk medicine and Western medicine) this is called "complementary health care." Some clinics in California are now delivering this type of care. Physicians and nurse practitioners work cooperatively with indigenous (folk) health practitioners (herbists, *curanderos*), or in some cases use herbs for certain symptoms or illnesses.

Traditional Health Beliefs.   Most of the Latino health beliefs are based on assumptions and traditions that have evolved over centuries. In the blending of older European, Spanish-Catholic, and Indian traditions, three basic aspects of Mexican and Latin American traditional folk health concepts and practices emerge. One aspect is concerned with the specific health beliefs and practices. A second aspect consists of a set of ritualistic acts that are believed to improve health. And lastly, the use of folk practitioners or *curanderos* has evolved (Gonzales, 1976).

Folk medicine does not treat symptoms of disease conditions alone. Folk medicine views the sick person as a whole psychobiocultural and spiritual being in relationship to the natural and supernatural environments. Whereas Western medicine focuses on epidemiology and pathophysiology, Latino folk medicine focuses on holistically treating the person.

Mexican-American.   Basic to Chicano health beliefs and practices are the health philosophies and ideologies of the culture that circumscribes these beliefs and practices. Dorsey and Jackson (1976) write that the basis for many health beliefs derives from notions about the importance of maintaining equilibrium. Human beings are viewed holistically, as being in harmony and unity with the natural and supernatural environments. Health is a result of maintenance of this natural state of balance between humans and the natural and supernatural worlds. Illness and disease stem from a loss in homeostasis or balance.

Preventive beliefs and rituals are exercised to promote this balance. Prayers, relics, faith, herbs, and spices are all used to ward off disease or to prevent complications of long-term illness. Two examples of the Chicano's concern with maintaining balance are in the consumption of hot and cold foods and in prenatal health practices. To achieve the necessary balance in the body, foods thought of as "hot" (heavy foods, meats, fatty or spicy foods) are eaten with "cold" foods (vegetables, ice cream), which are considered soothing and fresh to the body. Because pregnancy is seen as a delicate time when imbalances occur easily that can cause great harm to the fetus, the practice of the mother's wearing keys on the night of the lunar eclipse is thought to be protective. Mothers are also urged to maintain good diets, exercise, and take herbs and teas recommended by the *yerbero* (herbalist) or health leader in the family, thus maintaining the delicate balance during the months of pregnancy (Dorsey & Jackson, 1976).

In addition to disease being caused by "imbalances," disease also may be inflicted on an individual as a form of supernatural punishment for wrongdoing (Clark, 1970). Folk illnesses can be caused by a variety of circumstances, although most folk illnesses are believed to be intimately related to faulty social relationships (Herrera & Wagner, 1974; Prattes, 1973).

Some of the specific folk health beliefs, as expressed in form of folk illnesses, are the following.

Mal de ojo (bad or evil eye) is believed to be a result of excessive admiration or desire on the part of another. *Mal de susto* (illness from fright) is a syndrome believed to be the result of an emotionally traumatic experience. *Empacho* (indigestion) is believed to be caused by food clinging to the wall of the stomach in the form of a ball. *Caida de la mollera* (fallen fontanel) is the one illness that is felt to affect children only and is attributed to a child's being dropped and as the result of a fall. *Mal puesto* (sorcery) is considered to arise as a consequence of one of three kinds of social relationships: (1) a lover's quarrel, (2) unrequited love, or (3) as a reflection of invidiousness between individuals or nuclear families (Falicov, 1996; Herrera & Wagner, 1974).

Castro (1978) reports that unacculturated Mexican-American clients see mental illness as a "dreaded affliction." When a person becomes mentally ill, he or she loses the respect of friends and extended family and is viewed as no longer fit to have children or raise a family. The person is socially ostracized and believed to have offended God in some way or to be under the influence of a "hex." The mentally ill person's nuclear family feels social disgrace, but continues to love and feel compassion for him or her, in spite of the belief that the individual will never be the same again. Thus for the Mexican-American, mental illness is perhaps one of the most difficult health phenomena with which to cope or for which to seek professional help.

The Process of Seeking Health Care.

Typically in the traditional lower-class family, when an individual becomes ill, he or she usually consults the health expert in the family and tries to cure the illness with home remedies (prayers, diet, herbal remedies). If this does not relieve the symptoms depending on the type of health problem, he or she may consult a physician, folk practitioner, or sometimes both. Of the folk practitioners, the *yerbero* and then the *curandero* are usually consulted. The types of healing or remedies prescribed are reflective of the healer's perceptions of etiology. In folk medicine, all healing is geared toward restoring the necessary equilibrium or preventing disequilibrium. There are specific household remedies, such as those for being wet and chilled and those for menstruation. Spiritualistic practices are also appropriate for helping with illness considered supernatural in origin. Prayers and ritualistic activities are performed by *espiritualistas*, family, and patient. Herbs are extensively used for treating a multitude of illnesses, some of which have been found scientifically to have great benefit (Dorsey & Jackson, 1976).

Recent studies of Hispanic folk health practices demonstrate that Hispanic-Americans who use folk medicine do not rely entirely on folk prescriptions for cure, but consider them an important adjunct in expediting solutions to various health problems (Herrera & Wagner, 1974; Mikhail, 1994) or as appropriate for certain folk illnesses (Mikhail, 1994).

Folk Healers.   Clark (1970), an anthropologist, explains why traditionally oriented Mexican-American people may consider folk healers to be vital for meeting their health needs.

> Folk healers are not professionals in the sense that they have formal training in the art of medicine or earn their living by their practice; they are members of the community who are regarded as specialists because they have learned more of the popular medicinal lore of culture than have other barrio people; use language which patients understand and vocabulary familiar to patients; never dictate what must be done, advise the patient what she or he considers appropriate. (p. 207)

There are several levels and types of folk practitioners in most Latino communities, as described below.

Yerbero(a).   The herbalist is an expert in the source, purposes, and derivatives of herbs and spices useful for cure and prevention of disease. As a grower and distributor of herbs, as well as a teacher about their uses, the *yerbero(a)'s* position in the community is one of respect and esteem. Patients will often try family remedies first, herbs from the *yerbero* second, and a visit to the *curandero* and/or physician third (Dorsey & Jackson, 1976).

Curandero(a).   The *curandero(a)* is the most respected and specialized of folk healers in the Mexican-American community (Kuipers, 1995). The following characteristics of *curanderismo* have been noted: (1) *curanderos* are chosen through divine calling and live in the community; (2) they usually have their practice in their home and their reputation is established by their successes; (3) if respectable, they will not try to cure someone who is incurable, criti-

cally ill, or "hexed" (under the influence of a witch or magic); (4) most prescribe prayers, teas, poultices, and herbs; and (5) they do not charge fees, but do accept donations from families (Dorsey & Jackson, 1976; Prattes, 1973).

Espiritualisto(a).   This person is a spiritualist who has the ability to analyze dreams and fears, foretell the future, and treat some supernatural and magical diseases (those caused by *brujos*).

Brujo(a).   The *brujo(a)* is skilled in the use of magic and witchcraft and can cast spells or hexes on individuals, as well as remove those cast by other magicians. They are honored out of fear rather than admiration (Dorsey & Jackson, 1976).

Most of these above descriptions of health care practices and beliefs are those of Mexican-Americans. Central Americans tend to have similar practices and beliefs. Puerto Ricans, however, have some differences in their health beliefs and practices. Folk diseases are somewhat different. In addition, treatments for hot and cold diseases (food, medicines) are categorized as "hot," "cold," and "cool." Some Puerto Ricans believe in spirits and spiritualism. *Santerias*, similar to *espiritualistos*, are folk healers who use spiritual means for healing. The origins of the *Santerias* were in Nigeria and health practices were brought to the Americas in the 1500s during the slavery period (Spector, 1991).

Access to and Attitudes About Western Health Care

In spite of an increasing reliance on physicians and "scientific health care," especially among second- and third-generation Latinos, significant barriers to utilization of health care still exist. Many Latinos work in the secondary job market, characterized by low wages, poor working conditions, and limited or no health care insurance. Access to Western health care has also been problematic for many Latinos due to the problems associated with language barriers and cultural differences between Anglos and Latinos. Lack of access fuels underuse of health services, misuse of emergency rooms, and delayed treatment, i.e., waiting until the illness is more serious (Zambrana et al., 1995). A definite barrier to use of health care services by Hispanic-American families is the widespread lack of health insurance benefits. Valdez (1991), in a large study of Latino access to health care, found that 37 percent of Mexican-Americans are not covered for medical care, as compared to 10 percent of Anglos. Another of these barriers is the cultural tradition that "suggests that bad health, though unpleasant, is something that one endures" (Bullough & Bullough, 1982, p. 79). Moreover, when a Hispanic-American is in need of medical assistance, he or she is expected to turn to the family first in order to have these needs met. Only when familial resources have been exhausted or under unusual circumstances is it acceptable for the traditional Latino to seek outside help (Bullough & Bullough, 1982).

Mexican-Americans generally tend to dread illness and hospitalization more than Anglos do. Perhaps this is due to higher mortality rates or the poorer health the Chicanos experience. Certainly the family cannot afford the huge medical expenses. The estrangement Latinos often feel when dealing with the health care system also contributes to their apprehension of being sick, injured, or hospitalized (Herrera & Wagner, 1974).

Many authors have mentioned that Latino feelings about health providers and the "scientific" or Western health care systems are usually negative. There are several reasons for this:

1. Health providers use their own medical jargon, which is incomprehensible to poor Latino clients.

2. Fee-for-service arrangements between doctors and clients result in feelings of stiffness and mistrust.

3. The provider's ignorance and arrogance regarding Latino's traditional beliefs and practices make families feel alienated and uncertain (Farge, 1975; Herrera & Wagner, 1974).

4. Latinos generally object to clinical, cold, objective attitudes of physicians and nurses and to their concept of efficiency, which involves a time orientation that values speed and results rather than getting to know the patient.

In contrast to the above literature that portrays Hispanic-Americans as being negative about Anglo health care, Friedman (1985) in a study of 27 Latino families who had a child with cancer, found the parents to be overwhelmingly positive about their health care providers. Not only were parents satisfied with the ongoing care they and their children were receiving, but they also expressed confidence in their doctors and nurse practitioners. They saw these providers as "healers" who were very helpful in assisting them to cope with their child's illnesses.

Family Stress and Coping

Hispanic-American families collectively are likely to experience a greater number of major stressors when compared to Anglo families. Certainly poverty, discrimination, cultural conflicts, the immigration experience, social and geographical mobility, and language barriers are primary sources of stress. Substandard housing, inadequate health care and education, and poor employment opportunities are widespread. Immigrant families are identified as a very high risk group in terms of being candidates for family instability and individual health problems (Zambrana et al., 1995).

Based on the Hispanic-American family literature, seeking of social support from the extended family, and of spiritual support, appear to be the two central culturally derived family coping strategies.

Family Support.   Previous studies have empirically demonstrated that the Latino extended family is stronger and more active in providing both instrumental and emotionally supportive assistance than the Anglo family, and thus serves as an important family coping strategy (Sotomayor, 1991). This was empirically confirmed in a study by Friedman (1985). Friedman predicted that there would be differences in family coping between Anglo and Latino families. To examine this hypothesis she sampled 28 Anglo and 27 Latino families that had a child with childhood cancer. Friedman's (1985) findings demonstrate that the extended family, especially secondary kin, and religion are a significantly more important family coping strategies of Latino families than of Anglo families.

A well-articulated system of linked nuclear family households exist through which Hispanic-American families meet their various life needs. Clearly established patterns of reciprocal help and mutual aid are found between and among extended family members (Mirandé, 1977; Vega et al., 1983). This system offers assistance and feelings of security. An example of reciprocity is seen when a poor family becomes too large to support all of its members and, as a result, a child or some of the children are raised by grandparents, uncles, or aunts.

Spiritual Support.

Religion, prayer, and reliance on God and saints appear to be more important to Latinos than to Anglos. In Friedman's study, Latino parents reported that "God, prayers, and faith" were the most important way Latino families coped with their child's cancer. In terms of the predominant religion among Hispanic-American families, 95 percent are Catholic. Mexican Catholicism, it should be noted, varies from American Roman Catholicism. Mexican Catholicism is described as a blend of both Catholicism and pre-Cortesian Indian beliefs and ideology (Kruszewski et al., 1982). The basic Catholic premise that God governs one's life and ultimately takes it from us, permeates the traditional Hispanic attitude toward illness.

Fatalism/Passive Appraisal.

The extent to which Latino families employ fatalism as a passive appraisal type of coping strategy is not entirely clear in the literature, and certainly has been controversial, due to the early anthropological studies that stereotyped all Mexican-Americans as being fatalistic. Yet, Mirowsky and Ross (1984) and Neff and Hoppe (1993) did find a greater tendency for Latinos to be fatalistic than Anglos, especially among those Latinos with a stronger ethnic heritage. Fatalism can be looked at as implying a sense of vulnerability and lack of control in the presence of adversity, or as an adaptive response to uncontrollable life situations (Neff & Hoppe, 1993).

Contrast With Anglo Families.

In Friedman's (1985) study, Anglos reported that spousal support, helpfulness of friends and neighbors, and obtaining medical information were more important family coping strategies. In addition to these apparent ethnic differences, social class of parents also made a difference in family coping patterns. For example, spousal support was reported as a more helpful way of coping by both the middle-class Latinos and Anglos—who generally have more of a companionship type of marriage than lower- or working-class individuals have.

Vega and associates (1986) also studied ethnic differences (Anglo and Latino) in family coping—in the areas of family cohesion and family adaptability. When comparing families with respect to these two patterns, they found no significant ethnic differences. Both the Latino and Anglo families appeared to be functioning within healthy boundaries in terms of cohesion and adaptability.

One of the major considerations pertaining to culturally derived family coping strategies is the concern about what happens to a family when culturally derived coping strategies are not available. Researchers speculate that the consequences of the Latino family being heavily reliant on family support (and usually not on support from friends or neighbors) may have adverse effects when the extended family is not present (Keefe et al., 1978; Vega et al., 1983). When these families do not have a local extended family network, they will usually be without other social supports, leaving them less able to cope with stress. Friedman (1985) confirmed the increased vulnerability to stress that Latino nuclear families, who were unsupported by extended families, experienced under the prolonged stress of childhood cancer. These families showed much greater familial strains (greater family conflict) and expressions of parental distress.

▶ FAMILY NURSING PRACTICE IMPLICATIONS

Chapter 8, which addresses sociocultural assessment and intervention, discusses general family nursing interventions in working with culturally diverse families. Based on Latino culturally patterned beliefs and practices, as well as family characteristics, family nursing practice implications specific to the Latino family are discussed in this concluding section.

Interactions with Latino families need to be respectful, friendly, and warm, with sensitivity shown toward clients' feelings and their need to maintain their dignity. Avoiding direct confrontation with a traditional Hispanic-American family member and being alert to subtle, indirect messages are also important. A polite and mild disagreement from a client may actually mean a strong disagreement and hence should be clarified with the client in an nonthreatening manner.

In addition, because the Latino tends to respect authority figures and look at health care professionals in this light, attempting to form an egalitarian partnership type of nurse–client relationship may not be most effective. The Hispanic client may feel more comfortable with a hierarchical relationship and a structured instructive approach.

Family nurses, particularly those in community health and primary care, need to be alert to and understanding of the social environmental problems and institutional discriminatory barriers faced by less acculturated, poor Hispanic-American families (Gallegos, 1991). When referring families who have experienced these barriers to different service agencies, coordinating and streamlining referrals and intake procedures as much as possible will minimize confusion and ensure better outcomes. It is well to remember that other family problems may supersede the resolution of health problems. Helping a family tackle their other health-related problems, often by making well-coordinated referrals, may leave the way open for the family to engage in solving their primary health concerns.

Applying knowledge about the traditional Hispanic-American family structure, the family nurse should be sensitive to the role and expectations of different family members, such as the authority of the parents, especially the father, and the grandparents, especially the grandmother in the area of health care and child rearing. Family nurses should not expect a Latino client to make a significant health decision until he or she has a chance to consult with family members. For client compliance, the entire family needs to feel positive about the health decision and feel that the recommended treatment will work. The importance of the family members' mutual responsibility should be recognized. Family health professionals should make an effort to consult with those family members who have authority in the family group. Meeting with the extended family members to discuss a seriously or chronically ill family member's diagnosis and treatment plan is often an excellent way to bring the family into the health care planning and decision-making process.

Evaluating the extent to which a family subscribes to traditional folk or indigenous health practices and to Western health care should be part of a cultural assessment. As mentioned earlier, it is common for families to subscribe to both forms of health care, depending on the health problem and access to Western health care. The family nurse in community-based settings must be sensitive to the use of dual systems of health care. In fact, it is often necessary to ask a family whether they are trying any traditional Latino medical remedies. The family nurse should approach this issue in a respectful and understanding manner, rather than unwittingly hinting that Latino medical practices are inferior or unacceptable. If done properly, such a discussion will convey the nurse's cultural competence to the family, and will contribute to the therapeutic alliance between family and nurse (Hong, 1993; Hong, Lee, & Lorenzo, 1995). The family nurse should not interfere with non-Western health care practices as long as they are not detrimental to the client. In fact, when folk remedies are not harmful, support and encouragement of these in combination with Western health treatments (called complementary health care) shows respect for the clients' values, beliefs, and practices (Sheppard, 1990).

It is best to encourage the whole family or the extended family to adopt a new health program—such as dietary regimens or obtaining immunizations—rather than encouraging a sole individual to go it alone. People may be more influenced by what other significant family members say and do than by what the health care practitioner recommends. Monroe (1990) explains why many Latinos have not been getting the message about health promotive behavior.

> Health messages need to use traditional Latino family values . . . In effect, telling a Latino to exercise more and to eat a low-fat diet generally does not work if the implied short-term payoff is that a person will be thinner or feel better. Latinos, like American Indians, tend to see things more in a social context. . . . It's not all me, me, me. It's more of "How will that affect my family? I will live longer; therefore, my family will be better off." It is easy to see the effect of this lack of culturally appropriate health messages in the Latino community. (p. E1)

Planning programs to fit Latino cultural patterns and values is an extension of this latter suggestion. Because family involvement and participation work best, planning of family-oriented programs is recommended. Fostering of family-oriented rather than individually oriented self-care is another way of stating the above suggestion. Our own cultural bias may be for self-care and individual effort, but for the Latino who values familism, assisting the family to become competent makes more sense.

Family members, including the extended family, may want to take an active role in the treatment/rehabilitation of the ill member. It is important to allow all members of extended family to ask questions and participate in the treatment/rehabilitation as much as possible.

▶ study questions

1. What peoples constitute Hispanic-Americans? Which of these subgroups are most numerous in the United States?

2. Several important factors have adversely influenced the Latino family's integration into American society, even though some of these same factors may be "positive" for the family. Give three of these factors.

Are the following statements true or false?

3. Familism refers to the Mexican-American's propensity to marry early and have a family.

4. In the Chicano family the male and older person have both traditionally held positions of respect.

5. Male dominance in the Chicano family is widespread, the evidence indicating that the father-husband holds absolute power.

6. The institution of having *compadres* among Mexican-American families refers to the custom of having godparents. This custom is, however, declining as a result of acculturation.

7. Which of the following are criticisms that Latino family scholars and researchers have made about the early writings by social scientists?
   a. They are pejorative.
   b. They tend to describe the Latino family as homogeneous.
   c. The literature discusses only the middle-class family.
   d. They assume that acculturation will occur uniformly across all facets of family life.
   e. They view the family from a systems, ecological perspective.

8. For each of the following American central values, explain what the corresponding traditional Latino value is:

Area	American Core Value	Traditional Latino Value
Family	Americans see themselves as an individual first, a family member second.	
Work	Productivity and work are central and prominent values. Work often becomes an end rather than a means to an end.	
Materialism	Possession of material goods is a symbol of success. The greater the accumulation of goods, the greater the prestige.	
Time and punctuality	"Time is money." Punctuality is a moral value equated with being responsible.	
Interpersonal relationships	Americans value openness and directness in communication, as well as rationality versus emotional expressiveness.	

Are the following statements true or false?

9. The most profound structural change occurring in the Latino family today is the resurgence of the value of familism.

10. Democratic ideals and verbal facility in negotiation are taught at a young age in the Latino family.

11. The ethic of reciprocity in the Latino family has to do with the exchange that takes place between spouses when they role share.

12. Match the description of the folk healer with the type of folk healer.

    1. *Yerbero*   a. Herbalist.
    2. *Santeria*   b. Deals with supernatural illnesses.
    3. *Respecto*   c. Practices witchcraft or magic.
    4. *Espiritualisto(a)* d. Puerto Rican folk healer.
    5. *Brujo(a)*   e. Healer of folk illnesses in the
                                Chicano community.
    6. *Curandero(a)*   f. None of the above.

13. Fill in the name of each of the following common Mexican folk illnesses from this list of possibilities (mental illness, *empacho, susto, mal de ojo, mal puesto, caida de la mollera*).

a. "Bad eye," resulting from excessive admiration or desire on the part of another.

b. Disease given by God or a *brujo* as a hex or punishment on the patient.

c. Affliction caused by food adhering to the stomach wall in the form of a ball.

d. Fallen fontanels (in infants).

e. Sorcery.

f. Illness caused by fright or emotionally traumatizing experience.

14. Based on what is known of Latino families, and of families in general, identify which of the following practice suggestions would be most appropriate for which group (Latino family, A; all families, B).

a. Separation of hospitalized patient from family member(s) should be considered very carefully.

b. Client should not be expected to make a significant health care decision until he or she has had a chance to consult with the family.

c. It is best to attempt to have the whole family adopt a health promotion or maintenance program.

d. Other family problems may take precedence over health problems, and thus the health worker may have to help the family with its other problems in order for it to be able to resolve health needs.

e. Families need to be spoken to in terms and concepts they understand and suggestions need to appeal to their basic values.

f. An authoritative approach, whereby the health professional conveys expertise and confidence in his or her ability to "heal," is expected.

15. Identify two primary culturally derived family coping strategies of Mexican-Americans. Based on knowledge about culturally derived family coping strategies and an assessment of a Chicano's family's coping responses, state one practice implication.

▶ chapter 19 study answers

1. Mexican-American (most numerous, about 60 percent), Central and South American, Cuban, Puerto Rican.

2. List any three:

a. Language differences.

b. Religious differences.

c. Social class differences (large numbers of peasant agricultural workers and laborers migrated).

d. American discriminatory and segregation practices.

e. Mexican-American closeness with Mexico, so that Latinos can cross back and forth frequently. This consequently strengthens their ties to Mexico and reduces their need to become involved with some of the institutions within the United States.

3. False. (Familism refers to Latinos' deep identification with and commitment to their families.)

4. True.

5. False. (Evidence is that the father-husband probably never did hold absolute power, as a normative situation. Although male primary authority is declining, most Mexican-American families are still male dominant.)

6. True.

7. a, b, and d.

8.

Area	Traditional Latino Values
Family	Latinos see themselves as members of families first, as individuals second.
Work	Work is seen as a means (a necessity) in order to live. Other life experiences (social and emotional experiences) are valued more than work.
Materialism	Possession of goods and objects are necessary for living, not ends in themselves. Status and prestige are more likely derived from ability to intellectually and emotionally experience things. Social relationships and family are more important than accumulation of wealth.
Time and punctuality	Time is to be enjoyed. Punctuality does not have the moral overtones it does in American society.
Interpersonal relationships	Hispanic-Americans value the use of diplomacy and tactfulness. They are concerned about showing respect and are more elaborate, indirect, and emotionally expressive in their communications.

9. False. (The most profound change is the decline of the husband's/father's primary authority and the increase in egalitarianism.)

10. False. (Two major child-rearing patterns are that socialization is distinctly gender role related and that children are taught to respect father, older persons, and authority figures.)

11. False. (The ethic of reciprocity has to do with the system of mutual obligation, support, and assistance within the extended family.)

12. 1. a.
      2. d.
      3. f.
      4. b.
      5. c.
      6. e.

13. a. *Mal de ojo.*
    b. Mental illness.
    c. *Empacho.*
    d. *Caida de la mollera.*
    e. *Mal puesto.*
    f. *Susto.*

14. a. A.
    b. A.
    c. B.
    d. B.
    e. B.
    f. A.

15. Family coping strategies: seeking social support from extended family and seeking spiritual support.

    Practice implications:
    a. If culturally derived family coping strategies are not being used, explore possible use with family.
    b. Support family's coping strategies.
    c. If family does not have primary culturally patterned coping strategies available and is experiencing frustration because they are not available, attempt to assist family to obtain needed support/assistance. Also the family should be identified as at higher risk for adaptation problems.

The African-American Family

Marilyn M. Friedman

► learning objectives

1. Explain the criticism that is made about the early writings of social scientists with respect to the African-American family.

2. Briefly discuss the status of the African-American family in the 1990s, relative to social class differences and problems facing the black underclass.

3. Compare the family roles and power structure of black middle-class, working-class, and lower-class families.

4. Broadly describe differences in socialization and marital stability among middle-class, working-class, and lower-class African-American families.

5. Identify two traditional folk practitioners in black American communities in the past.

6. Recall two commonly seen responses of African-Americans when they initially utilize white health institutions.

7. Explain three health care practice implications based on African-American family values and coping strategies.

► HISTORICAL DEVELOPMENT OF THE AFRICAN-AMERICAN FAMILY

African-Americans are the largest racial/ethnic group in the United States. They are geographically and socioeconomically very diverse. Nevertheless, they share both cultural origins (coming from Africa centuries ago and enduring the legacy of slavery) and the necessity to manage the stress produced by discrimination and other social and institutional barriers.

In this chapter both African-American and black are used to describe this racial/ethnic group. The current literature addressing the black/African-American family also uses both terms interchangeably.

"The family is one of the strongest and most important traditions in the black community" (Franklin, 1988, p. 23). It is unclear as to how much of this tradition is part of the African legacy and how much was developed in the New World.

The development of the contemporary African-American family is overshadowed by the disastrous legacy of slavery. During the era of slavery, the black family existed only by the consent of the slave owner for the purposes of perpetuating the system and improving the slave owner's economic status. The black family was not autonomous or self-sufficient.

Slaves were able to construct a partial family unit when it suited the needs of the slave owners. These units often were mother centered, with the mother-child relationship primary and the husband-wife and father-child relationships tenuous (Rainwater, 1971).

▶ DEMOGRAPHIC PATTERNS OF AFRICAN-AMERICANS

African-Americans comprise approximately 12 percent of the American population, with over 81 percent now living in urban areas (U.S. Bureau of the Census, 1991a). The percentage of African-Americans in the population will rise slowly and in the year 2050 is projected to constitute 13.6 percent of the U.S. population (Rosenblatt, 1996) (see Table 8–1). Two striking developments have occurred within the black population in the United States since the civil rights movement of the 1960s. One is the emergence of an authentic, larger, and economically stronger middle class—better educated, better paid, better housed than for any group of African-Americans in the past (Gelman et al., 1988; Hutchinson, 1988). The other development is the emergence and growth of the black underclass (Taylor et al., 1990). In 1995, 29.3 percent of all black Americans were poor as compared to 11.2 percent of all white Americans (Fulwood, 1996) (see Fig. 19–2).

The black middle class grew to about 56 percent of all black wage earners in the 1980s. With a population estimated at 2.5 million, the black underclass is approximately three times larger than it was in the 1970s (Gelman et al., 1988). This group, as discussed in Chapter 8, generates a disproportionate share of the social pathology associated with living in a ghetto—poverty, unemployment, high welfare rates, high crime rates, gang warfare, drugs, dropouts, and teenage pregnancies. Poverty has hit black children particularly hard. For example, in 60 percent of African-American mother-headed families, children are poor. Black children are three times more likely to be poor than white children (see Table 8–4).

The opportunities of the 1960s and 1970s resulted in the underclass becoming isolated from the more educated and ambitious blacks who took advantage of opportunities to move to more middle-class or integrated neighborhoods and away from the ghet-tos. For the underclass left behind, the statistics in Table 20–1 bespeak their desperate condition.

With a growing proportion of African-Americans in poverty and the simultaneously rising proportion of African-Americans at the highest income levels (Malveaux, 1988), a polarity of economic extremes exists within the black community (Levy, 1988). It is important to emphasize this diverse complexion of black families in America. Despite the growing number and worsening status of the black underclass, the majority of African-Americans have experienced substantial economic improvements, although certainly more improvement is needed (for instance, the median black income is still only 57 percent of the median white income).

▶ TABLE 20–1

AFRICAN-AMERICAN FAMILIES: WIDENING ECONOMIC AND HEALTH DISPARITIES IN THE UNITED STATES

Evidence of the widening problems African-American families face:

- One-third of all African-American families live in poverty.
- African-Americans continue to make on the average about 57% of what white Americans make. Their real median income has not changed since 1969.
- A black man over 24 is twice as likely as a white man to be unemployed.
- The rate of unemployment for black youth is more than double that of white youth.
- Black children are three times as likely to live in poverty and in female-headed families than white children.
- Sixty percent of African-American children live in poverty.
- More than one in six black households live in dilapidated homes.
- Twenty percent of all African-American families live in public housing.
- College enrollment of African-Americans is dropping, often for economic reasons.
- A black baby is three times more likely than a white baby to have a mother who dies in childbirth or a mother who received no prenatal care.
- An African-American infant is twice as likely as a white American infant to die during the first year of life.
- Black teenagers and young adults are nearly five times as likely as their white counterparts to die of AIDS.

Source: Clinton (1995), Edelman (1997), Fulwood (1996), Schulte (1995).

Rise in Teenage Pregnancies and Single-Parent Families

The large and growing number of black teenage pregnancies and resulting single-parent families, which then live in poverty, is a major societal and family health concern. According to some sociologists (Meisler & Fulwood, 1989; Staples, 1985, 1989), the cause of the increased number of black single-parent families is the shortage of marriageable black males in the underclass.

Rising Number of African-American Men in Trouble

There is widespread concern about the declining status of black adult men in both the African-American and general community (Heady, 1996). Black males place at the bottom of nearly every social indicator—highest unemployment, highest infant mortality rate, lowest life expectancy, and poorest educated (Harris, 1990; Savage, 1990). Poverty is three times higher among black adult males than among their white male counterparts. In 1995, according to a national survey report (the "Sentencing Project"), 30 percent of young black men (20 to 29 years) are now under the supervision of the criminal justice system, and to add to this tragedy, young black men are murdered—almost always by other black men—at 10 times the rate of white men in the same age group (Brownstein, 1995). So bad is the black males' situation that the National Association for the Advancement of Colored People (NAACP) calls the black male an "endangered species." Hence, the large number of single-parent families is due, it is reasoned, not to the number of children born to young mothers (the fertility rate has remained about the same for blacks) but to the dearth of black marriages taking place.

▶ THE AFRICAN-AMERICAN FAMILY: A LEGACY OF VULNERABILITY AND RESILIENCE

Accounts of the African-American family portray two opposing pictures—one of incredible resilience (the family displaying resilience and adaptive coping strategies in the context of a harsh past and present environment) and the other of an endangered family with growing problems in race relations, living with racism and growing poverty (Greene, 1995; Ingrasia, 1993; Johnson, 1997).

Staples (1989), a noted family sociologist, brings into perspective the present and future status of African-American families. He summarizes the problems of the black family as being the same as in the past century. Problems are primarily poverty and racism.

Race relations continues to be a major barrier to integration of African-Americans; white and black Americans often see the same world in drastically different ways, and in spite of remarkable progress made in black and white relations, a considerable rift still exists. President Clinton, in addressing the University of Texas (1995), spoke of the responsibility of all Americans to acknowledge injustices and to help heal the division between the two races. He stated:

> White America must understand and acknowledge the roots of black pain. It began with unequal treatment first in law and later in fact. African Americans indeed have lived too long with a justice system that in too many cases has been and continues to be less than just. The record of abuses extends from lynchings and trumped-up charges to false arrests and police brutality. The tragedies of Emmett Till and Rodney King are bloody markers on the very same road. (p. A12)

Although the future of black middle-class families looks positive, the future of black families in the underclass looks dim. Black men continue to experience widespread problems as noted in Table 20–1, while black women and their roles are in a state of transition—paralleling some changes in American women generally (decreased fertility and greater liberation) (Staples, 1989).

▶ STATUS OF AFRICAN-AMERICAN FAMILIES: CRITICISM OF THE LITERATURE

There has been extensive criticism of both governmental reports and of the writings of social scientists about black families. The most controversy over governmental reporting was directed toward a report of Daniel P. Moynihan, then Assistant Secretary of Labor, who wrote a report that identified the black family with a "tangle of pathology" and with a deterioration of black society. He concluded that black families were falling apart, basing his conclusions on a myriad of statistical data showing such phenomena as numbers of absent fathers, children on welfare, and juvenile delinquency. This well-known, highly controversial report marked the beginning of the continuing debate and dialogue about the status of the black family, and more importantly, what/who was the victim and the cause. The real debate often centered around who was "to blame" for the multitude of problems besieging black lower-class families. Is it the family itself, the societal treatment of African-Americans, or a combination of both external and internal factors? (As we know from other studies, the most potent force for family behavior is external factors, particularly economic constraints.)

Although Moynihan pointed out that the societal treatment of blacks was ultimately to blame, this statement was hidden among the extensive evidence of the black family in trouble. His report also suggested that the black family itself, as a result of its weakening, possessed characteristics inimical to its welfare, as well as to the welfare of its family members and the black community. Moynihan identified the black family's matriarchal structure as a key contributor to the deterioration of the black family. Billingsley (1968) and other scholars on the black family disagreed. They see the black family as a resilient and adaptive system and maintain that black families survived their long journey from Africa to urban America by developing characteristic strength—chiefly a sense of extended family that provides support and nurture during crisis or parental absence (Billingsley, 1992; Greene, 1995; Hill, 1971).

In the past decades, controversy over who is to blame for the poor black family's multiple problems has created an atmosphere of defensiveness and not wanting to look squarely at the tremendous problems lower-class and underclass black families are facing. This is now changing. The black community, as well as health and social welfare scholars and practitioners, are closely examining the problems of the poor black family and proposing policy changes and strategies to counter some of the continuing and emergent problems (Edelman, 1997; Heady, 1996; Hill, 1997).

One of the significant points of clarification to come from the debate about the status of the black family is that the issues concerning the black family concern the black lower-class family. Notwithstanding the recognition that racism exists against all black Americans, the black middle-class family varies greatly from the lower-class and underclass family. It is similar to its white counterpart in family lifestyle and does not manifest the extensive strains of the poor black family.

The African-American family, regardless of social class status, has been repeatedly termed a matriarchal structure, forced into this family form because of the separation of husband and wife during slavery and more recently because of economic realities, welfare restrictions, and a lack of available, marriageable black men (almost one out of every three adult black males in their 20s is either in jail, on parole, or otherwise under the supervision of the criminal justice system (Clinton, 1995). But according to Billingsley (1992) and Willie (1976), this assertion does not properly account for the total range of black families in our society. First, 78 percent of adult black men and 70 percent of adult women work to support their families. Although still well below the proportion of two-parent white families with children, 41 percent of black families are two-parent families (Glick, 1993, 1997, U.S. Bureau of the Census figures cited).

During the last decade significant changes occurred in black families across the nation. The strong family tradition among blacks survived the slave system, discrimination, poverty, and hostile governmental and societal practices and attitudes. Since the 1960s, however, rapid urbanization and especially ghettoization, has had a devastating impact on many blacks who migrated to large cities from rural areas; black males were often unable to find work and governmental policies adversely affected black family strengths (Franklin, 1988). Truncated governmental programs have contributed to the deeper poverty and despair of many black and other ethnic peoples of color. Harriett McAdoo (1988), a black family scholar, asserts that "the need is even greater now to understand the economic situation, cultural patterns and socialization practices of black families" (p. 16).

The black family has adapted to the larger society in various ways, with the common experience of racial discrimination and economic adversity playing very significant roles. Billingsley (1992), a black sociologist, believes that the various structures and functions of black families have resulted largely as adaptive reactions to varying socio-economic conditions and stressors that threaten black families' survival.

Studies of African-American Families by Social Scientists

As with the Mexican-American family literature, there has also been extensive criticism of the writings of social scientists about the black family (Johnson, 1997). Dodson (1988) criticized black family literature as inconsistent, poorly conceptualized, and flawed in terms of research designs. Hill and co-workers (1993) cite the ubiquity of inadequate research perspectives that have guided African-American family research and social policy.

The early black family literature of the 1960s generally saw black families that deviated from mainstream white family lifestyles as deviant or pathological. Using the deficit theory (Peters, 1981), the root problem was often believed to reside within black families themselves. Social scientists and the media alike tended to view black families as homogeneous: poor and in trouble. A case of point is an analysis of black family articles published in the *Journal of Marriage and the Family* from 1939 to 1987 (Demos, 1990). In these articles sources of distortion were identified. A culture-of-poverty thesis was a prominent focus throughout the surveyed years and was an obvious source of distortion about the African-American family. This focus, encouragingly, has diminished considerably in recent years.

In the last decade or more a number of researchers (McAdoo, 1983; Peters, 1981; Staples, 1985) have looked at black families with a more positive theoretical perspective and also by social class (Billingley, 1992; Coner-Edwards & Spurlock, 1988; McAdoo, 1982). Having this more positive view, black family life is viewed from a cultural variant perspective (Johnson, 1997). This is also an ecological, systems perspective that views black families as viable, functional, and interacting within mainstream society. "This approach assumes that most Black families have developed patterns of behavior and child-rearing attitudes and practices which are appropriate to the values and constraints within their own lives" (Peters, 1981, pp. 73–74). Unique aspects of black life are not necessarily taken as reflections of pathology (Johnson, 1997).

One important deficiency among black American family literature is the paucity of research about blacks who come from diverse countries and cultures. Greater attention must be given to black American immigrant families who come from the West Indies, Central and South America, and Africa (Johnson, 1997).

▶ AFRICAN-AMERICAN FAMILY FORMS AND KINSHIP SYSTEM

Forty-six percent of all black families were nuclear two-parent families in 1990 (U.S. Bureau of the Census, 1993b) (see Fig. 1–4). Although the female-headed single-parent family is commonly seen (51 percent of all black families were single parent in 1991 according to the U.S. Bureau of the Census [1993]), the modal and ideal black family is the traditional nuclear two-parent family.

Extended Families

One of the distinctive characteristics of black families is the fact that a much higher proportion of black than white family households have extended family members living with them (Glick, 1997). Many of the 18 percent of black families that are not nuclear in form consist of groups of relatives such as grandparents and their grandchildren, brothers, sisters, and other relatives excluding parent–child sets living together (Glick, 1988a). Working-class and middle-class black families may have an older relative living in the home providing child care while both spouses work. In the poorer family, the more common pattern is of an older female relative bringing under her wing a younger woman and her children.

Three-generation households typically exist when there is no husband present. Most married couples have their own apartment or home.

One of the primary cultural patterns noted in the black family literature is the strong reliance on the extended and nuclear family (McAdoo, 1983). Parent–child bonds across the life course are very close (Taylor et al., 1988). Young black couples prefer to live near their families of origin. Strong kinship bonds are also evidenced by the high frequency with which African-American families take relatives (especially children under 18) into their households. Black families have developed their own network for the informal adoption of children (Hill & Shackleford, 1986). Babies born out of wedlock are frequently kept in the home; in 1978 fully 90 percent of such black children were reared by parents or relatives, whereas in white families only 33 percent of children born out of wedlock were kept in the home.

Historically the extended family served as a means of pooling meager resources. Today, especially among the poor, financial resources, food, emergency care, and child care are extensively shared among the extended family (Peters & Massey, 1983; Taylor et al., 1988). Child care is often provided by relatives. This is called "multiple mothering," meaning that grandmothers, aunts, cousins, close friends, or people considered as kin to the child's mother carry out parental roles. They provide emotional support, tangible child-care assistance, and alternative parent role models (Greene, 1995). The grandmother, especially the maternal grandmother, has been the most prominent provider of child care. Today, many of the grandmothers are very young themselves (between 27 and 39). A considerable number of these young grandmothers are feeling resistant to taking on another role—that of grandparenthood—because they still are involved in young adult roles themselves. Role overload has been identified as a problem with "off-timer" young grandmothers (Burton & Bengtson, 1985; Burton & de Vries, 1995).

Single-parent Families

Single-parent families are more numerous among African-Americans than other ethnic groups (see Fig. 1–4). In 1990, according to U.S. Bureau of Census 1993 data, 48.6 percent of all African-American families are mother-headed families. Another 2.4 percent are father-headed families. Of these single-parent families, two-thirds of births were to unmarried mothers in 1992 (U.S. Bureau of the Census, 1993). Never-married mother-headed families are most likely to be poor and often young. Fatherless families are generally more troubled economically and socially. Children who grow up without fathers are disadvantaged educationally, interpersonally, and psychologically. In many single-parent families, an extensive network of other family members, family friends, and neighbors participates in the rearing of and caring for the children (Greene, 1995).

► FAMILY VALUES AND COPING STRATEGIES

The black family's culturally derived values or ideology is basically conservative; that is, adult members believe in the traditional family structure, in church, hard work, and strong kinship bonds. However, for the poor some of these traditional values have not been realizable, particularly the value of the traditional family structure. It is important to recall here that values are the ideals or "what should be," and the real culture is "what actually is." There sometimes is a dissonance between culturally derived family values and the structural conditions in society, particularly for lower-class and underclass blacks. Staples (1985) describes this dissonance as being created because the black male is prevented from fulfilling his normative familial roles. The adaptation of family life that has occurred is seen in the dramatic increase in both households headed by women and out-of-wedlock births. The majority of adult women are not married and living with spouses. Moreover, two out of every three marriages end in divorce (the divorce rate for whites is also high, about 50 percent).

This analysis is presented to emphasize the point that sheer practical necessity often distorts one's values in everyday life and makes family values—what family members say is important—very different from actual behavior. Hence, some coping strategies—that is, how families respond to the demands placed upon them—are more prominently found in the working and middle-class families, and are discussed in those sections. Those coping strategies that are characteristic of African-Americans regardless of social class are addressed here.

The several core coping patterns common to African-Americans as identified in the black family literature are:

1. Strong religious commitment and participation.
2. Strong bond with and support from kin and friends.
3. Flexibility in family roles.

The widely cited major stressors are racism and oppression—which are felt irrespective of social class—and economic stressors. Included under economic stressors are the stressors of poverty, unemployment/underemployment; housing; and health care (Boyd-Franklin, 1993; McAdoo, 1983; Staples, 1989). Elaborations on the above coping strategies follow.

Strong Religious Commitment and Participation

A strong commitment to and participation in religion has served as a primary means of coping and decision making for both the black individual and family (Paniagua, 1994; Smerglia, Deimling, & Baresi, 1988). A religious orientation was a major aspect of the lives of Africans transported here as slaves. During the era of slavery the church played a vital role in helping black Americans cope with the oppression of slavery. It was through the church that blacks learned to use religion as a means to survive (Hill, 1971). Black churches today are descendants of the black church during slavery, where old-time religion and preaching were the mainstay of black family life (Pipes, 1997). Pipes (1988), in studying the old-time religion and preaching, explains that its purpose was to "stir up, to excite the emotions of the audience as a means for their escape from an impossible world" (pp. 55–56).

The black church is a central institution in African-American communities. In times of crisis, religion and the church-sponsored social services have been significant supportive elements in revitalizing hope for African-Americans (Ho, 1987). The church provides emotional, spiritual, intellectual, and social satisfaction. It is also an important avenue for gaining musical expression and leadership opportunities. Many black families identify elaborate church networks in which their minister and other church "sisters and brothers" are an important informal social network for the family and particularly for the older women members (Boyd, 1982). Hence, religion often plays a central role in family life, providing a powerful spiritual, social, and emotional resource (McGoldrick, 1993).

Strong Bonds and Support from Kin and Friends

Black families generally have a strong support system composed of kin and friends. As such, this social network represents crucial ways for families to cope. The kin and friendship help–exchange system supplements black families by sharing material, emotional, and social resources (Allen & Stukes, 1982) as well as emergency assistance (Taylor et al., 1988) and care for sick members, children, aging parents, and grandparents (Benin & Keith, 1995).

The genesis for strong kinship has been traced back to the traditional African culture (Nobles, 1974). The tradition survived the splitting up of families during slavery and has served to assist the family to deal with the harsh environment in such a way as to ensure survival, security, and self-esteem of its members. Black Americans need support and family involvement, conclude Taylor (1990) and Ellison (1990), who found in research on social support patterns of black Americans that higher levels of familial involvement and subjective family closeness were positively associated with greater family life satisfaction and personal happiness, respectively.

Black "extended families" are not necessarily drawn along "bloodlines" (Greene, 1995; Hill, 1971). There may be a number of nonkin people who function in important roles in families. It is common practice for long-time friends and neighbors to be brought into the family circle (Carrington, 1978). White (1972), in his study, observed that a number of "uncles, aunts, big mamas, boyfriends, older brothers and sisters, deacons, preachers, and others operate in and out of the African American home" (p. 45). Nonrelatives were often found to be as influential as relatives, according to one study of black social supports (Manns, 1988). African-Americans from lower-class backgrounds have been found to have a greater number of kin and nonkin in their social network than those from working- and middle-class backgrounds; the larger network serves to offset more adverse life experiences (Manns, 1988; McGoldrick, 1993).

Family Role Flexibility

Probably the most efficacious family coping strategy in terms of assisting the family to function effectively is the black family's role flexibility and shared decision making (McAdoo, 1988; Peters, 1981). The fluid interchanging of family roles emerged out of economic imperatives of black life (Ho, 1987). In most black families both parents have always had to work outside the home to make ends meet; hence, both parents shared the task of provider, as well as the domestic and child-care responsibilities. African-American women have worked outside the home for decades and still are more likely to combine child rearing and work (Benin & Keith, 1995). Thus, African-American men are not threatened by their wives' employment; having a working mate has fostered more egalitarian spousal relationships (Hines & Boyd-Franklin, 1996).

Although roles vary considerably between families, sharing of household and child-care tasks between spouses is more common than in white families (McAdoo, 1983). Older children in large families become responsible helpers, participating in caring for younger siblings and sometimes working part time to augment the family income. Family teamwork and cooperation are stressed.

Role flexibility within the nuclear and extended family is mobilized in times of crisis. For families experiencing problems such as separation, illness, hospitalization, death, substance abuse, or unemployment of a family member, being flexible in who does what in the family can make a difference between successful adaptation and maladaptation. Gathering information about the roles family members play, particularly when there is a crisis, should be part of the assessment process.

▶ FAMILY SOCIALIZATION PATTERNS

In African-American families, children are extremely important and valued. If the mother cannot handle them, extended kin will generally take a more active role in rearing and caring for the children (McGoldrick, 1993).

Research findings from ecologically oriented and comparative studies represent the most informative and enlightened types of child-rearing studies involving black Americans. In the ecologically oriented studies it is assumed that black families encourage the development of skills, abilities, and behaviors necessary to survive in their environment (Peters, 1997). In the comparative studies, relevant differences are examined using a relativistic perspective. In general, according to Peters (1997), black families are reported to be strong, functional, and flexible in their socialization practices. The values of sharing, reciprocity, collective actions, and cooperation are emphasized (McBridge, 1995).

Black Americans provide a home setting that is culturally different from that of white Americans.

Children are raised to adjust to the special stress of poverty (in the case of lower-class families) and discrimination, as well as the "ambiguity and marginality of living simultaneously in two worlds—the world of the Black community and the world of mainstream society" (Peters, 1981, p. 233). Greene (1995) explains that black parents must prepare their children to function adaptively within the dominant culture without internalizing the dominant culture's negative messages about African-Americans. Parents must teach their children to "make psychological sense out of their disparaged condition, deflect hostility from the dominant group and negotiate racial barriers under a wide range of circumstances" (Greene, 1995, p. 30).

Discipline techniques of black parents are reported in some child-rearing research studies to be more direct and strict, emphasizing obedience rather than being psychologically oriented. This stricter parenting style across social class lines is seen as a pragmatic and realistic adaptive practice necessary for survival in an inimical, harsh environment. Open communications and high levels of family support buffer parental strictness (Bartz & Levine, 1978). Also a high value is placed on getting along with others (Julian, McKenry, & McKelvey, 1994; Peters, 1997).

A blurring of gender roles was found by some researchers (the stress was on getting the job done rather than matching the job to the child's sex). Parents generally treat children of both sexes the same until early adolescence. At that time sex-based differences in socialization emerge.

There are clear differences in the responsibilities children are given depending on their birth order, with, for example, the oldest child having authority over the younger children and the firstborn receiving special preparation for a leadership role in the family (Lewis, 1975).

The oldest or an older child may be "parentified." This is especially so when both parents work, there are many children, or the family is mother headed. The child who assumes parental responsibilities may be developmentally unprepared and hence, the role becomes a stressor, or the parental child may successfully engage in that role and develop responsibility and maturity beyond his or her years (Minuchin, 1974).

Although child-rearing literature describes mothers' roles in terms of being child centered in their child rearing, very little is known about the role of the black father. What has primarily been written has focused on the negative impact of the absent black father (McAdoo, 1997). Where fathers are in the home, researchers have reported a greater sharing of housekeeping and nurturing of children than white fathers (McGoldrick, 1993). In comparative studies (comparing white, black, and other ethnic fathers), both black and white fathers are found to be predominantly nurturant, warm, and loving towards their children. Moreover, the most common interactional pattern of fathers and their children appears to be warm, nurturant, and loving (McAdoo, 1997). In several studies, African-American fathers evidenced greater interest and involvement in their children's socialization when compared to white, Asian, and Hispanic fathers (Julian et al., 1994; McAdoo, 1997).

Significant caretaking others (kin and nonkin) play an important role in encouraging educational and occupational achievement, according to a study of black achievers (Manns, 1997). These findings confirm that the child-rearing role is often a shared one—involving "multiple mothers" and significant others.

Maternal interactive behavior with children and other child-rearing practices are found to differ by social class. As discussed in Chapter 15, socialization practices of parents are molded by what they envision their children needing to adapt to the world as they see it. Because the worlds of the middle, working, and lower classes are so varied in terms of the skills and behaviors that are adaptive, it stands to reason then that child-rearing patterns would also differ. These differences will be addressed later.

▶ THE FAMILY HEALTH CARE FUNCTION

Historic Review

A brief review of historic African-American health practices is instructive for a comprehension of the present-day situation. After slavery and during the reconstruction period in the South, a rise in the use of folk remedies and the midwife or "granny" occurred (Kroska, 1985). As late as 1962 the black midwife was still delivering 42 percent of black babies in the state

of Mississippi (Harrison & Harrison, 1971). Their use in the South has been discontinued as a result of legal prohibitions. The use of the conjure doctor, voodoo or hoodoo man, or witch doctor—a practice brought from West Africa—also continued throughout the postemancipation period. Certain diseases were thought to be caused by God or the supernatural, one effect of which was to lead to the fatalism felt by many rural black Americans.

The use of conjure doctors, magical thought patterns, folk practices, and feelings of fatalism are all health attitudes that migrated north with poor black families. Immigrants from Haiti and Jamaica bring traditions of spiritualists, herbalists, and voodoo with them also. In some black ghettos today, some lower-class black families continue to use herb doctors, spiritualists, and faith healers. As medical care has become more accessible to black Americans, however, the use of folk medicine and practitioners has declined considerably. Particularly among the working and the middle classes, only isolated home remedies remain as reminders of the days of "grannies," conjure doctors, and folk health practices.

Use of Folk Medicine and Home Remedies Today

Folk medicine for a limited number of health problems has remained important in the urban ghettos and in the rural South. Low-income blacks commonly make use of patent medicines and home remedies, secure medical advice from friends, and are reluctant to seek professional health care. Often the poor black person will endure blatant symptoms of ill-health such as unexplained weight loss, abdominal pain, and frequent breathlessness without seeking care. In other words, for families of low socioeconomic status and/or families that feel socially and culturally alienated from available health care, the period of delay is longer. These families will generally exhaust all the home remedies known to kin and friends before feeling forced to turn to health care facilities for help.

Older women are the common repository of these folk remedies in today's black families. Bullough and Bullough (1982) explain that home remedies may have their origins in magical beliefs or have a logical, empirical basis. Two of the more common purely magical actions are putting a knife under the bed of a woman in labor to cut the pain and wearing amulets or charms to ward off disease. Empirical modalities include massage, heat, and tub baths for rheumatoid arthritis, and the application of poultices and the use of herb teas for colds.

Health Care Access Barriers

A considerable proportion of black Americans have serious problems obtaining health care. This is in large part due to the fact that many poor black Americans do not have health insurance or Medicaid. U.S. health statistics provide evidence of the inaccessibility of health care for many black Americans. Edelman (1988) writes that "black children are twice as likely as white children to have no regular source of health care, are more likely to be more seriously ill when they finally do see a doctor, and are five times as likely to have to rely on hospital emergency rooms or outpatient clinics for care" (pp. 286–287). Poor families avoid the expenses of preventive health care, and receive poorer and later prenatal care.

Because many African-Americans live in urban, crime-ridden, overcrowded ghettos with dilapidated housing (Edelman, 1997), the health of these individuals is adversely affected. Racism, poverty and unhealthy lifestyle patterns are contributory factors to the widening health disparity between the health status of white and black Americans (U.S. Department of Health and Human Services, 1993). The positive correlation between poor general health status and poverty and unsanitary, overcrowded, poor environments provides evidence of the negative impact of the environment on health (Stokes, 1974). Violence in these neighborhoods claims more young lives than any other health problem (Griffen, 1994).

Another reason why African-American clients may delay care is their feelings of discomfort and mistrust in going to a white health facility. New African-American patients sometimes feel strange, unwelcome, uncomfortable in, or mistrustful of white health facilities (Harrison & Harrison, 1971). There may have been so much difficulty working through the system to be cared for that a patient will come in assuming he or she is not going to be treated well (Monroe, 1989). These apprehensions and negative feelings lead some black clients to delay seeking health care.

▶ SOCIAL CLASS DIFFERENCES

To cope with the enormous sociocultural stresses of daily life—racism, discrimination, and economic distress—the African-American family has adapted by developing a variety of family structures, including the patriarchal, egalitarian, and matriarchal forms. The differences in family structure and function can best be understood when one looks at the social class differences. Sociologists Eshleman (1974) and Billingsley (1992) state that the most important variable in understanding the lifestyle of black families is social class. "Socioeconomic class stratification is an important, if not overlooked, dimension of African-American family life" (Billingsley, 1992, p. 57). The impact of socioeconomic status on family structure is seen in the statistics with respect to one- and two-parent families. In black families with incomes below the poverty line, only 20 percent of children live with both parents; while in black families where incomes are above the poverty line, three times more children live with both parents (U.S. Bureau of the Census, 1993).

A sense of peoplehood (common ethnic identity) is present among African-Americans regardless of socioeconomic status. Even though lower-class and upper-class black families exhibit dramatic differences in lifestyles and family life, they still share a common experience and ethnic identity that makes them feel as "one people," distinct from nonblack families, regardless of their social class similarity.

Billingsley (1992), a black family sociologist, has done the most work on black family social class characteristics. He has identified distinct social class strata in the African-American community. The social class strata are based primarily on family income and source of income, supplemented by educational, occupational, and lifestyle data. These strata include: (1) a small black *upper class* with high incomes and substantial wealth; (2) a *middle class*, primarily composed of skilled and professional white collar workers; (3) a *nonpoor working class*, comprised of unskilled and semiskilled workers above the poverty line; (4) the *working poor*, who are composed of workers with unskilled, low-paying jobs who are living below the poverty line; and (5) the *nonworking poor* who are made up of families where no members are working—described in the literature as the "underclass."

African-American Upper- and Middle-Class Families

In 1990 black middle-class and more affluent upper-class families comprised about 42 percent of all black families in the United States (Billingsley, 1992). Billingsley (1992) reported that the more affluent black upper class (those with family incomes over $50,000) increased from 6 to 14 percent from 1983 to 1990, a reflection of the growing number of well-educated black professionals. The black middle-class group is still growing also—from 25 percent in 1986 to 29 percent in 1990. In recent descriptions of the black middle class, Coner-Edwards and Edwards (1988) identify two categories of families, the "nouveau black middle-class" and the established black middle-class. The first group generally emerged into the middle class from the lower social classes during the window of opportunity of the 1960s and 1970s. The latter category of families includes descendants from middle-class and prominent families. These families appear to have a better sense of belonging than the nouveau black middle-class, who worry about loss of status and stability (Coner-Edwards & Edwards, 1988).

The black middle class is a diverse group, represented by a broad spectrum of income, occupational, and educational levels. They are usually skilled and professional white-collar workers and small business owners, whose education ranges from completion of high school through postdoctoral education.

Families tend to be nuclear in form, generally consisting of husband, wife, and two to three children. Because of their dual employment, cooperative work and team effort of husband and wife are needed. Thus many family tasks such as cooking, cleaning, and shopping are shared, and there is extensive adaptability or flexibility of roles. "Probably the best example of the liberated wife in American society is found in the black middle-class family. Spouses are partners out of economic necessity and have an egalitarian pattern of interaction" (Willie, 1976. p. 20). Egalitarian patterns include the sharing of decision making by spouses and more democratic communication patterns. Middle-class black families are more egalitarian than white middle-class families (Willie & Greenblatt, 1978).

The middle-class black family's value system and, consequently, its socialization patterns are largely congruent with those of the dominant culture (Coner-Edwards and Edwards, 1988). Value conflicts emerge as a continual problem, however, because black and white cultures have different value orientations (Benjamin, 1991). For the middle-class African-American there typically is extensive involvement in the nonblack world. This demands that middle-class blacks have the ability to live in two worlds simultaneously (termed being bicultural), managing dual sets of values, expectations, roles, ways of communicating and behaviors (Woodward, 1994).

Racist attitudes and practices are still commonly experienced by African-Americans within our institutions (e.g., work, education, the media, housing) (Benjamin, 1991; Woodward, 1994). Because middle-class black parents may not expect, because of discrimination, to get the full benefits for their efforts, they tend to be more protective of their children and act as a buffer between the outer world and the family, to help their children develop their potential while maintaining their self-esteem (Greene, 1995; McAdoo, 1983).

Social class variability in how black parents rear their children is seen. For instance, middle-class mothers are more vocal with their infants than are lower-class mothers. During later periods of development, middle-class parents are less coercive, restrictive, and arbitrary in their disciplining than lower-class parents. Middle-class parents use more reasoning, support, and communication of democratic approaches and less physical punishment with their children than do lower-class parents (Peterson & Rollins, 1987).

Recent research on the role of black fathers in socialization indicates that middle-income and affluent black fathers look much like their white counterparts in terms of their relationships with their children. John McAdoo (1997, 1988b) has noted that when economic status rises within the black family there is an increase in the active participation of black fathers in the socialization of their children. Most middle-class fathers are observed to be warm, nurturant, and loving in their interactions with their children. Some studies also report that black versus white fathers are more restrictive and controlling toward their children (McAdoo, 1997, 1988a).

Religion generally has a higher priority for black middle-class than for white middle-class families.

Parents tend to be active participants in church affairs, the church serving not only important emotional and spiritual needs but also as a central institution for black social life (Willie, 1976; McGoldrick, 1993).

Additionally, grandparents, older siblings, or extended family members usually play a more active role in the socialization process than in middle-class white families (Greene, 1995; Peters, 1997). It is interesting to note, however, that for upwardly mobile black families, connection with extended family members who have not moved up can be stressful or guilt-producing. A sense of responsibility and an obligation is felt toward those who assisted individuals in moving up or who have not moved up as they have (Coner-Edwards, 1988).

According to several black family scholars (McAdoo, 1983; Peters, 1997; Peters & Massey, 1983), the major stressor in black family life is the psychological and social pressures of racism in the everyday environment. This is termed "mundane extreme environmental stress" in some of the literature (Peters & Massey, 1983). In addition, paralleling large divorce rates in the general U.S. population, marital instability is quite prevalent among the black middle class, posing a stress on all members of the family (Billingsley, 1992).

African-American Nonpoor Working-Class Families

According to 1990 U.S. Bureau of the Census figures (Billingley, 1992), the nonpoor working class have been numerically and sharply declining beginning in the 1980s. In 1969, 42 percent of African-Americans were classified as nonpoor working class, while in 1986, 34 percent were so classified, and in 1990, only 31 percent were classified as nonpoor working class. The primary cause of this erosion in the nonpoor working class is found in the larger society. The shift from a manufacturing economy to a service economy has reduced the number of factory and manufacturing jobs and created low-paying service jobs (Billingsley, 1992).

These families tend to be nuclear households, but usually have more children than do middle-class families. There is also a greater likelihood that a relative or boarder may be part of the household. Both parents generally hold jobs. Men tend to work in semiskilled factory, restaurant, or janitorial positions and women are frequently employed at a similar level in community institutions. The parents have often not completed high school, but they desire more education for their own children, and encourage the more motivated children to go to college. Couples usually marry early and begin a family very soon after marriage.

Willie (1976) indicates that the relationship between husband and wife usually takes on an egalitarian character, because cooperation for getting by and survival is a necessity. Hammond and Enoch (1976) confirmed that in their sample of 51 black working-class families, 60 percent of husbands and 57 percent of wives scored their marriage as equalitarian. Because husbands carry out traditional family roles, women generally have more economic control in matters pertaining to the home and children (Greene, 1995). Additionally, there is a tendency toward some flexibility concerning child-care tasks based on the sex of the child. Lastly, the mother also takes on the social liaison role, primarily with the school and the church.

Respectability is important among black working-class families, with the ownership of one's own home and the good character of one's children being important symbols of the attainment of this value. Of great significance is one's family. The size of the family may be a source of pride for the parents, as the bearing and rearing of children is considered to be an important responsibility. Working-class parents often make great personal sacrifices for their families and kinship relationships are strong (Willie, 1976; McGoldrick, 1993).

Again, religion and the church play a central role in the lives of these families. And the church is often second only to the home as the emotional center of black life (Fellows, 1972; Hines & Boyd-Franklin, 1996).

In regard to child rearing, parents raise their children to assure that they receive the skills and attitudes necessary to survive in the world as the parents perceive it. Thus respectfulness, obedience, conformity to rules, and being "good" are stressed. A strong work ethic exists. During childhood, children are assigned household chores as part of their family responsibility and are encouraged to seek away-from-home jobs for pay when old enough.

Fulfilling the affective functions in the family poses difficulties because of the long hours both parents usually work to provide the necessities of life. Most black working-class families have to give up doing things together as a whole family. Many husbands hold down two jobs, and it is not uncommon for spouses to work different shifts to cover child-care responsibilities (Billingsley, 1992; Willie, 1976).

African-American Lower-Class Families: The Working Poor and the Nonworking Poor

In 1990, the black lower-class family comprised about 31 percent of all black families (Billingsley, 1992). Of this 31 percent, 12 to 13 percent are working poor and 18 percent are nonworking poor. In 1995, the proportion of black American poor had declined slightly to 29.3 percent (see Fig. 19–2) (Fulwood, 1996). The proportion of African-American poor is three times higher than in the white lower class. Poor black families largely live in the urban inner-city poverty areas (Levy, 1988), where social isolation and all the consequences of poverty exist. Racial discrimination and economic adversity are reasons why African-American poor live in urban, inner city ghettos.

Black lower-class families can be divided up into those that represent the working poor and those in the nonworking poor, the underclass—a group remaining at the bottom of the social ladder and increasingly estranged from mainstream patterns and norms of behavior (Wilson, 1987). The black underclass increased considerably in size in the 1970s and 1980s due to economic changes and governmental programs. The underclass is described more fully in Chapter 8.

Most married couples have their own households, although poorer black households are much more likely to be single-parent families (Glick, 1997). It is common to find extended families also, consisting of the grandmother and the mother and her children when no husband is present. Moreover, lower-class black families generally have more children than either the poor white family or the working- or middle-class black family.

In the lower class, desertion and divorce are chief causes for family disruption, although single-parent families are usually not entirely devoid of a male presence. Often the mother will have a boyfriend

who visits frequently and acts as companion to the family. Boyfriends and biological fathers often play supportive roles, assisting mothers financially and emotionally (Staples, 1989). If a husband-father is present, he is often unemployed, with the mother on welfare or working in an unskilled job. Even when either spouse is working, the possibility of unemployment is a continual threat.

The primary feature of lower-class African-American families is their low-income status. Due to the families' impoverished state, they are coerced into making various adaptations, some of which are heavily criticized by the wider society. These adaptations include multigenerational living arrangements and taking in boarders or foster children for pay. Adult heterosexual relationships may involve both marital and parental responsibilities in the absence of marriage. Poor households sometimes forgo conventional morality in order to provide an expedient arrangement for earning sufficient money to live on. "The struggle among poor families is a struggle for existence" (Willie, 1976, pp. 95–98). Movement and instability are great in areas of jobs, residence, and relationships.

Adolescent girls and boys from poor black families tend to have sexual experiences at an early age and have children earlier than their counterparts in the working and middle classes. Premarital pregnancy, though not condoned, is accepted by the family after the fact, as is the belief that, although it may be desirable, it is not necessary to have a man around the house in order to have and raise a family. Many teenage mothers are not marrying today, but raising their children alone, usually with the help of the extended family and friends. Via the process of informal adoption, some young mothers arrange for their children to be raised by kinfolk (Staples, 1989).

Marriage is looked upon ambivalently and in many cases negatively by both sexes, because of the stresses and strains associated with family life (Rainwater, 1971). This ambivalence and negativity has a reality base. Much greater marital instability exists, generally due to economics (unemployment), and, in addition, affectional problems (extramarital relationships) are commonplace.

One of the prevailing myths or stereotypes about the black lower-class family is that it is matriarchal (female-dominated) in structure. There is much convincing evidence that among married couples in the black lower class this is not the case (Cromwell & Cromwell,

1978; Dietrich, 1975; Scanzoni, 1971; Staples, 1976). Dietrich (1975) asserts that matriarchy is not normative in the poor black family. "The study, relying on self-report data from eight samples of black wives in intact nuclear families, reported a predominance of egalitarian decision-making structures in every study population" (Cromwell & Cromwell, 1978, p. 750). Cromwell and Cromwell's (1978) study of lower-class black married couples in Kansas City also suggests that egalitarian decision making predominates.

Because a majority of lower-class African-American families are female-headed single-parent families, by definition these families are matrifocal. The mother makes most of the necessary decisions and has the greatest sense of responsibility for the family. There is intense loyalty between mothers and grandmothers and their children or grandchildren. Mothers extend every effort to assist their children, even into adulthood; and the grandparents often take on the child-care role and act as prime socializers. Strong loyalty and reciprocity also exists among siblings. The problem here is that when one is in need, all of the siblings are struggling too. Nevertheless, they share their already overcrowded living quarters and often give whatever assistance they can.

The family's values are distinct and different from the wider society's values, thus helping to create the malintegration of this group within and the stigmatization by society of the black lower class. A few selected values will be explained. Fatalism is a common value and one associated with poverty. African-American lower-class families learn to hope for little and expect even less. Men and women get sexually involved, but are afraid to trust and commit themselves to each other due to their experience of repeated disappointments. Dependency, rather than self-sufficiency, is an orientation—not really valued, but accepted as a reality and a way to "get by" (e.g., it is all right to lean on extended family and on society by receiving welfare). A lack of valuing the achievement and work ethic is apparent, as is the lack of valuing education and future planning. In this regard it must be remembered that family values are reality-based—a reflection of what families can aspire to and expect in life.

Irrespective of social class, kinspeople (grandmothers, aunts, cousins, older siblings) play a more active role in the socialization of African-American children than is true of white families (Hines & Boyd-Franklin, 1996). In lower-class three-generation maternal households, it is the grandmother who is expected to stay at home with the young children (infants and preschoolers), because the mother has the right to continue outside activities. Some young grandmothers are now resisting this role, however (Burton & Bengtson, 1985; Burton & de Vries, 1995).

Rainwater (1971) described the African-American lower-class family as having little sense of the awesome responsibility of caring for children that the middle-class parent experiences. Although the confinement of being home with infants and preschoolers is also difficult for black mothers and grandmothers, there is not the constant solicitousness that is seen when observing working- and middle-class mothers from various ethnic backgrounds care for their infants. "Multiple mothers" help defray the responsibility of 24-hour child rearing (Greene, 1995).

In single-parent poor homes the maternal household is generally run with a loose organization. Children learn at an early age to fend for themselves, especially if the family is large, with school-aged children beginning to shop, cook, go to bed and school on their own, and watch after themselves when mother is gone. Lower-class, three-generation maternal homes are busy with kin and friends coming and going at all times of the day and evening on an unplanned basis. This openness of the home, in part, may be a reflection of the mother's sense of impotence in facing the street system. Although the mother often tries to keep children away from the street when they are young, as they grow older it becomes increasingly futile, and she may finally give up, disengage, and let the children have their freedom. Black ghetto street life increasingly involves gangs, drugs, criminal activity, and lack of good role models (Billingsley, 1992; Griffin, 1994). Poor parents often disengage themselves from their school-age or adolescent son when they feel they are powerless to change the direction of their child's life.

▶ FAMILY NURSING PRACTICE IMPLICATIONS

In order to provide more culturally sensitive care, the following practice implications are suggested.

Replacing Stereotypes With Informed Knowledge

Stereotypes about the African-American family must be replaced with informed knowledge about cultural similarities and differences. Behavior that is not congruent with white middle-class standards should not be prejudged and negatively labeled as deviant or dysfunctional, but evaluated and viewed within the family's cultural and situational context (Billingsley, 1992; Mitchell, 1982).

Reevaluating Family Definitions and Use of Social Networks and Self-help Groups

Family nurses must redefine the family and abandon limiting notions that include only the legally bonded couple or nuclear family in their definition of family (Boyd, 1982). In family assessment and intervention, family nurses should incorporate important people who the family identifies in its social network into the nursing process.

In this regard, because the extended family often provides a substantial amount of direct assistance as well as emotional support, this family resource should be considered when working with families. For the older or disabled person, help from extended family is often an invaluable asset that makes the difference between the client having to be placed in a nursing home or cared for in the home. For the family with young children, the assistance of the extended family support system is a central family strength and should be capitalized on in counseling families.

The importance of the role of the older adult woman or grandmother in the family should be especially recognized in working with African-American families. Parent–child bonds usually exist across the life span and are of critical importance for the provision of assistance (Taylor et al., 1988). Grandmothers are often the repository of both child-care expertise and health remedies. They can serve as both a crucial asset and also as a stumbling block if their central role in health matters is not appreciated and they are not brought into important family health decision making.

Community-based family nurses can facilitate the formation of self-help groups. Murata (1995) recommends that family nurses take this approach in helping single parents with parenting. She suggests locating organizations such as churches within the African-American community to sponsor parenting groups. "Providing single mothers with the opportunity to meet to discuss family and childrearing concerns and to form friendships that provide social support can be important" (Murata, 1995, p. 59).

Because the church plays a vital role in the life of most African-Americans, a family's church may be an important resource to utilize in assisting families with serious or long-term health problems. This resource may be especially useful in helping women because they tend to show more involvement with church activities than African-American men. If tangible and emotional supports from a particular church are available, it may be advisable to include church members in family interviews or in health decision making and planning (Paniagua, 1994).

Assisting With Health-related Family Problems

Poor families, from any cultural group, have survival needs that often supercede the resolution of health problems. Family nurses should recognize that their role needs to be enlarged in order to assist families with their problems of greater priority. Only after these more pressing problems are resolved can any real energy be given to health needs (Boyd-Franklin, 1989). Improvement in educational, environmental, social service, and employment opportunities for poor black families is crucial in elevating their health status.

Promotion of Family-centered Health Regimens

In recognition of the powerful influence the family exerts on personal behavior, the whole family should be encouraged to adopt a new health-promotion program, if appropriate, rather than involving only the identified client.

Dealing With Client Discomfort and Mistrust

Health care professionals must be aware of the discomfort and alienation poor black families frequently feel toward white health care facilities. An African-American family's inactive or nonverbal participation during a first interaction with a health care provider may simply represent the family's initial discomfort or mistrust of the health care provider (Ho, 1987). Interactions need to be warm, sensitive, and respectful of clients' needs, beliefs, and feelings. Communicating respect is key to successfully engaging families and making them feel comfortable.

With regard to dealing with the black client's initial discomfort and mistrust, some of the ethnic family literature suggests that it is helpful, but not necessary, to have a health care professional be of the same cultural or racial background as the client. However, this is many times not possible or practical. Successful assessments and educational and counseling interventions are still accomplished with black families when the family nurse is of another cultural background and he or she is informed, empathetic, sensitive, and concerned.

Emphasizing Strengths and Empowerment

In working with African-American families, it is much more effective to emphasize the family's and family members' strengths than its deficits. Exploring the resources black families have (e.g., the church, the extended family, "multiple mothers," role flexibility, etc.) invites families to feel a greater sense of control, optimism, efficacy, and empowerment. This positive approach is especially crucial in working with black families because of their experiences with racism and discrimination (Paniagua, 1994).

► study questions

1. Which of the following are some of the frequent effects on the black family of slavery, racism, and economic disadvantage? (Mark true or false after each statement.)
   a. The black male's self-esteem is lowered.
   b. The wife becomes submissive to her husband and his primary authority.
   c. The self-fulfilling prophecy often occurs in the areas of education and employment.
   d. Health-seeking behaviors are exaggerated.
   e. A mother-centered family becomes a practical necessity.
   f. Traditional husband–wife family roles become rigidly defined.

2. When one examines recent demographic statistics related to the black family, which of the following problems appear to be important? (Select all appropriate answers.)
   a. Economic
   b. Parenting and child care
   c. Access to health care
   d. Employment

3. Match the following family attributes with the black family according to social class.

Family Attribute	Class
a. Respectability is an important value.	1. Middle class
b. Both parents are college-educated and work.	2. Working class

  c. Role sharing between husband and wife
     occurs extensively.
  d. More likely to be single-parent families
     and/or matrifocal.
  e. A strong achievement orientation is present.
  f. Has the largest family and largest number of
     relatives living in same household.
  g. Church is a central value and institution.
  h. Egalitarian power pattern exists.
  i. Values most incongruent with wider society.
  j. Long-term dependency on public assistance
     is common.
  k. Families are child centered.
  l. Mothers are more vocal in their interactions
     with their infants.
  m. Physical punishment is more frequently used.

3. Lower class
4. Underclass

4. African-American clients who are new to a white health facility often feel
   uncomfortable initially. What are some of the other feelings or behaviors
   that have been observed?
   a. Overly cooperative
   b. Mistrustful
   c. Demanding more of a say in their own care
   d. Careful to say "the right thing"
   e. Avoidance behaviors

5. Which of the following are criticisms that black family scholars and
   researchers have made about the early writings on the black family?
   a. The authors viewed the black family as being deviant.
   b. They tended to describe the black family as homogeneous.
   c. The literature was heavily biased in terms of the focus being on the
      black lower-class family.
   d. The writings disregarded the impact of external forces—societal insti-
      tutions—on the family.
   e. Authors viewed the family from a systems, ecological perspective.

6. The most striking development within the African-American family is
   (choose the best answer):
   a. The black family has become more assimilated and more egalitarian.
   b. The middle class has grown numerically and economically while the
      underclass has numerically increased but become more economically
      impoverished.
   c. The fertility rate of black women has increased but their marriage rate
      has decreased.
   d. Poor black families have moved into the cities and wealthy blacks have
      moved into the suburbs.

7. Identify the two traditional folk practitioners used in the past by African-
   American families.

8. Briefly describe three family nursing practice implications based upon black family literature.

► chapter 20 study answers

1. a. True.
    b. False.
    c. True.
    d. False.
    e. True.
    f. False.

2. All (a–d).

3. a. 2.
    b. 1.
    c. 1, 2, and 3.
    d. 3.
    e. 1 and 2.
    f. 3.
    g. 1, 2, and 3.
    h. 1, 2, and 3.
    i. 4.
    j. 4.
    k. 1, 2, and 3.
    l. 1.
    m. 3.

4. b and e.

5. a, b, c, and d.

6. b.

7. Conjure doctors and midwives or grannies.

8. a. Most basic is to abandon stereotypes and be informed and knowledgeable about black families and their cultural background.
    b. Who is in the family must be identified by the family. Family nurses should incorporate these family members into their assessment and interventions.
    c. Because black families typically have strong bonds between parent and child and with kin and long-time friends, assessment of the characteristics of these important social networks is recommended, as well as assisting families to effectively use these social support resources.

d. Assisting poor families with pressing health-related problems first to free them to attend to their health problems.
e. Promotion of family-centered health regimens and programs.
f. Realizing the meaning of black clients' initial responses to new health care facilities and/or health providers, and responding in client interactions with empathy, sensitivity, respect, and feelings of concern.
g. Emphasizing family strengths and family empowerment.

The Asian-American Family

George K. Hong and Marilyn M. Friedman

1. Identify what population groups constitute Asian-Americans and explain the changing demographic pattern relative to the Asian-American population in the United States today.

2. Identify which groups of Asian-Americans are high-risk groups due to their higher levels of distress and explain the reason for their distress.

3. Explain how Filipino-Americans differ in their historical legacy from the other Asian-American populations.

4. Identify the three religious/philosophic belief systems that have pervasively shaped traditional Asian core values. Give an example of how one of these religious/philosophic belief systems has influenced Asian family or health beliefs or practices.

5. Name three traditional core values of Asian families and state what implications these values have for family nursing practice.

6. Explain the value clash that occurs frequently between the younger and older generations in Asian-American immigrant families.

7. Describe briefly two ways in which the Asian-American family changes when it settles in the United States.

8. Explain how two important values, "saving face" and keeping interpersonal harmony, affect family communication patterns.

9. Describe two traditionally based socialization patterns among Asian-American families.

10. Identify three central tenets or concepts of traditional Eastern medicine.

11. Identify one widely used family coping strategy, as well as one individual (family member) coping strategy, utilized in traditional Asian-American families.

12. Explain the importance of assessing an Asian-American family's degree of acculturation.

13. Discuss three family nursing intervention guidelines pertinent to the care of traditional Asian-American families.

▶ DEMOGRAPHIC PATTERNS OF ASIAN-AMERICANS

Asian-Americans are one of the fastest-growing ethnic minority groups in the country. Their number more than doubled from about 1.5 million in the 1970 census to 3.5 million in the 1980 census; and doubled again to 7.3 million in the 1990 census (Gardner, Robey, & Smith, 1985; Min, 1995a). A large proportion of Asian-Americans reside in the states of California (39.1 percent), New York (9.5

547

percent), and Hawaii (9.4 percent) (Min, 1995a; U.S. Bureau of the Census, 1993b). However, in comparison to African-Americans and Hispanic-Americans who account for 12.1 percent and 9 percent of the U.S. population respectively, Asian-Americans are still a small minority, accounting for only 2.9 percent of the U.S. population (Min, 1995a, U.S. Bureau of the Census, 1993b). As such, Asian-Americans are often overlooked in the planning of health services and in the research literature.

The terms Asian-Americans or Asian and Pacific Islanders refer to people from diverse countries and cultures in Asia, the Indian subcontinent, and islands in the Pacific Ocean, including Samoa and Hawaii. Given this diversity, it is practically impossible to describe all the different groups in a single chapter. Thus, in this chapter, we will focus on five groups from the East Asian area, namely Chinese-Americans, Japanese-Americans, Korean-Americans, Vietnamese-Americans, and Filipino-Americans. These Asian-Americans share many cultural commonalities. They are also among the larger subgroups of Asian-Americans (see Table 21–1). Together they constitute the majority of Asian-Americans.

In this chapter, we will first examine each group's immigration history and demographic trends. This is followed by a discussion of their family characteristics and implications for family nursing.

Chinese-Americans

Chinese Americans are the largest group among the current Asian-American population. The term Chinese-Americans includes immigrants from mainland China, Taiwan, and Hong Kong. Their numbers totaled over 1.6 million in the 1990, and the majority of them are immigrants. For example, from 1980 to 1990, between 23,000 to 32,000 Chinese immigrants entered the United States each year (Min, 1995a). This number constituted about 40 to 50 percent of the Asian immigrants during that period. There are also ethnic Chinese who came to the United States via other countries such as Vietnam, Singapore, Indonesia, Malaysia, and other Southeast Asian countries. Officially, these immigrants are considered nationals of the country from which they emigrated, but many of them would identify themselves as Chinese in daily life.

The Chinese were among the first Asians to immigrate to the United States in large numbers (Uba, 1994; Wong 1988, 1995). A significant number of Chinese came in the early 1850s. By 1860, the Chinese population in the United States totaled 34,933 (Wong, 1988). Most of them were single men who sought work in the gold mines of California or the transcontinental railroad. During that time, China was in a period of political, social, and economic turmoil. Many of these early immigrants came from the poorer area of the country with a sojourner's mentality, hoping to earn and save up enough money for them to return to China to retire.

As Chinese immigration continued into the 1870s, anti-Chinese sentiment developed among the general U.S. population. This was fueled by real and imagined competition with white workers, as well as xenophobic and racist attitudes (Wong, 1995). A series of legislative measures was passed to discourage the Chinese from immigrating to the United States. (Uba, 1994; Wong,

▶ TABLE 21–1

ASIAN-AMERICANS IN THE UNITED STATES (1960—1990)

Total	1960	1970	1980	1990
Asian-Americans	877,934	1,429,562	3,500,439	7,273,662
Chinese	237,292	436,062	806,040	1,645,472
Filipino	176,310	343,060	774,652	1,406,770
Japanese	464,332	591,290	700,974	847,562
Korean	—	69,150	354,593	798,849
Vietnamese	—	—	261,729	614,547

Adapted from Gardner, Robey, & Smith (1985), Min (1995a), U.S. Bureau of the Census (1983, 1993b).

1995). This was exemplified in the Chinese Exclusion Act passed by Congress in 1882. It was the first and only immigration act to specifically target a particular nationality group for exclusion from the country. It severely restricted Chinese immigration and made immigrants ineligible for American citizenship (Uba, 1994; Wong, 1988, 1995). Moreover, up until the first half of the 20th century, 14 states had miscegenation laws prohibiting intermarriage with the Chinese (Lyman, 1974).

The anti-Chinese sentiment and immigration exclusion of the Chinese started to relax during and after World War II (Wong, 1988, 1995), as China was an ally of the United States fighting against the Japanese in Asia. The communist takeover of mainland China and establishment of the People's Republic of China in 1949 also resulted in many refugees who sought admission to the United States. In 1965, the United States finally overhauled its immigration policy and passed the Immigration and Naturalization Act, which created a more equitable format for immigration. This Act, which became effective in 1968, allowed most countries a quota of 20,000 immigrants per year in general, regardless of race or ethnicity (Wong, 1988, 1995). This made it possible for more Chinese immigrants to come to the United States. The 1965 Act emphasized family reunification and favored people with professional and technical skills. Family members of immigrants could now come to the United States to join their family. Also, people with specific skills could apply for immigration and bring their nuclear families with them. As contrasted with early immigrants who had to immigrate as individuals and were forced to leave their families behind, Chinese immigrants could now immigrate as family groups, or by virtue of family ties. Thus the number of Chinese-Americans increased dramatically from 436,062 in 1970 to 806,040 in 1980.

In the 1980s the People's Republic of China loosened its tight emigration policy and made it easier for Chinese living on the mainland to come to the United States. About the same time, the Taiwan government also made it easier for its people to invest overseas and emigrate. Both of these factors further contributed to the rapid growth of the Chinese-American population, which again doubled to over 1.6 million in 1990. Of these, 69.3 percent are foreign born (Min, 1995a; U.S. Bureau of the Census, 1993a).

In terms of economic status, the median family income of Chinese-Americans is $41,316, as com-

pared to $37,152 for white Americans. However, while only 7.0 percent of white Americans are at the poverty level, 11.1 percent of Chinese-American families are at that level (Min, 1995a; U.S. Bureau of the Census, 1993a, 1994). These percentages are reflective of the socioeconomic diversity among Chinese-Americans, who are the most economically polarized group of all Asian-Americans (Min, 1995a).

In trying to understand Chinese culture, one must be aware that China is a vast country, slightly larger than the United States, but five times more populous. There are regional differences in dialects spoken and local customs (Hong & Ham, 1994). Many of the early immigrants were from Toisan, a rural area in the Province of Canton (now called Guangdong). Thus the Toisan dialect is commonly spoken by the long-time residents of the U.S. Chinatowns. Cantonese, another common Chinese dialect in the United States, is spoken by many immigrants who came in the 1970s and 1980s, many of them from Hong Kong or from mainland China via Hong Kong. In the newer Chinese communities, Mandarin is a common dialect. It is spoken by immigrants from mainland China and Taiwan, both of which have been promoting Mandarin as the official dialect for a number of decades. Many of these immigrants came in the 1980s. It should be noted that while there are different Chinese dialects or spoken languages, the written Chinese language is the same regardless of the dialects. The dialects are like different pronunciations of the same written word. Thus if a clinic has to post notices or mail letters in Chinese, the dialects will not be an issue. We will discuss other aspects of Chinese culture later.

Japanese-Americans

The Japanese did not immigrate to the United States in significant number until the 1880s (Kitano, 1988; Nishi, 1995; Uba, 1994). Like the Chinese, most of the early Japanese immigrants were single young men seeking work as laborers. Many went to work as farmers on the plantations in Hawaii, and later in California and other areas of the West Coast. By 1902, there were more than 30,000 Japanese immigrants in Hawaii, comprising about 75 percent of the sugarcane labor force in the islands (Min, 1988). The Japanese immigrants also faced the same wave of anti-Asian sentiments that prevailed in the United States from the late 18th century onwards. However, unlike China, Japan was a strong military power at that time. Thus the U.S. government was more reserved in enacting discriminatory legislation against the Japanese (Nishi, 1995). Still, the Immigration Act of 1924 made it practically impossible for all Asians, including the Japanese, to immigrate to the United States.

Anti-Japanese sentiment reached its peak during World War II. From 1942 to 1945, over 110,000 Japanese-Americans on the West Coast were interned in camps located in isolated areas (Kitano, 1988; Nishi, 1995). These camps were secured by armed guards and barbed wires, and routines of daily life were controlled by government directives. It was a major disruption to the traditional family and community life of Japanese-Americans.

While immigration restrictions loosened after the passing of the Immigration and Naturalization Act of 1965, the increase in numbers of Japanese immigrants has not been as dramatic as for other Asian groups. Instead of being new immigrants, most Japanese-Americans today are descendants of Japanese immigrants who came to the United States before 1924 (Uba, 1994). As shown in Table 21–1, Japanese-Americans were originally the largest subgroup among Asian-Americans, totalling 464,332 in 1960. But by 1980, their numbers were surpassed by both Chinese- and Filipino-Americans. From 1980 to 1990, the numbers of Japanese-Americans only increased from 700,974 to 847,562, unlike many other groups, which more than doubled their numbers during the same period. According to the 1990 census, only 32.3 percent of Japanese-Americans are foreign born, as compared to 63.1 percent of all Asian-Americans who are foreign born (Min, 1995a; U.S. Bureau of the Census, 1993a).

This slow rate of emigration is most likely the result of Japan's political stability and economic strength in the recent decades. Unlike other Asian countries such as China, Korea, and Vietnam, Japan has not experienced any major war or social/political upheaval since World War II. Thus there is less of a motive for its population to emigrate. Currently, Japanese-Americans are the most affluent group of Asian-Americans. Their median family income is $51,550, and only 3.4 percent of their families are at the poverty level (Min, 1995a; U.S. Bureau of the Census, 1993a).

Japanese-Americans often categorize themselves into generation groups. Issei refers to first-generation immigrants who were born in Japan. Nisei, or second generation, refers to American-born children of the immigrants. Sansei, the children of the Nisei, are the third generation. Currently, most of the Japanese-Americans are Nisei, Sansei, or younger generations, as compared to other Asian-Americans, most of whom are first-generation immigrants. Typically, because of their greater exposure to American culture, the Sansei and Yonsei (fourth generation) tend to be more Americanized than the Nisei, and the Nisei more Americanized than the Issei. However, as with other immigrants, the degree of cultural identification varies with the individual. A Sansei who was raised in an area with a large Japanese community is more likely to be more identified with Japanese culture than a Sansei, or even Nisei, who grew up in a white community (Kitano, 1988). Thus we have to be careful in applying cultural concepts when we work with different Japanese-American individuals.

Korean-Americans

Following the Chinese and the Japanese, Korean-Americans were the next group of Asian immigrants to enter the United States. The official immigration of Koreans began during 1903–1905, when 7226 Koreans came. They were recruited by the Hawaiian sugarcane plantation owners to offset the Japanese presence in the labor force (Min, 1988). However, the Japanese government was a major military power at that time. In response to the appeal of the Japanese laborers, the Japanese government forced the Korean government to stop emigration to the United States. The U.S. Immigration Act of 1924 further stopped immigration of Koreans and other Asians. Koreans did not resume immigration to the United States in significant numbers until after World War II.

In 1950, the Korean War broke out, which lasted until 1953. North Korea and the People's Republic of China, both communist powers, fought against South Korea and the U.S.–led United Nation forces. This military upheaval, as well as the close ties between South Korea and the United States, fueled another wave of immigration. Korean war brides, or women married to U.S. military personnel, and orphans adopted by U.S. parents were two major groups of immigrants at that time (Min, 1988, 1995a). The Immigration Act of 1965 later made it easier for Koreans and others to immigrate to the United States. While today South Korea has a strong economy, its relationship with North Korea is still a volatile issue. This political uncertainty is one of the factors that has continued to fuel Korean emigration.

In sum, the Korean-American population grew drastically from about 8000 before 1950 to 69,150 in 1970 (Gardner, Robey, & Smith, 1985). As shown in Table 21–1, by 1980, it had grown to 354,593, and then more than doubled to 798,849 in 1990. As such, most Korean-Americans are immigrants who came to the United States after 1965. According to the 1990 census, 72.7 percent of the Korean-American population are foreign born (Min, 1995a; U.S. Bureau of the Census, 1993a). Most of the families are composed either entirely of immigrant members, or of immigrant parents and American-born children. In comparison to Chinese- or Japanese-Americans, third- or younger-generation Korean-Americans are relatively few. Economically, Korean-Americans are one of the less-affluent groups among Asian-Americans. Their median family income is $33,909, and 14.7 percent of their families are at the poverty level (Min, 1995a; U.S. Bureau of the Census, 1993a).

Filipino-Americans

In contrast with other Asian-Americans, Filipino-Americans emigrated from a country that had experienced strong Western influence and had strong political ties with the United States. Indeed, the Philippines can be described as the most Westernized country in Asia (Agbayani-Siewert & Revilla, 1995; Min, 1995a). The Philippines was a Spanish colony from the middle of the 16th century to 1898. Thus, the Filipino culture was strongly influenced by Spanish culture. For example, the Philippines is the only Asian country in which Roman Catholicism is the majority religion. Today, over 80 percent of Filipinos are Roman Catholics (Agbayani-Siewert & Revilla, 1995; Min, 1995a). In 1898, the United States won the Spanish-American War, and the Philippines was ceded to the United States. It remained a U.S. colony until 1946 when it became independent. During this period, the American political and cultural influence permeated the Philippines. This impact still continues to the present time, especially in Philippine economic, political, and educational institutions (Agbayani-Siewert & Revilla, 1995; Min, 1995a).

Filipinos began to immigrate to the United States in large numbers around 1909 (Agbayani-Siewert & Revilla, 1995; Uba, 1994). Like the Japanese and Korean immigrants before them, most were farm laborers seeking work in the plantations of Hawaii. In the next two decades, over 100,000 Filipinos came to the United States, first to Hawaii, and later to California and other parts of the country. However, in the 1930s, Congress began to exclude Filipinos by limiting their immigration to 50 persons per year. This virtually stopped the immigration of Filipinos. There are few descendants of the early immigrants, since many of them never married or had children (Uba, 1994). The immigration restrictions started to loosen after World War II. However, significant Filipino immigration did not occur until the Immigration Act of 1965 made it easier for them to immigrate. The majority of the current Filipino-American population consists of immigrants or children of immigrants who came to the United States after 1965. According to the 1990 census, 65 percent of Filipino-Americans are foreign born (Min, 1995a; U.S. Bureau of the Census, 1993a). The close ties between their country and the United States is a major factor contributing to Filipino immigration here. Also, because of their greater exposure to American culture, most Filipino-Americans, in general, find it easier to accommodate to American life than other Asian immigrants (Agbayani-Siewert & Revilla, 1995; Uba, 1994). As seen in Table 21–1, by 1980, Filipino Americans had become the second-largest Asian-American group. In 1990, their populations totaled over 1.4 million. Filipino-Americans are also one of the more affluent groups among Asian-Americans. Their median family income is $46,698, and only 5.2 percent of their families are at the poverty level (Min, 1995a; U.S. Bureau of the Census, 1993a).

Vietnamese-Americans

The Vietnamese were among the newest groups of Asians to immigrate to the United States in significant numbers. Unlike other Asian-American groups discussed earlier, most Vietnamese-Americans were refugees who left their homeland in chaotic and traumatic situations at the end of the Vietnam War in 1975. These Vietnamese refugees, together with Cambodians and Laotians from neighboring countries, are often grouped together and called Southeast Asian refugees, or Indochinese refugees, as that part of Asia is also known as Indochina. The Vietnamese were the largest subgroup of Southeast Asian refugees.

The Vietnamese refugees left their homeland in different waves. The first wave fled at the end of the Vietnam War to escape persecution by the North Vietnamese communists. In 1975 alone, 130,000 Southeast Asian refugees, most of them Vietnamese, came to the United States (Uba, 1994). The second mass exodus occurred from 1978 to 1979 when the communist government sought to eliminate the influential Chinese business community by forcing the ethnic Chinese Vietnamese to leave. These refugees were known as the "boat people," as they were compelled to leave in crowded fishing boats. They often drifted about, many perishing in the open sea, as neighboring countries, already inundated with refugees, refused to accept them (Rumbaut, 1995). In 1975, the communists also took control of Cambodia, establishing a radical and oppressive regime that caused many to flee for their lives. This was followed by other military and political turmoil, such as the Vietnam invasion of Cambodia in late 1978. Thus, throughout the late 1970s to 1980s, many Southeast Asian refugees continued to leave by boat or by land (Rumbaut, 1995; Tran, 1988; Uba, 1994). Due to the large number of refugees, many countries simply refused to assist them, claiming that they were economic refugees seeking economic opportunities, rather than political refugees escaping for their life and freedom. Most of the refugees had to spend months, and often years, enduring destitute conditions in refugee camps, before they were officially screened and granted asylum. The United States was among a dozen or so countries that would accept them (Rumbaut, 1995; Tran, 1988).

In 1979, the Vietnamese government agreed with the United Nations High Commissioner for Refugees to allow Vietnamese nationals to leave the country and join their immediate families who had left earlier. This created a more orderly wave of emigration. At the same time, the U.S. government also agreed to allow its former employees in Vietnam to immigrate (Rumbaut, 1995; Tran, 1988). This further facilitated the immigration of Vietnamese to the United States. As seen in Table 21–1, by 1980, the Vietnamese-American population had grown to 261,729, and this more than doubled to 614,547 in 1990. According to the 1990 census, 79.9 percent of Vietnamese-Americans are foreign born (Min,

1995a; U.S. Bureau of the Census, 1993a). While the initial policy of the U.S. government was to resettle the Vietnamese refugees throughout the country, 45 percent of them eventually relocated to California, making it the state with the largest Vietnamese-American population (Min, 1995a; Rumbaut, 1995). It should be noted that ethnic Chinese Vietnamese refugees are considered Vietnamese-Americans in their official documents, while in everyday life, they would identify themselves as Chinese. These Chinese Vietnamese-Americans are a source of newcomers to Chinese-American communities.

As refugees, many Vietnamese-Americans, as well as Cambodian- and Laotian-Americans, have personally experienced the violence and turmoil of war and escape. Many of them left behind family members, possessions, and careers in order to start their life anew. The long waits for asylum proceedings in refugee camps literally put their lives on hold, without any certainty that they would be accepted by a host country. Because this is a painful trauma that has lasting effects on most people, we must be sensitive to the impact of the clients' refugee experience when we work with this population. Since most of them fled their country of origin with few or no possessions, Vietnamese-Americans are the lowest income group among Asian-Americans. According to the 1990 census data, their median family income was $30,550, with 23.8 percent of their families living at or below the poverty level (Min, 1995a; U.S. Bureau of the Census, 1993a).

▶ CULTURAL CHARACTERISTICS OF ASIAN-AMERICAN FAMILIES: COMMONALITIES AND DIVERSITY

In spite of their diversity, the Asian-American groups discussed in this chapter share many common cultural characteristics. This is due to geographical proximity and the historical interactions among their countries of origin. Thus, China, Japan, Korea, and Vietnam all share a cultural heritage that was strongly influenced by Confucianism, Buddhism, and Taoism. This distinguishes them, as a group, from Western or mainstream American culture, which is dominated by the Judeo-Christian tradition.

In this regard, we can discuss the general cultural elements of these Asian-Americans collectively.

Filipino culture, from a sociopolitical perspective, differs from these Asian cultures because of the 500 years of Spanish influence, and more recently, the 50 years of U.S. influence. Yet, it still retains many characteristics in common with other Asian cultures. In a sense, Filipino culture may be seen as a mixture of Western cultures, especially Spanish culture, and Asian cultures, including the indigenous Filipino culture.

In exploring the cultural characteristics of Asian families, we have to be aware of the differences between the normative or traditional culture and the contemporary culture. For example, the contemporary culture practiced in the cosmopolitan urban centers of Asia like Hong Kong, Tokyo, or Taipei, is more westernized than the culture practiced in the rural areas, which tends to be closer to traditional culture. There are also socioeconomic class and generational differences among Asian-Americans in regard to their assimilation to mainstream American or Western culture. For example, middle- and upper-class Asian-Americans, particularly those who received their higher education in the United States, are more likely to be culturally assimilated than working-class Asian immigrants. American-born Asian-Americans, having a greater exposure to mainstream culture in their formative years, are more likely to be culturally assimilated than their foreign-born immigrant parents. This cultural gap is often a source of stress or conflict in the Asian-American family (Hong, 1989, 1996).

Aside from these general group differences, we have to be aware of individual differences in cultural identification, which can be seen on a continuum. For example, there are some immigrants who will try to become integrated into mainstream culture as fast as they can, while there are second- or further-generation Asian-Americans who are strongly identified with their cultural roots and wish to retain this rich legacy. There are others who are bicultural in the sense that they can comfortably switch between mainstream culture and Asian culture, depending on the environment or social setting. Still others might feel alienated, sensing that they do not belong to either world (Hong, 1996). Thus, the following discussion of specific cultural characteristics of the Asian-American family should be used judiciously.

▶ FAMILY STRUCTURAL CHARACTERISTICS

Although Asian-American families constitute diverse minority groups in the United States, they have many cultural elements in common, especially when we look at their family and psychosocial characteristics (Hong, 1988; Hong & Ham, 1994). Their culturally derived values differ significantly from the dominant American value system (Min, 1995a). Thus, the commonalities will be emphasized, with description of some of the major differences among the various Asian-American families also pointed out.

The following discussion is based on both empirical findings and observational writings of Asian families in both Asia and the United States. Much less literature is available on contemporary Asian-American families, particularly for certain groups such as Filipino-American and Southeast Asian-American families. Uba (1994), in her review of the literature on Asian-American families, warns readers that there are serious limitations in Asian-American family research, as well as large gaps in our knowledge about particular Asian-American groups, as noted above. In addition to findings sometimes being based on small convenience samples with no comparison groups, data may also have been collected decades ago.

Family Values and Beliefs

Influence of Eastern Religious and Philosophical Beliefs.   One of the core cohesive elements of Asian cultures, with the partial exception of the Philippines, is their common world view. This world view is based on the Eastern religions and philosophies of Confucianism, Taoism, and Buddhism. In contrast, in Western culture the common world view is based on the Judeo-Christian legacy (Henderson, 1989; Hong, 1993). These three Eastern religions/philosophies have pervasively shaped the core values that Asian-American families to varying degrees hold. Thus, as a foundation to our discussion of Asian-American values, the three major Eastern religions/philosophies are first briefly described.

Confucianism.   Confucianism is based on the teachings of Confucius (circa 551–479 BC), a Chinese sage. It is a philosophic system of ethics, education, statesmanship, and religion designed to produce a "righteous person" who possesses self-knowledge, self-respect, sincerity, kindness, and honesty (Henderson, 1989). Under Confucianism, duties and obligations related to social interactions are clearly defined, giving rise to much of the prescribed family relationships and behavior. The family is central in Confucian thought and the norms and values of Confucianism form the basis of much of traditional Asian family life (Meredith & Abbott, 1995). Over the centuries, Confucianism exerted a strong influence and became embedded into Chinese and other Asian cultures. It should be noted that while Confucius is later venerated as a saint by some people, Confucianism is basically a philosophy, a way of life and a world view, rather than a religion.

Taoism. Taoism is a philosophy founded by the Chinese philosopher Lao-Tzu (also called Laozi), who lived around the 6th to 4th century BC. Many scholars believed he was a contemporary of Confucius. Taoism emphasizes intuition, simplicity, and the attainment of profound insight through the ability to perceive "Tao," the primal cause in daily activities and surroundings. Taoism states that people can find harmony and peace by being good to all things, being humble, simple, and peaceful, avoiding honors and distinctions, and enjoying the forces of nature (Henderson, 1989).

In the 3rd century AD, Zhang Leng founded the religion of Taoism. He based it on the philosophy of Taoism, but instituted religious rituals and alchemy, emphasizing the cultivation of elixirs or potions for immortality. The Taoist religion asserts that it is following the teachings of Lao-Tzu, and venerates him as one of its saints or deities. However, the Taoist philosophy does not embrace the rituals and many of the beliefs of the Taoist religion. Thus Taoism the philosophy is different from Taoism the religion. In general, many concepts common to both are deeply embedded in the cultures of China and other Asian countries.

Taoism, both the philosophy and the religion, is often associated with the concepts of *yin* and *yang*, which have gained considerable attention in the West. While these concepts were part of Taoism, they were actually of even more ancient origin. Moreover, they were probably present in Chinese medical thought long before the time of Lao-Tzu. *Yin* is the feminine, negative, dark, and cold energy.

Yang is the masculine, positive, light, and warm energy. The balance of *yin* and *yang* is the key to harmony and peace. As applied to health, balance or good health is maintained by proper diet, avoidance of strong emotions, and the use of appropriate herbs. This belief is the basis of Chinese or Eastern medicine, a system of care that focuses on prevention as well as care (Henderson, 1989; Spector, 1991).

Buddhism. Buddhism grew out of Hinduism in India. It was founded by Siddhartha Gautama, the Buddha (circa 560–480 BC). Adherents of Eastern religions of Hinduism and Buddhism seek maximum human development (Henderson, 1989). Buddha taught that the human condition is embedded in fear, suffering, disease, and death. As Henderson (1989) explains, "The wise person realizes this and looks for a way to resolve it. . . . Buddha's message focuses on the experiences or path that leads to liberation for the human condition" (p. 70). Self-knowledge and love and universal goodwill are two primary virtues of Buddhism. Buddhism teaches that the best path to self-knowledge is through proper conduct, self-control, humility, generosity, and mercy.

Buddhism spread from India into China during the first century AD, and became a popular religion. Over the centuries, Buddhism in China has developed into various schools by incorporating many elements of Chinese culture and thought adapted from Confucianism and Taoism. From China, Buddhism spread to Japan and later to Korea. In Japan, some schools of Buddhism incorporated elements of Shintoism, an indigenous Japanese religion. In summary, there are different schools of Buddhist thought in different Asian countries (Henderson, 1989). However, the average lay follower may not be cognizant of such distinctions.

The influences of the philosophies/religions of Confucianism, Taoism, and Buddhism are deeply ingrained in Asian cultures. Thus, whether or not an Asian overtly identifies with these systems of thought/belief, he or she inadvertently follows their prescriptions, which are often synonymous with cultural norms/values. Similarly, in the United States today, these philosophies/religions still influence the family life of many Asian-Americans regardless of their religion. Indeed, one must be careful not to stereotype the religious affiliations of Asian-Americans. For example, while the Chinese in Asia are typically considered to be Buddhist by default, ethnic Christian churches play a very active role in many Chinese-American communities here (Hong & Ham, 1994). This also applies to Korean-Americans (Min, 1995c), and, of course, to Filipino-Americans whose country of origin is predominately Roman Catholic (Agbayani-Siewert & Revilla, 1995).

Asian-American Core Values

Asian-American families hold traditional Asian values to varying degrees. It may be, however, that only a few Asian-Americans adhere to all the traditional values identified here Table 21–2 provides a comparison of Eastern and Western core values.

Familism. Familism refers to the centrality of the family, family relationships, and family responsibilities. There is a strong belief in the importance of the family over the individual. The needs of the individual, therefore, are subordinated to those of the family. The cultural focus is on the family rather than

on the individual as in Western culture (Chung, 1991; Hong, 1988, 1995). Familism applies to the nuclear family as well as to the extended family and the entire kinship network.

Filial Piety. Filial piety, referring to respect for parents, grandparents, and other significant elders, is a highly cherished value in traditional Asian families. It prescribes that children should repay their parents' love and care by caring for them in their old age. Reflective of the value of filial piety, immigrant families often sponsor their own parents to come to the United States. Filial piety is a basic foundation upon which the traditional Asian family is built (Chung, 1991; Henderson, 1989; Meredith & Abbott, 1995).

Respect for the Elderly. Respect for the elderly is seen in the deference given to older family members, both living and deceased (Chung, 1991; Min, 1995b). The traditional practice of ancestor worship is a ritual that manifests the value of respecting the elderly.

► TABLE 21–2

COMPARISON OF EASTERN AND WESTERN VALUES

Eastern Values	Western Values
Harmony with nature.	Mastery of nature.
Conformity.	Competition.
Smooth, harmonious interpersonal relationships. Conflict avoidance, restraint, self-control.	Assertion of one's thoughts and feelings.
Consensus, assumption of the "middle position."	Dissensus acceptable (holding of a different position).
Indirect, nonverbal expression of ideas, thoughts, and feelings.	Open, direct expression of thoughts, ideas, and feelings.
Tradition and continuity.	Change, innovation, progress.
Respect for older persons.	Adulation of youth and youthfulness.
Hierarchical positions and status. Respect for authority.	More egalitarianism in status and in relationships.
Cyclical concept of time.	Specific points, schedule, clocks.
Collective orientation and group accomplishments.	Individual orientation and self-accomplishments.
Familism.	Individualism.
Interdependence.	Independence.

Adapted from Stauffer (1995), Ho (1992), Chung (1991).

Respect for Authority.

Traditionally Asian-American values also stress respect for authority figures, including teachers and health professionals (Chung, 1991; Uba, 1994). Respect is displayed in the home by emphasizing obedience to parents.

Interdependence and Reciprocity.

The value of interdependence is seen in relationships within and outside the family—with friends, neighbors, employers, and fellow employees. The ethic of reciprocity and collective obligation is an inherent part of interdependency. Asian-Americans are to a much greater extent than Euro-Americans group oriented, with a strong sense of duty and social responsibility (Chung, 1991; Hong, 1989; Min, 1995b).

Interpersonal Harmony.

The value of maintaining harmony is also central in traditional Asian-American families (Uba, 1994). Maintaining peaceful and agreeable relationships by accommodation, compromise, conformity, and other nonconfrontational means, is the way in which harmony is achieved. In most Asian cultures, it is socially unacceptable to be aggressive or confrontational. Suffering without complaining or suffering quietly is connected to the value/norm of "exhibiting dignity."

Avoidance of Disagreement and Conflict.

The norm of self-control, restraint in emotional expression, and retaining smooth interpersonal relations is widely held in contrast to the focus on individuality that characterizes Western cultural norms (Chung, 1991; Meredith & Abbott, 1995). As part of this interpersonal value and norm, disagreement and conflict is avoided, while conformity and compromise (taking the "middle position") are emphasized.

Saving Face.

There is a high value on *saving face* or maintaining one's respect and status. Typically one loses face when one has failed to carry out a socially appropriate role/behavior. Losing face is often viewed as not merely a personal shame, but also a family shame, for the behavior of each family member is a reflection on the whole family. Family honor is widely emphasized. Therefore, there is great pressure to behave properly so as to not bring shame on the family. Shame, then, is a major social control mechanism (Chung, 1991; Shon & Ja, 1982).

Fatalism.

Acceptance of one's fate is a widely held belief in Asian cultures. Rather than being seen as a negative life adjustment, it is a pragmatic way of coping with life's vicissitudes. Instead of challenging a situation or unfortunate event, traditional Asian-Americans may accept the event/situation as a given condition of their fate (Henderson, 1989).

Education/Achievement Orientation.

Asian-American families generally place a high value on education. There is research demonstrating that Asian-American parents stress achievement in their children more than Euro-Americans do (Uba, 1994). Families are often willing to undergo substantial financial hardship to support their children who are receiving a good education. Moreover, the scholastic success of Asian children is well recognized. For instance, in a survey of 1400 Southeast Asian refugee families, Caplan, Choy, and Whitmore (1992) found that the families of school-aged children played a pivotal role in their children's academic success.

Strong Work Ethic.

In traditional Asian cultures, both educational and occupational achievement are highly valued (Min, 1995b). This is related to the cultural emphasis on fulfilling one's obligation to the family and to society by being educated and productive. Asian-Americans usually work longer hours than Americans in general. For instance, Korean-American immigrant men and women, many of whom own small family businesses, work long hours. Korean-American women worked on the average of 75.5 hours/week in job and household work, according to a New York City survey. Korean-American men worked long hours too (63.5 hours/week), but 12 hours less per week than their wives because they did not share the household tasks (Min, 1995c).

Family Role and Power Structure

In the traditional Asian family, age, gender, and generational status are the primary determinants of family roles and power. Most basic, relative to the Asian family, is that it is patriarchal, with the exception perhaps of the Filipino family. Family roles are clearly defined. Males, particularly the father and eldest son, have the most dominant positions. Traditionally, the father maintains an authoritative, strict, and dignified relationship to the family (Uba, 1994). He is the leader, provider, and disciplinarian of the family. Traditionally, power is passed on from father to eldest son.

Traditionally, wives and daughters are in subordinate positions. They are expected to respect and obey their husbands, husband's parents, or fathers, if unmarried (Hsu, 1971; Meredith & Abbott, 1995). A traditional Asian-American wife-mother devotes herself to the care of her husband, children, and home (Henderson, 1989).

Sons and older persons are more valued in traditional Asian families than are daughters and younger members. Sons are more valued because they will carry on the family name and will care for their elderly parents. The oldest son is most respected (Shon & Ja, 1982). Older siblings command respect and are typically addressed as "older sister," "second oldest brother," and so on, rather than by name. Older siblings are expected to be role models to younger siblings (Uba, 1994). Grandparents have a position of honor by virtue of their older and parental status (Hong, 1989).

Asian-American families are on the average larger in size than white American families. For instance, 59 percent of white American families in 1990 consisted of 1 to 2 persons, while the same percentage of Chinese-American families consisted of 3 to 7 persons (Wong, 1995).

A major power and control issue or problem in immigrant Asian-American families is the clash between traditional (Eastern) and modern (Western) values. The literature describes cultural conflicts between parents and children, and to a lesser extent, between spouses (Detzner, 1992; Hong, 1989, 1996). Children socialized in U.S. schools are taught to be independent, individualistic, and egalitarian in relationships. When Asian-American children and youth bring home these Western notions to immigrant parents whose values and beliefs are of deference, obedience, interdependency, familism, and so on, conflict between the generations often ensues. Conflict between immigrant spouses may also occur as Asian-American women begin working outside the home or otherwise become more Westernized, and consequently challenge the authoritarian, dominant position of their husbands (Detzner, 1992).

The traditional Asian family is multigenerational, extending vertically to include older generations, even those who are deceased, and horizontally to include living relations through fourth cousins. One's ancestors are remembered and respected.

The traditional Asian family is often patrilocal, with the married couple living in the same household with the husband's parents. This pattern is changing in the urbanized or industrialized areas where the size of housing units and job mobility often make it impractical for the extended family to live in the same household. In addition, when families migrated from Asia to the United States, their extended families often did not accompany them. Thus, not only was the large extended family network reduced, but also the patrilocal household pattern was not possible (Hong, 1995; Hong & Ham, 1992).

Family Communication Patterns and Processes

The core Asian values are seen in the characteristic ways in which traditional Asian-Americans communicate. Given the high value placed on interpersonal harmony, avoidance of disagreement and conflict, and "saving face," more indirect, subtle, and nonverbal expression of thoughts and feelings is seen. In contrast, Euro-Americans favor more direct, open, and straightforward expression of thoughts and feelings (Hong, 1989; Locke, 1992).

Among traditional Asian-Americans, emphasis is placed on avoiding offending others and being socially sensitive. Family members are encouraged to refrain from expressing their feelings when they could potentially disrupt family harmony. Instead of overtly disagreeing when differences between persons exist, traditional Asian-Americans may verbalize their thoughts in a mild or circumventive manner. Family members are much less inclined to express directly their disagreements to an authority figure such as a health professional. For example, a more acceptable, less confrontational way of disagreeing is for the client to say: "Some people say that I can do it this way . . . [instead of your way]," making the disagreement less personal and more polite (Hong, 1989, p. 16).

In the traditional Asian-American home, clearly defined roles of dominance and respect rule out argument and negotiation. Communication is typically one way, from parent to child. Direct messages predominate and two-way communication is more brief and perfunctory, e.g., talking about safe subjects (Locke, 1992; Uba, 1994). Traditional, clearly defined family roles may promote stability and security, but they may also promote emotional distance between father and children and limit the avenues to express and resolve problems.

A reliance on nonverbal communication also enhances smooth, harmonious relationships because disapproval is communicated in a manner that is not as divisive and oppositional as verbal challenges (Uba, 1994). For instance, a family member may convey displeasure or disapproval by giving other members subtle looks that signal his or her feeling.

Uba (1994) explains that there is a clustering of behaviors that involve a particular kind of "reserve, reticence, deference and humility" (p. 17). Manifestations of these behavior patterns include a hesitancy to speak up in class, particularly to openly contradict a teacher, and a hesitancy to dominate a conversation.

Communication behaviors that show the values of self-control, self-discipline, and ability to delay gratification and suppression of expression of negative and positive emotions are also commonplace among traditional Asian-Americans (Uba, 1994). Asian-American patients may be silent and uncomplaining about their pain and symptoms; behaviors which are, as noted, manifestations of the above values.

In many immigrant Asian-American families, there may be more limited family communication than in Euro-American families, not only because of cultural factors, but also because of a language gap between parents and children, i.e., children increasingly use English at home, while parents being monolingual, only use their native language. This language gap further reduces communication and creates emotional distance between parents and children (Hong, 1989, 1996; Yu & Kim, 1983).

▶ FAMILY FUNCTIONAL CHARACTERISTICS

The Family Affective Function

Parent–child attachment bonds are described in the Asian-American family literature. Generally children

feel emotionally closer to their mothers than their fathers according to Shon and Ja (1982). One major factor for this closeness is the mother's role in nurturing and rearing the children. Traditionally, the mother's most important bond may be to her children, especially the eldest son, rather than to her husband, whereas the husband's strongest bond is often to his own mother (Uba, 1994).

Asian-American family research has also found that Asian-American families are generally more cohesive than Euro-American families (Uba, 1994). These families tend to have strong commitment to family, tend to live closer to parents, feel more obligated to their parents and interact more frequently with them (Uba, 1994). The cohesion generally found in Asian-American families is rooted in the value of familism, interdependency, and filial piety. Cohesion is also a familial response to outside pressures to the family, such as the pressure of coping with immigration to a new society and coping with racism.

Family Socialization Function

Traditionally, acceptable norms for behavior are clearly defined and very much shaped by the teachings of Confucius, especially by his emphasis on the values of filial piety and veneration of age. Social order in the family is maintained by keeping the proper order of relationships between parents and children, older and younger persons, and husband and wife (Locke, 1992). These relationships are hierarchical and taught to children at an early age. The family exerts a great deal of control over children who are expected to be devoted to and rely on their family (Uba, 1994). There is also a strong emphasis placed on preserving family honor as indicated under the discussion of saving face. Shame, guilt, and appeals to family obligation and social responsibility are used by parents as socialization control techniques to mold children's behavior and attitudes (Locke, 1992).

Respect for educated persons and the importance of a child's education are stressed in Confucianism and reflect core Eastern values. In fact, Min (1995b) considers the emphasis on children's education to be probably the most salient feature of child socialization. Because of the centrality of education in the minds of parents, the pressure that Asian-American families exert on their children to excel in school is high (Locke, 1992). Julian, McKenry, and McKelvey (1994) also found that Asian-American parents tended to emphasize self-control, as well as doing well in school.

According to Uba (1994), a number of studies show that Asian-American mothers tend to be more restrictive about their children's independence than do Euro-American mothers. Asian-American mothers supervise their children more closely and expect them to be independent at a later age. Parents are more likely to demonstrate love and affection indirectly, such as by sacrificing for their children so that they may receive a good education, rather than directly through hugs and kisses (Hong, 1989; Shon & Ja, 1982).

In many immigrant Asian-American families it is common to find relatively strict discipline and control of children when compared to Euro-American families (JWK International, 1978, cited in Uba, 1994). It appears, however, that as mothers become acculturated, their control, strictness, and close supervision diminish (Uba, 1994).

The ways in which parents discipline and punish their children also change after families have settled in the United States. Immigrant Asian families sometimes find that what was acceptable in their country of origin may not be acceptable in the United States. An example of an unacceptable child-rearing practice that parents are being forced to change is the following. In Southeast Asia, coin rubbing, a medical treatment, is used to treat certain illnesses. Because this therapy bruises the skin, school authorities have reported children with this type of bruising to child protective agencies as possible cases of abuse. Different child-rearing rules and laws have left some immigrant Asian families confused and unsure of their parental skills and authority (Bemak, Chung, & Bornemann, 1996; Hong & Hong, 1991).

Evidence that families do change in their child-rearing as part of their adaptation to a new country was found in a large national survey conducted by Julian, McKenry, and McKelvey (1994). These researchers compared parenting across cultural groups in the United States and found differences in child-rearing between Hispanic-Americans, Asian-Americans, African-Americans, and whites to be much less than expected when socioeconomic status was controlled for.

Asian-American fathers appear to have a limited role in child-rearing, although recent studies of Korean-American families show this is changing (Huang & Ying, 1989). Fathers' role in child-rearing is particularly minimal when children are infants (Suzuki, 1985).

Family Health Care Function

Little is written in the literature about how the family fulfills the health care function. The mother and other women in the home are the caregivers. In seeking Western health care, treatment may be delayed because of the high value placed on self-control, not complaining about pain, and suppression of feelings. Once recognized as being ill, however, the ill family member receives a great deal of care and concern and is encouraged to assume a dependent role within the family (Chan, 1992).

Traditional Asian health care beliefs and practices are Chinese in origin, with the exception of Filipino culture where indigenous medical beliefs and practices are based primarily on Malaysian culture. Chinese medicine teaches that health is a state of spiritual, psychological, and physical harmony. Violating this harmony or balance causes illness and disease. A central concept in preventing and treating diseases is *holism*. Holistic Chinese medicine recognizes the interrelatedness of structures within the human body, as well as the need to integrate the human body with the external environment. The onset, evolution, and alteration of an illness are assessed within the context of the patient's environment (Spector, 1991). The *yin–yang* polar, oppositional energies, powers that regulate the universe and the human body, must be in balance for health to be maintained (Chang, 1995). Therefore, illness is the disharmony of *yin* and *yang*, the vital energy, leading to pathology, with excesses in one and deficiencies in the other.

Traditionally, there is a respect for the human body. Good nutrition, rest, calm emotions, and exercise are seen as important in maintaining the proper balance needed for promoting health.

In Chinese medicine, acupuncture, massage, cupping, moxibustion, skin scrapping, and herbal remedies are widely used to treat illness (Chang, 1995). Their purpose is to restore the proper balance of *yin* and *yang*. The ginseng root is the most famous of all herbs. It is used to treat a large variety of illnesses and to stimulate better general health.

A fuller description of *yin* and *yang*—their locations within the human body and their functions—as well as the Chinese ways of preventing, diagnosing, and treating illness can be found in Rachel Spector's *Cultural Diversity in Health and Illness* (3rd ed., 1991). An excellent bibliography of books and articles on Chinese medicine are also listed there.

Because traditional Asian-Americans have a deep respect for their bodies and are used to Chinese medicine, they may be upset by some of Western medicine's intrusive modalities, such as intrusive diagnostic tests, particularly drawing blood and surgical treatments. Many traditional Asian-Americans refuse surgery except under the most dire circumstances (Spector, 1991).

Asian-Americans often use both Western and Chinese medical services (predominantly herbal medicine). For instance, a Chinese-American may treat minor and chronic illnesses with Chinese medicine and acute and serious problems with Western medicine (Liu, 1986). Asian-Americans may also use both herbal medicines and Western medicines concurrently for the same condition (Chang, 1995). This is especially common when they are dealing with a chronic or serious illness that Western medicine has little hope of curing (Hong, 1993, 1995).

Traditional Asian-Americans will tend to underutilize medical services for economic reasons. Mental health services are also underutilized because of cost, but probably more importantly, because of the shame and stigma that mental illness attaches to both the individual and his or her family (Hong, 1988). The belief that mental disorders are not preventable or treated effectively, as well as the belief that self-help is the means for handling psychosocial problems also are factors that curtail the use of mental health services by traditional Asian-American families (Kitano & Maki, 1996).

▶ FAMILY COPING STRATEGIES AND PROCESSES

Discussion of family coping patterns among Asian-American families has to be inferred from the literature on traditional cultural values, as no literature on this topic could be located. From the core cultural values identified earlier, family coping consists of pulling together (cohesiveness) and seeking and receiving direct assistance and support from the extended family. Immigrant families may be cut off from their social support system when they migrate to the United States. Sometimes only one side of the extended family is here or only the nuclear family migrates. This isolation from the family's social support system is often stressful because it eliminates a significant traditional way Asian families cope. Health professionals need to be informed of community resources to help families utilize these resources to fill some of the vacuum that the family social support system often fulfilled (Hong, 1988, 1989).

Seeking social and financial support from self-help community groups has also been mentioned as a way of coping for Asian-American families. Many Asian-American communities have organizations targeted at helping new immigrants and other less acculturated Asian-Americans who have difficulty accessing mainstream agencies. Acceptance of one's fate (fatalism) may also serve as a way for family members to cope with family stressors over which they have no control (Henderson, 1989).

When considering which Asian-American families are in the high-risk group for distress and dysfunction, probably the group that has experienced the greatest stress in more recent years is from the Southeast Asian countries of Vietnam, Laos, and Cambodia, particularly those who came as refugees rather than immigrants (Stauffer, 1995). The difference between these two categories is that refugees migrate because of fear of persecution and often have had very traumatic experiences in their native country and in their migration to the United States. Immigrants, in contrast, migrate to the United States primarily because of economic or personal reasons. For example, Link and Dohrenwend (1980) found that in their large sample of Southeast Asian refugees, respondents reported levels of severe distress that were three times greater than that found among the American population in general.

A common way of coping with interpersonal and intrapersonal stress and conflict is through somatization (Hong, Lee, & Lorenzo, 1995). Psychosomatic problems are cited widely as a common way of seeking help. Because suppression of emotions is emphasized, however, there may be silent forbearance of one's suffering and pain (Morrow, 1987).

▶ INFLUENCE OF ACCULTURATION ON FAMILY STRUCTURE AND FUNCTIONS

As succeeding generations of Asian-Americans became more acculturated, family structural and functional patterns correspondingly change. Moreover, Asian-American families, in response to both structural factors in society, such as immigration policies, and racism, continually undergo change. In spite of the growth in acculturation with each succeeding generation, a dominant theme in the literature is the dynamic tension that exists between Eastern tradition and Western modernity (Hong, 1996; Hong & Ham, 1994; Mirandé, 1991).

Gender roles are changing rapidly as women join the workforce and are exposed to American core values and life. With increased labor force participation, Asian-American women's power in the family also increases and correspondingly, the husband's dominance diminishes. Research, however, still demonstrates systematic cultural biases favoring males (Pedersen et al., 1996).

A study conducted by Huang and Ying (1989) provides evidence of the types of gender role changes occurring in families. They found that among more acculturated Korean-American families, gender-specific differences in child-rearing were not so glaring as in the past. They reported that in their sample, most Korean-American fathers were helping with child rearing, an "unknown" practice in the past. Moreover, in acculturated Asian-American families, the researchers speculated that even though the husband-father may still be the family spokesperson and leader in public, behind the scenes the wife often has considerable decision-making power (Huang & Ying, 1989).

The role of the elder generation (the grandparents) in the Asian-American family is also changing with acculturation. Hong (1989) points out that grandparents, who are honored by virtue of their status, may have diminished say in family decision-making, especially when their children are financially independent.

The problem most discussed in the counseling literature about Asian-Americans is the effect of acculturation on the children of immigrant families and the resultant generational gap and conflict. The clash of values between parents who retain their traditional values and the children (particularly adolescents) who take on the American values of independence, individualism, and assertiveness, is a commonly cited problem that brings Asian-American children to the attention of school and community counselors (Hong, 1989, 1996; Hong & Ham, 1992; Pedersen et al., 1996). Conflict between parents and adolescents in Korean-American communities is a case in point. Here, according to Min (1995c), value conflicts, combined with a language barrier between immigrant parents who speak Korean and children who speak English, build dysfunctional distance between parents and their adolescent children. Adolescents who are having trouble coping at home often act out at school and in the community. School counselors working with Korean-American high school students in Los Angeles report that cutting class, skipping school, fighting, running away from home, and joining gangs are common problems of troubled Korean-American youth (Min, 1995c).

The concept of generational changes is important also when discussing acculturation. In the Japanese-American family literature, family life among third- and fourth-generation Japanese-American families is much more westernized. For example, the family patterns and marital division of work of the Sansei (third generation) very closely resemble the American pattern (Kitano, 1988). Moreover, fewer Japanese-American families are likely to hold traditional values because they have lived in the United States for so long (Uba, 1994).

▶ FAMILY NURSING PRACTICE IMPLICATIONS

Family Nursing Assessment

Two factors should be taken into consideration in assessing an Asian-American family. These factors are the family's culture and their environment (Hong, 1989).

Culture.   Culture, as a factor for assessment, pertains to the cultural issues relevant to a particular family. The family nurse needs to consider to what extent the characteristics of Asian families described in this chapter are applicable to this family. Also, to what extent does a family member, or the family as a whole, identify with their culture of origin or with mainstream American culture? Different families, as well as members within a family, may differ in their cultural identification. Rather than there being a discrete dichotomy between Asian and mainstream American cultures, a continuum exists with an infinite number of positions present which individuals and families may take.

Given the diversity in cultural identification, the family nurse should approach an Asian-American family with a flexible attitude and refrain from stereotyping. However, if the family nurse is unsure of how to approach the family in an interview, he or she should take a conservative approach and avoid going against the cultural norms such as ignoring the traditional family hierarchy or being confrontive.

In working with traditional Asian-American families, attempting to form an egalitarian partnership type of nurse–client relationship may not be most effective. The Asian-American client may feel more comfortable with a hierarchial relationship due to Asian norms of deference to authority and modesty with superiors (Marsella, 1993).

A cultural assessment also includes evaluating how strongly a family subscribes to traditional Asian health/medical practices versus Western practices. As mentioned earlier, it is common for immigrant Asian-Americans to subscribe to both forms of practices, and the practitioner must be sensitive to this. In fact, it is often necessary to ask a family whether they are trying any traditional Asian medical remedy. The family nurse should approach this issue in a respectful and understanding manner, rather than unwittingly hinting that Asian medical practices are nonmainstream, inferior, or unacceptable. If done properly, such a discussion will convey the nurse's cultural competence to the family, and will be a major contribution to the therapeutic alliance (Hong, 1993; Hong, Lee, & Lorenzo, 1995).

In working with a family, the family nurse should also be alert to the possible differences in cultural identification among family members, such as that between parents and children. In this situation, the nurse might, at times, defer to the cultural beliefs of the active decision-makers of the family. At other times, the nurse might have to identify the cultural conflict as an issue and help the family arrive at a consensus or compromise in planning interventions.

Environment.

Environment, as a factor for assessment, refers to the extent to which a family is encountering social/environmental problems. Is the family in financial hardship? Is an immigrant Asian-American family suffering from the loss of their traditional social support network, which was left behind in their country of origin? Are language and lack of familiarity with U.S. institutions interfering with their access to health services? For refugee Asian-Americans, to what degree is their past trauma affecting their current adjustment? An evaluation of these issues will be very useful in formulating realistic goals for working with the family.

In assessing an Asian-American family, the family nurse should be aware that many new immigrants are preoccupied with the tasks of basic survival. They have to adjust to a new social environment, settle in new jobs, new neighborhoods, make new friends, and develop a new social network. For some, it may take years, or even a lifetime, before they feel psychologically secure.

A serious health problem of a family member is a major burden for an immigrant family that is adjusting to a new environment. Some family members might try to deny or minimize the problem. Others may harbor repressed anger towards the person with the illness for bringing "additional trouble" upon the family. On the other hand, the person with the illness might experience feelings of guilt for "being the burden" (Hong, 1995). These are feelings that family nurses should carefully consider in their assessment.

Family nurses must be empathic to the obstacles refugee Asian-Americans have encountered before being allowed to enter the United States. Many refugee families may not want to attract any "government" attention again. They are often reluctant to discuss their family history or trauma with a stranger, especially one who is from a public or government agency. In these situations, the nurse needs to reassure the family before discussing any of these issues, and proceed slowly and sensitively.

Stephan Jiang (1995), Executive Director of the Association of Asian and Pacific Islanders Community Health Organization, sums up some of the key assess-

► TABLE 21–3

KEY QUESTIONS TO ASK ASIAN-AMERICAN CLIENTS AS PART OF HEALTH ASSESSMENT

- What language or languages do you speak?
- Do you use any traditional healing methods?
- How long have you and your family lived in this country?
- How do you identify your nationality and ethnicity?

Adapted from Jiang (1995).

ment issues by delineating several questions, which he recommends be part of a clinician's health assessment (Table 21–3). The answers to these key questions will help clinicians both to avoid stereotyping and to develop an individualized plan of care for Asian-American clients. He also suggests that when making recommendations for a particular health problem the client be asked, "Is that different from what you expect?" (p. 3).

Family Nursing Interventions

Based on the discussion in this chapter, the following are principles that will guide the formulation of culturally sensitive interventions for Asian-American families:

1. Given the family structure and hierarchy in Asian cultures, family nurses should be sensitive to the role and expectations of different family members, such as the authority of parents, especially the father. Extended family members, if available, might need to be involved along with the nuclear family. In addition, familism suggests that family members are likely to be more concerned with their mutual responsibilities than are typical mainstream American family members.

2. Considering the cultural norms governing communication and social interactions, family nurses should avoid direct confrontation with the family. In addition, they must be alert to the subtle, indirect messages sent by a client. A polite and mild disagreement from the client may actually mean a strong disagreement. When in doubt, clarify the communication in a nonthreatening manner.

3. Family nurses need to be sensitive to the stigma and shame often associated with chronic illness and mental disorder. They need to be empathic to the possible anger or guilt experienced by different family members who might feel that the illness is an "added" problem for an immigrant family that is already stressed by basic survival needs.

4. As research and clinical observations attest, many first-generation Asian-Americans follow both traditional Asian medical practices and Western medicine. This is especially true when families are dealing with a serious or chronic illness that Western medicine has little hope of curing. Family nurses should not interfere with these practices as long as they are not detrimental to the client or in conflict with the prescribed care. If unsure, consulting with practitioners who are familiar with the culture is often helpful.

5. Family health professionals need to be alert to the social/environmental problems and institutional barriers faced by less-acculturated Asian-American families. If a family needs to be referred to different agencies for service, there is a need for the family nurse to coordinate and streamline referral/intake procedures to minimize confusion and ensure compliance.

6. Family nurses should be sensitive to the trauma experienced by refugee Asian-Americans. This is a lifelong psychological burden for many families and individuals.

7. Last but not least, it is important to remember that Asian-Americans differ in their cultural practices. In addition, they differ in their identification with Asian and mainstream American cultures. Family nurses must avoid stereotyping a family. When in doubt about a cultural issue, discussing one's questions with the family itself or with professionals who are familiar with the culture is often critical to providing culturally competent family health care.

► study questions

1. What peoples constitute Asian-Americans?

2. What is the current demographic pattern with respect to Asian-Americans in the United States today?

3. Filipino-Americans differ from the other four largest groups of Asian-Americans in the following ways (indicate all correct answers):
   a. Their history includes about 500 years of Spanish colonization.
   b. Their country of origin is described as the most westernized in Asia.
   c. The majority of Filipinos are Catholic.

4. Select three core values of traditional Asian-American families and link a family nursing practice implication to each of these core values.

5. Describe the value clash that often occurs between children and their parents in Asian-American immigrant families.

6. When the Asian-American immigrant family settles in the United States, which of the following changes typically occur(s) in family life?
   a. Children work two jobs and often drop out of school early.
   b. Women enter the labor market and, because of their employment, have more power in the family.
   c. Patrilocality is often not possible or practical, so in these cases nuclear families live in separate households.

7. "Saving face" in Asian culture influences communication patterns in the following way(s):
   a. Communication is more indirect and subtle.
   b. Disagreements may be expressed in a circumventive manner.
   c. Communication is usually polite and respectful.
   d. Mistakes are never acknowledged or communicated.

8. Socialization of children in traditional Asian-American families, when compared with socialization in mainstream American families, involves:
   a. An emphasis on filial piety and veneration of age.
   b. Children are taught to be independent at an early age.
   c. The family exerts greater control over children's behavior.
   d. The importance of education is stressed in the family.

9. Which of the following are central tenets/key concepts in Eastern medicine?
   _____ Physical assessment.
   _____ Balance.
   _____ Holism.
   _____ *yin–yang*.
   _____ The value of mastery.

_____ Health promotion.
_____ Surgical intervention.
_____ Vital energy.
_____ Use of herbs.
_____ Psychotherapy.
_____ Talk therapy.

10. Which of the following family coping strategies would most likely be used among traditional Asian-American families?
    a. Self-reliance
    b. Use of humor in problem solving
    c. Seeking spiritual support
    d. Seeking social support from extended family network

11. Discuss three general intervention guidelines pertinent to working with traditional Asian-American families.

► chapter 21 study answers

1. Asian-Americans, also called Asian and Pacific Islanders, are people from countries and cultures in Asia, the Indian subcontinent, and the Pacific Ocean islands, including Somoa and Hawaii. The three largest Asian-American population groups in the United States are Chinese-Americans, Filipino-Americans, and Japanese-Americans (Asian Indians outnumber Korean- and Vietnamese-Americans).

2. Changing demographic pattern: Asian-Americans are proportionally the fastest-growing ethnic minority group in the United States.
   Current population figures: Asian-Americans constitute nearly 3 percent of the U.S. population.

3. All (a, b, and c).

4. Refer to Table 21–2. Depending on the values selected, many practice implications can be identified.

5. The value clash refers to the clash between traditional (Eastern) and modern (Western) values. Cultural conflicts are observed between parents and children. Children are socialized in U.S. schools to be independent, individualistic, and egalitarian in relationships. Immigrant parents were socialized in their native country to be deferent, interdependent, respectful of authority and parents, and familistic. Thus, conflict often ensues between the two generations.

6. b and c.

7. a, b, and c.

8. a, c, and d.

9. Balance, holism, *yin–yang*, health promotion, vital energy, use of herbs.

10. d.

11. Any of these guidelines are appropriate:
    - Be sensitive to family roles and expectations, e.g., family hierarchy.
    - Include relevant family members in health decisions.
    - Avoid direct confrontation with family.
    - Be sensitive to possible stigma and shame felt by family members when chronic illness and/or mental disorder is(are) present.
    - Do not interfere with family using Eastern medicine unless it is detrimental or in conflict with Western medical regimen.
    - Aid family in addressing their environmental stresses and problems, such as acting as advocate, coordinator, and referral agent for needed services.
    - Individualize care and do not come with preconceptions of what an Asian-American family is like.

The Friedman Family Assessment Model (Long Form)

The following guidelines represent a collation and abbreviation of the assessment questions/areas that appear at the end of Chapters 6 and 8 to 17, beginning with the assessment of identifying and environmental data, continuing through the assessment of structural and functional dimensions, and concluding with an assessment of family stress and coping. After each broad heading, a footnote alerts the reader as to where the related family theory and further discussion of assessment areas may be found.

The Friedman Family Assessment Model consists of six broad categories:

1. Identifying data
2. Developmental stage and history
3. Environmental data
4. Family structure
5. Family functions
6. Family stress and coping

Each category contains numerous subcategories. Nurses assessing families should decide which subcategories are particularly relevant (after a basic screening type assessment) so that these can be explored in more depth during family visits/encounters. Not all the subcategory assessment areas may need to be assessed—the depth and breadth of assessment is dependent on the family's goals, problems, and resources, as well as the nurse's role in working with the family.

▶ IDENTIFYING DATA

Foundational data that describe the family in basic terms are included in this section.

1. **Family Name**[1]
2. **Address and Phone**[1]
3. **Family Composition**[1]: To gather this information either a table such as Table A–1, or a family genogram (see Fig. 8–2), may be used. To use the table format, after the adult family members, record oldest child first, followed by each succeeding child in order of birth. Include any other related or nonrelated members of household next. If there are extended family members or friends who are considered to be family members, although not living in household, include them also at end of listing. The relationship of each family member to each other, as well as birthdate, birthplace, occupation, and education, should be specified.
4. **Type of Family Form**[1]
5. **Cultural (Ethnic) Background**[2] (including extent of acculturation): In describing this, use the following criteria as guideposts for determining family's cultural and religious orientation and extent of acculturation.
   5.1. Family's or family members' stated ethnic background (self-identified)?

► TABLE A–1

FAMILY COMPOSITION FORM

Name (Last, First)	Gender	Relationship	Date/Place Of Birth	Occupation	Education
1. (Father)					
2. (Mother)					
3. (Oldest child)					
4.					
5.					
6.					
7.					
8.					

5.2. Language(s) spoken in home? Do all family members speak English?

5.3. Country of origin as well as length of time family has lived in the United States (what generation are family members, relative to their immigration status)?

5.4. The family's social network (from the same ethnic group)?

5.5. Family residence (part of an ethnically homogeneous neighborhood)?

5.6. Religious, social, cultural, recreational, and/or educational activities (are they within the family's cultural group)?

5.7. Dietary habits and dress (traditional or westernized?)

5.8. Home decor (signs of cultural influences)?

5.9. Presence of traditional or "modern" family roles and power structure?

5.10. The portion(s) of the community the family frequents—the family's territorial complex (is it within the ethnic community primarily)?

5.11. The family's use of health care services and practitioners. Does the family visit folk practitioners, engage in traditional folk health practices, or have traditional indigenous health beliefs?

6. **Religious Identification**

6.1. What is the family's religion?

6.2. Do family members differ in their religious beliefs and practices?

6.3. How actively involved is the family in a particular church, temple, or other religious organization?

6.4. What religious practices does the family engage in?

6.5. What religiously based beliefs or values appear central in the family's life?

7. **Social Class Status**[3] (based on occupation, education, and income):

Estimate the family's social class, based on the three above indicators.

Economic Status

Who is (are) the breadwinner(s) in the family?

Does the family receive any supplementary funds or assistance? If so, what are they (from where)?

Does family consider their income to be adequate? How does the family see itself managing financially?

Social Class Mobility[3]

8. **Family's Recreational or Leisure-time Activities**[4] Suggested assessment areas per-

what for fun

taining to the family recreational or leisure-time activities include:

8.1. Identifying the family's activities— what types and how often do these activities occur?

8.2. Listing the leisure-time activities of family subsystems (spouse subsystem; parent–child subsystems; and sibling subsystems).

8.3. Exploring the family members' feelings about the family's leisure-time/recreational activities.

▶ DEVELOPMENTAL STAGE AND HISTORY OF FAMILY[5]

9. Family's present developmental stage.

10. The extent to which the family is fulfilling the developmental tasks appropriate for the present developmental stage.

11. The family's history from inception through present day, including developmental history and unique health and health-related events and experiences (divorces, deaths, losses, etc.) that happened in the family's life.

12. Both parents' families of origin (what life in family of origin was like; past and present relations with parents of parents).

▶ ENVIRONMENTAL DATA[6]

Environmental data covers the family's universe—from consideration of the smallest area such as aspects of home to the larger community in which the family resides.

13. **Characteristics of Home**[6]

13.1. Describe the dwelling type (home, apartment, rooming house, etc.). Does family own or rent its home?

13.2. Describe the home's condition (both the interior and exterior of house). House interior would include number of rooms and types of rooms (living room, bedrooms, etc.), their use and how

they are furnished. What is the condition and adequacy of furniture? Is there adequate heating, ventilation, and lighting (artificial and daylight)? Are the floors, stairs, railings, and other structures in adequate condition?

13.3. In the kitchen, assess the water supply, sanitation, and the adequacy of refrigeration.

13.4. In bathrooms, observe sanitation, water supply, toilet facilities, presence of towels and soap. Do family members share towels? In bathtub, are there grab bars?

13.5. Assess the sleeping arrangements in the house. Are they adequate for family members, considering their age, relationships, and their special needs?

13.6. Observe the home's general state of cleanliness and sanitation. What are the family's hygiene and cleanliness practices? Are there any infestations of vermin (interior especially) and/or sanitation problems due to presence of pets?

13.7. Are there signs of flaking, old paint (possible source for lead poisoning) which young children might be exposed to?

13.8. Identify the family's territorial unit. Are they comfortable driving out of their neighborhood to use resources/services?

13.9. Evaluate the privacy arrangements and how the family feels about the adequacy of its privacy.

13.10. Evaluate the home's presence or absence of safety hazards.

13.11. Evaluate the adequacy of waste and garbage disposal.

13.12. Assess the family members' overall satisfaction/dissatisfaction with their housing arrangements. Does the family consider the home adequate for its needs?

14. **Characteristics of Neighborhood and Larger Community**[6]

14.1. What are the physical characteristics of the immediate neighborhood and the larger community?

Type of neighborhood/community (rural, urban, suburban, intercity).

Types of dwellings (residential, industrial, combined residential and small industry, agrarian) in neighborhood.

Condition of the dwellings and streets (well kept up, deteriorating, dilapidated, being revitalized).

Sanitation of streets, home (cleanliness, trash and garbage collected, etc.).

Problems with traffic congestion?

Presence and types of industry in neighborhood.

Are there air, noise, or water pollution problems?

14.2. What are the demographic characteristics of the neighborhood and community?

Social class and ethnic characteristics of residents.

Occupations and interests of families.

Density of population.

Recent changes in neighborhood/community demographically.

14.3. What health and other basic services and facilities are available in the neighborhood and community?

Marketing facilities (food, clothing, drug store, etc.).

Health agencies (clinics, hospital, emergency facilities).

Social service agencies (welfare, counseling, employment).

Laundromat services for those families in need.

Family's church or temple.

14.4. How accessible are the neighborhood and community schools and what is their condition? Are there busing and integration problems which affect the family?

14.5. Recreational facilities.

14.6. Availability of public transportation. How accessible (in terms of distance, suitability, hours, etc.) are these services and facilities to the family?

14.7. What is the incidence of crime in the neighborhood and community? Are there serious safety problems?

15. **Family's Geographical Mobility**[6]

15.1. How long has the family lived in the area?

15.2. What is the family's history of geographical mobility?

15.3. From where did the family move or migrate?

16. **Family's Associations and Transactions with Community**[6]

16.1. *Who* in the family uses *what* community services or is known to what agencies?

16.2. How frequently or to what extent do they use these services or facilities?

16.3. What is the family's territorial patterns–communities or areas frequented?

16.4. Is the family aware of community services relevant to its needs, such as transportation?

16.5. How does family feel about groups or organizations from whom it receives assistance or with whom it relates?

16.6. How does the family view its community?

17. **Family's Social Support System or Network**[7]:

Who helps family in time of need for assistance, support, counseling, family activities (babysitting, transportation, etc.)?

17.1. *Informal:* Family's ties with friends, neighbors, relatives (kin), social groups, employers, employees.

Who are they and what is the nature

of their relationship (the quality of the relationships)?

The family ecomap illustrated in Figure 8–4 is useful for assessing this area as it graphically depicts the family's relationships and interactions with its immediate environment. The family genogram (Fig. 8–2) also provides information on family social support.

17.2. *Formal:* Family's relationships with health care and related agencies.

▶ FAMILY STRUCTURE

18. **Communication Patterns**[8]

18.1. In observing the family as a whole and/or the family's set of relationships, how extensively are functional and dysfunctional communication used? Diagram or give examples of recurring patterns.

How firmly and clearly do the members state their needs and feelings?

To what extent do members use clarification and qualification in interacting?

Do members elicit and respond favorably to feedback or do they generally discourage feedback and exploration of an issue?

How well do members listen and attend when communicating?

Do members seek validation from one another?

To what degree do members use assumptions and judgmental statements in interaction?

Do members interact in an offensive manner to messages?

How frequently is disqualification utilized?

18.2 How are emotional (affective) messages conveyed in the family and within the family subsystems?

How frequently are these emotional messages conveyed?

What types of emotions are transmitted within the family subsystems? Are negative, positive, or both types of emotions transmitted?

18.3. What is the frequency and quality of communication within the communication network and familial sets of relationships?

Who talks to whom and in what usual manner?

What is the usual pattern of transmitting important messages? Does an intermediary exist?

Are messages sent that are appropriate for the developmental age of the members?

18.4. Are the majority of messages of family members congruent in content and instruction? (Include observations of nonverbal messages.) If not, who manifests what kind of incongruency?

18.5. What types of dysfunctional processes are seen in the family communication patterns?

18.6. What areas are closed off to discussion that are important issues to the family's wellness or adequate functioning?

18.7. How do the following factors influence family communication patterns:

- The context/situation.
- The family life cycle stage.
- The family's cultural background.
- Gender differences in family.
- Family form.
- Family's socioeconomic status.
- The family's unique miniculture.

19. **Power Structure**[9]

Power Outcomes

19.1. Who makes what decisions? Who has the last "say" or "who wins?"

19.2. How important are these decisions or issues to the family?

More specific questions might include: Who budgets, pays bills, decides how money is to be spent? Who decides on how to spend an evening or what friends or relatives to visit?

Who decides on changes in jobs or residence?

Who disciplines and decides on child's activities?

Decision-making Process

19.3. What specific techniques are utilized for making decisions in the family and to what extent are these utilized (e.g., consensus; accommodation-bargaining; compromising or coercion; de facto)? In other words, *how* does the family make its decisions?

Power Bases. The various bases or sources of power are legitimate power/authority and a variation of it, "helpless" power; referent power; expert power or resources power; reward power; coercive power; informational power (direct and indirect); affective power; and tension management power.

19.4. On what bases of power do the family members make their decisions?

Variables Affecting Family Power

19.5. Recognizing the existence of any of the following variables will help the assessor interpret family behavior from which family power can be assessed.
   •The family power hierarchy.
   •Type of family form.
   •Formation of coalition(s).
   •Family communication network.
   •Social class status.
   •Family life cycle stage.
   •Ethnic and religious background.
   •Situational contingencies.
   •Person variables (members' ages, gender, interpersonal skills).
   •Spouses' emotional interdependency and commitment to the marriage.

Overall Family System and Subsystem Power

19.6. From your assessment of all the above broad areas, are you able to deduce whether family power can be characterized as dominated by wife or husband, child, grandmother, etc.; egalitarian–syncratic or autonomic; leaderless or chaotic? The family power continuum can be used for a visual presentation of your analysis.

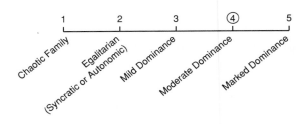

Family Power Continuum: If dominance is found, who is the dominant one?

19.7. To determine the overall power pattern, asking a broad, open-ended question is often illuminating (asking both spouses and children if feasible), examples of which are given below.

Who usually has "last say" or makes the decisions about important issues?

Who is really in charge and why (getting at bases for power)?

Who runs the family?

Who wins the important arguments or issues?

Who usually wins out if there is a disagreement?

Who gets his or her way when parents/spouses disagree?

Are family members satisfied with how decisions are made and with who makes them (i.e., the present power structure)?

20. **Role Structure**[10]

Formal Role Structure

20.1. What formal positions and roles do each of the family members fulfill? Describe how each family member carries out his or her formal roles.

20.2. Are these roles acceptable and consistent with family members' expectations? In other words, do role strain or role conflict exist?

20.3. How competently do members feel they perform their respective roles?

20.4. Is there flexibility in roles when needed?

Informal Role Structure

20.5. What informal or covert roles exist in family? Who plays them and how frequently or consistently are they enacted? Are members of the family covertly playing roles different from those which their position in the family demands that they play?

20.6. What purpose does the presence of the identified covert or informal role(s) serve?

20.7. Are any of the informal roles dysfunctional to the family or family members in the long run?

20.8. What is the impact on the person(s) who play this (these) role(s)?

Analysis of Role Models (when role problems are present)

20.9. Who were (or are) the models that influenced a family member(s) in his or her early life, who gave him or her the feelings and values about growth, new experiences, roles, communication techniques?

20.10. Who specifically acted as role model for the mates in their roles as parents, and as marital partners, and what were they like?

20.11. If the informal roles are dysfunctional in the family, who enacted these roles in previous generations?

Variables Affecting Role Structure

20.12. Social class influences: How does social class background influence the formal and informal role structure in the family?

20.13. Cultural influences: How is the family's role structure influenced by the family's ethnic and religious background?

20.14. Developmental or life cycle stage influences: Are the present role behaviors of family members developmentally appropriate?

20.15. Situational events: Changes in family member's health status. How have health problems affected family roles? What reallocation of roles/tasks have occurred? How have family members who have assumed new roles adjusted? Any evidence of role stress or role conflicts? How has the family member with the health problem reacted to his or her change or loss of role(s)?

21. **Family Values**[11]

21.1. Use of "compare and contrast" method is suggested (with values of either dominant culture, family's reference group—ethnic group with whom they identify—or both).

American Core Values/Family Values
Productivity
Work ethic
Materialism
Individualism
Education
Consumption ethic
Progress and mastery over environment
Future time orientation
Efficiency, orderliness, practicality
Rationality
Democracy, equality, and freedom
"Doing orientation"
Patriarchal authority
The family's interests
The family as a haven
Health

21.2. Is there congruence between the family's values and the family's reference group and/or the wider community?

21.3. Is there congruence between the family's values and each family members' values?

21.4. How important are these identified values to the family?

21.5. Are these values consciously or unconsciously held?

21.6. Are there any value conflicts evident within the family itself?

21.7. How does the family's social class, ethnic background, degree of acculturation, generational differences, and geographical setting (urban, suburban, or rural) influence its values?

21.8. How do the family's values affect family health status?

▶ FAMILY FUNCTIONS

22. Affective Function[12]
Family Need–Response Patterns

22.1. To what extent do family members perceive the needs of the other individuals in the family?
Are parents (spouses) able to describe their children's and mate's needs and concerns?
How sensitive are family members in picking up cues regarding other's feelings and needs?

22.2. Are each member's needs, interests, differentness respected by the other family members?
Does a mutual respect balance exist (do they show mutual respect toward each other)?
How sensitive is the family to each individual's actions and concerns?

22.3. To what extent are the recognized needs of the family members being met by the family? What is the process for emotional release (unburdening) in the family? For questions 22.1, 22.2, and 22.3, it is suggested that a list of the family members be included with their needs (as perceived by family members) and the extent to which these needs are being met by the family.

Mutual Nurturance, Closeness, and Identification

22.4. To what extent do family members provide mutual nurturance and support to each other?

22.5. Is a sense of closeness and intimacy present among the sets of relationships within the family?
How well do family members get along with each other?
Do they show affection toward each other?

22.6. Does mutual identification, bonding, or attachment appear to be present? (Empathetic statements, concerns about other's feelings, experiences, and hardships are all indicative.) To answer questions 22.4, 22.5, and 22.6, an attachment diagram is very helpful (see Fig. 14–1).

Separateness and Connectedness

22.7. How does the family deal with the issues of separateness and connectedness?
How does the family help its members want to be together and maintain cohesiveness (connectedness)?
Are opportunities for developing separateness available and are they appropriate for the age and needs of each of the family members?

23. Socialization Function[13]

23.1. Assess family's child-rearing practices in the following areas.
• Behavior control, including discipline, reward and punishment.
• Autonomy and dependency.
• Giving and receiving of love.
• Training for age-appropriate behavior (social, physical, emotional, language, and intellectual development).

23.2. How adaptive are the family's child-rearing practices for its particular family form and situation?

23.3. Who assumes responsibility for the child-care role or socialization function? Is this function shared? If so, how is this managed?

23.4. How are the children regarded in this family?

23.5. What cultural beliefs influence the family's child-rearing patterns?

23.6. How do social class factors influence child-rearing patterns?

23.7. Is this a family that is at high risk for child-rearing problems? If so, what factors place the family at risk?

23.8. Is the home environment adequate for children's needs to play (appropriate to children's developmental stage)? Are age-appropriate play equipment/toys present?

24. **Health Care Function**[14]

24.1. Family's health beliefs, values, and behaviors:
What value does the family assign health? Health promotion? Prevention?
Is there consistency between family health values as stated and their health actions?
What health-promoting activities does the family engage in regularly? Are these behaviors characteristic of all family members or are patterns of health-promoting behavior highly variable among family members?
What are the family's health goals?

24.2. Family's definition of health–illness and their level of knowledge:
How does the family define health and illness for each family member? What clues provide this impression, and who decides?
Can the family observe and report significant symptoms and changes?
What are the family members' sources of health information and health advice?

How is health information and advice transmitted to family members?

24.3. Family's perceived health status and illness susceptibility:
How does the family assess its present health status?
What present health problems are identified by the family?
To what serious health problems do family members perceive themselves vulnerable?
What are the family's perceptions of how much control over health they have by taking appropriate health actions?

24.4. Family dietary practices:
Does the family know food sources from the food guide pyramid?
Is the family diet adequate? (A 3-day food history record of family eating patterns is recommended.)
Who is responsible for the planning, shopping, and preparation of meals?
How are the foods prepared?
How many meals are consumed per day?
Are there budgeting limitations? Food stamps usage?
What is the adequacy of storage and refrigeration?
Does mealtime serve a particular function for the family?
What is the family's attitude toward food and mealtimes?
What are the family's snack habits?

24.5. Sleep and rest habits:
What are the usual sleeping habits of family members?
Are family members meeting sleep requirements appropriate for their age and health status?
Are regular hours established for sleeping?
Do family members take regular naps or have other means of resting during the day?

Who decides when children go to sleep?

Where do family members sleep?

24.6. Physical activity and recreation:

Are family members aware that active recreation and regular aerobic exercise are necessary for good health?

What types of recreational and physical activities do family members engage in regularly? Are these activity patterns representative of all family members or only certain members?

Do usual daily work activities allow for physical activity?

24.7. Family drug habits:

What is the family's use of alcohol, tobacco, coffee, cola, or tea?

Do family members take drugs for recreational purposes?

How long has (have) family member(s) been using alcohol or other recreational drugs?

Is the use of tobacco, alcohol, or prescribed/illicit drugs by family members perceived as a problem?

Does the use of alcohol or other drugs interfere with the capacity to carry out usual activities?

Do family members regularly use over-the-counter or prescription drugs? Does the family save drugs over a long period of time and reuse?

Are drugs properly labeled and in a safe place away from young children?

24.8. Family's role in self-care practices:

What does the family do to improve its health status?

What does the family do to prevent illness/disease?

Who is (are) the health leader(s) in the family? Who makes the health decisions in the family?

What does the family do to care for health problems and illnesses in the home?

How competent is the family in self-care relative to recognition of signs and symptoms, diagnosis, and home treatment of common, simple health problems?

What are the family's values, attitudes, and beliefs regarding home care?

24.9. Medically based preventive measures:

What are the family's history and feelings about having physicals when well?

When were the last eye and hearing examinations?

What is the immunization status of family members?

24.10. Dental health practices:

Do family members use fluoridated water, or is a daily fluoride supplement prescribed for the children?

What are the family's oral hygiene habits in regard to brushing and flossing after meals?

What are the family's patterns of simple sugar and starch intake?

Do family members receive regular preventive professional dental care including education, periodic x-rays, cleaning, repair, and (for children) topical or oral fluoride?

24.11. Family health history:

What is the overall health of family members of origin and marriage (grandparents, parents, aunts, uncles, cousins, siblings, and offspring) over three generations? Establish whether there is presently or in the past a history of genetic or familial diseases—diabetes, heart disease, high blood pressure, stroke, cancer, gout, kidney disease, thyroid disease, asthma and other allergic states, blood diseases, or any other familial diseases.

Is there a family history of psychiatric or emotional problems or suicide?

Are there any present or past environmentally related family diseases?

24.12. Health care services received:

From what health care practitioner(s) and/or health care agency(ies) do the family members receive care?

Does provider(s) or agency(ies) see all members of the family and take care of all their health care needs?

24.13. Feelings and perceptions regarding health care services:

What are the family's feelings about the kinds of health care services available to it in the community?

What are the family's feelings and perceptions regarding the health care services it receives?

Is the family comfortable, satisfied, and confident with the care received from its health care providers?

Does the family have any past experience with family health nursing services? What are the family's attitudes and expectations of the role of the nurse?

24.14. Emergency health services:

Does the agency or physician the family receives care from have an emergency service?

Are medical services by current health providers available if an emergency occurs?

If emergency services are not available, does the family know where the closest available (according to their eligibility) emergency services are for both the children and adults in the family?

Does the family know how to call for an ambulance and for paramedic services?

Does the family have an emergency health plan?

24.15. Source of payment:

How does the family pay for services it receives?

Does the family have a private health insurance plan, Medicare, or Medicaid; or must the family pay for services fully or partially?

Does the family receive any free services (or know about those for which it is eligible)?

What effect does the cost of health care have on the family's utilization of health services?

If the family has health insurance (private, Medicare, and/or Medicaid), is the family informed about what services are covered, such as extent of coverage for preventive services, special medical equipment, home visits?

24.16. Logistics of receiving care:

How far away are health care facilities from the family's home?

What modes of transportation does the family use to get to them?

If the family must depend on public transportation, what problems exist in regard to hours of service and travel time to health care facilities?

▶ FAMILY STRESS AND COPING[15]

25. **Stressors and Strengths:** What stressors (both long- and short-term and socioeconomic and environmental) are being experienced by the family?

Are you able to estimate the duration and strength of the family's stressors?

What strengths counterbalance these stressors?

Is the family able to handle the usual stresses and strains of daily life?

26. Is the family able to act based on a realistic and objective appraisal of the stressful situation?

27. **Coping Strategies:** How does the family react to stressful situations (what coping strategies are used)?

What coping strategies has the family employed to deal with what types of problems?

Do family members differ in their ways of coping with their present problem? If so, how?

What are the family's inner coping strategies?

Family group-reliance.

Use of humor.

Sharing of feelings, thoughts, and activities (maintaining cohesiveness).

Controlling the meaning of the problem/reframing.

Joint problem solving. (What are problem-solving abilities of various family members?)

Role flexibility.

Normalizing.

What are the family's external coping strategies?

Seeking and using of information.

Maintaining linkages with the broader community (general external involvement).

Seeking social support (both formal and informal support systems).

Seeking spiritual support.

28. What dysfunctional adaptive strategies has the family used or is the family using? If there are signs of any of the following dysfunctionalities, record their presence and how extensively they are used:

- Scapegoating.
- Use of threat.
- Family myth.
- Triangling.
- Pseudomutuality.
- Authoritarianism (submission to marked dominance).
- Alcohol and/or drug abuse.
- Family violence (spouse, child, elder, parent, or sibling abuse).
- Child neglect.

▶ FOOTNOTES

1. Chapter 8.
2. Chapter 8.
3. Chapter 8.
4. Chapter 8.
5. Chapter 6.
6. Chapter 9.
7. Chapters 8 and 17.
8. Chapter 10.
9. Chapter 11.
10. Chapter 12.
11. Chapter 13.
12. Chapter 14.
13. Chapter 15.
14. Chapter 16.
15. Chapter 17.

B

The Friedman Family Assessment Model (Short Form)

The following form is shortened for ease in assessing the O'Shea family (Appendix C) and other families. If you are not sure what data should be covered in each of the assessment areas below, please refer to Appendix A for the long form, where more detailed questions/areas are presented, or refer to the related chapters where both content and assessment areas are addressed.

Before using the following guidelines in completing family assessments, two words of caution are noted: First, not all areas included below will be germane for each of the families visited. The guidelines are comprehensive and allow depth when probing is necessary. The student should not feel that every subarea needs be covered when the broad area of inquiry poses no problems to the family or concern to the health worker. Second, by virtue of the interdependence of the family system, one will find unavoidable redundancy. For the sake of efficiency, the assessor should try not to repeat data, but to refer the reader back to sections where this information has already been described.

▶ IDENTIFYING DATA

1. **Family Name**
2. **Address and Phone**
3. **Family Composition**

See Table B–1 or Figures 8–1 and 8–2 (family genogram).

4. **Type of Family Form**
5. **Cultural (Ethnic) Background**
6. **Religious Identification**
7. **Social Class Status**
8. **Family's Recreational or Leisure-time Activities**

▶ DEVELOPMENTAL STAGE AND HISTORY OF FAMILY

9. **Family's Present Developmental Stage**
10. **Extent of Family Developmental Tasks Fulfillment**
11. **Nuclear Family History**
12. **History of Family of Origin of Both Parents**

▶ ENVIRONMENTAL DATA

13. **Characteristics of Home**
14. **Characteristics of Neighborhood and Larger Community**
15. **Family's Geographical Mobility**
16. **Family's Associations and Transactions With Community**

▶ TABLE B–1

FAMILY COMPOSITION FORM

Name (Last, First)	Gender	Relationship	Date/Place Of Birth	Occupation	Education
1. (Father)					
2. (Mother)					
3. (Oldest child)					
4.					
5.					
6.					
7.					
8.					

17. **Family's Social Support System or Network**
Ecomap, Figure 8–4, is helpful here. Family Genogram, Figure 8–2, is also useful here.

▶ FAMILY STRUCTURE

18. **Communication Patterns**
Extent of Functional and Dysfunctional Communication (types of recurring patterns)
Extent of Emotional (Affective) Messages and How Expressed
Characteristics of Communication Within Family Subsystems
Extent of Congruent and Incongruent Messages
Types of Dysfunctional Communication Processes Seen in Family
Areas of Open and Closed Communication
Familial and Contextual Variables Affecting Communication

19. **Power Structure**
Power Outcomes
Decision-making Process
Power Bases
Variables Affecting Family Power
Overall Family System and Subsystem Power
(Family Power Continuum Placement)

20. **Role Structure**
Formal Role Structure

Informal Role Structure
Analysis of Role Models (optional)
Variables Affecting Role Structure

21. **Family Values**
Compare the family to American or family's reference group values and/or identify important family values and their importance (priority) in family.
Congruence Between the Family's Values and the Family's Reference Group or Wider Community
Congruence Between the Family's Values and Family Member's Values
Variables Influencing Family Values
Values Consciously or Unconsciously Held
Presence of Value Conflicts in Family
Effect of the Above Values and Value Conflicts on Health Status of Family

▶ FAMILY FUNCTIONS

22. **Affective Function**
Family's Need–Response Patterns
Mutual Nurturance, Closeness, and Identification
Family attachment diagram, Figure 14–1, is helpful here.
Separateness and Connectedness

23. **Socialization Function**
Family Child-rearing Practices

Adaptability of Child-rearing Practices for Family Form and Family's Situation

Who Is (Are) Socializing Agent(s) for Child(ren)?

Value of Children in Family

Cultural Beliefs That Influence Family's Child-rearing Patterns

Social Class Influence on Child-Rearing Patterns

Estimation About Whether Family Is at Risk for Child-rearing Problems and If So, Indication of High Risk Factors

Adequacy of Home Environment for Children's Needs to Play

24. **Health Care Function**

Family's Health Beliefs, Values, and Behavior

Family's Definitions of Health–Illness and Their Level of Knowledge

Family's Perceived Health Status and Illness Susceptibility

Family's Dietary Practices

Adequacy of family diet (recommended 3-day food history record).

Function of mealtimes and attitudes toward food and mealtimes.

Shopping (and its planning) practices.

Person(s) responsible for planning, shopping, and preparation of meals.

Sleep and Rest Habits

Physical Activity and Recreation Practices (not covered earlier)

Family's Drug Habits

Family's Role in Self-care Practices

Medically Based Preventive Measures (physicals, eye and hearing tests, and immunizations)

Dental Health Practices

Family Health History (both general and specific diseases—environmentally and genetically related)

Health Care Services Received

Feelings and Perceptions Regarding Health Services

Emergency Health Services

Source of Payments for Health and Other Services

Logistics of Receiving Care

▶ FAMILY STRESS AND COPING

25. **Short- and Long-term Familial Stressors and Strengths**

26. **Extent of Family's Ability to Respond, Based on Objective Appraisal of Stress-producing Situations**

27. **Coping Strategies Utilized** (present/past)

    Differences in family members' ways of coping

    Family's inner coping strategies

    Family's external coping strategies

28. **Dysfunctional Adaptive Strategies Utilized** (present/past; extent of useage)

Case Study of the O'Shea Family*

The O'Shea family was referred to the community health nurse, Ms. Bell, by the county hospital's maternity service for the following reasons. "Mrs. O'Shea has expressed the desire to learn about family planning. She also needs a referral for postpartum and well-baby care." The following information was included in the referral: Mary—age 35; gravida VII, para V, miscarriages II. Delivered newborn son, Daniel—born 11/3 (5 days ago); birth weight—7 lbs, 2 oz; length—19 inches; hypertension during pregnancy; normal labor and delivery; mother's postpartum status and stay was normal, bonding well with infant.

▶ FIRST HOME VISIT

During Ms. Bell's first home visit, the father and two oldest children were at work and school. From her conversation with the mother and her observations of the home and family members, the following family data were obtained from the nurse's notes. Family: Patrick, father—age 43; Mary, mother—age 35 (looks older, tired, and overweight); Joseph, son—age 6; Maureen, daughter—age 5; Betty, daughter—age 4; Richard, son—age 3; and Daniel, son—age 1 week. Pat works as a butcher in his father's small grocery store located in same neighborhood a mile away from home. Mary's parents are Kate

(mother), age 70, in good health; and Bill (father), who died 2 years ago from heart problems. Patrick's parents are Marian (mother), age 72, who has osteoarthritis of hips and spine; and Pat (father), age 78, who suffers from back problems due to all the lifting he's done in the grocery business.

The family lives in an older wooden, three-bedroom flat in the Maplewood district—an Irish neighborhood—located 5 miles from a New England city with a population of 300,000. The immediate neighborhood is ethnically and socially homogeneous (working class) and residential, although located very near to a heavily industrialized factory district.

The family's home is rented from a cousin for $800 per month and is sparsely furnished, with a minimum of furniture in each room. The kitchen is clean, containing a small refrigerator and stove. There is one bathroom with toilet and bathtub. The parents have their own room, which they presently share with the newborn (who has a new bassinet the women's group at the parish donated). The girls, Maureen and Betty, have their own bedroom with a double bed, while the boys share the other bedroom, having twin beds and a small chest of drawers. A few area carpets are noted, but few decorations—with the exception of the children's school photos and a photo of the Irish coast on the living room wall and Catholic religious articles in the parent's room and dining room. Curtains matching the tablecloth hung in the

---

* Genevieve Monahan revised Appendix C for the third edition.

dining room, a wedding gift from Mary's mother to them when they were married. A color television set was the centerpiece of the living room. The mother said the home was adequate for their needs, although it was getting smaller with the arrival of another baby.

The outside of the house needs painting but was not cluttered and in fair repair. It was noted, however, that the stairs leading up to the front porch were loose, and there was no railing or lighting. A few children's toys were scattered around the backyard.

Mary was talkative and responsive to questions. When Ms. Bell explained that she had come because of a referral from the county hospital where Mrs. O'Shea had delivered her last baby, Mary was pleased that the nurse had been contacted to visit her. She offered the nurse a cup of coffee as they talked in the living room.

NURSE: How are you managing since you have been home from the hospital with your new baby?

MARY: Not too bad, but it sure is harder with five than with four, and being older doesn't help. I just don't have the energy to get up at night and feed Daniel.

NURSE: What kinds of help are you getting?

MARY: My mother came over the first day I was home and Pat's mother came over 2 days ago. They helped by cooking and cleaning up the house a little, and looking after the children. I also have a sister nearby who goes shopping for me sometimes.

NURSE: Anyone else?

MARY: No, that's about it, except for a neighbor and the women from my church, who told me to call if I needed anything. But I wouldn't want to bother them.

NURSE: What about your husband?

MARY: Pat helps a bit with the children, especially with getting them into bed at night. It's hard for him to do much

more than that after working all day. Besides, he's pretty conservative and still holds to women being in charge when it comes to taking care of the children. He thinks that if I do need more help it should come from my mother or sister. Pat would usually rather spend his free time playing football or meeting his friends for a beer at the local bar.

NURSE: Is this the way it's been with the other children too—you handling most things by yourself?

MARY: Yes, I'll just have to "offer it up" to the Lord.

NURSE: How have you managed to keep everything going?

MARY: I'm pretty well organized, and I learned quite a bit from my mother about managing a household.

NURSE: Have you found ways to save your energy?

MARY: Mainly it's a question of sleeping when the baby does, letting the other kids watch TV, and not worrying about the housecleaning.

NURSE: Sounds like a good list of priorities. Your health, children, and baby are certainly more important than housework. Is there anything that is important and needs doing that you can't handle?

MARY: Nothing immediately—my family lives here and they help—but I am very worried about getting pregnant again and having more children. I didn't think I would have the need to ask about family planning—I was planning for Richie to be my last. I had two miscarriages since him—1 and 2 years ago—and the doctors told me that I definitely shouldn't have any more children because my blood pressure gets so high. I discussed the problem with our priest, who then spoke to my husband about the rhythm method, but I guess he didn't get the right instructions. Since then, my girlfriends tell me that's not a very good method anyway.

NURSE: So you and your husband have decided not to have more children?

MARY: I'm not sure how Pat feels about it. I told him just yesterday that this was the end of kids for me, and he just looked and listened without a comment—and then just walked into the kitchen and got himself a beer. I can't talk to that man—that's the problem! When he has something on his mind, he sure lets me hear about it. But when I'm talking it's like I'm nagging or like it's not any of his concern.

I think he's torn because he knows how hard our lives would be if we have more, but he's a very devout man and really follows the teaching of the church on this. I'm not sure what he'll say in the end.

NURSE: Would you be willing to tell me a bit more about your marriage?

MARY: Well, we were married when I was 28 and he was 36. I guess that's been 7 years. As you can see, babies started coming pretty quickly after that—one a year until now, including the two miscarriages. We both knew each other from the parish and our parents both live in the neighborhood. We both graduated from Catholic high schools in the neighborhood. After high school Pat went to work in his father's grocery store, was in the service for 3 years, and then when his older brother stopped working for his father, Pat got the job of being butcher in the store—been doing that for his father 4 years now. I worked as a clerk in an electronics factory before we got married. I really liked it there and made a lot of friends at the factory.

I started seeing Pat 3 years after I finished high school, and we went together 5½ years before he asked me to marry him. I was afraid I was going to be an old maid like some of my friends were. Sure was a lot easier being single though, but my family and friends were always hinting and pressuring me to "tie the noose around Patrick."

NURSE: Overall, how would you describe your marriage to Pat?

MARY: Hard work a lot of the time. I always feel like I'm really working at getting along and keeping things on an even keel.

NURSE: Has it always been that way? What was it like in the beginning and after the children came?

MARY: (looking at the nurse with a tired, disappointed expression on her face, and sadness in her eyes): I think our marriage started out all wrong—not that it was so different from any of my friends' and cousins' or sisters' marriages—but it was just not like the marriages I read about in the papers and magazines and see on television. I was raised a strict Catholic, in an Irish school and parish. My grandparents came over from Ireland during the depression. Pat's folks also are Irish, and his father came over here as a teenager and worked in construction until he could save enough to buy a small grocery store—the one he has now. We didn't know much about sex except what we heard from our friends. Our parents never mentioned it, and the nuns certainly never brought it up. Things have changed a lot since then. But we were raised in a time when you didn't have relations until your wedding night. I'm ashamed to say this, but I never really liked having sex that much. It hasn't been the way I thought it would be when I was young. Pat seems to enjoy it pretty well, though I'm not sure.

NURSE: Have you ever discussed it with him?

MARY: Not really. Every time I try I get mortified and then worry that I would hurt his feelings if I told him. Besides, what good would it do?

NURSE: Do you ever talk to your sisters, mother, or friends about it?

MARY: Only my sister and one girlfriend, and they both have the same frustrations. My sister tells me that there are books you can read to make sex more pleasurable—but it seems unnatural to make a study of it like that. Besides, one of the first things I ever learned about it was from my friend's mother, who said it was something you just put up with in marriage.

We used to go out to the movies or friends' homes together—and talk more. But, after the children came we grew apart. Don't misunderstand me, we wanted the children and were happy to see them born, but somehow the demands in raising them caused problems between us. Now we don't talk much, except about the children and money problems—we're always just barely making it through the month. Pat spends more and more time with the boys. You know, going to football, baseball, and basketball games or spending time at the bar. And when he's home, he's really not home. I can't get him to do anything around the house. When I ask him to do something he looks at me as if I'm imposing on him and I'm making his life difficult. When I try to talk to him about problems, he'll say: "Don't bother me with that now. Can't you see that I'm tired. I'll do something about it tomorrow." And tomorrow never comes.

NURSE: I appreciate your sharing so much about your concerns and experience with Pat and the children. You mentioned feeling a little overwhelmed since Daniel's birth and worried about finances. You told me that you've decided that you don't want any more children, and it sounds like you wish that your relationship with Pat was closer, like when you were first married. I would like to offer my support and information, and to work together with you to look at options you have for your concerns.

Ms. Bell then outlined ways that she could help Mary, and asked Mary which problem bothered her most. She then asked permission to make another home visit to meet the rest of the family.

The first visit also consisted of discussing the newborn, Daniel, and Mary's physical health status. Ms. Bell planned to return in a week with information for her on clinic services for the baby and on family planning and postpartum care and follow-up.

▶ SECOND HOME VISIT

During the second home visit 1 week later, the nurse came at 3:30 P.M. when the children were home from school. Patrick was expected home for part of visit (he returned from work at 4:00 P.M.). After discussing Mary's and Daniel's health and giving Mary appointments for the baby clinic and Mary's postpartum examination at the local health center, the nurse spoke briefly about family planning and asked Mary if she felt that this could be discussed with her husband. Mary agreed, although she did not seem sure about how her husband would react to a woman talking to him about such an intimate subject. However, when Ms. Bell suggested that this might be a way to help both of them talk more directly about this delicate subject, she seemed to reconsider her previous hesitancy and said she thought it would be a good idea.

Before talking with the parents about family planning, Ms. Bell asked them for a brief health history of each of the children and was able to observe and elicit data related to parent–child relationships, parenting roles, and child rearing. She noted that Mary was very warm and cuddly with newborn Daniel. Mary held him close, handled him gently, and appeared relaxed and confident in his care and sensitive to his basic needs. Pat, in contrast, looked proudly at Daniel, but did not hold him, and according to Mary did not get involved in his physical care (nor did he with any of the other children when they were babies).

Both mother and father were warm and Mary physically quite affectionate with Richard, age 3. She seemed quite indulgent with him, letting him "have his way" and giving him a lot of freedom to run around and play.

With the older children—Betty, 4; Maureen, 5; and Joseph, 6—there was not the same permissiveness as observed with Richard. Mary said, "They are older and so need to be more responsible." All three older children were fairly quiet around the nurse. They spoke when spoken to, but otherwise talked quietly with each other or listened. The parents agreed that Joseph is the mother's favorite, and said he is too serious and has problems handling himself sometimes, becoming bossy and wanting to take over. Betty was identified as the father's favorite, "since she is petite, very sweet, and looks like Pat's mother."

The parents believe in children behaving and showing respect for their elders and carrying out their responsibilities, even if at these ages they are not expected to do much. The father spanks the children with the palm of his hand on their buttocks if they misbehave. He explained by saying, "None of these newfangled ideas about disciplining for us." It was noticed that children were asked to do several things— pick up the toys from the floor and help their mother. Both Maureen and Betty acted immediately, while Joseph ignored and then refused until his father yelled at him. No positive reinforcement followed when the children did obey. Maureen and Betty seemed pleased to have a new baby brother, while Richard was jealous of the baby and has been more demanding since the baby's arrival. The parents understand, though, that he feels displaced and jealous and that he needs more parental attention during this time. Joseph states he does not like the new baby.

When asked about each of the children and what they were like, the mother led the conversation although the father chimed in about Joseph and Betty. The descriptions are given in Table C–1. Ms. Bell asked Mary to have the children play in another room and then raised the issue of family planning.

NURSE: Mary, would you be willing to share with Pat our discussion about family planning?

MARY: Yes. Like I tried to tell you Pat, I'm at the end of my rope. I don't want to get pregnant again and I want to look into some kind of family planning method.

NURSE: Pat, I'd like to know how you feel about this.

PAT: I was a little surprised she would bring this up with you, but since she did, I guess we can talk about it. I have felt that my wife is taking things in her own hands—complaining all the time about her life and seeing her job as such a burden. My mother had seven children, and I never heard her complain. It would be very difficult for us if we had another baby—but I can't see any way around it. If the good Lord wants her to have more, then I think she'll just have to accept them and manage with what we have.

NURSE: Does that mean that religiously you're against any form of family planning?

PAT: Well not exactly. I know that Catholics are not all of the same mind on this issue and that many of them do things to prevent pregnancy. I won't say that my mind is completely closed, but that I have serious questions about it. We tried that rhythm method, but it didn't seem to work.

NURSE: Mary, would you like to say something about this?

MARY: Well, I just can't go on like this. Something has got to be done. You ought to stay home some day, Pat,

► TABLE C–1

THE O'SHEA PARENTS' DESCRIPTIONS OF THEIR CHILDREN

	Mother's Description	Father's Description
Joseph, age 6	He's a bright, independent child. Joseph is the leader of the children at home and school and likes to take over. I try to give him some responsibilities for caring for his sisters and brothers, but have to watch that he doesn't get too bossy. I'm able to talk to Joseph more than the other children. He's a sensitive child and listens to me. I know I'm a little protective of him, but that's just because we're so close to each other.	Joseph is always arguing and wanting his own way. My wife spoils him. He's going to grow up thinking he'll be the President by the time he's 35. He needs to be put in his place by my wife.
Maureen, age 5	Maureen is a helpful child who likes to help me. She is an easy child to raise. She's quiet, likes to play alone, and doesn't cause any trouble. Maureen follows her brother Joseph all the time when they play together.	She's great fun.
Betty, age 4	Betty knows how to get people to like her. She's a "people pleaser"—can act cute and sweet when it is in her favor. She needs special watching, however, as she can pull the wool over one's eyes very quickly with her sweet and cunning ways.	The father acts disgusted with his wife's statement and responds by saying: "That's not true. She is a sweet, affectionate little sweetheart. You're just jealous because we have a special relationship."
Richard, age 3	He's always into everything! Very active and inquisitive. I try to let him have a lot of freedom to run around in the house, otherwise he gets so bottled up that he shouts, screams, and makes the rest of us miserable.	He's at the age where we really have to keep an eye on him.

and just see what raising this many kids is like.

PAT: But our mothers found a way to do it. . . .

MARY: Yes, but things are so much more expensive now, and they never had a choice, but I do. I would like to find out more about what is available and really look into family planning methods.

NURSE: Pat, what's the benefit you see in having more children? Your wife feels it's hard for her to manage now and that further pregnancies are dangerous for her.

PAT: I didn't say I wanted any more. I just said that she's pretty lucky and she doesn't know it. I suppose our family is big enough, but we can't depend on "Russian roulette," I mean the rhythm method, to solve our problem.

NURSE: Do you understand the problem your wife has in having more children now? I mean the hypertension during pregnancy, which has grown worse with each succeeding pregnancy?

PAT: Not really. (Nurse explains the problem and how pregnancy makes problem worse.)

Ms. Bell then asks the spouses if they have discussed their problem or family planning methods with their priest and family doctor, and then suggest that they do this together, because neither priest nor doctor has been approached to discuss the problem. She gives a basic overview of family planning methods that are available, including natural family planning, and gives them a booklet on family planning for more information. Ms. Bell acknowledges their progress in discussing a sensitive subject and encourages them to request further information as needed. She then asks permission to make a follow-up visit.

▶ THIRD HOME VISIT

As the spouses speak to each other and with the nurse, the nurse makes the following observations regarding Pat and the couple's relationship.

Pat seems easygoing, verbal, and quite a conversationalist—as long as he controls the flow. He likes to be the center of attention and loses interest if Mary is talking; in this case, jumping in to refocus attention on himself. He expresses an interest in getting some help for his wife from his mother, but feels that helping himself is "not his job." He says that Mary and his mother don't get along too well together, however, there being too much competition between the two of them. According to Mary, Pat's mother caused tremendous tension during their engagement and early years of marriage. She had bitter arguments with her husband about his mother, but as the mother-in-law finally began to accept the reality of her son's marriage, their problems subsided.

In terms of the marital relationship, there appeared to be no expression of love or affection either physically or verbally. Their relationship was characterized by a lack of empathy or two-way communication between them. One received the impression that Mary was there to meet the needs of her husband, but that he had no similar responsibility to her. Pat expected her to serve him, care for the home and children, and manage with the limited funds he allotted her weekly for groceries and other home and child expenses.

While Pat was present, Mary took little part in the discussions, except when asked direct questions. She acted very self-effacing and subservient in his presence, except when she voiced the opinion that he should spend time with the children to see what it was really like.

Pat did communicate to the children that they should have respect for Mary—because she was their mother. However, in his own communications with her, he did not express much respect. Most communications were in the form of commands, with few requests or room for feedback from his wife. When Mary spoke to him, he seemed to tune her out. Most of the time he halfheartedly agreed that she was right and that he would follow through on such matters as making appointments with the priest and the doctor, which he then failed to do.

The children and parents were quite talkative concerning the recent Thanksgiving holiday and other happy events. With pleasant subjects, all of the family contributed verbally to family conversations. Unpleasant subjects or angry statements were cut off, such as Joseph's reaction to the new baby, or minimized, such as the mother's feelings of being burdened by too many children. It was also noted that the children spoke directly to their mother, but only indirectly to their father. If they had a request, they would ask their mother to ask their father for permission.

When asked what activities the family engaged in together, Mary reported that family visiting is their most popular and frequent activity. "Movies and eating out are beyond our reach. I like taking the kids to the park, but Patrick doesn't like coming. I go to Mass regularly and so does Pat. We don't travel much—our close relatives live in town and we can't afford traveling much on Pat's salary. Pat's car isn't very dependable. Groceries, clothing, and the usual household items we buy at Pat's father's store. The shopping center is about a half-mile from here."

In terms of friendships, Mary states that she has a few old high school friends whom she still sees occasionally and that Pat sees his friends at sports events or the local bar. But Pat and Mary have no couple friends with whom they engage in social activities.

Ms. Bell asked the couple how they liked the community. Both the parents related that this was the only community and neighborhood they had ever lived in and said, "We like it here. We know where everything is. All of the storekeepers and neighbors are old friends and acquaintances." The family, having lived in the community for many years, was familiar with the community agencies, health centers, and private doctors in town. Up until recently, they used a nearby hospital for children's emergency care; and a family doctor, a general practitioner, for all the health care that they needed, such as maternity and pediatric care. But the parents did not go in for checkups (Pat never had a physical examination as far as Mary knew), although Mary did have a physical with each pregnancy. Children are only seen when they are sick, with the exception of well-baby care at the health center when they were infants and for immunizations during infancy and preschool periods.

Two months ago, Pat received group medical insurance through his father's store (the father just arranged for it), so their choice of health care was expanded. The family doctor is an older physician whom the family has seen for years. His charges are very low, but Mary feels he is getting too old to keep up with all he needs to know. She used the county hospital to deliver Daniel, because they were not covered by medical insurance at that time and could not raise the money for a private hospital. Now they will have to pay the county back in small payments until their bill is taken care of.

With their expanded health insurance benefits Mary and Pat asked for information regarding regular health care services they might be eligible for. After a bit of prodding from Mary, Pat asked how he might get a physical exam. He also expressed concern about his slow, but steady weight gain, or "gut" since he stopped playing sports.

Dental care for the family has been close to nonexistent. It is obtained at a private neighborhood dental clinic. The mother took Joseph in once when he complained of a toothache.

One of his baby teeth had to be filled. The other children have not been seen. Pat and Mary go in when they have problems, and brush their teeth twice a day after meals. Mary is teaching Joseph to brush his teeth now, too.

When Ms. Bell did a nutritional survey of the family, she found that their diet consisted of a lot of starches, mainly potatoes and breads primarily at every meal. Their diet was basically American, with certain Irish specialties included —stews and boiled dinners. The family made little use of fruit or fruit juices, except for bananas, apples when in season, and canned peaches— and occasionally apple or orange juice. One vegetable, in addition to potatoes, was usually eaten with the evening meal, and casseroles, stews, and processed food such as frozen dinners, pizza, chicken pies, and macaroni and cheese were frequently served for dinner. Salads were infrequently eaten; soups were served about every other night, especially in the colder months. The weights of the children were within normal limits, but both parents were 10 to 20 percent overweight (visually) for their height. There were no food allergies among any of the family members, according to their mother.

Their diet for yesterday (excluding Daniel) was:

Breakfast	Cold cereal and whole milk
	Toast—1 to 2 pieces for Joseph, Mary, and Pat
	Coffee—2 cups (parents)
Snacks	Crackers for children (3 to 4 apiece) and milk
	Coffee—mother
Lunch	Soup (tomato)
	Dish of mashed potatoes and butter
	Canned peaches
	Milk
	(Husband and Joseph not home)
Snacks	None
Dinner	Stew with meat (½ lb), carrots, potatoes, and celery
	White cake
	Milk—children
	Coffee—wife
	Beer—husband

Because having adequate money for food was mentioned as a monthly concern, Mary was asked whether she received food stamps. When she said she did not, information on the program was provided. The nurse also learned that the family had very little left over each month and that 2 years ago Pat borrowed $2000 from his father to buy a used car (without Mary's knowledge) and still had not been able to pay his father back.

With Ms. Bell's encouragement Mary discussed with Pat her desire to work part time to increase the family income. She mentioned that her mother and sister both offered to take care of the children so that she could do so. They agreed that along with family planning this would be an area for further discussion.

The family associates with several organizations in the community: the parish church and school primarily. The family can walk to both, because they are only five blocks away. The health department, the family doctor, and the family dental clinic are also visited. In addition, the bars Pat frequents, the stores they shop in, and Pat's father's grocery store are all community places and people with whom friendly ties exist. Mary makes all the contacts with church, school, dentist, and doctors. The family's relationships with church, teachers, doctor, health center, dentists, and emergency room seem to have been good. There is public transportation available when family needs it, but Mary drives Pat to work on days that she needs the car, because taking the children with her on the bus is not easy.

Stemming from Mary's extensive experience in raising children and taking them to doctors, she seems to have a good, basic understanding of how to handle common minor illness and injuries. She also is able to explain what to do when more serious injuries occur or symptoms appear. She uses over-the-counter medicines such as aspirin, Tylenol, first-aid medications, Sudafed, and milk of magnesia carefully and correctly and keeps medicines in a safe place out of the reach of the children.

Neither she nor her husband watch their diet or weight or engage in regular exercise. Although Mary was never active (except doing housework), Pat was very active in sports until recently. For relaxation Mary watches TV and thinks her husband uses TV and socializing at the bar as ways of relaxing.

When the initial family assessment was completed Ms. Bell discussed her observations with Mary to identify which issues or concerns she felt were most amenable to change and could be worked on by the entire family.

Appendix D presents a family assessment and family care plan for this family.

D

Family Nursing Process Example: The O'Shea Family*

1. **Family Name:** O'Shea.
2. **Address:** Maplewood district, New England city.
3. **Family Composition:** See Table D–1 and Figure D–1.
4. **Type of Family Form:** Two parent, intact nuclear.
5. **Cultural (Ethnic) Background:** The family is Irish-American and to a large extent unacculturated (Connery, 1968). This conclusion derives from Mary's clearly stated ethnic and religious preferences; the fact that family's social network is from the same ethnic/religious group; the family has resided in same ethnically homogeneous neighborhood for life; visits to extended family and church activities seem to be central activities; family roles and power structure are in keeping with traditional structures within Irish families; home decor is lacking of much visual art and the presence of religious objects is indicative of family's culture and religious orientation; and family stays primarily within ethnic neighborhood.
6. **Religious Identification:** Family actively involved in Catholic religious practices and belief system: attends Mass regularly, consults priest on matters of importance, belief in family and children stressed.

7. **Social Class Status:** Father is sole breadwinner.
   Economic status: Family sees its income as marginal; nevertheless, it is steady. Based on the father's occupation, income (estimated only), and education of parents, family is part of working class.
   Social mobility: The parents of the O'Sheas were poor, and thus Pat feels he, Mary, and the children are more fortunate. In fact, however, the family's history does not indicate much, if any, upward mobility. Actually, with more children the standard of living within their own nuclear family has probably declined.
8. **Family's Recreational or Leisure-time Activities:** Whole family visits extended families together (their most frequent family activity). Mother takes children to park to play. No travel, movies, or eating out because of finances and car's poor condition. Mary and Pat do not go out as couple by themselves or with friends.
9. **Family's Present Developmental Stage:** Family is in the stage of a family with school-aged children because of the age of the oldest child.
10. **Extent to Which Family Is Fulfilling Family Developmental Tasks:** Family appears to be meeting the family members needs for adequate housing, space, privacy, and safety.

---

* Genevieve Monahan revised Appendix D in the third edition.

► TABLE D–1

O'SHEA FAMILY COMPOSITION

Name	Gender	Relationship	Age	Place of Birth	Occupation	Education
O'Shea, Patrick	M	Father	43 years	Maplewood district	Butcher	High school graduate
O'Shea, Mary	F	Mother	35	Same	Housewife	High school graduate
O'Shea, Joseph	M	Son	6	Same	Student	In first grade
O'Shea, Maureen	F	Daughter	5	Same	Student	In kindergarten
O'Shea, Betty	F	Daughter	4	Same	—	—
O'Shea, Richard	M	Son	3	Same	—	—
O'Shea, Daniel	M	Son	5-day-old infant	Same	—	—

Mother is adequately socializing children (see discussion of socialization function). Mother feeling strained in attempting to integrate new child member into family due to her role overload.

Maintenance of satisfactory parent–child relationships, but decline in satisfaction by wife in marital relationship.

11. **Family's History:** Parents both lived in same neighborhood and went to same church. Went together 5½ years before marriage. During engagement and early years of marriage, sex was an uncomfortable area and later awkward and unsatisfying, reported the wife. Wife feels this has created a lack of closeness between them. Both parents expected children and wanted them, with the exception of the last, which Mary did not want but now accepts warmly.

12. **Parents' Families of Origin:** Father's family: Father came over from Ireland as teenager. Worked for construction companies and saved his money until he could buy the grocery store he now owns. Raised family in same neighborhood in a strict Catholic fashion. Mother's family: Her grandparents came over from Ireland

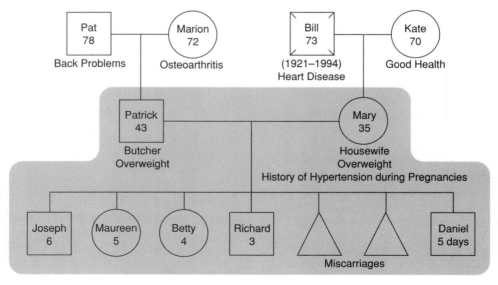

Figure D–1. O'Shea family genogram.

during the depression for economic reasons. Raised as Catholic in same neighborhood as family now resides. Both Mary's and Pat's families were mentioned as being poor while they were growing up. No mention of what life with their respective families of origin was like.

13. **Characteristics of Home:** Three-bedroom, older wooden house rented from cousin for $800 per month. Outside of house: fair condition, needs paint, loose stairs, and no outside lighting or railing present. Inside of house: minimally furnished. Living room has a color TV. Dining room has lace curtains and tablecloth, a wedding present from Mary's mother. Parents have own bedroom, presently shared with newborn who has a bassinet. The boys have one bedroom, while the girls share the other. Adequate sleeping arrangements in home. Minimal decorations, but several Catholic religious objects and photos of the children were noted. Kitchen contains small refrigerator and stove. One bathroom with toilet and bathtub. Common towels used. Mary considers the house just adequate for their needs now, but becoming more crowded because of the new baby. Safety hazards: outside loose stairs, no railings or outside light.

14. **Characteristics of Neighborhood and Larger Community:** Neighborhood (Maplewood district) is residential and composed of Irish working-class families. Neighborhood is near industrial area and 5 miles from center of city of 300,000 located in New England. Family likes closeness and familiarity of neighborhood, though worried about influx of members of minority groups nearby and rise in crime in the past several years. Family uses Pat's father's grocery store and a nearby shopping center (half mile away) for most of its shopping needs. Family's church and church school located five blocks away. Public transportation available, but Mary has access to husband's car when needed.

15. **Family's Geographical Mobility:** Family members have lived in the same community and neighborhood for all their lives.

16. **Family's Associations and Transactions With Community:** The family is known in parish church and school. Parents go to mass regularly and seem to have close trusting relationship with Father O'Neal. Women's group at church donated bassinet for new baby. Mother acts as liaison with school. Family also relates to the family doctor (although Mary wants to change physicians), family dental clinic, and children's hospital emergency room. In addition to receiving community health nursing visits, mother has taken children to well-baby clinic and for immunizations at the local health department. Family seems to stay primarily within its neighborhood.
Family not aware of food stamp program (which was explained to Mary).

17. **Family's Social Support Network**
Informal Systems
Family, especially parents on both sides and mother's sister, seem to be quite helpful. Pat's father employs son in his grocery store as butcher and loaned him $2000 for purchase of a car. Pat's mother helped with housework and children when Mary came home from hospital. (Although relations with wife were conflictual during early days of marriage, they are improved but still competitive, according to Pat.) Mary's mother also helped with house and children after Mary returned from hospital and Mary's sister went shopping for her. In addition to her sister, Mary has neighbors she talks to sometimes about her problems. And Pat has his buddies at the tavern that he relates to frequently (the degree of their support is unknown, however).
Formal Systems
Family has ties with priest, doctor, community health nurse, and teachers.

▶ FAMILY STRUCTURE

18. **Communication Patterns**
Extent of Functional and Dysfunctional Communication (types of recurring patterns):

Dysfunctional communication used between husband and wife.

a. Husband gives commands and makes requests without giving opportunity for feedback

b. Wife voices problems and husband minimizes them (does not validate or accept that her problems are real).

c. Wife voices concerns or asks husband's assistance, but he tunes her out, walks away, belittles her, or agrees with her and says he'll follow through, but does not (incongruency). Pat does not listen to Mary when she is communicating her needs to him.

d. Mary, in turn, does not express herself in some intimate areas due to cultural values and, possibly, fear of rejection. She probably does not directly express her needs in many areas.

e. Neither partner states needs and feelings clearly, except in case of Mary's expressed desire to curtail pregnancies.

f. Rules underlying communication patterns include the following: (1) don't question the status quo and tradition; (2) things are the way they are and complaining won't help or change things (powerless, fatalistic outlook); (3) closedness—husband doesn't want wife becoming exposed to any outside influences.

Extent of Affective Messages and How Expressed: Affective messages are not expressed openly (or privately according to Mary) between spouses. Mary is warm and affectively responsive to Daniel and Richard. She is also verbally warm and close to son Joseph. Father is verbally (and physically?) affectionate to daughter Betty. Pleasant emotions are more openly expressed, whereas negative emotions (anger, talk about unpleasant events) are inhibited. Evidently, family rules exist that prohibit expression of these latter emotions.

Characteristics of Family Communication Network: Children make requests of father through mother. Little direct involvement and communication between father and children (except Betty–father relationship). Quality of communication between spouses poor and limited in scope (mainly regarding children and money problems) and quality (see dysfunctional patterns). Interactions are distant and unsatisfying to wife.

Areas of Closed Communications: Between spouses: inner feelings and perceptions, especially sexual feelings and thoughts.

Familial and Contextual Variables Affecting Communication: Cultural variables are important for this family. Men and women live in different worlds in traditional Irish culture. Roles and worlds are separate, and sexes typically do not learn to communicate intimately with each other. Nor is expression of affection or warmth toward spouse seen as acceptable in public. Sex is riddled with guilt and ignorance, making it difficult for some Irish couples to generate and retain close affective bonds. Socioeconomic stressors (marginal incomes and economic hardships) make family role enactment, housing, and fulfilling of family functions more onerous.

19. **Power Structure**

Power Outcomes

Husband decides major purchases (car, for example).

Wife is delegated (or relegated) sole roles of housekeeper and child rearer, and allotted a certain portion of paycheck to cover home and family expenses.

Husband in charge of distribution of funds.

Husband in charge of calling priest and doctor to initiate appointment with them.

Decision-making Process: Husband uses his formal position of dominance to influence family decisions. Process used is accommodation. He seemed to be compromising with wife, under pressure of community health nurse, when he agreed to discuss family planning health problems with priest and doctor and attempt to come up with an effective plan to prevent further pregnancies; but because he has not followed through in making appointments, one can question his sincerity in this case. May use de facto process in these cases; by doing nothing he has made a decision.

Power Bases: Father-husband maintains legitimate power or authority, granted to him culturally by virtue of his position in family. Mother has referent power (position of mother is exalted in the Catholic Church), which is more salient in her relationships with her children than it is in her relationship with her husband. Both parents have reward and coercive power over children, and husband has reward/coercive power over his wife, although no description of his using this is evident.

Variables Affecting Family Power Characteristics: Wife's position as go-between in family communication network and as implementer of family decisions should give her increased power; there is no evidence that it is being exercised, however.

Interpersonal resources: The wife's hesitancy and fear to speak out more often and confront husband reduces what power she does/could have.

Social class/cultural and life cycle factors: Marital expectations that are commonly found in working class predominate. These same marital and family role and power expectations are characteristic of traditional Irish family life. Life cycle of family reduces wife's power and increases husband's power, because wife is burdened with day-to-day household and childcare responsibilities and has no time or energy to exercise whatever influence/power she has.

```
      1        2        3       ④        5
      |--------|--------|--------|--------|
  Chaotic  Egalitarian  Mild   Moderate  Marked
  Family  (Syncratic or  Dominance  Dominance  Dominance
          Autonomic)
```

Overall Family Power

Moderate dominance seen (father dominant), with some dissatisfaction of this situation expressed by wife.

20. **Role Structure**

Formal Role Structure

Pat: Father and husband. He acts as sole provider for family, and is leader of family. Does not see his position as involving a companionship, recreational, or therapeutic role, however, and only occasionally does he help with the child-care role (when he feels like it). Marital roles enacted, although constricted, appear consistent with his expectations of marital roles.

Mary: Mother and wife. She acts as the homemaker (not shared), involving cooking, shopping, and cleaning home; enacts the child-care role (not shared to any real extent); the recreational role (taking children to park to play). No therapeutic role or companion role enacted in marriage. Sexual role inadequate. Wife has expressed disappointment that the therapeutic role is not present and that the sexual role is unsatisfying (distant communications, no enjoyment in sexual relationship). Wife appears to have some expectations of Pat that are more consistent with American middle-class ideas of marriage, although she seems also resigned to the fact that Pat's traditional expectations of both of their positions in the family are fairly stable and not likely to be changed. She enacts the roles needed to complement husband's role expectations of her, while at the same time trying to limit her family roles in future to some extent by having no more children. Mary definitely shows some role strain in trying to handle child care and all the other mother-wife roles by herself, as well as the possibility that she might return to part-time work.

Joseph: Older son and brother to siblings.
Maureen: Older daughter and sister to siblings.
Betty: Younger daughter and sister to siblings.

Richard: Younger son and brother to siblings.

Daniel: Youngest (baby) son and brother to siblings.

Informal Role Structure

Pat: Leader; distant one (does not get involved in family life); unconcerned one (does wife see him in this way or is this the way she expects husbands to act?)

Mary: Subservient one; go-between role (between children and their father); martyr?

Joseph: Leader of the children, mother's favorite and perhaps confidant, because mother cannot confide in and share affectively with husband. Serious one.

Maureen: Cooperative, compliant one. Follower.

Betty: Sweet one. "People-pleaser" role. Mother perceives her to play cute, manipulative role, whereas father defends her sweetness as being genuine and not manipulative. Father's favorite. Mary is perhaps threatened by husband's affections toward Betty.

Richard: Active one (with explosive temper if exploration and freedom are restricted).

Daniel: No comments by parents.

Variables Affecting Role Structure:

Social class influences: Working-class families are likely to be more traditional in terms of marital roles. Being Irish-American and fairly unacculturated affects family roles. Traditional Catholic background reinforces patriarchal family structure. The family developmental stage and presence of five small children make wife dependent on husband as sole breadwinner, which further increases his dominance and her dependency.

21. **Family's Values:** In comparing the O'Sheas' values with American and traditional Irish and Irish-American values, the O'Sheas' values are definitely much more in keeping with the traditional Irish values and the working-class values of today. Productivity and success are not primary values. Pat has worked for his father since graduation from high school, except for time he was in the Armed Services. Mary worked in an electronics factory after graduation and until the first child was born. The work ethic and materialism do not seem central in family's life. The family does not value individualism, but familism and the ethic of reciprocity (assisting one's family and church) is salient, as is the value of doing one's duty and playing expected family roles (conformity). Education is not highly valued, nor is progress, change, and mastery; conservatism and fatalistic thinking assume greater importance. No long-term plans were expressed, except Mary's ardent plans to prevent further pregnancies and desire to return to part-time employment. Equality and individual freedom are not inferred to be important values either. The "doing orientation" does not fit this family. Time is not carefully allotted and used. Much of Pat's time outside of work is spent in recreational pursuits (spectator sports and social drinking with friends). Health care and practices are not of prime importance to family.

There appears to be a conflict in values, to some degree, between Mr. and Mrs. O'Shea. Mary obviously feels caught between the values of American society and those of traditional Irish culture that govern family roles, power relationships, and communication. She is trying—not very effectively—to assert herself with her husband, demonstrating the value of egalitarianism, individualism, and progress. Pat retains the old traditional values, as stated above. This directly affects the health status of the family, by creating strain in the marital relationship.

22. **Affective Function**

Family Need–Response Patterns

Pat: For the most part, he does not make any of his socioemotional needs known to his wife or children; therefore, they are presumably not adequately met in family. (Perhaps his needs are met through work and socializing with friends at sports events and tavern.) He does, however, make his needs for affection and warmth known to daughter Betty, who responds in a sweet, affectionate manner toward him.

Mary: Expressed problem of not being able to talk to husband and of not feeling emotionally close to him. He does not respond to her needs to communicate and does not empathize with her feelings regarding the responsibilities she assumes. Her son Joseph meets some of her socioemotional needs, because she feels she can talk to him, whereas Pat is not available to meet her needs.

Joseph (age 6): Has need to handle things, lead, and be assertive. His mother gives him this opportunity; Pat feels his son's behavior is inappropriate and feels he should be put in his place. The younger children follow him. Becomes rebellious or bossy when his needs to be assertive are frustrated.

Maureen (age 5): Expresses need to cooperate with and help her mother; emulates mother's behavior and roles. Mary gives her the opportunity to fulfill these needs.

Betty (age 4): Expresses need to please people and be liked. Mother sees this as a way to "get her way" (a form of manipulation). Father sees this need as genuine, and she is his favorite. He responds to Betty's sweetness, reinforcing her behavior and need to please.

Richard (age 3): Richard has a need to explore and be autonomous. Mary realizes this and responds by letting him run around the house and explore. Also has need for extra attention because of arrival of new baby, which parents understand and are responding to.

Daniel (age 1 to 3 weeks): Needs to trust and have his basic physiological and affectional needs met. These are being fulfilled ably by the mother.

Mutual Nurturance, Closeness, and Identification: Adequate between mother and Joseph, Maureen, Richard, and Daniel.

Maybe attenuated between Mary and Betty, because Mary may feel threatened by her husband's favoritism and diversion of affections to Betty.

Adequate between father and Betty and father and Richard (?). Remainder of father's relationships with children are distant, and father is relatively uninvolved. Inadequate between Mary and Pat. Mutual identification involving closeness and nurturance are weak, hence spousal bonds are weak also. She expresses need for greater closeness, whereas he does not express these needs.

Separateness and Connectedness: Not discussed here to any extent. It will become an issue with Joseph soon, because he is assertive, has leadership qualities and needs, and will increasingly wish to individuate. At present conformity and connectedness are valued much more highly than separateness.

23. **Socialization Function**

Family Child-rearing Practices: Observations limited. Pat advocated old-fashioned child rearing, not "new-fangled" methods. Believes in punishment, respect, and obedience. However, he has a minimal role in implementation, so that Mary may undermine some of his wishes regarding child rearing. From their behavior the children show they have been taught that "children should be seen but not heard" when adults are talking. Mary is very warm and physically affectionate, permissive, and tolerant when children are younger, but when they become preschoolers (age 4 up), she and Pat expect more self-restraint, self-discipline, respect, and obedience. Also could be seen that boys are allowed to be more assertive and aggressive than the girls of family (sex-linked socialization practices are evident).

Adaptibility of Child-rearing Practices for Family's Situation: They appear adaptive in that children are being raised to live in the world as the parents see and experience it. This involves the need to be respectful, obedient, and conforming, and for boys and girls to know their appropriate sex roles and behavior.

Who Is the Socializing Agent? The mother predominantly, but father's influence also present, albeit more indirect. School teachers and priest, in addition to kin, are also socializing agents in children's lives and will become increasingly important as the children age.

Value of Children: They were wanted and accepted. Children appear to be highly valued. Children are highly cherished in the Catholic religion and Irish-American families. Being a mother is the central role for Mary; however she now feels the "burden" of having so many children to care for.

24. **Health Care Function**

Family's Health Beliefs, Values, and Behaviors: Preventive care for children (except for immunizations) is not given; mother did receive physicals with each pregnancy, hence her health maintenance behaviors are more consistent than her husband's. Pat expressed concern about his steady weight gain and "gut" since he stopped playing sports.

Family's Definition of Health–Illness and Level of Knowledge: By taking children and herself to a physician or clinic when they are not visibly ill means that she acknowledges that health is more than just being able to function or a state of feeling well. Wife is health leader and decides when children are ill and in need of health services. Mother has good basic understanding of how to handle common minor illnesses and injuries. She also knows what to do when more serious injuries occur or symptoms appear.

Family Members' Perceived Health Status: Unknown.

Family Dietary Practices: Adequacy of family diet: From data regarding the family the information was inserted into a food history record (Table D–2) to the extent possible.

Caloric Intake: Adequate, although husband and wife are a little overweight (children's weights are within normal limits). Data obtained via visual inspection only. Cultural food assessment: Stews and boiled dinners prepared. Extensive use of potatoes (the Irish staple); otherwise diet is basically American.

Typicality of 24-hour Diet: This report is typical. Mary said that their diet contains little fruit or fruit juices, except for bananas, apples (in season), and canned peaches—and occasionally apple or orange juice. One cooked vegetable besides potatoes is served at dinner each evening. Soups are eaten three to four times per week; salads are infrequently eaten.

Food Allergies: None noted.

Function of mealtimes and their attitudes toward food and mealtime: Not noted.

Shopping practices and person responsible: Mary goes to nearby shopping center and Pat's father's grocery store. She has budgetary limitations and just barely gets by each month. She does not use food stamps but is interested in applying to obtain them.

Refrigerator and Stove: Functioning and adequate, though small. Wife is totally responsible for planning, shopping, and preparation of meals.

Sleep and Rest Habits: Sleeping patterns not noted. Mary stated she used TV for relaxing and that Pat does same, in addition to going over to the bar to socialize and drink for the purposes of relaxation.

Physical Activity and Recreation Practices: Parents do not have regular exercise program for themselves. It is not mentioned as to whether they believe this is a necessity for health maintenance. Wife gets a moderate amount of physical activity doing housework and child-care activities. Husband used to be active in sports but is not presently. He stands at his job (as butcher).

► TABLE D-2

FAMILY FOOD HISTORY RECORD

Meal	Food Served	Quantity	Individual Differences
Breakfast	Cold cereal	1 bowl	All family ate cereal
	Milk	½ cup for cereal	
	Toast, 1 or 2 pieces		Parents only
	Coffee	1 cup	Parents
	Milk	1 cup	Children
Snacks	Crackers	3 or 4 crackers	Children
	Milk	1 glass	
	Coffee	1 cup	Mother
Lunch	Tomato soup	1 bowl	Joseph, Maureen, and
	Mashed potatoes	½–1 cup	father not home
	and butter	1 tbsp	
	Canned peaches	½ cup	
	Milk	1 cup	
Snacks	None		
Dinner	Stew: containing		All ate stew, but children
	meat	¼ cup	had smaller servings
	carrots	½ cup	
	potatoes	½ cup	
	celery	¼ cup	
	White cake	1 slice	All family
	Milk	1 cup	Children
	Coffee	1 cup	Wife
	Beer	1 cup	Husband
Snacks	Cookies		

Family's Drug Habits: Husband drinks alcohol (type and amount unknown); socializing at bars is a frequent and central activity for him.

Both parents drink coffee (2 to 3 cups per day noted).

Tobacco is not used.

It is not mentioned whether use of alcohol is considered a problem.

Family's use of prescription and over-the-counter drugs:

Use of prescription drugs not noted.

Use of over-the-counter drugs directed by Mary. She uses cold medicines (Sudafed, etc.), gastrointestinal medicines (milk of magnesia, etc.), first-aid medications, and aspirin correctly and carefully. She also stores medicines in a safe cabinet away from children's reach.

Family's Role in Self-care Practices: See prior comments. Also administers medications carefully and correctly.

Medically Based Preventive Measures: Children (except when infants) and adults do not have periodic physical examinations.

No information on recency or on vision/hearing examinations or immunization status of family members.

Dental Health Practices: Nutritional: breads and some desserts noted in diet. No candy noted.

Brushing Teeth: Parents brush teeth two times a day after meals. Joseph is being taught to brush teeth. Other children have not started brushing teeth yet.

Use of fluoride: Not mentioned.

No dental check-ups and cleanings. Family visits family dental clinic in neighborhood when dental problems arise. Joseph has had one cavity filled (baby tooth). Parents have been to dentist on a problem basis only. Children other than Joseph have not been seen by a dentist.

Family Health History: No information included.

Health Services Received: Receive pediatric and maternity services from family doctor. Last baby, Daniel, delivered at county hospital because family could not raise necessary funds for private hospital and did not have health insurance at the time. They are now covered by husband's employment, however. Receive well-baby care and immunizations through health department. Pat had never been seen by doctor for physical examinations to Mary's knowledge.

Perceptions/Feelings Regarding Health Care: Family physician (long-time family doctor) is liked, but because family has medical insurance now, Mary would like to switch doctors. Stayed with above physician because his rates were low; but he is old, and Mary is afraid he is not up-to-date in his practice. Mary and Pat asked for information on regular health care services that health insurance covers.

No comments regarding health department services or dental services.

Emergency Health Services: Family uses children's hospital in community when emergency care is needed for children. No mention of where parents go or would go if emergency arose.

Source of Payment: Family has had to assume total expense of medical and dental care up to now. Recently received group health insurance through Pat's father's business (the grocery store). No dental insurance mentioned. Provisions of health insurance not known.

Logistics of Receiving Care: No problems noted. Care has been accessible and mother has car for transportation.

► FAMILY COPING

25. **Short-term Stressors:**
    a. Recent addition to family (Daniel), causing need to reallocate resources and relationships in family.
    b. Wife's potential to become pregnant again (lack of family planning).
    c. Richard's sibling rivalry and acting-out behaviors, although this does not seem to be a serious stressor.
    d. Role overload and strain experienced by mother due to the arrival of another baby and heavy household and child-care responsibilities.

Long-term Stressors:
    a. Economic: Marginally adequate income ("barely gets by every month") and two outstanding debts to pay off: car and hospital bills. With new baby and inflation, economic problems may increase.
    b. Marital: Lack of communication between husband and wife.
    c. Role strain of wife (role overload). Mary's role strain appears not to be recognized as burden by Pat and is minimized as a problem within their cultural/religious orientation.
    d. Threat of future pregnancies (short- and long-term stressor).
    e. Value conflicts between Irish-American subculture and American majority culture.

Strengths That Counterbalance Stressors:
Family has several strong assets that counterbalance to a moderate extent the above family stressors:
    a. Husband's steady job (stable provider).
    b. Mary's ability and willingness to work and Mary's mother's offer to provide infant care.
    c. Permanency of residence. Family knows neighborhood and community, familiar with resources. They like neighborhood's cohesiveness and are well integrated into neighborhood.

d. Social support system of family is moderately strong. Extended family present and assistance available and partially utilized. Also, neighbors and friends were mentioned as helpful. Church and church school are important resources to family.

e. Health status of family members appears adequate to good with no obvious problems except Mary's hypertension during pregnancies mentioned.

f. Adequate housing and furnishings at present.

g. Adequate health care (except preventive), nutritional practices, and health resources (health services and insurance).

26. **Family's Ability to Base Decisions on Objective Appraisal of Stress-Producing Situation:** Role overload (role strain) experienced by Mary and her expressed need to prevent further pregnancies are the two stress-producing situations occurring during nurse's visits. Mary seems to be able to appraise situations realistically, but Pat denies the significance of her concerns and strains. As a family they have not taken action yet on wife's concerns because Pat was supposed to call the priest and doctor for appointments but has neglected to do so. As a family, parents have not worked together to appraise problems objectively and solve them.

27. **Family's Reaction to Stressors: Functional Coping Strategies Utilized (Present and Past):** The family uses their social support system of extended family and church primarily to assist them in time of need. Inner coping resources are not mentioned as means for dealing with stressors. The family is able to meet the usual stresses and strains of daily life, largely through the efforts of Mary, who is the central figure in the family. Mary and Pat, albeit more reluctantly, are seeking information about health care services.

28. **Dysfunctional Adaptive Strategies Utilized (Past and Present):** First, the family does not use its inner resources adequately to deal with stressors. There is no "pulling together," increased cohesiveness, or sharing of feelings and thoughts during periods of greater demand. Pat goes his own way rather than pitching in as part of the family team. The more overt dysfunctional coping mechanism that can be identified is that of authoritarianism, coupled with an element of neglect. Interestingly enough, this pattern is an exaggeration of the traditional Irish or Irish-American pattern. The stance may be taken that Pat uses his position of dominance too extensively, however, because through his authoritarianism and neglect (his minimal involvement with family life) he stifles the growth and quality of their marital relationship, as well as reduces the quality of his relationship with his children (except with Betty). Moderate husband dominance occurs where feelings and input are often not solicited or received from family members, especially the wife. This coping pattern affects the family unit, its subsystems, and the individual family members adversely (Table D–3).

▶ OTHER FAMILY NURSING DIAGNOSES GENERATED FROM O'SHEA ASSESSMENT

- Father–child relationships weak (except for Betty).
- Nutritional deficiencies: Insufficient use of vegetables and fruits, especially ones containing vitamin C; lack of sufficient iron in diet.
- Inadequate dental hygiene and care: Brushing for Maureen and Betty; examinations for whole family.
- Lack of exercise program for the spouses.
- Home safety hazards: No lighting or railings on outside steps. Stair boards loose.

▶ FURTHER ASSESSMENT DATA NEEDED

- Perceived health status of family members.
- Health insurance benefits.
- Family's knowledge regarding how to locate another family physician.
- Family's knowledge of accessible emergency rooms for adults.
- Eye/hearing examinations and immunization status of family members.
- Family medical history.
- Roles: role models of parents.
- Environmental exposure to pollutants from industrial area nearby.
- Spouses' feelings about their sexual relationship and attitudes about counseling.
- Husband's drinking pattern and consumption of alcohol.

FAMILY NURSING CARE PLAN AND FURTHER ASSESSMENT NEEDED

Family Nursing Diagnoses Including Contributing Factors	Signs and Symptoms (Identifying Characteristics)	Further Assessment Data Needed	Goals	Interventions	Evaluation
1. Altered marital and parental role performance (role strain/overload) related to arrival of another baby, heavy child-care responsibilities, and inadequate family coping patterns.	No companion role present (couple does not do things together). Wife expresses feelings of being overburdened.	Do spouses wish to do leisure time activities together?	*Short-term:* Spouses will be able to discuss wife's concerns and their relationship and roles.	Discuss with the couple the stress and role strain they are experiencing with the arrival of the new baby.	To be completed after intervention. Would look at goals to determine to what degree these have been achieved.
			Long-term: Spousal relationship (subsystem) will be strengthened by enlarging number of	Help them redefine or reframe the problem as a family problem, not a mother-wife problem.	
Variables Cultural and religious values and norms regarding marital roles and adult roles for women and men. Life cycle of family: high demands being placed on both parents at this stage of family's life. Socioeconomic position: marginal income, limited education, constricted world.	Therapeutic role inadequate. Husband does not listen to wife's concerns. Lack of communication except for money and some of children's problems and sexual roles unsatisfying, according to wife.	Does husband feel there is a problem with communication? Does husband feel that sexual roles are problem and an area for improvement? Would wife feel that this is an area she would be too embarrassed to have discussed?	roles involved in marital positions (companion, therapeutic, and perhaps sexual) and by improving communications.	Encourage them to share their concerns about their growing responsibilities and the financial strain. Encourage greater use of existing support system (e.g., grandmothers and aunt) to have more leisure time together. Assist the couple to explore options for leisure time that would be satisfying for both of them.	

(Continued)

▲ TABLE D-3 *(Continued)*

FAMILY NURSING CARE PLAN AND FURTHER ASSESSMENT NEEDED

Family Nursing Diagnoses Including Contributing Factors	Signs and Symptoms (Identifying Characteristics)	Further Assessment Data Needed	Goals	Interventions	Evaluation
				Open up discussion with couple about Mary's interest in obtaining part-time job and support her efforts to obtain information.	
				Assist couple to discuss and clarify their roles, expectations of each other, their communications with each other, to open up avenues for modification of their roles/communication to create more functional patterns.	
				Assist couple to identify internal coping mechanisms (e.g., humor) or joint problem solving that could be utilized to reduce stressors.	
				Discuss with Pat his willingness to take on some responsibilities with child care and child rearing if Mary returns to part-time work.	

Variables	Assessment	Goals	Interventions	Evaluation
Life cycle of family: high demands being placed on both parents at this stage of family's life. Socioeconomic position: marginal income, limited education, constricted world.	Mates do not "pull together" (become cohesive and reliant on own resources during periods of high demand on family). Assess couple's, especially husband's, willingness and readiness to explore ways of strengthening marital relationship.		Support exploration of child care resources/options (aunt or children's grandmother). Explore the couple's perceived need and interest in marital counseling and in receiving information on marital and sexual relationships. Initiate referral(s) if need and interest are present. Suggest they discuss family/marriage with priest. See if couple can obtain new, enlightened information and guidance on family planning and marriage. Socioeconomic: Refer to food stamp program.	To be completed after intervention. Would look at goals to determine to what degree these have been achieved.
2. Alteration in health maintenance: Ineffective family planning.	Wife's hypertension during pregnancies and potential harm to health from subsequent pregnancy. Pregnancies in family have not been planned. How do family's priest and physician feel about family planning for couple? What is couple's relationship with physician and priest? Are they the most appropriate resources to refer couple to?	*Short-term:* Couple will be able to accurately describe the types of family planning methods available and acceptable to them (within their cultural/religious belief system).	Help couple explore feelings regarding limiting family, effects of having additional children on family. Assist couple to problem solve in making and carrying out decision in this area (resources, who will follow up with contacting them, etc.).	
Variables History of high fertility, pregnancies every year.	Mother does not want more children—strain on herself, budget, housing, etc.	Couple will be able to explore their thoughts and feelings about	Refer family to health and religious resources (if needed)	

(Continued)

▲ TABLE D-3 (Continued)

FAMILY NURSING CARE PLAN AND FURTHER ASSESSMENT NEEDED

Family Nursing Diagnoses Including Contributing Factors	Signs and Symptoms (Identifying Characteristics)	Further Assessment Data Needed	Goals	Interventions	Evaluation
History of hypertension during pregnancies. Cultural/religious influences on family planning. Weak spousal relationship (lack of spousal communication).	Family-planning methods inadequate (not a problem at present, but will be soon). Husband is not sufficiently empathetic with wife's concerns regarding having no more children and passively accepts unplanned pregnancies.		having no more children. Husband will understand wife's concerns and see problem as a family problem. *Long-term:* Couple will successfully use family planning method(s) to prevent further pregnancies.	as part of problem-solving process. Follow-through with spouses after they have met with physician and priest to discuss any questions, thoughts, or areas where further information is needed, making sure they have sufficient knowledge about family planning methods that were recommended.	
3. Health-seeking behaviors (expressed desire for improvement in preventive health care behavior).	Preventive health services are accessible and family has new health insurance benefits. None of the family has had regular preventive dental or medical examinations.	What benefits are included under new health insurance policy? Knowledge of age-appropriate preventive health care practices. Immunization status of children.	*Short term:* Couple will be able to identify preventive health care services under their new health insurance policy. *Long term:* Family will make full and regular use of all medical and dental benefits eligible for under health insurance benefits. All family members will receive preventive medical examinations	Review with couple their health insurance policy and determine preventive health care benefits. Explain the importance of preventive medical and dental examinations. Refer to low-cost community services for care not covered by insurance policy (e.g., dental).	To be completed after intervention. Would look at goals to determine to what degree these have been achieved.

Assessment		Goals	Interventions
		allowed by health insurance policy. *Short-term:* Spouses All family members will receive dental checkup and cleaning. Will perform other age-appropriate preventive health behavior (e.g., immunizations, safety, stress management, and self-examinations)	Review preventive health care practices that would be beneficial for family group as well as for each member of the family. To expand and reinforce knowledge, provide health education materials regarding age appropriate preventive health care practices. Refer family members, as needed, to community resources for preventive health behavior modification (e.g., health education programs and self-help groups).
Parents are both overweight with no regular exercise program.	What kind of physical exercise would couple be willing to participate in? Level of physical activity of children.	Parents will initiate a regular exercise program.	Support husband's concern about need to exercise and positive efforts couple makes to get information or start exercise program.
Diet—more fat in diet than recommended. Insufficient fruits and vegetables.	Willingness to alter diet.	Family will alter diet to reduce fat and increase fruits and vegetables.	Compliment parents on the positive aspects of their family diet and encourage them to increase positive dietary patterns.
Husband's use of alcohol by report of wife.	Extent of husband's alcohol use.		Encourage parents' efforts to improve diet.

609

References

Aamodt, A. M. (1978). Culture. In A. L. Clark (Ed), *Culture, childbearing and health professionals*. Philadelphia: Davis.

Abernathy, W. J., & Schrems, E. L. (1971). *Distance and health services—Issues of utilization and facility choice for demographic strata* (Research Paper No. 19). Palo Alto, CA: Stanford University Graduate School of Business.

Ackerman, N. (1966). *The psychodynamics of family life*. New York: Basic Books.

Adams, B., & Adams, D. (1990). Child care and the family. In National Council on Family Relations, *2001: Preparing families for the future* (pp. 18–19). Minneapolis, MN: Bolger Publications.

Adams, B. N. (1971). *The American family*. Chicago: Markham Publishing.

———. (1980). *The family. A sociological interpretation*. Boston: Houghton Mifflin.

Aday, L. A., & Eichhorn, R. (1972). *The utilization of health services: Indices and correlates—A research bibliography* (Publication No. [HSM] 73-3003). Washington, DC: Department of Health, Education and Welfare, National Center for Health Services Research and Development.

Agbayani-Siewert, P., & Revilla, L. (1995). Filipino Americans. In P. G. Min (Ed.), *Asian Americans: Contemporary trends and issues* (pp. 134–198). Thousand Oaks, CA: Sage.

Agnew, R., & Huguley, S. (1989). Adolescent violence toward parents. *Journal of Marriage and the Family, 51* (3), 699–711.

Ahrons, C. R. (1980, Nov.). Redefining the divorced family. A conceptual framework. *Social Work*, 437–441.

Ahrons, C. R., & Perlmutter, M. S. (1982). The relationship between former spouses: A fundamental subsystem in the remarriage family. In J. C. Hansen & L. Messinger (Eds.), *Therapy with remarried families*. Rockville, MD: Aspen.

Ainsworth, M. D., et al. (1966). *Deprivation of maternal care*. New York: Schocken.

Aldous, J. (1974). The making of family roles and family change. *Family Coordinator, 23* (2), 232–237.

———. (1978). *Family careers: Developmental change in families*. New York: Wiley.

———. (1996). *Family careers: Rethinking the developmental perspective*. Thousand Oaks, CA: Sage.

Alexander, J. S., Younger, R. E., Cohen, R. M., & Crawford, L. V. (1988). Effectiveness of a nurse-managed program for children with chronic asthma. *Journal of Pediatric Nursing, 3*, 312–317.

Allen, C. E. (1994). Families in poverty. *Nursing Clinics of North America, 29* (3), 277–393.

Allen, K. R., & Demo, D. H. (1995). The families of lesbians and gay men: A new frontier in family research. *Journal of Marriage and the Family, 57*, 111–127.

Allen, W. R., & Stukes, S. (1982). Black family lifestyles and the mental health of black Americans. In F.V. Munoz & R. Endo (Eds.), *Perspectives on minority group mental health* (pp 45–51). Washington, DC: University Press of America.

Alpenfels, E. J. (1969). Cancer in situ of the cervix: Cultural clues to reactions. In L. R. Lynch (Ed.), *The cross-cultural approach to health behavior*. Cranbury, NJ: Fairleigh Dickinson University Press.

American Academy of Pediatrics. (1995). *Caring for your school age child. Ages 5 to 12*. New York: Bantam Books.

American Association of Retired Persons. (1990). *A profile of older Americans, 1990*. Washington, DC: AARP.

———. (1993). *A profile of older Americans, 1992*. Washington, DC: AARP.

American Cancer Society. (1996). *Cancer facts and figures—1996*. Atlanta, GA: ACS.

American Dental Association. (1988). *Seal out decay*. Chicago: ADA Division of Communications.

American Nurses Association. (1980). *Social policy statement*. Kansas City, MO: ANA.

———. (1985). *The scope of practice of the primary health care nurse practitioner*. Kansas City, MO: ANA.

———. (1986). *Standards of home health nursing practice*. Kansas City, MO: ANA.

———. (1987). *Standards of practice for the primary health care nurse practitioner*. Kansas City, MO: ANA.

———. (1988). *Rehabilitation nursing: Scope of practice.* Kansas City, MO: ANA.

———. (1991). *Standards of clinical nursing practice.* Kansas City, MO: ANA.

———. (1992). *Nursing's agenda for health care reform.* Washington, DC: ANA.

———. (1994). *Statement on psychiatric–mental health clinical nursing practice and standards of psychiatric–mental health clinical nursing practice.* Kansas City, MO: ANA.

———. (1995a). *Nursing's social policy statement.* Kansas City, MO: ANA.

———. (1995b). *Scope and standards of gerontological nursing practice.* Kansas City, MO: ANA.

American Nurses Association, Council of Community Health Nurses. (1986). *Standards of community health nursing practice.* Kansas City, MO: ANA.

American Nurses Association, Division on Maternal and Child Health Nursing Practice. (1983). *Standards of maternal and child health nursing practice.* Kansas City, MO: ANA.

American Nurses Association, Division on Psychiatric–Mental Health Nursing Practice. (1982). *Standards of psychiatric and mental health nursing practice.* Kansas City, MO: ANA.

American Nurses Association Task Force on Case Management. (1988). *Nursing case management.* Kansas City, MO: ANA.

Ames, K. (1992, March 23). Domesticated bliss: New laws are making it official for gay and live-in couples. *Newsweek,* 40.

Anderson, K., & Tomlinson, P. (1992). The family health system as an emerging paradigmatic view for nursing. *Image, 23* (1), 57–63.

Anderson, K. E. (1972). *Introduction to communication theory and practice.* San Jose, CA: Cummings.

Anderson, K. H. (1994). The relationship between family sense of coherence and family quality of life after illness diagnosis: Collective and consensus views. In H. McCubbin, E. Thompson, A. Thompson, & J. Fromer (Eds.), *Sense of coherence and resiliency: Stress, coping and health* (pp. 169–187). Madison, WI: University of Wisconsin-Madison, System Center for Excellence in Family Studies.

Anderson, R., & Carter, I. (1974). *Human behavior in the social environment—A social systems approach.* Chicago: Aldine.

Andrews, M. M. (1995). Transcultural nursing care. In M. M. Andrews & J. S. Boyle (Eds.), *Transcultural concepts in nursing care* (2nd ed.) (pp. 49–96). Philadelphia: Lippincott.

Andrews, M. M., & Boyle, J. S. (Eds.). (1995). *Transcultural concepts in nursing care* (2nd ed.). Philadelphia: Lippincott.

Aneshensel, C. S., Pearlin, L. I., Mullan, J. T., Zarit, S. H., & Whitlatch, C. J. (1995). *Profiles in caregiving: The unexpected career.* San Diego: Academic Press.

Angel, R. (1985). The health of the Mexican origin population. In R. De La Garza, et al. (Eds.), *The Mexican American experience: An interdisciplinary anthology* (pp. 410–426). Austin, TX: University of Texas Press.

Antonovsky, A. (1979). *Health, stress and coping.* San Francisco: Jossey-Bass.

———. (1987). *Unraveling the mystery of health: How people manage stress and stay well.* San Francisco: Jossey-Bass.

———. (1994). The sense of coherence: An historical and future perspective. In H. McCubbin, E. Thompson, A. Thompson, & J. Fromer (Eds.), *Sense of coherence and resiliency: Stress, coping and health* (pp. 3–21). Madison, WI: University of Wisconsin-Madison, System Center for Excellence in Family Studies.

Antonovsky, A., & Sourani, T. (1988). Family sense of coherence and family adaptation. *Journal of Marriage and the Family, 50,* 79–92.

Araji, S. K. (1977). Husbands' and wives' attitude—Behavior congruence of family roles. *Journal of Marriage and the Family, 39* (2), 311–321.

Archer, S., & Fleshman, R. (1975). *Community health nursing.* North Scituate, MA: Duxbury Press.

Ardell, D. (1982). *Fourteen days to a wellness life-style.* Mill Valley, CA: Whatever Publishers.

———. (1977). *High level wellness—An alternative to doctors, drugs and disease.* Emmaus, PA: Rodale Press.

Ardell, D., & Newman, A. (1977). Health promotion—Strategies for planning. *Health Values: Achieving High Level Wellness, 1* (3), 100.

Armentrout, G. (1993). A comparison of the medical model and the wellness model: The importance of knowing the difference. *Holistic Nursing Practice, 7* (4), 57–62.

Arnette, J. K. (1996). Physiological effects on chronic grief: A biofeedback treatment approach. *Death Studies, 20,* 59–72.

Artinian, N. T. (1989). Family member perceptions of a cardiac surgery event. *Focus on Critical Care, 16* (4), 301–308.

———. (1994). Selecting a model to guide family assessment. *Dimensions of Critical Care Nursing, 14* (1), 4–16.

Association for the Care of Children's Health. (1989). Conference Announcement. Washington, DC: ACCH.

Auger, J. R. (1976). *Behavioral systems and nursing.* Englewood Cliffs, NJ: Prentice-Hall.

Austin, R. (1985). Attitudes toward old age: A hierarchical study. *The Gerontologist, 25* (4), 431–434.

Avioli, P. S. (1989). The social support functions of siblings in later life: A theoretical model. *American Behavioral Scientist, 33,* 45–57.

Aylmer, R. C. (1988). The launching of the single young adult. In B. Carter & M. McGoldrick (Eds.), *The changing family life cycle* (pp. 191–208). New York: Gardner Press.

Baca-Zinn, M. (1981). Sociological theory in emergent Chicano perspectives. *Pacific Sociological Review, 24* (2), 255–272.

Backett, E. M., Davies, A. M., & Petros-Barvazian, A. (1984). *The risk approach in health care.* Geneva, Switzerland: World Health Organization.

Bahnson, C. B. (1987). The impact of life-threatening illness on the family and the impact of the family on illness: An overview. In M. Leahey & L. M. Wright (Eds.), *Families and life-threatening illness* (pp. 26–44). Springhouse, PA: Springhouse Corporation.

Baier, M. (1987). Case management with the chronically mentally ill. *Journal of Psychosocial Nursing, 25* (6), 17–20.

Baker, T. (1985). Introduction to sleep and sleep disorders. *Medical Clinics of North America, 69,* 1123–1151.

Balswick, J. O., & Balswick, J. P. (1995). Gender relations and marital power. In B. B. Ingoldsby & S. Smith (Eds.), *Families in multicultural perspective* (pp. 297–320). New York: Guilford Press.

Bandura, A. (1977). *Social learning theory.* Englewood Cliffs, NJ: Prentice-Hall.

Banks, L. J. (1992). Counseling. In G. M. Bulechek & J. C. McCloskey (Eds.), *Nursing interventions. Essential nursing treatments* (2nd ed.) (pp. 279–303). Philadelphia: Saunders.

Barber, B. K., & Thomas, D. L. (1986). Dimensions of fathers' and mothers' supportive behavior: The case for physical affection. *Journal of Marriage and the Family, 48* (4), 783–794.

Baringer, F. (1990, Aug. 30). Census data show sharp rural losses. *The New York Times,* pp. 1, B12.

Baringer, F. (1991, March 11). Census shows profound change in racial make-up of nation. *The New York Times,* p. 1.

Barnett, R. C., & Baruch, M. (1987). Determinants of fathers' participation in family work. *Journal of Marriage and the Family, 49* (1), 29–40.

Barnett, T., Fatis, M., Sonnek, D., & Torvinen, J. (1992). Treatment satisfaction with an asthma management program: A "five"-year retrospective assessment. *Journal of Asthma, 29,* 109–116.

Barnum, B. J. S. (1994). *Nursing theory: Analysis, application, and evaluation* (4th ed.). Philadelphia: Lippincott.

Barth, R. P. (1990). Theories guiding home-based intensive family preservation services. In L. M. Tracy & C. Booth (Eds.), *Reaching high risk families: Intensive family preservations in human services.* Hawthorne, NY: Aldine de Gruyter.

Bartz, K. W., & Levine, B. S. (1978). Childrearing by Black parents: A description and comparison to Anglo and Chicano parents. *Journal of Marriage and the Family, 40,* 709–720.

Bass, D., & Noelker, L. (1987). The influence of family caregivers on elders' use of in-home services: An ex-panded conceptual framework. *Journal of Health and Social Behavior, 28,* 184–196.

Bassuk, E. L., & Rubin, L. (1987). Homeless children: A neglected population. *American Journal of Orthopsychiatry, 57* (2), 279–286.

Bassuk, K. L. (1990). The problem of family homelessness. In E. L. Bassuk, R. W. Carmen, L. F. Weinrek, & M. M. Herzig (Eds.), *Community care for homeless families* (p. 7). Washington, DC: Interagency Council on the Homeless.

Bateson, G. (1958). *Naven* (2nd ed.). Stanford, CA: Stanford University Press.

———. (1972). *Steps to an ecology of the mind.* New York: Ballantine.

———. (1979). *Mind and nature.* New York: Bantam Books.

Bateson, G., Jackson, D. D., Haley, J., & Weakland, K. J. (1963). A note on the double bind—1962. *Family Process, 2,* 154–161.

Battiste, H. B. (1975). Family myths. In S. Smoyak (Ed.), *The psychiatric nurse as a family therapist.* New York: Wiley.

Baumann, B. (1961). Diversities in conceptions of health and physical fitness. *Journal of Health and Human Behavior, 2* (1), 40.

Baumrind, D. (1978). Parental disciplinary patterns and social competency in children. *Youth and Society, 9,* 239–276.

———. (1985). Familial antecedents of adolescent drug use: A developmental perspective. In C. Jones & R. Battjes (Eds.), *Etiology of drug abuse: Implication for prevention.* NIDA Research Monograph. Washington, DC: U.S. Government Printing Office.

———. (1994). The social context of child maltreatment. *Family Relations, 43,* 360–368.

———. (1996). Parenting. The discipline controversy revisited. *Family Relations, 45,* 405–414.

Baxter, K. (1996, Sept. 6). Blazing trails between clashing cultures. *Los Angeles Times,* p. E1.

Beavers, W. (1977). *Psychotherapy and growth: A family systems perspective.* New York: Brunner/Mazel.

Beavers, W. R., & Hampson, R. B. (1990). *Successful families. Assessment and intervention.* New York: Norton.

———. (1993). Measuring family competence. In F. Walsh (Ed.), *Normal family processes* (2nd ed.) (pp. 73–95). New York: Guilford Press.

Beck, M., et al. (1990, July 16). Trading places. *Newsweek,* 48–54.

Becker, M. H. (1972). The health belief model and personal health behavior. *Health Education Monographs, 2,* 326–327.

———. (1974). *The health belief model and personal health behavior.* Thorofare, NJ: Charles B. Slack.

Becvar, D. S., & Becvar, R. J. (1996). *Family therapy: A systemic integration.* Boston: Allyn & Bacon.

Bell, J. (1995). Wanted: Family nursing interventions. *Journal of Family Nursing, 1* (4), 355–358.

Bell, J. M. (1996). Advanced practice in family nursing: One view. *Journal of Family Nursing, 2* (3), 244–248.

Bell, R. (1971). *Marriage and family interaction.* Homewood, IL: Dorsey Press.

Bell, R., & Vogel, E. F. (1968). *A modern introduction to the family.* New York: Free Press.

Bellah, R. N., Madsen, L., Sullivan, W. M., Swidler, A., & Tipton, S. M. (1986). *Habits of the heart: Individualism and commitment in American life.* New York: Harper & Row.

Belsky, J. (1995). A nation (still) at risk? *National Forum, 75* (3), 36–38.

Belsky, J., & Isabella, R. (1985). Marital and parental child relationships in family of origin and marital change following the birth of a baby: A retrospective analysis. *Child Development, 56,* 342–349.

Bemak, F., Chung, R. C., & Bornemann, T. H. (1996). Counseling and psychotherapy with refugees. In P. B. Petersen, J. G. Braguns, W. J. Lonner, & J. E. Trimble (Eds.), *Counseling across cultures* (pp. 243–265). Thousand Oaks, CA: Sage.

Benedek, E. (1978, Dec. 8). *Spousal Abuse.* Paper presented at the 1978 Winter Scientific Session of the American Medical Association, Las Vegas, Nevada. Reported by Nelson, H. Abused wives cling to hope, doctors say. *Los Angeles Times,* pp. 1, 18.

Benedict, R. (1938). Continuities and discontinuities in cultural conditioning. *Psychiatry, 1,* 168.

———. (1976). Continuities and discontinuities in cultural conditioning. In P. J. Brink (Ed.), *Transcultural nursing. A book of readings.* Englewood Cliffs, NJ: Prentice-Hall.

Bengtson, V. N. (1985). Diversity in symbolism in grandparental roles. In V. Bengtson & T. Robertson (Eds.), *Grandparenthood* (pp. 11–25). Newbury Park, CA: Sage.

Bengtson, V., Mangen, D., & Landry, P. (1987). Intergenerational linkages. In H. Garms, E. M. Hoerning, & A. Schaeffer (Eds.), *Intergenerational relationships.* New York: J. Hogrefe.

Bengtson, V., & Robertson, T. (Eds.). (1985). *Grandparenthood.* Newbury Park, CA: Sage.

Benin, M., & Keith, V. M. (1995). The social support of employed African American and Anglo mothers. *Journal of Family Issues, 16* (3), 275–297.

Benne, K. D., & Sheats, P. (1948). Functional roles of group members. *Journal of Social Issues, 4* (Spring), 41.

Benner, P. (1984). *From novice to expert.* Menlo Park, CA: Addison-Wesley.

Berardo, F. M. (1988, Dec.). The American family. *Journal of Family Issues, 8* (4), 426–428.

Berkanovic, E. (1976). Behavioral science and prevention. *Preventive Medicine, 5,* 93.

Berkey, K. M., & Hanson, S. M. H. (1991). *Pocket guide to family assessment and intervention.* St. Louis: Mosby.

Bernal, G., & Shapiro, E. (1996). Cuban families. In M. McGoldrick, J. Giordano, & J. K. Pearce (Eds.), *Ethnicity and family therapy* (2nd ed.) (pp. 155–168). New York: Guilford Press.

Bernard, J. (1972). *The future of marriage.* New York: Bantam.

Berne, A. S., Dato, C., Mason, D. J., & Rafferty, M. (1990). A nursing model for addressing the health needs of homeless families. *Image, 22* (1), 8–13.

Berriesi, C. M., Ferraro, K. F., & Hobey, L. L. (1984). Environmental satisfaction, sociability and well-being among urban elderly. *International Journal of Aging and Human Development, 18* (4), 277–284.

Besmer, A. (1967). Economic deprivation and family patterns. In L. M. Irelan (Ed.), *Low-income life styles.* Washington, DC: U.S. Department of Health, Education, and Welfare.

Bete, C. (1976). *Don't worry about home accidents.* Greenfield, MA: Channing Bete Co.

Bianchi, S. M. (1995). The changing demographic and socioeconomic characteristics of single parent families. In S. H. Hanson, M. L. Heims, D. J. Julian, & M. B. Sussman (Eds.), *Single parent families: Diversity, myths and realities* (pp. 71–97). New York: Haworth Press.

Biddle, B. J., & Thomas, E. J. (1966). *Role theory: Concepts and research.* New York: Wiley.

Biegel, D. E., Sales, E., & Schulz, R. (1991). *Family caregiving in chronic illness.* Newbury Park, CA: Sage.

Bild, B. R., & Havighurst, R. (1976). Senior citizens in great cities: The case of Chicago. *The Gerontologist, 16* (1), 63.

Billingsley, A. (1968). *Black families in white America.* Englewood Cliffs, NJ: Prentice-Hall.

———. (1992). *Climbing Jacob's ladder.* New York: Simon and Schuster.

Birenbaum, L., Robinson, M. A., Phillips, D., Stewart, B., & McCown, D. (1990). The response of children to the dying and death of a sibling. *Omega, 20* (3), 213–228.

Black, B. (1974). *Families in crisis: Assessment and nursing intervention.* Los Angeles, CA: Intercampus Nursing Project, California State University, Los Angeles.

Blattner, B. (1981). *Holistic nursing.* Englewood Cliffs, NJ: Prentice Hall.

Blau, P. M. (1977). *Heterogeneity and inequality: A pragmatic theory of social structure.* New York: Free Press.

Blood, R. O. (1969). *Marriage* (2nd ed.). Glencoe, IL: Free Press.

Blood, R. O., & Wolfe, D. M. (1960). *Husbands and wives: The dynamics of married living.* Glencoe, IL: Free Press.

Bloom, B. S. (1956). *Taxonomy of educational objectives handbook: Cognitive domain.* New York: David McKay.

Blumer, H. (1962). Society as symbolic interaction. In A. Rose (Ed.), *Human behavior and social processes.* Boston: Houghton-Mifflin.

Blumstein, P., & Schwartz, P. (1983). *American couples.* New York: Morrow.

———. (1991). Money and ideology: Their impact on power and the division of household labor. In R. L.

Blumberg (Ed.), *Gender, family, and economy: The triple overlap* (pp. 261–288). Newbury Park, CA: Sage.

Bobak, I. M., Jensen, M. D., & Zalar, M. D. (1989). *Maternity and gynecologic care. The nurse and family* (4th ed.). St. Louis: Mosby.

Bodman, D. A., & Peterson, G. W. (1995). Parenting processes. In R. D. Day, K. R. Gilbert, B. H. Settles, & W. R. Burr (Eds.), *Research and theory in family science* (pp. 205–225). Pacific Grove, CA: Brooks/Cole.

Boehm, S. (1992). Patient contracting. In G. M. Bulechek & J. C. McCloskey (Eds.), *Nursing interventions. Essential nursing treatments* (2nd ed.) (pp. 425–433). Philadelphia: Saunders.

Bolton, F. G., & Bolton, S. R. (1987). *Working with violent families.* Newbury Park, CA: Sage.

Bomar, P. J. (Ed.). (1996). *Nurses and family health promotion* (2nd ed.). Philadelphia: Saunders.

Bomar, P. J., & McNeely, G. (1996). Family health nursing role: Past, present and future. In P. J. Bomar (Ed.), *Nurses and family health promotion* (2nd ed.) (pp. 3–21). Philadelphia: Saunders.

Booth, A., & Cowell, J. (1976, Sept.). Crowding and health. *Journal of Health and Social Behavior, 17,* 218.

Boss, P. (1988). *Family stress management.* Newbury Park, CA: Sage.

Boss, P. G., Doherty, W. J., La Rossa, R., Schumm, W. R., & Steinmetz, S. K. (Eds.). (1993). *Sourcebook of family theories and methods: A contextual approach.* New York: Plenum.

Bossard, J. H., & Boll, E. S. (1956). *The large family system: An original study in the sociology of family behavior.* Philadelphia: University of Pennsylvania Press.

Bott, E. (1957). *Family and social networks.* London: Tavistock.

Boulding, E. (1976). Familism and the creation of futures. In E. Eldridge & N. Meredith (Eds.), *Environmental issues: Family impact.* Minneapolis, MN: Burgess.

Bowdler, J. F., & Barrell, L. M. (1987). Health needs of the homeless. *Public Health Nursing, 4* (3), 135–140.

Bowen, G. L., Desimone, L. M., & McKay, J. K. (1995). Poverty and the single mother family: A macroeconomic perspective. In S. Hanson, M. Heims, D. Julian, & M. Sussman (Eds.), *Single parent families: Diversity, myths and realities* (pp. 115–142). New York: Haworth Press.

Bowen, M. (1960). Family concept of schizophrenia. In D. D. Jackson (Ed.), *Etiology of schizophrenia.* New York: Basic Books.

———. (1976). Theory in the practice of psychotherapy. In P. J. Guerin (Ed.), *Family therapy* (pp. 42–90). New York: Gardiner Press.

———. (1978). *Family therapy in clinical practice.* New York: Aronson.

Bower, F. L. (1977). *The process of planning nursing care* (2nd ed.). St. Louis: Mosby.

Bower, K. (1992). *Case management by nurses.* Washington, DC: American Nurses Publishing.

Bowlby, J. (1966). *Maternal care and mental health.* New York: Schocken.

———. (1977). The making and breaking of affectional bonds. *British Journal of Psychiatry, 133,* 201–210.

Bowling, A., & Windsor, J. (1995). Death after widow(er)-hood: An analysis of mortality rates up to 13 years after bereavement. *Omega, 31* (1), 35–49.

Boyd, N. (1982). Family therapy with black families. In E. E. Jones & S. J. Korchin (Eds.), *Minority mental health* (pp. 227–249). New York: Praeger.

Boyd-Franklin, N. (1989). *Black families in therapy.* New York: Guilford Press.

———. (1993). Race, class and poverty. In F. Walsh (Ed.), *Normal family processes* (2nd ed.) (pp. 361–376) New York: Guilford Press.

Boyum, L. A., & Parke, R. D. (1995). The role of family emotional expressiveness in the development of children's social competence. *Journal of Marriage and the Family, 57* (Aug.), 593–608.

Bozett, F. W. (1987). Family nursing and life-threatening illness. In M. Leahey & L. M. Wright (Eds.), *Families and life-threatening illness.* Springhouse, PA: Springhouse Corporation.

Bozett, F. W., & Gibbons, R. (1983). The nursing management of families in the critical care setting. *Critical Care Update, 10,* 22–27.

Bradburn, N. M. (1970). *The structure of psychological well-being.* Chicago: Aldine.

Braden, C. J. (1984). *The focus and limits of community health nursing.* Norwalk, CT: Appleton & Lange.

Bradt, J. O. (1988). Becoming parents: Families with young children. In B. Carter & M. McGoldrick (Eds.), *The changing family life cycle* (2nd ed.) (pp. 235–254). New York: Gardner Press.

Bramlett, M. H., Gueldener, S. H., & Sowell, R. R. (1990). Consumer-centric advocacy: Its connection to nursing frameworks. *Nursing Science Quarterly, 3,* 156–161.

Bray, J. H., Berger, S. H., & Boethel, C. L. (1994). Role integration and marital adjustment in stepfather families. In K. Pasley & M. Ihinger-Tahlman (Eds.), *Stepparenting: Issues in theory, research, and practice.* Westport, CT: Greenwood Press.

Brazelton, T. B. (1989, Feb. 13). Working parents. *Newsweek,* 66–70.

Briggs, K., Hubbs-Tait, L., Culp, R., & Blankemeyer, M. (1995). Perceiver bias in expectancies for sexually abused children. *Family Relations, 44,* 291–298.

Brink, P. (1976). *Transcultural nursing.* Englewood Cliffs, NJ: Prentice-Hall.

Broderick, C. B. (1971). Behind the five conceptual frameworks: A decade of development in family theory. *Journal of Marriage and the Family, 33,* 129–159.

———. (1990). Family process theory. In J. Sprey (Ed.), *Fashioning family theory* (pp. 171–206). Newbury Park, CA: Sage.

———. (1993). *Understanding family process.* Newbury Park, CA: Sage.

Brody, E., Litvin, S., Hoffman, C., & Kleban, M. (1992a). Differential effects of daughter's marital status on their parental experiences. *The Gerontologist, 32,* 58–67.

———. (1992b). On having a "significant other" during the parent care years. *Journal of Applied Gerontology, 14* (2), 131–149.

Brody, E., & Schoonover, C. B. (1986). Patterns of parent-care when adult daughters work and when they do not. *The Gerontologist, 26* (4), 372–381.

Brody, E. M. (1985). Parent care as a normative family stress. *The Gerontologist, 25,* 19–29.

———. (1995). Prospects for family caregiving: Response to change, continuity, and diversity. In R. A. Kane & J. D. Penrod (Eds.), *Family caregiving in an aging society: Policy perspectives.* Thousand Oaks, CA: Sage.

Brody, E. M., Litvin, S. J., Kleben, M. H., & Hoffman, C. (1990, Nov.). *Differential Effects of Daughters' Marital Status on Their Parent Care Experiences.* Paper presented at the 43rd Annual Meeting of the Gerontological Society of America, Boston, MA.

Brody, G. H. (1994). Family processes and adolescent development. An introduction to a special issue. *Family Relations, 43,* 359.

Broering, J. (1993). The adolescent, health and society: From the perspective of the nurse. In S. Millstein, A. Petersen, & E. Nightingale (Eds.), *Promoting the health of adolescents: New directions for the twenty-first century* (pp. 151–155). New York: Oxford University Press.

Bronfenbrenner, U. (1969). The changing American child— A speculative analysis. In R. L. Coser (Ed.), *Life cycle and achievement in America* (pp. 1–20). New York: Harper & Row.

———. (1974). The origins of alienation. *Scientific American, 231,* 53.

———. (1979). *The ecology of human development: Experiments by nature and design.* Cambridge, MA: Harvard University Press.

Bronstein, P., Clauson, J., Stoll, M. F., & Abrams, C. L. (1993). Parenting behavior and children's social, psychological, and academic adjustment in diverse family structures. *Family Relations, 42,* 268–276.

Bronstein, P., & Cowan, C. P. (1988). *Fatherhood today: Men's changing role in the family.* New York: Wiley.

Brooks-Gunn, S., & Chase-Lansdale, P. (1995). Adolescent parenthood. In M. H. Bornstein (Ed.), *Handbook of parenting Vol 3: Status and social conditions of parenting* (pp. 113–149). Hillsdale, NJ: Erlbaum.

Brooks-Gunn, S., & Paikoff, R. (1993). Sex is a gamble, kissing is a game: Adolescent sexuality, conception, and pregnancy. In S. P. Millstein, A. Peterson, & E. O. Nightingale (Eds.), *Promoting the health of adolescents: New directions for the twenty-first century* (pp. 180–208). New York: Oxford University Press.

Brothers, J. (1990, June 20). Testing parental philosophies. *Los Angeles Times,* p. E4.

Brown, G. W., & Harris, T. (1978). *Social origins of depression.* New York: Free Press.

Brown, M. A., & Waybrant, K. M. (1988). Health promotion, education, counseling, and coordination in primary health care nursing. *Public Health Nursing, 5* (1), 16–23.

Brown, S. L. (1978). Functions, tasks, and stresses of parenting: Implications for guidance. In L. E. Arnold (Ed.), *Helping parents help their children.* New York: Brunner/Mazel.

Brownstein, R. (1995, Nov. 6). Why are so many black men in jail? Numbers in debate equal a paradox. *Los Angeles Times,* p. A5.

Brubaker, T. H. (1983). *Family relationships in later life.* Beverly Hills, CA: Sage.

———. (1985). *Later life families.* Beverly Hills, CA: Sage.

Bruce, B. (1994). *Nurses' Perceptions and Practices of Family-centered Care.* Paper presented at the Third International Family Nursing Conference, May 25–28, 1994, Montreal, Quebec, Canada.

Bruhn, J., & Cordova, F. D. (1978). A developmental approach to learning wellness behavior (Part II). Adolescence to maturity. *Health Values: Achieving High Level Wellness, 2* (1), 20.

Buckley, W. (1967). *Sociology and modern systems theory.* Englewood Cliffs, NJ: Prentice-Hall.

Bulechek, C. M., & McCloskey, J. C. (Eds.). (1992). *Nursing interventions: Essential nursing treatments* (2nd ed.). Philadelphia: Saunders.

———. (1994). Nursing interventions classification (NIC) defining nursing care. In J. C. McCloskey & H. K. Grace (Eds.), *Current issues in nursing* (4th ed.) (pp. 129–135). St. Louis: Mosby.

Bulger, M. W., Wandersman, A., & Goldman, C. R. (1993). Burdens and gratifications of caregiving: Appraisal of parental care of adults with schizophrenia. *American Journal of Orthopsychiatry, 64,* 255–265.

Bullough, V., & Bullough, B. (1982). *Health care for the other Americans.* Norwalk, CT: Appleton & Lange.

Bullrich, S. (1989). The process of immigration. In L. Combrinck-Graham (Ed.), *Children in family contexts* (pp. 482–501). New York: Guilford Press.

Bumpass, L., & Sweet, S. (1991). Family experiences across the life course: Differences by cohort, education and race/ethnicity (NSFH, Working Paper No. 42). Madison, WI: Center for Demography and Ecology.

Bumpass, L., Sweet, S., & Cherlin, A. (1991). The role of cohabitation in declining rates of marriage. *Journal of Marriage and the Family, 53,* 913–927.

Burden, D. S. (1986). Single parents and the work setting: The impact of multiple job and homelife responsibilities. *Family Relations, 35* (1), 37–43.

Burgess, A. W. (1978). *Nursing: Levels of intervention.* Englewood Cliffs, NJ: Prentice-Hall.

Burgess, E. W., Locke, H. J., & Thomas, M. M. (1963). *The family* (3rd ed.). New York: American Book.

Burns, K. (1996). A new recommendation for physical activity as a means of health promotion. *Nurse Practitioner, 21* (9), 18–28.

Burr, W., Day, R., & Bahr, K. (1993). *Family science.* Pacific Grove, CA: Brooks/Cole.

Burr, W., Klein, S., Burr, R., Doxey, C., Harker, B., Holman, T., Martin, P., McClure, R., Parrish, S., Stuart, D., Taylor, A., & White, M. (1994). *Reexamining family stress: New theory and research.* Thousand Oaks, CA: Sage.

Burr, W. R. (1970). Satisfaction with various aspects of marriage over the life cycle. *Journal of Marriage and the Family, 32* (1), 29.

———. (1973). *Theory construction and the sociology of the family.* New York: Wiley.

———. (1995). Using theories in family science. In R. D. Day, K. R. Gilbert, B. H. Settles, & W. R. Burr (Eds.), *Research and theory in family science* (pp. 73–90). Pacific Grove, CA: Brooks/Cole.

Burrell, N. A. (1995). Communication patterns in stepfamilies. In M. A. Fitzpatrick & A. L. Vangelisti (Eds.), *Explaining family interactions* (pp. 290–309). Thousand Oaks, CA: Sage.

Burton, L. (1992). Black grandparents rearing children of drug-addicted parents: Stress, outcomes, and social needs. *The Gerontologist, 32,* 744–751.

Burton, L., & Bengtson, V. (1985). Black grandmothers: Issues of timing and continuity of roles. In V. L. Bengtson & J. F. Robertson (Eds.), *Grandparenthood* (pp. 61–78). Newbury Park, CA: Sage.

Burton, L., & deVries, C. (1995). Challenges and rewards: African-American grandparents as surrogate parents. In L. M. Burton (Ed.), *Families and aging.* Amityville, NY: Baywood.

Bushy, A. (1990). Rural determinants in family health: Considerations for community nurses. *Family and Community Health, 12* (4), 29–38.

Bussell, D. A., & Reiss, D. (1993). Genetic influences on family processes. The emergence of a new framework for family research. In F. Walsh (Ed.), *Normal family processes* (2nd ed.) (pp. 161–181). New York: Guilford Press.

Butler, R. N., & Lewis, M. I. (1982). *Aging and mental health: Positive psychosocial and biomedical approaches.* St. Louis: Mosby.

Byng-Hall, J. (1988). Scripts and legends in families and family therapy. *Family Process, 27,* 167–179.

———. (1995, March). Creating a secure family base: Some implications of attachment theory for family therapy. *Family Process, 34,* 45–58.

Calfie, D. (1994). *Going it alone. A closer look at grandparents parenting grandchildren.* Washington, DC: American Association of Retired Persons.

Campbell, A., et al. (1976). *The quality of American life.* New York: Russell Sage.

Canino, I. A., & Spurlock, J. (1994). *Culturally diverse children and adolescents: Assessment, diagnosis, and treatment.* New York: Guilford Press.

Cantor, M. (1983). Strain among caregivers: A study of experience in the United States. *The Gerontologist, 23,* 597–604.

Caplan, G. (1964). *Principles of preventive psychiatry.* New York: Basic Books.

———. (1970). *The theory and practice of mental health consultation.* New York: Basic Books.

———. (1974). *Support systems and community mental health.* New York: Behavioral Publications.

———. (1976). The family as a support system. In G. Caplan & M. Killilea (Eds.), *Support systems and mutual help.* New York: Grune & Stratton.

Caplan, N., Choy, M. H., & Whitmore, J. K. (1992). Indochinese refugee families and academic achievement. *Scientific American* (Feb.), 36–42.

Caplin, M. S., & Sexton, D. L. (1988). Stresses experienced by spouses of patients in a coronary care unit with myocardial infarction. *Focus on Critical Care, 15* (5), 31–40.

Caplow, T. (1968). *Two against one. Coalitions in triads.* Englewood Cliffs, NJ: Prentice-Hall.

Carey, R. (1989). How values affect the mutual goal setting process with multiproblem families. *Journal of Community Health Nursing, 6* (1), 7–14.

Carlsen, H. J. (1976). The recreational role. In F. I. Nye (Ed.), *Role structure and analysis of the family* (Vol. 24). Beverly Hills, CA: Sage.

Carmel, S., Anson, O., Levenson, A., Bonneh, D., & Maoz, B. (1991). Life events, sense of coherence, and health: Gender differences on the kibbutz. *Social Science and Medicine, 32,* 1089–1096.

Carney, P. (1992). The concept of poverty. *Public Health Nursing, 9* (2), 74–79.

Carpenito, L. J. (1987). *Handbook of nursing diagnoses* (2nd ed.). Philadelphia: Lippincott.

———. (1989). *Handbook of nursing diagnoses* (3rd ed.). Philadelphia: Lippincott.

———. (1995). *Handbook of nursing diagnoses* (6th ed.). Philadelphia: Lippincott.

Carrington, R. W. (1978). The Afro-American. In A. L. Clark (Ed.), *Culture, childbearing, and health professionals.* Philadelphia: Davis.

Carruth, A. K. (1996). Development and testing of the Caregiver Reciprocity Scale. *Nursing Research, 45* (2), 92–97.

Carter, E. A., & McGoldrick, M. (Eds.). (1989). *The changing family life cycle: A framework for family therapists* (2nd ed.). New York: Gardner Press.

Cary, A. H. (1996). Case management. In M. Stanhope & J. Lancaster (Eds.), *Community health nursing. Promoting health of aggregates, families, and individuals* (pp. 357–373). St. Louis: Mosby.

Casas, J. M., & Vasquez, M. J. T. (1996). Counseling the Hispanic. In P. B. Pedersen, J. G. Draguns, W. J. Lonner, & J. E. Trimble (Eds.), *Counseling across cultures.* (4th ed.) (pp. 146–176). Thousand Oaks, CA: Sage.

Casavantes, E. (1970, Winter). Pride and prejudice: A Mexican American dilemma. *Civil Rights Digest, 3,* 22.

Casey, B. (1996). The family as a system. In P. J. Bomar (Ed.), *Nurses and family health promotion: Concepts, assessment, and interventions* (2nd ed.). Philadelphia: Saunders.

Casey, B. A. (1989). The family as a system. In P. J. Bomar (Ed.), *Nurses and family health promotion* (pp. 37–46). Baltimore: Williams & Wilkins.

Castro, E. M. (1978). The Mexican American: How his culture affects his mental health. In R. A. Martinez (Ed.), *Hispanic culture and health care.* St. Louis: Mosby.

Castro, J. (1991, Nov. 25). Condition: Critical. *Time,* 32–42.

Caudill, W. (1975, April). The individual and his nexus. In L. Nader & T. W. Maretzi (Eds.), *Cultural illness and health.* Washington, DC: American Anthropological Association.

Cavan, R. S. (1969). *The American family.* New York: Crowell.

Center for Health Economics Research. (1993). *Access to health care. Key indicators for policy.* Waltham, MA: Center for Health Economics Research.

Centers, R., Raven, B. H., & Rodrigues, A. (1971, April). A conjugal power structure. A re-examination. *American Sociology Review, 36,* 245–263.

Chan, S. (1992). Families with Asian roots. In E. W. Lynch & M. J. Hanson (Eds.), *Developing cross-cultural competence. A guide for working with young children and their families* (pp. 181–257). Baltimore: Paul H. Brooks.

Chang, K. (1995). Chinese Americans. In J. N. Giger & R. E. Davidhizar (Eds.), *Transcultural nursing: Assessment and intervention* (2nd ed.) (pp. 395–414). St. Louis: Mosby.

Chavez, N. (1986). Mental health services delivery to minority populations: Hispanics—a perspective. In M. Mirandé & H. Kitano (Eds.), *Mental health research and practice in minority communities.* Rockville, MD: National Institute of Mental Health.

Cherlin, A., & Furstenberg, F. F. (1985). Styles and strategies of grandparenting. In V. Bengtson & J. F. Robertson (Eds.), *Grandparenthood* (pp. 97–116). Beverly Hills, CA: Sage.

———. (1986). *The new American grandparent: A place in the family a life apart.* New York: Basic Books.

Cherry-Loveland, C. J. (1989). Family health promotion and health protection. In P. J. Bomar (Ed.), *Nurses and health promotion* (pp. 13–25). Baltimore: Williams & Wilkins.

Chesler, M. A., & Barbarin, D. A. (1987). *Childhood cancer and the family.* New York: Brunner/Mazel.

Chess, S. (1983). Basic adaptation to successful parenting. In V. J. Sasserath (Ed.), *Minimizing high-risk parenting* (pp. 5–11). Skillman, NJ: Johnson & Johnson Baby Products.

Chicago Tribune Staff. (1986). *The American milestone. An examination of the nation's permanent underclass.* Chicago: Contemporary Books.

Children's Defense Fund (1995). *State of America's children—1995 Year Book.* Washington, DC: Children's Defense Fund.

Chilman, C. S. (1966). *Growing up poor* (Publication No. 13). Washington, DC: Department of Health, Education and Welfare, Welfare Administration (U.S. Government Printing Office).

———. (1978, April). Habitat and American families: A social–psychological overview. *Family Coordinator, 27,* 106–109.

———. (1988). Never-married, single, adolescent parents. In C. S. Chilman, E. W. Nunnally, & F. M. Cox (Eds.), *Variant family forms.* Newbury Park, CA: Sage.

Chilman, C. S., Nunnally, E. W., & Cox, F. M. (1988). *Families in trouble—Chronic illness and disability.* Beverly Hills, CA: Sage.

Chrisman, M., & Fowler, M. D. (1980). The system-in-change model for nursing practice. In J. Riehl & C. Roy (Eds.), *Conceptual models for nursing practice* (pp. 74–102). New York: Appleton-Century-Crofts.

Chung, D. (1991). Asian cultural commonalities: A comparison with mainstream American culture. In S. Furuto, R. Biswas, D. Chung, & F. Ross-Sheriff (Eds.), *Social work practice with Asian Americans* (pp. 27–44). Newbury Park, CA: Sage.

Clark, A. L. (1966). Adaptation problems and the expanding family. *Nursing Forum, 5,* 98.

Clark, M. (1970). *Health in the Mexican-American culture: A community study.* Berkeley, CA: University of California Press.

Clark, M. J. (1984). *Community nursing: Health care for today and tomorrow.* Reston, VA: Reston Publishing Co.

Clawson, J. (1996). A child with chronic illness and the process of family adaptation. *Journal of Pediatric Nursing, 11,* 52–61.

Clemen, S. (1977). Concepts of culture and value clarification. In S. Clemen & M. Gregerson (Eds.), *Family and community health nursing: A workbook.* Ann Arbor, MI: The University of Michigan Media Library.

Clemen-Stone, S., Eigsti, D., & McGuire, S. L. (1987). *Comprehensive family and community health nursing* (2nd ed.). New York: McGraw-Hill.

Cleveland, E. J., & Longaker, W. D. (1972). Neurotic patterns in the family. In G. Handel (Ed.), *The psychosocial interior of the family* (2nd ed.) (pp. 159–185). Chicago: Aldine-Atherton.

Cleveland, M. (1980). Family adaptation to traumatic spinal cord injury: Response to crisis. *Family Relations, 29,* 558–565.

Cline, C. L. (1996, Spring). Five variations in the marriage theme: Types of marriage formation. *Bulletin of Family Development, 3,* 10.

Clinton, B. (1995, Oct. 17). We are one nation, one family indivisible. *Los Angeles Times,* p. A12.

Cobb, S. (1976). Social support as a moderator of life stress. *Psychosomatic Medicine, 38,* 300–314.

Coddy, B. (1975). The therapist was a gringa. In S. Smoyak, (Ed.), *The psychiatric nurse as a family therapist.* New York: Wiley.

Cogswell, B. E. (1975). Variant family forms and life styles: Rejection of the traditional nuclear family. *The Family Coordinator, 24,* 391–394.

Cohen, S., & Syme, S. L. (1985). Issues in the study of social support. In S. Cohen & L. S. Syme (Eds.), *Social support and health* (pp. 3–20). New York: Academic Press.

Cohn, H. D., & Lieberman, E. J. (1974). Family planning and health. *American Journal of Public Health, 3,* 226–230.

Coleman, J. S. (1962). *The adolescent society.* Glencoe, IL: Free Press.

Coleman, M., Ganong, L. H., & Goodwin, C. (1994). The presentation of stepfamilies in marriage and family textbooks. A reexamination. *Family Relations, 43,* 289–297.

Colley, K. D. (1978). Growing up together: The mutual respect balance. In L. E. Arnold (Ed.), *Helping parents help their children.* New York: Brunner/Mazel.

Coner-Edwards, A. F., & Edwards, H. E. (1988). Introduction. In A. F. Coner-Edwards & J. H. Spurlock (Eds.), *Black families in crisis. The middle class.* New York: Brunner/Mazel.

Coner-Edwards, A. F., & Spurlock, J. H. (Eds.). (1988). *Black families in crisis. The middle class.* New York: Brunner/Mazel.

Connery, D. S. (1968). *The Irish.* New York: Simon & Schuster.

Connors, H. R. (1988, April). Nurse case management. NAMFE: A three year perspective. *Kansas Nurse,* 8–9.

Conover, T. (1993, Sept. 19). The United States of asylum. *New York Times Magazine,* pp. 56–58, 74–78.

Constantine, L. L. (1986). *Family paradigms: The practice of theory in family therapy.* New York: Guilford Press.

Cooley, C. H. (1909). *Social organization.* New York: Scribners.

Coontz, S. (1995). The way we weren't. The myth and reality of the "traditional" family. *National Forum, 75* (3), 11–14.

———. (1996, May–June). Where are the good old days? *Modern Maturity,* 36–53.

Corless, I., Germino, B., & Pittman, M. (Eds.). (1994). *Dying, death, and bereavement: Theoretical perspectives.* Boston: Jones & Bartlett.

Corless, I., Germino, B., & Pittman, M. (1995). *A challenge for living: Dying, death, and bereavement.* Boston: Jones & Bartlett.

Corrales, R. G. (1975). Power and satisfaction in early marriage. In R. F. Cromwell & D. H. Olson (Eds.), *Power in families* (pp. 196–215). New York: Sage.

Coser, L. A. (1956). *The functions of social conflict.* Glencoe, IL: Free Press.

Courtney, R. (1995). Community partnership primary care: A new paradigm for primary care. *Public Health Nursing, 12* (6), 366–373.

Cowan, C. P., & Cowan, P. A. (1988). Who does what when partners become parents: Implications for men, women and marriage. *Marriage and Family Review, 12,* 105–131.

Cowan, C. P., Cowan, P. A., Heming, G., & Miller, N. B. (1991). Becoming a family: Marriage, parenting, and family development. In P. A. Cowan & M. Hetherington (Eds.), *Family transitions.* Hillsdale, NJ: Erlbaum.

Craft, M. J., & Willadsen, J. A. (1992). Interventions related to family. *Nursing Clinics of North America, 27* (2), 517–529.

Cromwell, R. E., & Olson, D. H. (1975). Introduction. In R. E. Cromwell & D. H. Olson (Eds.), *Power in families* (pp. 2–3). New York: Sage.

Cromwell, R. E., & Ruiz, R. A. (1979). The myth of macho dominance in decision-making within Mexican and Chicano families. *Hispanic Journal of Behavioral Science, 1* (4), 355–373.

Cromwell, V. L., & Cromwell, R. E. (1978, Nov.). Perceived dominance in decision-making and conflict resolution among Anglo, Black and Chicano couples. *Journal of Marriage and the Family, 40,* 749–759.

Cronkite, R. C. (1977). The determinants of spouses: Normative preferences for family roles. *Journal of Marriage and the Family, 39,* 575–585.

Crooks, C. E., Iammarino, N. K., & Weinberg, A. D. (1987). The family's role in health promotion. *Health Values, 11* (2), 7–12.

Crosbie-Burnett, M. (1994). Remarriage and recoupling. In P. C. McHenry & S. J. Price (Eds.), *Families and change: Coping with stressful events.* Thousand Oaks, CA: Sage.

Crosby, J. F., & Jose, N. L. (1983). Death: Family adjustment to loss. In C. R. Figley & H. I. McCubbin (Eds.), *Stress and the family. Vol. II: Coping with catastrophe* (pp. 76–89). New York: Brunner-Mazel.

Cuber, J. F., & Harroff, P. B. (1965). *The significant Americans: A study of sexual behavior among the affluent.* New York: Appleton-Century-Crofts.

Curran, D. (1983). *Traits of a healthy family.* Minneapolis, MN: Winston Press.

Curtin, L. (1979). The nurse as advocate: A philosophical foundation for nursing. *Advances in Nursing Science, 1,* 1–10.

Dadds, M. R. (1995). *Families, children and the development of dysfunction.* Thousand Oaks, CA: Sage.

Daka-Mulwanda, V., Thornburg, K. R., Filbert, L., & Klein, T. (1995). Collaboration of services for children and families. A synthesis of recent research and recommendations. *Family Relations, 44,* 219–223.

Dalgas-Pelish, P. L. (1993). The impact of the first child on marital happiness. *Journal of Advanced Nursing, 18,* 437–441.

Daniel, L. (1986). Family assessment. In B. B. Logan & C. E. Dawkins (Eds.), *Family-centered nursing in the community* (pp. 183–208). Menlo Park, CA: Addison-Wesley.

D'Antonio, W. V. (Ed.). (1983). Family, life, religion, and societal values and structure. In W. V. D'Antonio & J. Aldous (Eds.), *Families and religions.* Beverly Hills, CA: Sage.

D'Antonio, W. V., & Aldous, J. (1983). Introduction. In W. V. D'Antonio & J. Aldous (Eds.), *Families and religions.* Beverly Hills, CA: Sage.

Darling, R., & Darling, J. (1982). *Children who are different: Meeting the challenges of birth defects in society.* St. Louis: Mosby.

Davies, B. (1995). Sibling bereavement research. In I. Corless, et al. (Eds.), *A challenge for living* (pp. 173–202). Boston: Jones & Bartlett.

Davies, B., Spinetta, J., Martinson, I., McClowry, S., & Kulenkamp, E. (1986). Manifestations of levels of functioning in grieving families. *Journal of Family Issues, 7* (3), 297–313.

Davis, C., Haub, C. & Willette, J. L. (1988). U.S. Hispanics: Changing the face of America. In E. Acosta-Belen & B. R. Sjostrom (Eds.), *The Hispanic experience in the U.S.* (pp. 3–56). New York: Praeger.

Davis, F. (1963). *Passage through crisis: Polio victims and their families.* New York: Bobbs-Merrill.

Davis, K. (1940). The sociology of parent–youth conflict. *American Sociology Review, 5,* 523.

Davis, O. S. (1978). Nursing approach to the postpartum family. In M. L. Moore (Ed.), *Realities in childbearing.* Philadelphia: Saunders.

Davis, R., & Voegtle, K. (1994). *Culturally competent health care for adolescents.* Chicago: American Medical Association.

Day, A. T., & Day, L. H. (1993, Sept.). Living arrangements and successful aging among ever-married American white women 77–87 years of age. *Aging and Society, 13* (3), 365–387.

Day, J. C. (1992). Population projection of the United States, by age, sex, race, and Hispanic origin: 1992 to 2050. *Current Population Reports* (pp. 25–1082). Washington, DC: Bureau of the Census.

DeFrain, J., Le Masters, E. E., & Schroff, J. A. (1991). Environment and fatherhood: Rural and urban influences. In F. W. Bozett & S. M. H. Hanson (Eds.), *Fatherhood and families in cultural context* (pp. 162–186). New York: Springer.

Dell Orto, A. E. (1988). Respite care: A vehicle for hope, the buffer against desperation. In P. W. Power, A. E. Dell Orto, & M. S. Gibbons (Eds.), *Family interventions throughout chronic illness and disability* (pp. 265–284). New York: Springer.

Demos, J. (1970). *A little commonwealth: Family life in Plymouth Colony.* New York: Oxford University Press.

Demos, V. (1990, Aug.). Black family studies in the Journal of Marriage and the Family and the issue of distortion. A trend analysis. *Journal of Marriage and the Family, 52* (3), 603–612.

deShazer, S. (1991). *Putting difference to work.* New York: Norton.

Detzner, D. F. (1992). Life histories: Conflict in Southeast Asian refugee families. In J. F. Gilgun, K. Daly, & G. Handel (Eds.), *Qualitative methods in family research* (pp. 85–102). Newbury Park, CA: Sage.

Deutcher, I. (1964). The quality of post-parental life: Definitions of the situation. *Journal of Marriage and the Family, 26,* 52.

Diaz-Guerrero, R. (1975). *Psychology of the Mexican culture and personality.* Austin, TX: University of Texas Press.

Dickinson, D., Clark, C. M. F., & Swaford, M. J. G. (1988). AIDS nursing care in the home. In A. Lewis (Ed.), *Nursing care of persons with AIDS/ARC* (pp. 215–237). Rockville, MD: Aspen.

Dickinson, G. E., & Leming, M. R. (1995). *Understanding families. Diversity, continuity and change* (2nd ed.). Forth Worth, TX: Harcourt Brace College.

Diekelmann, N. (1977). *Primary health care of the well adult.* New York: McGraw-Hill.

Dietrich, K. T. (1975). A re-examination of the myth of black matriarchy. *Journal of Marriage and the Family, 37* (2), 367–374.

Dilworth-Anderson, P., & McAdoo, H. P. (1988, July). The study of ethnic minority families: Implications for practitioners and policy makers. *Family Relations, 37* (3), 265–267.

Diosy, L. L. (1956). Socioeconomic status and participation in the poliomyelitis vaccine trial. *American Sociological Review, 21,* 185.

Doak, C. C., Doak L. G., & Root, J. H. (1996). *Teaching patients with low literacy skills* (2nd ed.). Philadelphia: Lippincott.

Dodson, J. (1988). Conceptualizations of black families. In H. P. McAdoo (Ed.), *Black families* (2nd ed.) (pp. 77–88). Newbury Park, CA: Sage.

Doherty, W. J. (1988). Implications of chronic illness for family treatment. In C. S. Chilman, E. W. Nunnally, & F. M. Cox (Eds.), *Chronic illness and disability* (pp. 193–210). Newbury Park, CA: Sage.

_____. (1992). Linkages between family theories and primary health care. In R. Sawa (Ed.), *Family health care* (pp. 30–39). Newbury Park, CA: Sage.

_____. (1995).Boundaries between parent and family education and family therapy. *Family Relations, 44,* 353–358.

Doherty, W. J., & Baird, M. A. (1983). *Family therapy and family medicine.* New York: Guilford Press.

_____. (Eds.). (1987). *Family-centered medical care: A clinical casebook.* New York: Guilford Press.

Doherty, W. J., Boss, P. G., LaRossa, R., Schumm, W. R., & Steinmetz, S. K. (1993). Family theories and methods. A contextual approach. In P. G. Boss, W. J. Doherty, R. LaRossa, W. R. Schumm, & S. K. Steinmetz (Eds.), *Sourcebook of family theories and methods. A contextual approach* (pp. 3–30). New York: Plenum.

Doherty, W. J., & Campbell, T. L. (1988). *Families and health.* Newbury Park, CA: Sage.

Donaldson, M., Yordy, K., & Vanselow, N. (1994). *Defining primary care: An interim report.* Washington, DC: National Academy Press.

Donaldson, S. K., & Crowley, D. M. (1978). The discipline of nursing. *Nursing Outlook, 26,* 113–120.

Donnelly, E. (1990). Health promotion, families and the diagnostic process. *Family and Community Health, 12* (4), 12–20.

Dorfman, L., & Rubenstein, L. (1993). Paid and unpaid activities and retirement satisfaction among rural seniors. *Physical and Occupational Therapy in Geriatrics, 12* (1), 45–63.

Dorsey, R. R., & Jackson, J. Q. (1976). Cultural health traditions: The Latino/Chicano perspective. In M. Branch (Ed.), *Providing safe care to ethnic people of color* (pp. 41–79). New York: Appleton-Century-Crofts.

Dougherty, M. C. (1975). A cultural approach to the nurse's role in health planning. In B. E. Spradley (Ed.), *Contemporary community nursing* (pp. 439–445). Boston: Little, Brown.

Douvan, E., & Adelson, J. (1966). *The adolescent experience.* New York: Wiley.

Draguns, J. G. (1996). Humanly universal and culturally distinctive. In P. B. Pedersen, J. G. Draguns, W. J. Lonner, & J. E. Trimble (Eds.), *Counseling across cultures* (4th ed.) (pp. 1–20). Thousand Oaks, CA: Sage.

Drotar, D., Crawfor, P., & Bush, M. (1984). The family context of childhood chronic illness: Implications for psychosocial intervention. In M. C. Eisenberg, L. C. Sutkin, & M. A. Jansen (Eds.), *Chronic illness and disability through the life span. Effects on self and family* (pp. 103–132). New York: Springer.

Duffy, M. (1988). Health promotion in the family: Current findings and directives for nursing research. *Journal of Advanced Nursing, 13,* 109–117.

Duncan, D. F., & Gold, R. S. (1986, May/June). Reflections: Health promotion. What is it? *Health Values, 10* (3), 47–49.

Dunn, H. L. (1961). *High-level wellness.* Arlington, VA: Beatty.

Duvall, E. M. (1977). *Marriage and family development* (5th ed.). Philadelphia: Lippincott.

Duvall, E. M., & Miller, B. L. (1985). *Marriage and family development* (6th ed.). New York: Harper & Row.

Dyer, W. (1973). Working with groups. In A. Reinhardt & M. Quinn (Eds.), *Family-centered community nursing.* St. Louis: Mosby.

Easley, M., & Epstein, N. (1991). Coping with stress in a family with an alcoholic parent. *Family Relations, 40,* 218–224.

Ebersole, P., & Hess, P. (1994). *Toward healthy aging, human needs and nursing response* (4th ed.). St. Louis: Mosby.

Edelman, C., & Mandle, C. L. (1986). *Health promotion throughout the life span.* St. Louis: Mosby.

Edelman, M. W. (1987). *Families in peril.* Cambridge, MA: Harvard University Press.

_____. (1988). An advocacy agenda for black families and children. In H. P. McAdoo (Ed.), *Black families* (2nd ed.) (pp. 286–295). Newbury Park, CA: Sage.

_____. (1997). An advocacy agenda for Black families and children. In H. P. McAdoo (Ed.), *Black families* (3rd ed.) (pp. 323–333). Thousand Oaks, CA: Sage.

Edgerton, R., Karon, M., & Fernandez, I. (1970). Curanderismo in the metropolis: The diminishing role of folk psychiatry among Los Angeles Mexican Americans. *American Journal of Psychotherapy, 24,* 124–134.

Elder, G. (1974). *Children of the great depression.* Chicago: University of Chicago Press.

Elias, M. (1987, Nov.). Role strained couples. *American Health,* pp. 58–60.

Eliason, M. (1996). Lesbian and gay family issues. *Journal of Family Nursing, 2* (1), 10–29.

Elkind, D. (1988). *The hurried child.* Reading, MA: Addison-Wesley.

_____. (1994). *Ties that stress. The new family imbalance.* Cambridge, MA: Harvard University Press.

Elkins, C. P. (1984). *Community health nursing—Skills and strategies.* Bowie, MD: Brady.

Ell, K., & Northen, H. (1990). *Families and health care.* New York: Aldine de Gruyter.

Elliott-Binns, D. P. (1973). An analysis of lay medicine. *Journal of the Royal College of General Practice, 23,* 255.

Ellis, A. & Grieger, R. (1977). *Handbook of rational emotive therapy*. New York: Springer.

Ellis, V. (1995, March 1). Report finds California children's quality of life in decline. *Los Angeles Times*, pp. A3, A19.

Ellison, C. G. (1990). Family ties, friendships, and subjective well-being among black Americans. *Journal of Marriage and the Family, 52* (3), 298–310.

Ellman, B., & Taggart, M. (1993). Changing gender norms. In F. Walsh (Ed.), *Normal family processes* (pp. 377–404). New York: Guilford Press.

Elmer-Dewitt, P. (1990, Fall). The great experiment. *Newsweek*, 73–75.

Engebretson, J. (1994). Folk healing and biomedicine: Culture clash or complementary approach? *Journal of Holistic Nursing, 12* (3), 240–250.

Epstein, N. B., Bishop, D. S., & Baldwin, L. M. (1982). McMaster model of family functioning: A view of the normal family. In F. Walsh (Ed.), *Normal family processes* (pp. 115–141). New York: Guilford Press.

Epstein, N. B., Bishop, D., Ryan, C., Miller, I., & Keitner, G. (1993). The McMaster model: View of healthy family functioning. In F. Walsh (Ed.), *Normal family processes* (2nd ed.) (pp. 138–160). New York: Guilford Press.

Epstein, Y. M. (1981). Crowding and human behavior. *Journal of Social Issues, 37* (1), 126–131.

Erikson, E. H. (1950). *Childhood and society*. New York: Norton.

————. (1959). *Identity and the life cycle. Psychological issues*, Vol. I. New York: International Universities Press.

————. (1963). *Childhood and society* (2nd ed.). New York: Norton.

Erickson, R. J., & Gegas, V. (1991). Social class and fatherhood. In F. W. Bozett & S. M. H. Hanson (Eds.), *Fatherhood and families in cultural context* (pp. 114–137). New York: Springer.

Eshleman, J. R. (1974). *The family: An introduction*. Boston: Allyn & Bacon.

Evans, C. J. (1991). Description of a follow-up program for childbearing families. *Journal of Obstetric, Gynecologic, and Neonatal Nursing, 20* (2), 113–118.

Evashwick, C., Nay, J., & Siemon, J. E. (1985). *Case management: Issues for hospitals*. Chicago: Hospital Research and Educational Trust.

Falicov, C. J. (1982). Mexican families. In M. McGoldrick, J. Pierce, & J. Giordano (Eds.), *Ethnicity and family therapy*. New York: Guilford Press.

————. (1988). Learning to think culturally. In D. C. Breunlin & R. C. Schwartz (Eds.), *Handbook of family therapy, training and supervision*. New York: Guilford Press.

————. (1996). Mexican families. In M. McGoldrick, J. Giordano, & J. K. Pearce (Eds.), *Ethnicity and family therapy* (2nd ed.) (pp. 169–182). New York: Guilford Press.

Falloon, I. R. H. (1991). Behavioral family therapy. In A. S. Gurman & D. P. Kniskern (Eds.), *Handbook of family therapy*. New York: Brunner/Mazel.

The Family Connection. (1996, June 25). How California can fight teen pregnancy. *Los Angeles Times*, p. A21.

Family Service America. (1984). *The state of families, 1984–1985*. New York: Family Service of America.

Farberow, N. L., Gallagher-Thompson, D., Gilewski, M., & Thompson, L. (1992). Changes in grief and mental health of bereaved spouses of older adult suicides. *Journal of Gerontology, 47* (6), 357–366.

Farge, E. J. (1975). *La Vida Chicano: Health care attitudes and behaviors of Houston Chicanos*. San Francisco: R & E Research Associates.

Fast, I., & Cain, A. C. (1966). The stepparent role: Potential for disturbances in family functioning. *American Journal Orthopsychiatry, 36*, 485.

————. (1991). Spouses' experiences during pregnancy and the postpartum: A program of research and theory development. In A. Whall & J. Fawcett (Eds.), *Family theory development in nursing: State of the science and art*. Philadelphia: Davis.

Fawcett, J. (1991). Spouses' experiences during pregnancy and postpartum: A program of research and theory development. In A. Whall & J. Fawcett (Eds.), *Family theory development in nursing: State of the science and art*. Philadelphia: Davis.

————. (1995). *Analysis and evaluation of conceptual models of nursing* (3rd ed.). Philadelphia: Davis.

Fawcett, J. & Downs, F.S. (1992). *The relationship of theory and research*. Philadelphia: Davis.

Feiring, C., & Lewis, C. (1984). Changing characteristics of the U.S. family. In M. Lewis (Ed.), *Beyond the dyad* (pp. 59–89). New York: Plenum.

Feldman, F., & Scherz, F. (1967). *Family social welfare*. New York: Atherton.

Feldman, H. (1961). The development of the husband–wife relationship. Unpublished study supported in part by the National Institute of Mental Health.

————. (1969). *Parent and Marriage: Myths and Realities*. Paper read at the Merrill-Palmer Institute Conference on the Family, November 21.

————. (1971). The effects of children on the family. In A. Michel (Ed.), *Family issues of employed women in Europe and America* (pp. 107–125). Leiden, Netherlands: E. J. Brill.

Fellows, D. K. (1972). *A mosaic of America's ethnic minorities*. New York: Wiley.

Ferree, M. M. (1987). Family and job for working class women: Gender and class systems seen from below. In N. Gerstel & H. Gross (Eds.), *Families and work* (pp. 289–301). Philadelphia: Temple University Press.

Ferreira, A. J. (1963). Family myth and homeostasis. *Archives of General Psychiatry, 9*, 457.

Fife, B. L. (1985). A model for predicting the adaptation of families to medical crisis: An analysis of role integration. *Image, 17* (4), 108–112.

Figley, C. (Ed.). (1995). *Compassion fatigue: Coping with secondary traumatic stress disorder in those who treat the traumatized.* New York: Brunner/Mazel.

Figley, C. R. (1989). *Helping traumatized families.* San Francisco: Jossey-Bass.

Filsinger, E. E. (1983). *Marriage and family assessment.* Newbury Park, CA: Sage.

Fine, M. (1992). Families in the United States: Their current status and future prospects. *Family Relations, 41,* 430–435.

Fine, M. A., Donnelly, B. W., & Voydanoff, P. (1986). Adjustment and satisfaction of parents: A comparison of intact, single parent and stepparent families. *Journal of Family Issues, 7,* 391–404.

Finley, N. J. (1989). Theories of family labor as applied to gender differences in caregiving for elderly parents. *Journal of Marriage and the Family, 51* (1), 79–86.

Fischer J. & Wampler R. (1994). Abusive drinking in young adults: Personality type and family role as moderators of family-of-origin influences. *Journal of Marriage and the Family, 56,* 469–479.

Fisher, K. (1987, August). Quality assurance: Case management. *Quality Review Bulletin,* 287–290.

Fisher, L., & Ransom, D. C. (1995). An empirically derived typology of families: 1. Relationships with adult health. *Family Process, 34,* 161–181.

Fishman, H. C. (1985). Diagnosis and context: An Alexandrian quartet. In R. L. Ziffer (Ed.), *Adjunctive techniques in family therapy.* New York: Grune & Stratton.

Fitting, M., Rabins, P., Lucas, M. J., & Eastham, J. (1986). Caregivers for demented patients: A comparison of husbands and wives. *The Gerontologist, 26,* 248–252.

Fitzpatrick, M. A., & Ritchie, L. D. (1993). Communication theory and the family. In P. G. Boss, W. J. Doherty, R. LaRossa, W. R. Schumm, & S. K. Steinmetz (Eds.), *Sourcebook of family theories and methods: A contextual approach* (pp. 565–585). New York: Plenum.

Fitzpatrick, S. B., Coughlin, S. S., & Chamberline, J. (1992). A novel asthma camp intervention for childhood asthma among urban blacks. *Journal of the National Medical Association, 84* (3), 233–237.

Flacks, R. (1971). *Youth and social change.* Chicago: Markham.

Flannery, R., Perry, C., Penk, W., & Flannery, G. (1994). Validating Antonovsky's sense of coherence scale. *Journal of Clinical Psychology, 50,* 575–577.

Flaskerud, J. (1984, Sept.). Mental health—The culture component. *California Nurse,* 4.

Foley, V. D. (1986). *An introduction to family therapy* (2nd ed.). Orlando, FL: Grune & Stratton.

Folkman, S., Lazarus, R. S., Dunkel-Schetter, C., De Longis, A., & Gruen, R. J. (1986). The dynamics of a stressful encounter: Cognitive appraisal, coping and encounter-outcomes. *Journal of Personality and Social Psychology, 50,* 992–1003.

Follen, M. A., Johnson, D., & Kronenwetter, S. (1994). Family interventions in a critical care setting. In *Program and Abstracts of the Third International Family Nursing Conference.* Montreal, Canada, May 25–28, 1994.

Ford, L. (1979). The development of family nursing. In D. P. Hymovich & M. U. Barnard (Eds.), *Family health care.* New York: McGraw-Hill.

Forrest, J. (1981). The family. The focus for health behavior generation. *Health Values: Achieving High Level Wellness, 5* (4), 138–144.

Fraley, A. M. (1992). *Nursing and the disabled. Across the life span.* Boston: Jones and Bartlett.

Francis, G. M., & Munjas, B. A. (1976). *Manual of socialpsychologic assessment.* New York: Appleton-Century-Crofts.

Franklin, J. H. (1988). A historical note on black families. In H. P. McAdoo (Ed.), *Black families* (2nd ed.) (pp. 23–26). Newbury Park, CA: Sage.

Freeman, D. S. (1992). *Multigenerational family therapy.* New York: Haworth Press.

Freeman, R. B. (1970). *Community health nursing practice.* Philadelphia: Saunders.

Frey, M., & Sieloff, C. (Eds.). (1995). *Advancing King's systems framework and theory of nursing.* London: Sage.

Friedemann, M. L. (1989). Closing the gap between grand theory and mental health practice with families. Part 1. *Archives of Psychiatric Nursing, III* (Feb.), 10–19.

————. (1993a). Closing the gap between grand theory and mental health practice with families. In G. Wegner & R. Alexander (Eds.), *Readings in family nursing* (pp. 41–56). Philadelphia: Lippincott.

————. (1993b). The concept of family nursing. In G. D. Wegner & R. J. Alexander (Eds.), *Readings in family nursing* (pp. 13–22). Philadelphia: Lippincott.

————. (1995). *The framework of systemic organization.* Thousand Oaks, CA: Sage.

Friedman, D. B. (1957). Parent development. *California Medicine, 86,* 25.

Friedman, M. (1985). *Family stress and coping among Anglo and Latino families with childhood cancer.* Unpublished PhD dissertation, University of Southern California.

————. (1986). *Family nursing: Theory and assessment* (2nd ed.). Norwalk, CT: Appleton & Lange.

————. (1987). Intervening with families of school-aged children with cancer. In M. Leahey & L. M. Wright (Eds.), *Families and life-threatening illness* (pp. 219–234). Springhouse, PA: Springhouse Publishing.

————. (1990). Transcultural family nursing: Application to Latino and Black families. *Journal of Pediatric Nursing, 5* (3), 214–222.

Friedman, M. M. (1992). *Family nursing: Theory and practice* (3rd ed.). Norwalk, CT: Appleton & Lange.

Friedman, M. M., & Ferguson-Marshalleck, E. (1996). Sociocultural influences on family health. In S. Hanson & S. Boyd (Eds.), *Family health care nursing: Theory, practice & research* (pp. 81–98). Philadelphia: Davis.

Fulwood, S. (1996, Sept. 27). Income shows 1st rise since 1989 as poverty falls. *Los Angeles Times,* pp. A1, A16.

Furstenberg, F. F., & Nord, C. W. (1985). Parenting apart: Patterns of childrearing after marital disruption. *Journal of Marriage and the Family, 47* (4), 893–904.

Gable, S., Ernic, K., & Belsky, J. (1994). Co-parenting within the family system. Influences on children's development. *Family Relations, 43,* 380–386.

Gadow, S. (1980). Existential advocacy: Philosophical foundations of nursing. In S. Spicker & S. Gadow (Eds.), *Nursing images and ideals.* New York: Springer.

Gagne, P. (1992). Appalachian women: Violence and social control [Special issue]. *Journal of Contemporary Ethnography, 20,* 387–415.

Gallegos, J. S. (1991). Culturally relevant services for Hispanic elderly. In M. Sotomayor (Ed.), *Empowering Hispanic families: A critical issue for the 90's* (pp. 173–190). Milwaukee, WI: Family Service America.

Galvin, K. M., & Brommel, B. J. (1986). *Family communication: Cohesion and change* (2nd ed.). Glenview, IL: Scott, Foresman.

Ganong, L., Coleman, M., & Fine, M. (1995). Remarriage and stepfamilies. In R. D. Day, K. R. Gilbert, B. H. Settles, & W. R. Burr (Eds.), *Research and theory in family science* (pp. 287–303). Pacific Grove, CA: Brooks/Cole.

Garcia, J. M. (1993). *The Hispanic population in the U.S.: March, 1992* (U.S. Bureau of Census, Current Population Reports, P20-465 RV). Washington, DC: Government Printing Office.

Garcia-Preto, N. (1996). Latino families: An overview. In M. McGoldrick, J. Giordano, & J. K. Pearce (Eds.), *Ethnicity and family therapy* (2nd ed.) (pp. 141–154). New York: Guilford Press.

Gardner, R. W., Robey, B., & Smith, P. C. (1985). Asian Americans: Growth, change, and diversity. *Population Bulletin, 40* (4). Washington, DC: Population Reference Bureau.

Garner, M. K. (1978). Our values are showing: Inadequate childhood immunization. *Health Values: Achieving High Level Wellness, 2* (3), 129.

Geba, B. (1985). *Being at leisure, play at life.* La Mesa, CA: Leisure Science Systems International.

Gecas, V., & Seff, M. A. (1991). Families and adolescents: A review of the 1980's. In A. Booth (Ed.), *Contemporary families. Looking forward, looking back* (pp. 208–225). Minneapolis, MN: National Council on Family Relations.

Gecas, V. (1976). The socialization and child care roles. In F. I. Nye (Ed.), *Role structure and analysis of the family.* Vol. 24. Beverly Hills, CA: Sage.

———. (1979). The influence of social class on socialization. In W. R. Burr, R. Hill, F. I. Nye, & I. L. Reiss (Eds.), *Contemporary theories about the family. Vol. I* (pp. 365–404). New York: Free Press.

Geismar, L. L., & La Sorte, B. (1964). *Understanding the multiproblem family.* New York: Association Press.

Gelcer, E. (1986). Dealing with loss in the family context. *Journal of Family Issues, 7* (3), 315–335.

Gelles, R. J. (1980). Violence in the family: A review of research on the seventies. *Journal of Marriage and the Family, 42* (4), 873–885.

———. (1990). Methodological issues in the study of family violence. In G. R. Patterson (Ed.), *Family social interaction. Content and methodology issues in the study of aggression and depression* (pp. 49–74). Hillsdale, NY: Erlbaum.

Gelles, R. J., & Maynard, P. E. (1987). A structural family systems approach to intervention in cases of family violence. *Family Relations, 36* (3), 270–275.

Gelman, D., et al. (1985, July 15). Playing both mother and father. *Newsweek,* 42–50.

———. (1988, March 7). Black and white in America. *Newsweek,* 18–23.

Gendell, M., & Siegel, J. S. (1996). Trends in retirement age in the United States, 1955–1993 by sex and race. *Journal of Gerontology, 51B* (May) 3.

George, L., & Gwyther, L. (1986). Caregiver well-being: A multidimensional examination of family caregivers of demented adults. *The Gerontologist, 26* (3), 253–259.

Germain, C. P. (1992). Cultural care: A bridge between sickness, illness, and disease. *Holistic Nursing Practice, 6* (3), 1–9.

Gershwin, M. W., & Nilsen, J. M. (1989). Healthy families. In C. L. Gilliss, B. L. Highley, B. M. Roberts, & I. M. Martinson (Eds.), *Towards a science of family nursing* (pp. 77–91). Menlo Park, CA: Addison-Wesley.

Gerson, W. M. (1960). Leisure and marital satisfaction of college married couples. *Marriage and Family Living, 22,* 360–361.

Giger, J. N., & Davidhizar, R. E. (1995). *Transcultural nursing: Assessment and intervention* (2nd ed.). St. Louis: Mosby.

Gilbert, D., & Kahl, J. A. (1993). *The American class structure.* Belmont, CA: Wadsworth.

Giles-Sims, J., Straus, M. A., & Sugarman, D. B. (1995). Child, maternal, and family characteristics associated with spanking. *Family Relations, 44,* 170–176.

Gilford, R. (1984). Contracts in marital satisfaction throughout old age: An exchange theory analysis. *Journal of Gerontology, 39,* 325–333.

Gilligan, C. (1982). *In a different voice.* Cambridge: Harvard University Press.

Gilliss, C. L. (1984). Reducing family stress during and after coronary artery bypass surgery. *Nursing Clinics of North America, 19* (1), 103–111.

———. (1989a). *Family Nursing Research, Theory, & Practice: Our Challenges*. Presentation at the National Conference on Family Nursing, Sept. 15, Portland, Oregon.

———. (1989b). Why family health care and What is family nursing? In C. L. Gilliss, B. L. Highley, B. M. Roberts, & I. M. Martinson (Eds), *Toward a science of family nursing* (pp. 3–8, 64–73). Menlo Park, CA: Addison-Wesley.

———. (1991). Family nursing research. *Image, 23* (1), 19–22.

Gilliss, C. L., & Davis, L. L. (1993). Does family intervention make a difference? An integrative review and meta-analysis. In S. L. Feetham, S. B. Meister, J. M. Bell, & C. L. Gilliss (Eds.), *The nursing of families: Theory, research, education and practice* (pp. 259–265). Newbury Park, CA: Sage.

Gilliss, C. L., Rose, D. B., Hallburg, J. C., & Martinson, I. M. (1989). The family and chronic illness. In C. L. Gilliss, B. L. Highley, B. M. Roberts, & I. M. Martinson (Eds.), *Toward a science of family nursing* (pp. 287–299). Menlo Park, CA: Addison-Wesley.

Gilliss, C. L., Sparacino, P. S. A., Gortner, S. R., & Kenneth, H. Y. (1985). Events leading to the treatment of coronary artery disease: Implications for nursing care. *Heart & Lung, 14* (4), 350–356.

Gladding, S. T. (1995). *Family therapy: History, theory, and practice*. Englewood Cliffs, NJ: Prentice-Hall.

Glasser, P., & Glasser, L. (1970). *Families in crisis*. New York: Harper & Row.

Glenn, M. L. (1987). *Collaborative health care: A family-oriented model*. New York: Praeger.

Glick, P. C. (1988a). Demographic pictures of black families. In H. P. McAdoo (Ed.), *Black families* (2nd ed.) (pp. 111–132). Newbury Park, CA: Sage.

———. (1988b). Fifty years of family demography: A record of social change. *Journal of Marriage and the Family, 50* (4), 861–873.

———. (1989). The family life cycle and social change. *Family Relations, 38* (2), 123–129.

———. (1994). American families: As they are and were. In A. S. Skolnick & J. H. Skolnick (Eds.), *Family in transition* (8th ed.) (pp. 91–104). New York: HarperCollins College.

———. (1997). Demographic pictures of African American families. In H. P. McAdoo (Ed.), *Black families* (3rd ed.) (pp. 118–138). Thousand Oaks, CA: Sage.

Godwin, D. D., & Scanzoni, J. (1989). Couple consensus during marital joint decision-making: A context, process, outcome model. *Journal of Marriage and the Family, 51* (4), 943–956.

Goering, P. N., Wasydlenki, D. A., et al. (1988). What difference does case management make? *Hospital and Community Psychiatry, 39* (3), 272–276.

Goldenberg, I., & Goldenberg, H. (1996). *Family therapy. An overview* (4th ed.). Monterey, CA: Brooks/Cole.

———. (1990). *Counseling today's families*. Pacific Grove, CA: Brooks/Cole.

Goldfried, M. & Sobocinski, D. (1975). The effect of irrational beliefs on emotional arousal. *Journal of Consulting and Clinical Psychology, 43,* 504–510.

Goldner, V. (1985). Feminism and family therapy. *Family Process, 24,* 31–47.

Gonzales, E. (1976). The role of Chicano folk beliefs and practices in mental health. In C. A. Hernandez, M. J. Haug, & N. N. Wagner (Eds.), *Chicanos—Social and psychological perspectives* (2nd ed.). St. Louis: Mosby.

Gonzalez, G. (1991). Hispanics in the past two decades, Latinos in the next two: Hindsight and foresight. In M. Sotomayor (Ed.), *Empowering Hispanic families: A critical issue for the '90s* (pp. 1–19). Milwaukee, WI: Family Service America.

Goode, W. J. (1964). *The family*. Glencoe, IL: Free Press.

———. (1971). *Introduction to the contemporary American family*. Chicago: Quadrange.

Goodman, E. (1978, June 25). America's war against its children makes monsters of all of us. *Los Angeles Times*, p. 4.

Goodspeed, H. E. (1975). Scapegoating: A process continuing when parents divorce. In S. Smoyak (Ed.), *The psychiatric nurse as a family therapist*. New York: Wiley.

Gordner, S. (1980). Nursing science in transition. *Nursing Research, 29,* 80–83.

Gordon, M. (1976). Nursing diagnoses and the diagnostic process. *American Journal of Nursing, 76,* 1298.

———. (1978). *The American family*. New York: Random House.

———. (1982). Historical perspective. The national group for classification of nursing diagnoses. In M. J. Kim & D. A. Moritz (Eds.), *Classification of nursing diagnoses*. New York: McGraw-Hill.

———. (1985). *Manual of nursing diagnoses—1984–1985*. New York: McGraw-Hill.

Gordon, M. M. (1964). *Assimilation in American life*. New York: Oxford University Press.

Gordon, T. (1970). *Parent effectiveness training*. New York: Wyden.

Gorman, G. (1975). New families, new marriages. In S. Smoyak, (Ed.), *The psychiatric nurse as a family therapist*. New York: Wiley.

Gottfried, A. E., & Gottfried, A. W. (1994). *Redefining families: Implications for children's development*. New York: Plenum.

Gottlieb, B. H. (1983). *Social support strategies: Guidelines for mental health practice*. Beverly Hills, CA: Sage.

Gottlieb, D., & Ramsey, C. (1964). *The American adolescent.* Homewood, IL: Dorsey Press.

Gottman, J. (1995, Nov.). *Predictors of Divorce: Narrow Therapy.* Presentation made at the annual convention of the National Council on Family Relations, Portland, Oregon.

Gottman, J., Notarius, C., Gonso, J., & Markman, H. (1977). *A couples guide to communication.* Champagne, IL: Research Press.

Graedon, T. F. (1985). A transcultural approach to nursing practice. In J. E. Hall & B. R. Weaver (Eds.), *Distributive nursing practice. Systems approach to community health* (3rd ed.) (pp. 315–331). Philadelphia: Lippincott.

Grau, L. (1984, Nov./Dec.). Case management and the nurse. *Geriatric Nursing,* 372–375.

Gray, V. (1996). Family self-care. In P. J. Bomar (Ed.), *Nurses and family health promotion: Concepts, assessment, and interventions* (2nd ed.). Philadelphia: Saunders.

Grebler, L., Moore, J. W., & Guzman, R. C. (1970). *The Mexican-American people: The nation's second largest minority.* New York: Free Press.

Green, M. (1994). *Bright futures. Guidelines for health supervision of infants, children and adolescents.* Arlington, VA: National Center for Education in Maternal and Child Health.

Greenblatt, J., Gfroerer, J., & Melnick, D. (1995, Dec. 1). Increasing morbidity and mortality associated with abuse of methamphetamines—United States, 1991–1994. *Morbidity and Mortality Weekly Report, 44,* 47.

Greene, B. (1995). African American families. *National Forum, 75* (3), 29–32.

Greiner, D. S., & Demi, A. S. (1995). Family therapy. In B. S. Johnson (Ed.), *Child, adolescent, and family psychiatric nursing* (pp. 358–368). Philadelphia: Lippincott.

Greydanus, D. E. (Ed.). (1991). *Caring for your adolescent* (American Academy of Pediatrics Publication). New York: Bantam Books.

Griffin, J. L. (1994, Feb. 14). Black health risks unique. *The Oregonian,* p. A2.

Grimes, M. L. (1996). Middle class morality: Postures towards the poor. *National Forum, 76* (3), 3–4.

Grotevant, H. D., & Carlson, C. I. (Eds.). (1989). *Family assessment: A guide to methods and measures.* New York: Guilford Press.

Gudykunst, W. B. (1991). *Bridging differences: Effective intergroup communicaton.* Newbury Park, CA: Sage.

Gurin, J. (1985, Oct.). Families: A personal way to get unstuck. *American Health,* 39–41.

Gurin, J., & Harris, T. G. (1987, March). Taking charge: The happy health-confidants. *American Health,* 53–57.

Haber, R. (1987). Friends in family therapy: Use of a neglected resource. *Family Process, 26* (June), 269–281.

Hagestad, G. O. (1988). Demographic change and the life course: Some emerging trends in the family realm. *Family Relations, 37* (4), 405–410.

Hajal, F. (1990). Family scapegoating in the life and works of Karen Blixen. *Journal of the American Academy of Psychoanalysis, 18,* 626–643.

Haley, J. (1976). *Problem-solving therapy.* San Francisco: Jossey-Bass.

———. (1980). *Leaving home.* New York: McGraw-Hill.

Hall, A., & Wellman, B. (1985). Social networks and social support. In S. Cohen & S. L. Syme (Eds.), *Social support and health* (pp. 23–41). New York: Academic Press.

Hall, J., & Weaver, B. (1974). Crisis: A conceptual approach to family nursing. In J. Hall & B. Weaver (Eds.), *Nursing of families in crisis* (pp. 3–9). Philadelphia, Lippincott.

Hallen, L. L. (1978). Family systems theory in psychiatric intervention. *American Journal of Psychiatry, 74* (3), 463.

Hammer, T. J., & Turner, P. H. (1985). *Parenting in contemporary society.* Englewood Cliffs, NJ: Prentice-Hall.

Hammond, J., & Enoch, J. (1976). Conjugal power relations among Black working class families. *Journal of Black Studies, 7* (1), 107–127.

Handel, G. (1972). *The psychosocial interior of the family* (2nd ed.). Chicago: Aldine Atherton.

Hanson, S. M. H., & Boyd, S. T. (Eds.). (1996a). *Family health care nursing: Theory, practice and research.* Philadelphia: Davis.

———. (1996b). Family nursing: An overview. In S. M. H. Hanson & S. T. Boyd (Eds.), *Family health care nursing: Theory, practice and research* (pp. 5–37). Philadelphia: Davis.

Hanson, S. M. H., & Bozett, F. H. (Eds.). (1985). *Dimensions of fatherhood.* Newbury Park, CA: Sage.

———. (1987). Fatherhood and changing family roles. *Family and Community Health, 9* (4), 9–21.

Hanson, S. M. H., & Kaakinen, J. R. (1996). Family health assessment. In M. Stanhope & J. Lancaster (Eds.), *Community health nursing* (pp. 497–520). St. Louis: Mosby.

Hanson, S. M. H., & Mischke, K. (1996). Family health assessment and intervention. In P. J. Bomar (Ed.), *Nurses and family health promotion* (2nd ed.) (pp. 165–202). Philadelphia: Saunders.

Harburg, E., Erfurt, J. C., Chape, G., & Havenstein, L. S. (1973). Socioecological stressor areas and Black–White blood pressure. Detroit. *Journal of Chronic Diseases, 26,* 595–611.

Hardwick, P. (1991). Families and the professional network: An attempted classification of professional network actions which can hinder change. *Journal of Family Therapy, 13,* 187–205.

Hardy, M. E., & Conway, M. (1978). *Role theory: Perspectives for health professionals.* New York: Appleton-Century-Crofts.

Hardy, M. E., & Hardy, W. L. (1988). Role stress and role strain. Managing role strain. In M. E. Hardy & M. Conway (Eds.), *Role theory: Perspectives for health professionals* (pp. 159–255). Norwalk, CT: Appleton & Lange.

Hareven, T. K. (1987). Historical analysis of the family. In M. B. Sussman & S. K. Steinmetz (Eds.), *Handbook of marriage and the family* (pp. 37–57). New York: Plenum Press.

Harris, L., et al. (1975). *The myths and reality of aging in America.* Washington, DC: National Council on Aging.

Harris, R. (1990, July 10). Blacks: Grim statistics considered threat to race. *Los Angeles Times,* pp. A1, A25.

———. (1991, May 14). A generation of innocents carries drug abuse scars. *Los Angeles Times,* pp. A1, A18, A19.

Harris, S. E. (1975). Negativity as a major communication pattern in a family. In S. Smoyak (Ed.), *The psychiatric nurse as a family therapist* (pp. 210–216). New York: Wiley.

Harris, T. G. (1984). From hedonism to health. *American Health, 3* (2), 54–56.

Harris, T., & Gurin, J. (1985, March). The new eighties lifestyle: Look who's getting it all together. *American Health,* 42–47.

Harrison, A. O., et al. (1994). Family ecologies of ethnic minority children. In G. Handel & G. G. Whitchurch (Eds.), *The psychosocial interior of the family* (4th ed.) (pp. 187–209). New York: Aldine de Gruyter.

Harrison, I. E., & Harrison, D. S. (1971). The Black family experience and health behavior. In C. Crawford (Ed.), *Health and the family* (pp. 175–199). New York: Macmillan.

Hartman, A. (1978). Diagrammatic assessment of family relationships. *Social Casework, 59,* 456–476.

Hartman, A., & Laird, J. (1983). *Family-centered social work practice.* New York: Free Press.

Hartrick, G., Lindsey, A. E., & Hills, M. (1994). Family nursing assessment: Meeting the challenge of health promotion. *Journal of Advanced Nursing, 20,* 85–91.

Harvath, T. A., Stewart, B. J., & Archibold, P. G. (1994). *Third International Family Nursing Conference, Program and Abstracts,* May 25–28, Montreal, Canada.

Harwood, A. (1981). Guidelines for culturally appropriate health care. In A. Harwood (Ed.), *Ethnicity and medical care* (pp. 482–507). Cambridge, MA: Harvard Press.

Haug, M., Belgrove, L., & Jones, S. (1992). Partner's health and retirement adaptation of women and their husbands. *Journal of Women and Aging, 4* (3), 5–29.

Hawkes, G. R., & Taylor, M. (1975, Nov.). Power structure in Mexican and Mexican-American farm labor families. *Journal of Marriage and the Family, 37* (4), 807–811.

Hawkins, A. J., Marshall, C. M., & Meiners, K. M. (1995). Exploring wives' sense of fairness about family work. *Journal of Family Issues, 16* (6), 693–721.

Hawkins, J., Weisberg, C., & Ray, D. (1980). Spouse differences in communication style. Preference, perception, behavior. *Journal of Marriage and the Family, 42* (3), 585–593.

Haydon, D. F. (1987). The family and health/fitness. *Health Values, 11* (2), 36–39.

Hayes-Battista, D. (1990, April 26). *Creating Health Policy in Multi-cultural California.* Paper presented at a statewide conference of the California Coalition for the Future of Public Health, Los Angeles, CA.

Haywood, M. D., & Liu, M. C. (1992). Men and women in their retirement years: A demographic profile. In M. Snizovcz, D. J. Ekerdt, & D. H. Vinick (Eds.), *Families and retirement* (Sage Focus ed.) Newbury Park, CA: Sage.

Hazzard, M. (1971). An overview of systems theory. *Nursing Clinics of North America, 6,* 385–393.

Heady, M. (1996, May 15). Holistic plan urged to aid Black males. *Los Angeles Times,* p. A12.

Health Resources and Services Administration. (1990). *Health status of the disadvantaged* (Publication No. HRSP-DV 90-1). Washington, DC: U.S. Government Printing Office.

Healy, A., Keesee, P. D., & Smith, B. S. (1985). *Early services for children with special needs: Transactions for family support.* Iowa City, IA. Division of Developmental Disabilities, University Hospital School, Dept. of Pediatrics.

Heinrich, K. (1996). Family sexuality. In P. J. Bomar (Ed.), *Nurses and family health promotion* (2nd ed.) (pp. 284–302). Philadelphia: Saunders.

Heller, P. L. (1976). Familism scale: Revalidation and revision. *Journal of Marriage and the Family, 38* (2), 423–429.

Henderson, A. A., & Brouse, A. J. (1991). The experiences of new fathers during the first three weeks of life. *Journal of Advanced Nursing, 18,* 293–298.

Henderson, G. (1989). *A practitioner's guide to understanding indigenous and foreign cultures.* Springfield, IL: Charles C. Thomas.

Herberg, P. J. (1995). Theoretical foundations of transcultural nursing. In M. M. Andrews & J. S. Boyle (Eds.), *Transcultural concepts in nursing care* (2nd ed.) (pp. 3–96). Philadelphia: Lippincott.

Herbst, P. G. (1954). Conceptual framework for studying the family: Family living regions and pathways, family-living patterns of interaction. In O. A. Oeser & S. B. Hammond (Eds.), *Social structure and personality in a city.* New York: Macmillan.

Hernandez, M. (1996). Central American families. In M. McGoldrick, J. Giordano, & J. K. Pearce (Eds.), *Ethnicity and family therapy* (2nd ed.) (pp. 214–223). New York: Guilford Press.

Herrera T., & Wagner, N. N. (1974). Behavioral approaches to delivering health services in a Chicano community. In A. Reinhardt & M. Quinn (Eds.), *Family-centered community nursing.* St. Louis: Mosby.

Herzog, E., & Sudia, C. E. (1973). Children in fatherless families. In B. M. Caldwell & M. N. Ricutti (Eds.), *Review of child development research,* Vol. 3. Chicago: University of Chicago Press.

Hickey, T. (1988). Self-care behavior of older adults. *Family and Community Health, 11* (3), 23–32.

Hilgenberg, C., Liddy, K. G., Standerfer, J., & Schraeder, C. (1992). Changes in family patterns six months after a myocardial infarction. *Journal of Cardiovascular Nursing, 6* (2), 46–56.

Hill, M. S. (1988). Marital stability and spouses' shared time. *Journal of Family Issues, 9* (4), 427–451.

Hill, R. (1949). *Families under stress.* New York: Harper & Row.

———. (1958). Social stresses on the family: Generic features of families under stress. *Social Casework, 39,* 139–150.

———. (1965). *Challenges and resources for family development. Family mobility in our dynamic society.* Ames, IA: Iowa State University.

———. (1970). Interdependence among the generations. *Family development in three generations* (Chap. 2). Cambridge, MA: Schenkman.

———. (1986). Life cycle stages for types of single parent families: Of family development theory. *Family Relations, 35* (1), 19–29.

Hill, R., & Hansen, D. (1960). The identification of conceptual frameworks utilized in family study. *Marriage and Family Nursing, 22* (4), 299–311.

Hill, R., Katz, A. M., & Simpson, R. L. (1957). An inventory of research marriage and family behavior: A statement of objectives and progress. *Marriage and Family Living, 19,* 89–92.

Hill, R. B. (1971). *The strengths of black families.* New York: Emerson-Hall.

———. (1981). *Economic policies and black progress: Myths and realities.* New York: National Urban League.

———. (1997). Social welfare policies and African American families. In H. P. McAdoo (Ed.), *Black families* (3rd ed.) (pp. 349–363). Thousand Oaks, CA: Sage.

Hill, R. B., Billingsley, A., Engram, E., et al. (1993). *Research on the African American family. A holistic perspective.* Westport, CT: Auburn House.

Hill, R. B., & Schackleford, S. (1986). The black family revisited. In R. Staples (Ed.), *The black family. Essays and studies* (3rd ed.) (pp. 194–200). Belmont, CA: Wadsworth.

Himmelstein, D., & Woolhandler, S. (1994). *The national health program book: A source guide for advocates.* Monroe, ME: Common Courage Press.

Hines, P. M., & Boyd-Franklin, N. (1996). African American families. In M. McGoldrick, J. Giordano, & J. K. Pearce (Eds.), *Ethnicity and family therapy* (2nd ed.) (pp. 66–84). New York: Guilford Press.

Ho, M. K. (1987). *Family therapy with ethnic minorities.* Newbury Park, CA: Sage.

———. (1992). *Minority children and adolescents in therapy.* Springfield, IL: Charles C. Thomas.

Hobart, C. (1987). Parent–child relations in remarried families. *Journal of Family Issues, 8* (3), 259–277.

Hobbes, T. (1947). *Leviathan.* New York: MacMillan (Original work published in 1651).

Hobbs, D. F., & Cole, S. P. (1976). Transition to parenthood: A decade replication. *Journal of Marriage and the Family, 38* (March), 723–731.

Hoffer, J. (1996). Family communication. In P. J. Bomar (Ed.), *Nurses and family health promotion* (2nd ed.) (pp. 94–106). Philadelphia: Saunders.

Hofferth, S. L. (1984). Kin networks, race, and family structure. *Journal of Marriage and the Family, 46* (4), 791–806.

Hofferth, S. L., & Phillips, D. A. (1987). Child care in the U.S., 1970–1995. *Journal of Marriage and the Family, 49* (3), 559–571.

Hoffman, L. (1981). *Foundations of family therapy: A conceptual framework for system change.* New York: Basic Books.

Hoffman, L. W. (1977, Aug.). Changes in family roles, socialization, and sex differences. *American Psychologist, 32,* 644.

Hogan, M. J. (1990). Economic issues and the family. In National Council for Family Relations, *2001: Preparing families for the future* (pp. 14–15). Minneapolis, MN: National Council for Family Relations.

Hogan, M. J., Buchler, C., & Robinson, B. (1984). Single parenting: Transitioning alone. In H. I. McCubbin & C. R. Figley (Eds.), *Stress and the family, Vol. I: Coping with normative transitions.* New York: Brunner/Mazel.

Hogue, C. G. (1977). Support systems for health promotion. In J. Hall & B. Weaver (Eds.), *Distributive nursing practice: A systems approach to community health.* Philadelphia: Lippincott.

Hollingshead, A. B. (1949). *Elmstown's youth.* New York: Wiley.

———. (1950). Class differences in family stability. *Annals of the American Academy of Political and Social Science, 272.*

Holman, A. M. (1979). *Finding families.* Beverly Hills, CA: Sage.

———. (1983). *Family assessment: Tools for understanding and intervention.* Beverly Hills, CA: Sage.

Holmes, T. (1956). Multidiscipline studies of tuberculosis. In P. Spacer (Ed.), *Personality stress of tuberculosis.* New York: International University Press.

Holmes, T. H., & Rahe, R. H. (1967). The social readjustment rating scale. *Journal of Psychosomatic Research, 1,* 213–218.

Hong, G. K. (1988). A general family practitioner approach for Asian American mental health services. *Professional Psychology: Research & Practice, 19,* 600–605.

———. (1989). Application of cultural and environmental issues in family therapy with immigrant Chinese Americans. *Journal of Strategic and Systemic Therapies, 8,* 14–21.

———. (1993). Synthesizing Eastern and Western psychotherapeutic approaches. In J. L. Chin, J. H. Liem, M. D. Ham, & G. K. Hong (Eds.), *Transference and empathy in Asian American psychotherapy: Cultural values and treatment needs.* Westport, CT: Praeger.

———. (1995). Cultural considerations in rehabilitation counseling for Asian Americans. *National Association of Rehabilitation Professionals in the Private Sector Journal, 10* (2), 59–65.

———. (1996). Culture and empowerment: Counseling services for Chinese American families. *The Journal for the Professional Counselor, 11* (1), 69–80.

Hong, G. K., & Ham, M. D. (1992). Impact of immigration on the family life cycle: Clinical implications for Chinese Americans. *Journal of Family Psychotherapy, 3* (3), 27–40.

———. (1994). Psychotherapy and counseling for Chinese Americans: Curriculum and training issues. *Bulletin of the Hong Kong Psychological Society, 32/33,* 5–19.

Hong, G. K., & Hong, L. K. (1991). Comparative perspectives on child abuse and neglect: Chinese versus Hispanics and Whites. *Child Welfare, LXX* (4), 463–475.

Hong, G. K., Lee, B. S., & Lorenzo, M. K. (1995). Somatization in Chinese American clients: Implications for psychotherapeutic services. *Journal of Contemporary Psychotherapy, 25* (2), 89–104.

Honigman, J. I. (1967). *Personality in culture.* New York: Harper and Row.

Honig, M. (1996). Retirement expectations: Differences by race, ethnicity, and gender. *The Gerontologist, 36* (3), 373–382.

Horwitz, A. (1993). Adult siblings as sources of social support for the severely mentally ill: A test of the serial model. *Journal of Marriage and the Family, 54,* 233–241.

House, J. S., & Kahn, R. L. (1985). Measures and concepts of social support. In S. Cohen & S. L. Syme (Eds.), *Social support and health* (pp. 83–108). Orlando, FL: Academic Press.

Houseknecht, S. K. (1987). Voluntary childlessness. In M. B. Sussman & S. K. Steinmetz (Eds.), *Handbook of marriage and the family.* New York: Plenum Press.

Howell, M. C. (1975). *Helping ourselves: Families and the human network.* Boston: Beacon Press.

Hsu, F.L.K. (1971). *The challenge of the American dream: The Chinese in the U.S.* Belmont, CA: Wadsworth.

Huang, L.N., & Ying, Y.W. (1989). Chinese American children and adolescents. In J. T. Gibbs, L. N. Huang, et al. (Eds.), *Color of color. Psychological interventions with minority children* (pp. 30–66). San Francisco: Jossey-Bass.

Hughes, R., & Perry-Jenkins, M. (1996). Social class issues in family life education. *Family Relations, 45,* 175–182.

Hunter, J. D. (1994). The family and the culture war. In A. S. Skolnick & J. H. Skolnick (Eds.), *Family in transition* (8th ed.) (pp. 537–547). New York: HarperCollins College.

Hunter, K., & Bryant, B. (1994). Pharmacist provided education and counseling for managing pediatric asthma. *Patient Education and Counseling, 24,* 127–134.

Hupcey, J., & Morse, J. (1995). Family and social support: Application to the critically ill patient. *Journal of Family Nursing, 1,* 257–280.

Hutchinson, E. (1988, Feb. 28). Black America: Tale of two nations., *Los Angeles Times,* Part IV, pp. 3, 6.

Hutchison, I. W. (1975). The significance of marital status for morale and life satisfaction among low-income elderly. *Journal of Marriage and the Family, 35,* 2, 287.

Hymovich, D. P., & Barnard, M. U. (1979). *Family health care.* New York: McGraw-Hill.

Ingoldsby, B. B. (1995a). Family origin and universality. In B. B. Ingoldsby & S. Smith (Eds.), *Families in multicultural perspective* (pp. 83–96). New York: Guilford Press.

———. (1995b). Poverty and patriarchy in Latin America. In B. B. Ingoldsby & S. Smith (Eds.), *Families in multicultural perspective* (pp. 335–351). New York: Guilford Press.

Ingrasia, M. (1993, Aug. 30). Endangered family. *Newsweek,* 17–25.

Inkeles, A. (1977). Paper presented to the American Sociological Association, Washington, DC, in September, 1977. Cited in *Los Angeles Times,* September 20, 1977, Part I, pp. 1, 10.

Irelan, L. M. (1972). *Low income life styles.* US Department of HEW, Social and Rehabilitation Services. Washington, DC: U.S. Government Printing Office.

Jackson, D. (Ed.). (1969). *Communication, marriage, and the family.* Palo Alto, CA: Science and Behavior Books.

Jackson, D., & Lederer, W. (1969). *Mirages of marriage.* New York: Norton.

Jackson, D. D. (1965a). The study of the family. *Family Process, 4* (1), 1–20.

———. (1965b). Family rules: Marital quid pro quo. *Archives of General Psychiatry, 12,* 589–594.

Jackson, J. (1966). A conceptual and measurement model for norms and roles. *Pacific Sociological Review, 9,* 35–38.

Jackson, M. P., & McSwane, D. Z. (1996). Homelessness as a determinant of health. *Public Health Nursing, 9* (3), 185–192.

Jacob, T. (1992). Family studies of alcoholism. *Journal of Family Psychology, 5,* 319–338.

Jacob, T., & Tennenbaum, D. L. (1988). *Family assessment: Rationale, methods, and future directions.* New York: Plenum Press.

Jahoda, M. (1958). *Current concepts of positive mental health. Joint Commission on Mental Illness and Health,* Monograph No. 1. New York: Basic Books.

Jaramillo, P. T., & Zapata, J. T. (1987). Roles and alliances with Mexican-American and Anglo families. *Journal of Marriage and the Family, 49* (4), 727–735.

Janosik, E. H., & Green, E. (1992). *Family life.* Boston: Jones & Bartlett.

Janosik, E. H., & Miller, J. R. (1980). *Family-focused care.* New York: McGraw-Hill.

Jayaratne, S. (1978). Behavioral intervention and family decision-making. *Social Work, 23,* 24.

Jellinek, P. S. (1988, Summer). Case-managing AIDS. *Issues in Science and Technology,* 59–63.

Jenkins, K. W. (1995). Communication in families. In R. Day, K. R. Gilbert, B. H. Settles, & W. R. Burr (Eds.), *Research and theory in family science* (pp. 171–185). Pacific Grove, CA: Brooks/Cole.

Jensen, D. P. (1985). Patient contracting. In G. M. Bulechek & J. C. McCloskey (Eds.), *Nursing interventions. Treatment for nursing diagnoses* (pp. 92–98). Philadelphia: Saunders.

Jiang, S. (1995, Summer). Recognizing Asian communities: Differences key to providing care. *National Health Service Corps in Touch* (Newsletter) (p. 3). Chevy Chase, MD: U.S. Public Health Service.

John, D., Shelton, B. A., & Luschen, K. (1995). Race, ethnicity, and perceptions of fairness. *Journal of Family Issues, 16* (3), 357–379.

Johnson, C. L. (1975). Authority and power in Japanese-American marriage. In R. E. Cromwell & D. H. Olson (Eds.), *Power in families* (pp. 182–196). New York: Sage.

Johnson, L. B. (1997). Three decades of black family empirical research. Challenges for the 21st century. In H. P. McAdoo (Ed.), *Black families* (3rd ed.) (pp. 94–113). Thousand Oaks, CA: Sage.

Johnson, P. B. (1974). *Social power and sex-role stereotyping.* PhD Dissertation, University of California, Los Angeles.

Johnson, R. (1984). Promoting the health of families in the community. In M. Stanhope & J. Lancaster (Eds.), *Community health nursing* (pp. 330–360). St. Louis: Mosby.

Johnson, S. H. (1986). Introduction and role theory strategies. In S. H. Johnson (Ed.), *Nursing assessment and strategies for the family at risk. High-risk parenting* (2nd ed.) (pp. 1–12, 388–401). Philadelphia: Lippincott.

Johnson, S. K., Craft, M., Titler, M., Halm, M., Kleiber, C., Montgomery, L. A., Megivern, K., Nicholson, A., & Buckwalter, K. (1995). Perceived changes in adult family members' roles and responsibilities during critical illness. *Image, 27* (30), 238–243.

Johnston, M., & Sarty, M. (1977). *Ethnic Differences in Sex Stereotyping by Mothers: Implications for Health Care.* Paper presented to 1977 World Congress on Mental Health, Vancouver, BC, Canada, Aug. 1977.

Joint Commission on Accreditation on Community Mental Health Service Programs. (1976). *Standards for community mental health centers. Balance service system.* Chicago: Joint Commission on the Accreditation of Hospitals.

Jonas, S. (1996). Exercise. In S. Woolf, S. Jonas, & R. Lawrence (Eds.), *Health promotion and disease prevention in clinical practice* (pp. 176–192). Baltimore: Williams & Wilkins.

Jones, K. C. (1994). Managed care: The coming revolution in home health care. *Journal of Home Health Care Practice, 6* (2), 1–11.

Jones, S. L. (1980). *Family therapy. A comparison of approaches.* Bowie, MD: Brady.

Jones, S. L., & Dimond, M. (1982). Family theory and family therapy models. Comparative review with implications for nursing practice. *Journal of Psychosocial Nursing and Mental Health Services,* 12–19.

Julian, T. W., McKenry, P.C., & McKelvey, M. W. (1994). Cultural variations in parenting: Perceptions of Caucasian, African-American, Hispanic & Asian-American parents. *Family Relations, 43* (1), 30–37.

Juni, S. (1995). Triangulation as splitting in the service of ambivalence. *Current Psychology: Developmental, Learning, Personality, Social, 14,* 91–111.

JWK International Corporation. (1978). Summary and recommendations of conference on Pacific and Asian American families and HEW-related issues. Annandale, VA: JWK International Corporation.

Kagan, J. (1978). The parental love trap. *Psychology Today, 12* (3), 58–59.

Kahana, E., Kahana, B., Johnson, J. R., Hammand, R. J., & Kercher, K. (1994). Developmental challenges and family caregiving: Bridging concepts and research. In E. Kahana, D. E. Biegel, & M. L. Wykle (Eds.), *Family caregiving across the lifespan.* Thousand Oaks, CA: Sage.

Kahn, A. M. (1990). Coping with fear and grieving. In I. M. Lubkin (Ed.), *Chronic illness: Impact and intervention* (pp. 179–199). Boston: Jones & Bartlett.

Kalish, R. A. (1975). *Late adulthood: Perspectives on human development.* Monterey, CA: Brooks/Cole.

Kandzari, J. H., & Howard, J. R. (1981). *The well family: A developmental approach to assessment.* Boston: Little, Brown.

Kane, C. F. (1988). Family social support: Toward a conceptual model. *Advanced Nursing Science, 10* (2), 18–25.

Kane, R. (1988). Case management: Ethical pitfalls on the road to high-quality managed care. *Quality Review Bulletin, 14,* 161–166.

Kane, R., & Kane, R. (1989). *Long-term care.* New York: Springer.

Kane, R. L., Kasteler, J. M., & Gray, R. M. (1976). *The health gap.* New York: Springer.

Kang, R., Barnard, K., & Oshio, S. (1994). Description of the clinical practice of advanced practice nurses in family-centered early intervention in two rural settings. *Public Health Nursing, 11* (6), 376–384.

Kanter, R. M. (1978). Jobs and families: Impact of working roles on life. *Children Today, 7,* 13.

Kantor, D., & Lehr, W. (1975). *Inside the family: Toward a theory of family process.* San Francisco: Jossey-Bass.

Kantrowitz, B., & Wingert, P. (1990, Winter/Spring). Step by step. *Newsweek* (Special Issue), 24–37.

Kaplan, M. S., Adamek, M., & Johnson, S. (1994). Trends in firearm suicide among older American males: 1979–1988. *The Gerontologist, 34* (1).

Kardiner, A. (1945). *The psychological frontiers of society.* New York: Columbia University Press.

Kastenbaum, R. (1994). Alternatives to suicide. In D. Lester & M. Tallmer (Eds.), *Now I lay me down: Suicide in the elderly.* Philadelphia: Charles Press.

Katz, A. H., & Bender, E. I. (1976). *The strength within us.* New York: Franklin Watts.

Kay, M. A. (1978). The Mexican American. In A. L. Clark (Ed.), *Culture, childbearing and health professionals.* Philadelphia: Davis.

Kearney, J. A., & Yurick, C. M. (1996). Nurse to nurse referral: The role of the child psychiatric nurse consultant. *Journal of Pediatric Health Care, 10* (3), 115–120.

Keating, N., & Cole, P. (1980). What do I do with him 24 hours a day? *The Gerontologist, 20,* 84–89.

Keefe, S. E. (1981). Folk medicine among urban Mexican-Americans: Cultural persistence, change and displacement. *Hispanic Journal of Behavioral Science, 3* (1), 41–48.

———. (1984). Real and ideal extended familism among Mexican Americans and Anglo Americans: On the meaning of "close" family ties. *Human Organization, 43,* 65–70.

Keefe, S. E., Padilla, A. M., & Carlos, M. L. (1978). The Mexican-American extended family as an emotional system. In J. M. Casas & S. E. Keefe (Eds.), *Family and mental health in the Mexican-American community.* Los Angeles: Spanish-speaking Mental Health Research Center, UCLA.

Keeney, B. (1982). What is an epistemology of family therapy? *Family Process, 21,* 153–168.

Kell, D., & Patton, C. (1978). Reaction to induced early retirement. *The Gerontologist, 18,* 173–180.

Kelleher, K. (1996, Jan. 10). Who's minding the kids? *Los Angeles Times,* p. E3.

Kelly, J. R. (1978). Family leisure in three communities. *Journal of Leisure Research, 10* (1), 47–60.

Kelly, K. C., McClelland, E., & Day, J. M. (1992). Discharge planning. In G. M. Bulechek & J. C. McCloskey (Eds.), *Nursing interventions: Essential nursing treatments* (2nd ed.) (pp. 265–273). Philadelphia: Saunders.

Kemp, B. J. (1981). The case management model of human service delivery. *Annual Review of Rehabilitation, 2,* 212–238.

Kemper, P. (1988, April). The evaluation of the national long-term demonstration. *Health Services Research, 23* (1), 161–174.

Kendall, J. H. (1974). Maternal behavior one year after early and extended postpartum contact. *Developmental Medicine and Neurology, 16,* 172.

Kennedy, G. E. (1989). Involving students in participatory research on fatherhood. A case study. *Family Relations, 38* (4), 363–37.

Kerckhoff, R. K. (1976). Marriage and middle age. *Family Coordinator, 25* (1), 7–10.

Kerr, M. E., & Bowen, M. (1988). *Family evaluation: An approach based on Bowen theory.* New York: Norton.

Kessler, R. C. (1982). Life events, social supports, and mental health. In W. R. Gove (Ed.), *Deviance and mental illness.* Beverly Hills, CA: Sage.

Kick, I. (1996). Sleep and the family. In P. J. Bomar (Ed.), *Nurses and family health promotion* (2nd ed.) (pp. 245–263). Baltimore, MD: Williams & Wilkins.

Kidwell, J., Fischer, L., Dunham, R. M., & Baranowski, M. (1983). Parents and adolescents: Push and pull of change. In H. I. McCubbin & C. R. Figley (Eds.), *Stress and the family: Coping with normative transitions.* New York: Brunner/Mazel.

Kiecolt-Glaser, J. K., & Glaser, R. (1989). Caregiving, mental health and immune function. In E. Light & B. Lebowitz (Eds.), *Alzheimer's disease treatment and family stress* (DHHS Publication No. 89-1569) (pp. 310–320). Washington, DC: U.S. Government Printing Office.

Kievit, M. B. (1968). Family roles. In Rutgers School of Nursing, *Parent–child Relationships—Role of the nurse.* Newark, NJ: Rutgers University.

Kileen, M. R. (1995). Problems in parenting. In B. S. Johnson (Ed.), *Child, adolescent and family psychiatric nursing* (pp. 32–44). Philadelphia: Lippincott.

Killien, M. G. (1985). An environmental approach to nursing practice. In J. E. Hall & B. R. Weaver (Eds.), *Distributive nursing practice: A systems approach to community health* (2nd ed.) (pp. 259–277). Philadelphia: Lippincott.

Kim, M. J., McFarland, G. K., & McFarlane, A. M. (1995). *Pocket guide to nursing diagnoses* (6th ed.). St. Louis: Mosby.

Kindig, D. (1975). Interdisciplinary education for primary health care team delivery. *Journal of Medical Education, 50,* 102.

King, I. (1981). *Family therapy: A comparison of approaches.* Bowie, MD: Brady.

———. (1983). King's theory of nursing. In I. W. Clements & J. B. Roberts (Eds.), *Family health: A theoretical approach to nursing* (pp. 177–187). New York: Wiley.

———. (1987, May). *King's Theory.* Paper presented at Nursing Theories Conference, Pittsburgh, PA (Cassette recording).

King, K. B., Parrinelo, K. M., & Baggs, J. B. (1996). Collaboration and advanced practice nursing. In J. V. Hickey, R. M. Ovimette, & S. L. Venegoni (Eds.), *Advanced practice nursing* (pp. 146–162). Philadelphia: Lippincott.

Kingson, E. R., Hirshorn, B. A., & Cornman, J. M. (1986). *Ties that bind. The interdependence of generations.* Washington, DC: Seven Locks Press.

Kirschenbaum, H. (1977). *Advanced value clarification.* La Jolla, CA: University Associates.

Kirschling, J., Gilliss, C., et al. (1989). Persons who describe themselves as family nurses: Why they are, where they practice and what they do. Handout at presentation by the Special Interest Group, Family Nursing Continuing Education Project, Oregon Health Sciences University, at the National Family Nursing Conference, Sept. 1989. Portland.

Kirshling, J. M., Gilliss, C. L., Krentz, L., et al. (1994). "Success" in family nursing: Experts describe phenomena. *Nursing and Health Care, 15,* 186–189.

Kitano, H. H. L. (1988). The Japanese American family. In C. H. Mindel, R. W. Habenstein, & R. Wright, Jr. (Eds.), *Ethnic families in America* (pp. 258–275). New York: Elsevier.

Kitano, H. H., & Maki, M. T. (1996). Continuity, change and diversity: Counseling Asian Americans. In P. B. Pedersen, J. G. Draguns, W. J. Lonner, & J. E. Trimble (Eds.), *Counseling across cultures* (4th ed.) (pp. 124–145). Thousand Oaks, CA: Sage.

Kitson, G. C., Babri, F. B., Roach, M. J., & Placidi, K. S. (1989). Adjustment to widowhood and divorce. *Journal of Family Issues, 10* (1), 5–32.

Klaus, M. H., & Kendall, J. H. (1976). *Maternal–infant bonding.* St. Louis: Mosby.

Klein, D. M. (1983). Family problem-solving and family stress. In H. I. McCubbin, M. B. Sussman, & J. M. Patterson (Eds.), Social stress and the family (Special Issue). *Marriage and Family Review, 6* (1/2), 85–112.

Klein, D. M., & White, J. M. (1996). *Family theories: An introduction.* Thousand Oaks, CA: Sage.

Kleinman, A. (1980). *Patients and healers in the context of culture: An exploration of the borderland between anthropology, medicine, and psychiatry.* Berkeley, CA: University of California Press.

———. (1988). *The illness narratives: Suffering, healing, and the human condition.* New York: Basic Books.

Kleinman, A., Eisenberg, L., & Good, B. (1978). Culture, illness and care. Clinical lessons from anthropologic and cross-cultural research. *Annals of Internal Medicine, 88,* 251–258.

Klose, D. (1995). M. Scott Peck's analysis of human evil: A critical review. *Journal of Humanistic Psychology, 35* (3), 37–66.

Kluckholm, F. R. (1976). Dominant and variant value orientations. In P. Brink (Ed.), *Transcultural nursing.* Englewood Cliffs, NJ: Prentice-Hall.

Knafl, K. A., & Deatrick, J. A. (1986). Concept analysis: An analysis of the concept of normalization. *Research in Nursing and Health, 9* (3), 215–222.

Knapp, D. A., Knapp, D. E., & Engle, J. (1966). The public, the pharmacist and self medication. *Journal of the American Pharmacology Association, 56,* 460.

Knapp, M. (1984). *Interpersonal communication and human relationships.* Boston: Allyn & Bacon.

Knesek, G. (1992). Early versus regular retirement: Differences in measures of life satisfaction. *Journal of Gerontological Social Work, 19* (1), 3–34.

Knowles, M. (1973). *The adult learner: A neglected species* (2nd ed.). Houston, TX: Gulf Publishing.

Kobrin, F. E., & Goldscheider, G. (1978). *The ethnic factor in family structure and mobility.* Cambridge, MA: Ballinger.

Koenenn, C. (1997, March 16). Living legal. *Los Angeles Times,* p. E2.

Koerner, B. L., & Armstrong, D. M. (1984). Collaboration practice cuts cost of patient care: Study. *Hospitals, 58,* 52–54.

Kohlberg, L. (1970). Education for justice: A modern statement of the platonic view. In, *Moral education: Five lectures.* Cambridge, MA: Harvard University.

Kohn, M. L. (1969). Social class and parent–child relationships: An interpretation. In R. L. Coser (Ed.), *Life cycle and achievement in America* (pp. 21–42). New York: Harper Torchbooks.

———. (1977). *Class and conformity. A study of values* (2nd ed.). Chicago: University of Chicago Press.

Kohnke, M. F. (1982). *Advocacy: Risk and reality.* St. Louis: Mosby.

Koin, D. (1989). The effects of caregiver stress on physical health status. In E. Light & B. Lebowitz (Eds.), *Alzheimer's disease treatment and family stress* (DHHS Publication No. 89-1569) (pp. 245–266). Washington, DC: U.S. Government Printing Office.

Kollack, P., Blumstein, P., & Schwartz, P. (1985). Sex and power in interaction: Conversational privileges and duties. *American Sociological Review, 50,* 34–46.

Komarovsky, M. (1964). *Blue-collar marriage.* New York: Random House.

Koos, E. (1954). *The health of regionville.* New York: Columbia University Press.

Koshi, P. T. (1976). Cultural diversity in the nursing curricula. *Journal of Nursing Education, 15,* 14.

Kosik, S. H. (1972). Patient advocacy or fighting the system. *American Journal of Nursing, 72,* 694.

Kosten, T. R., Jacobs, S. C., & Kasl, S. V. (1985). Terminal illness, bereavement and the family. In D. C. Turk & R. D. Karns (Eds.), *Health, illness and families. A life span perspective* (pp. 311–334). New York: Wiley.

Koten, J. (1987, March 9). A once tightly knit middle class finds itself divided and uncertain. *Wall Street Journal,* Section 2, p. 25.

Kozol, J. (1990). The new untouchables. *Newsweek* (Special Issue on the 21st Century Family), Winter/Spring, 48–53.

Kranichfield, M. L. (1987). Rethinking family power. *Journal of Family Issues, 8* (1), 42–56.

Kroeber, A. L. (1948). *Anthropology.* New York: Harcourt, Brace.

Kroska, R. A. (1985). Ethnographic research method. A qualitative example to discover role of granny midwives in health services. In M. Leininger (Ed.), *Qualitative research methods in nursing.* New York: Grune & Stratton.

Krozy, R. E. (1996). Community health promotion. Assessment and intervention. In S. H. Rankin & K. D. Stallings (Eds.), *Patient education. Issues, principles, practices* (pp. 245–271). Philadelphia: Lippincott.

Kruszewski, A., Anthony, R., Hough, L., & Ornstein-Galicia, J. (1982). *Politics and society in the Southwest.* Boulder, CO: Westview Press.

Kub, J., & Steel, S. A. (1995). School health. In C. M. Smith & F. A. Maurer (Eds.), *Community health nursing: Theory and practice* (pp. 747–775). Philadelphia: Saunders.

Kuipers, J. (1995). Mexican Americans. In J. N. Giger & R. E. Davidhizar (Eds.), *Transcultural nursing: Assessment and intervention* (2nd ed.) (pp. 205–234). St. Louis: Mosby.

Kunst-Wilson, W., & Cronenwett, L. (1981). Nursing care for the emerging family: Promoting paternal behavior. *Research in Nursing and Health, 4,* 201–211.

Kus, R. J. (1985). Crisis intervention. In G. M. Bulechek & J. C. McCloskey (Eds.), *Nursing interventions: Treatments for nursing diagnoses* (pp. 277–287). Philadelphia: Saunders.

_____. (1992). Crisis intervention. In G. M. Bulechek & J. C. McCloskey (Eds.), *Nursing interventions. Essential nursing treatments* (2nd ed.) (pp. 179–190). Philadelphia: Saunders.

Kyle, M. (1995). Collaboration. In M. Snyder & M. P. Mirr (Eds.), *Advanced practice nursing* (pp. 169–181). New York: Springer.

Labonte, R. (1989). Community and professional empowerment. *Canadian Nurse, 3,* 23–30.

Lacey, K. (1989). Nutrition. In P. Swinford & J. Webster (Eds.), *Promoting wellness: A nurse's handbook.* Rockville, MD: Aspen.

Lackey, C., & Williams, K. (1995). Social bonding and the cessation of partner violence across generations. *Journal of Marriage and the Family, 57,* 295–305.

Laird, J. (1993). Lesbian and gay families. In F. Walsh (Ed.), *Normal family processes* (2nd ed.) (pp. 282–328). New York: Guilford Press.

Lamb, G. S., & Napadano, R. J. (1984). Physician–nurse practitioner interaction patterns in primary care practices. *American Journal of Public Health, 74,* 26–29.

Lamb, M. E. (1987). *The father's role: Cross-cultural perspectives.* Hillsdale, NJ: Erlbaum.

Lamers, E. (1995). Helping children during bereavement. In Lorless, I., et al. (Eds.), *A challenge for living* (pp. 203–220). Boston: Jones & Bartlett.

Lange, S. (1970). Transactional analysis and nursing. In C. Carlson (Ed.), *Behavioral concepts and nursing intervention.* Philadelphia: Lippincott.

Langius, A., & Björnvell, H. (1993). Coping ability and functional status in a Swedish population sample. *Scandinavian Journal of Caring Sciences, 7,* 3–10.

Langman, L. (1987). Social stratification. In M. B. Sussman & S. K. Steinmetz (Eds.), *Handbook of marriage and the family* (pp. 211–249). New York: Plenum Press.

LaRocca, S. (1978). An introduction to role theory for nurses. *Supervisor Nurse, 9* (12), 41–45.

LaRossa, R., & La Rossa, M. M. (1981). *Transition to parenthood. How infants change families.* Newbury Park, CA: Sage.

Larrabee, E. (1973). Comments to Loretta Ford's research. An ethnic perspective. *Community nursing research: Collaboration and completion.* Denver, CO: Western Institute of Higher Education Commission.

Larsen, D. (1989, Feb. 5). Elder abuse. *Los Angeles Times,* Part IV, p. 1.

Larsson, G., & Setterlind, S. (1990). Work load/work control and health: Moderating effects of heredity, self-image, coping, and health behavior. *International Journal of Health Sciences, 1,* 79–88.

Lasch, C. (1977). *Haven in a heartless world. The family besieged.* New York: Basic Books.

_____. (1979). *The culture of narcissism.* New York: Norton.

Lauver, D. (1980). Recognizing alternatives: A process for client centered health care. *Health Values: Achieving High Level Wellness, 4* (3), 134–138.

Lawton, M. P. (1980). *Environment and aging.* Monterey, CA: Brooks/Cole.

_____. (1985). Housing and the living environment of older persons. In R. Binstock & E. Shanas (Eds.), *Handbook of aging and the social sciences* (pp. 450–478). New York: Van Nostrand Reinhold.

Lazarus, R., Averill, J. R., & Opton, E. M. (1974). The psychology of coping. Issues in research and assessment. In G. R. Coelho, D. A. Harburg, & J. E. Adams (Eds.), *Coping and adaptation.* New York: Basic Books.

Lazlo, E. (1972). *The systems view of the world.* New York: George Braziller.

Leahey, M., & Harper-Jaques, S. (1996). Family–nurse relationships: Core assumptions and clinical practice. *Journal of Family Nursing, 2* (2), 133–151.

Leahy, K., Cobb, M., & Jones, M. (1977). *Community health nursing* (3rd ed.). New York, McGraw-Hill.

Leavell, H., Clark, E. G., Gurney, B., et al. (1965). *Preventive medicine for the doctor in his community: An epidemiologic approach* (3rd ed.) (pp. 19–28). New York: McGraw-Hill.

Leavitt, M. B. (1982). *Families at risk: Primary prevention in nursing practice.* Boston: Little, Brown.

Leddy, S., & Pepper, J. M. (1985). *Conceptual basis of professional nursing.* Philadelphia: Lippincott.

Lederer, W. J., & Jackson, D. D. (1968). *Mirages of marriage.* New York: Norton.

Lee, G. R. (1978). Marriage and morale in later life. *Journal of Marriage and the Family, 40* (1), 131.

_____. (1979). Effects of social networks on the family. In W. Burr, R. Hill, F. I. Nye, & I. L. Reiss (Eds.), *Contemporary theories about the family,* Vol. I. New York: Free Press.

Lee, G., & Lancaster, J. (1988). Conceptual models for community health nursing. In M. Stanhope & J. Lancaster (Eds.), *Community health nursing* (2nd ed.) (pp. 131–148). St. Louis: Mosby.

Lee, J. L., & Cohen, J. I. (1995). Collaboration: A concept analysis. *Journal of Advanced Nursing, 21,* 103–109.

Leeds, J. (1996, June 3). Poverty on rise for children of working poor. *Los Angeles Times,* pp. B1, B6.

Leininger, M. (1970). *Nursing and anthropology: Two worlds to blend.* New York: Wiley.

_____. (1974). Transcultural nursing; A promising subfield of study for nurses. In A. Reinhardt & M. Quinn (Eds.), *Family centered community nursing* (pp. 7–44). St. Louis: Mosby.

_____. (1976). *Transcultural health care issues and conditions.* Philadelphia: Davis.

_____. (1978). *Transcultural nursing: concepts, theories and practice.* New York: Wiley.

_____. (1995). Teaching transcultural nursing to transform nursing for the 21st century. *Journal of Transcultural Nursing, 6* (2), 2–3.

LeMasters, E. E. (1957). Parenthood as crisis. *Marriage and Family Living, 19* (2), 352.

_____. (1974). Parents without partners. In A. Skolnick & J. H. Skolnick (Eds.) *Intimacy, family and society.* Boston: Little, Brown.

Leonard, G. (1976, May 10). The holistic health revolution. *New West,* 43.

LeShan, E. J. (1973). *The wonderful crisis of middle age.* New York: McKay.

Leslie, G. R., & Korman, S. K. (1989). *The family in social context* (7th ed.). New York: Oxford University Press.

Lester, P. A. (1986). Teaching strategies. In S. H. Johnson (Ed.), *Nursing assessment and strategies for the family at risk. High-risk parenting* (2nd ed.) (pp. 415–433). Philadelphia: Lippincott.

Lesthaeghe, R. (1983, Sept.). A century of demographic and cultural change in Western Europe. *Population and Development Review,* 411–435.

Levac, A. M., Wright, L. M., & Leahey, M. (In press). Family assessment and intervention. In S. A. Fox (Ed.), *Primary health care of children.* St Louis, MO: Mosby.

Levin, L. S. (1977). Forces and issues in the revival of interest in self-care: Impetus for reduction in health care. *Issues in Self-care (Health Education Monographs), 5* (2), 116.

Levin, L. S., Katz, A., & Holst, E. (1976). *Self-care—Lay initiatives in health.* New York: Prodist Press.

Levin, R. J., & Levin, A. (1975, Sept.). Sexual pleasure. The surprising preferences of 100,000 women. *Redbook,* 51–58.

Levine, E. M. (1988). The realities of day care for children. *Journal of Family Issues, 8* (4), 451–454.

Levy, F. (1988, Feb. 28). Black America: Tale of two nations. *Los Angeles Times,* Part IV, pp. 3, 6.

Lewis, A., & Levy, J. S. (1982). *Psychiatric liaison nursing. The theory and clinical practice.* Reston, VA: Reston Publishing.

Lewis, D. (1975). The black family. Socialization and sex roles. *Phylon, 2,* 221–237.

Lewis, J. I., Beavers, W. R., Gossett, J. T., & Phillips, V. A. (1976). *No single thread: Psychological health in family systems.* New York: Brunner/Mazel.

Lewis, O. (1961). *Children of Sanchez.* New York: Random House.

Libman, J. (1988, Aug. 9). Growing up too fast. *Los Angeles Times,* Part V, p. 1.

Lidz, T. (1963). *The family and human adaptation.* New York: International Universities Press.

Lin, C. C., & Fu, V. R. (1990). A comparison of child-rearing practices among Chinese, immigrant Chinese, and Caucasian American parents. *Child Development, 61,* 429–433.

Lindgren, C. L. (1993, Spring). The caregiver career. *Image, 25* (3), 214–219.

Link, B., & Dohrenwend, B. P. (1980). Formulation of hypotheses about the true prevalence of demoralization. In B. P. Dohrenwend (Ed.), *Mental illness in the U.S.: Epidemiological estimates* (pp. 114–132). New York: Praeger.

Linnett, M. (1970). Prescribing habits in general practice. *Proceedings of the Royal Society of Medicine, 61,* 613–615.

Lipson, J. G. (1996). Culturally competent nursing care. In J. G. Lipson, S. L. Dibble, & P. A. Minarik (Eds.), *Cultural and nursing care.* San Francisco: University of California, San Francisco Nursing Press.

Litman, T. J. (1974). *Health care and the family: A three generational study.* Washington, DC: Division of Community Health Services and Medical Care Administration, U.S. Public Health Service.

Littlefield, V. M. (1977). Emotional considerations for the pregnant family. In J. P. Clausen, M. H. Flook, B. Ford, M. M. Green, & E. S. Popiel. (Eds.), *Maternity nursing today* (2nd ed.). New York: McGraw-Hill.

Litwak, E. (1972). Occupational mobility and extended family cohesion. In I. L. Reiss (Ed.), *Readings on the family system* (pp. 413–431). New York: Holt, Rinehart & Winston.

Litwak, E., Jessop, D. J., & Moulton, H. J. (1994). Optimal use of formal and informal systems over the life course. In E. Kahana, D. E. Biegel, & M. L. Wykle (Eds.), *Family caregiving across the lifespan.* Thousand Oaks, CA: Sage.

Liu, W. T. (1986). Health services for Asian elderly. *Research on Aging, 8* (1), 156–175.

Lobsenz, S. M. (1988, May). Tips for closer family ties. *Redbook.*

Locke, D. C. (1992). *Increasing multicultural understanding.* Newbury Park, CA: Sage.

Loe, H. (1988). Americans are smiling at fewer cavities. *Food insight reports.* Washington, DC: International Food Information Council.

Lopata, H. (1973). *Widowhood in an American city.* Cambridge, MA: Schenkman.

Los Angeles Times Editorial (1996, Aug. 11). Some revisionist thinking in the family values season. *Los Angeles Times,* p. M4.

Love, L. (1970). Process of role change. In C. Carlson (Ed.), *Behavioral concepts and nursing intervention.* Philadelphia: Lippincott.

Loveland-Cherry, C. (1988). Issues in family health promotion. In M. Stanhope, & J. Lancaster (Eds.), *Community health nursing* (2nd ed.). St. Louis: Mosby.

———. (1996). Family health promotion and health protection. In P. J. Bomar (Ed.), *Nurses and family health promotion* (2nd ed.) (pp. 22–35). Philadelphia: Saunders.

Lowenthal, M. F. (1972). Some potentialities of a life-cycle approach to the study of retirement. In F. M. Carp (Ed.), *Retirement.* New York: Behavioral Publications.

Lum, M. R. (1995). Environmental public health: Future direction, future skills. *Family and Community Health, 18* (1), 24–25.

Lum, M. R., Hibbs, B. F., Phillips, L., & Narkunas, D. M. (1996). Environmental health. M. Stanhope & J. Lancaster (Eds.), *Community health nursing* (4th ed.) (pp. 135–154). St. Louis: Mosby.

Lustig, M. W. (1988). Value differences in intercultural communication. In L. A. Samovar & R. E. Porter (Eds.), *Intercultural communication: A reader* (pp. 55–61). Belmont, CA: Wadsworth.

Lyman, S. (1974). *Chinese Americans.* New York: Random House.

MacElveen, P. M. (1978). Social networks. In D. C. Longo & R. A. Williams (Eds.), *Clinical practice in psychosocial nursing: Assessment and intervention.* New York: Appleton-Century-Crofts.

MacKay, D. (1968). The informational analysis of questions and commands. In W. Buckley (Ed.), *Modern systems research for the behavioral scientist.* Chicago: Aldine.

Macklin, E. D. (1988). Nontraditional family forms. In M. B. Sussman & S. K. Steinmetz (Eds.), *Handbook of marriage and the family* (pp. 317–353). New York: Plenum Press.

MacPhee, M., & Hoffenberg, E. (1996). Nursing case management for children with failure to thrive. *Journal of Pediatric Health Care, 10,* 63–73.

Madanes, C. (1991). Strategic family therapy. In A. S. Gurman & D. P. Kniskern (Eds.), *Handbook of family therapy* (Vol. II). New York: Brunner/Mazel.

Maddox, M. A., & Tillery, M. (1988). Elderly image seen by health care professionals. *Journal of Gerontological Nursing, 14* (11), 21–25.

Madsen, W. (1964). *The Mexican-American of South Texas.* New York: Holt-Reinhart & Winston.

Mahon, M., & Page, M. (1995). Childhood bereavement after the death of a sibling. *Holistic Nursing Practice, 9* (3), 15–26.

Malinski, V. M. (1987). Nursing science within the science of unitary human beings. In V. M. Malinski (Ed.), *Explorations on Martha Rogers' science of unitary human beings* (pp. 25–32). Norwalk, CT: Appleton & Lange.

Mallinchak, A. A., Wright, D., & Older, A. (1978, March/April). Americans and crime: The scope of victimization. *Aging,* 281–282.

Malveaux, J. (1988). The economic statuses of black families. In H. P. McAdoo (Ed.), *Black families* (2nd ed.) (pp. 133–147). Newbury Park, CA: Sage.

Mancini, J. A., & Orthner, D. K. (1988). The context and consequences of family change. *Family Relations, 37*(4), 363–366.

Manley, M. (1996). Tobacco use. In S. Woolf, S. Jonas, & R. Lawrence (Eds.), *Health promotion and disease prevention in clinical practice* (pp. 163–175). Baltimore: Williams & Wilkins.

Manns, W. (1988). Supportive roles of significant others in black families. In H. P. McAdoo (Ed.), *Black families* (2nd ed.) (pp. 270–283). Newbury Park, CA: Sage.

———. (1997). Supportive roles of significant others in African American families. In H. P. McAdoo (Ed.), *Black families* (3rd ed.) (pp. 198–213). Thousand Oaks, CA: Sage.

Mares, M. L. (1995). The aging family. In M. A. Fitzpatrick & A. L. Vangelisti (Eds.), *Explaining family interactions* (pp. 310–343). Thousand Oaks, CA: Sage.

Marin, G., & Marin, B. V. (1991). *Research with Hispanic populations*. Newbury Park, CA: Sage.

Marmor, J. (1988, Fall). Access to health care. A growing crisis. *UCLA public health* (pp. 1–5). Los Angeles: UCLA School of Public Health.

Marosy, J. P. (1994). Collaboration: A key to future success in long-term care. *Journal of Home Health Practice, 6* (2), 42–48.

Marsella, A. (1993). Counseling and psychotherapy with Japanese Americans: Cross-cultural considerations. *American Journal of Orthopsychiatry, 63,* 200–208.

Marshall, R. (1991). *The state of families, 3: Losing direction.* Milwaukee, WI: Family Service America.

Martell, L. L., & Imle, M. (1996). Family nursing with childbearing families. In S. M. H. Hanson & S. T. Boyd (Ed.), *Family health care nursing: Theory, practice and research* (pp. 215–236). Philadelphia: Davis.

Martin, J. P. (1987). Sustaining care of persons with AIDS. In J. D. Durham & F. L. Cohen (Eds.), *The person with AIDS: Nursing perspectives* (pp. 161–177). New York: Springer.

Martin, K. (1994). How can the quality of nursing practice be measured? In J. C. McCloskey & H. K. Grace (Eds.), *Current issues in nursing* (4th ed.) (pp. 342–349). St. Louis: Mosby.

Martin, K., & Scheet, N. (1992). *The Omaha system: Applications for community health nursing.* Philadelphia: Saunders.

Martinez, C. (1976). Community mental health and the Chicano movement. In C. A. Hernandez, M. J. Haug, & N. N. Wagner (Eds.), *Chicanos—Social and psychological perspectives* (2nd ed.). St. Louis: Mosby.

Martinez, E. A. (1988). Child behavior in Mexican American/Chicano families. Maternal teaching and child-rearing practices. *Family Relations, 37* (3), 275–280.

———. (1993). Parenting young children in Mexican American/Chicano families. In H. P. McAdoo (Ed.), *Family ethnicity. Strength in diversity* (pp. 184–195). Newbury Park, CA: Sage.

Martinez, R. A. (Ed.). (1978). *Hispanic culture and health care.* St. Louis: Mosby.

Maslow, A. (1954). *Motivation and personality.* New York: Harper & Row.

Matsui, W. T. (1996). Japanese families. In M. McGoldrick, J. Giordano, & J. K. Pearce (Eds.), *Ethnicity and family therapy* (pp. 268–280). New York: Guilford Press.

Mattessich, P. & Hill, R. (1987). Lifecycle and family development. In M. B. Sussman & S. K. Steinmetz (Eds.), *Handbook of marriage and the family* (pp. 437–469). New York: Plenum Press.

Maturana, H. (1978). Biology of language: The epistemology of reality. In G. Millar & E. Lenneberg (Eds.), *Psychology and biology of language and thought* (pp. 27–63). New York: Academic Press.

Maturana, H. R., & Varela, F. J. (1992). *The tree of knowledge: The biological roots of human understanding* (rev. ed.). Boston: Shambhala.

McAdoo, H. P. (1978). Minority families. In J. H. Stevens & M. Mathew (Eds.), *Mother/child; Father/child relationships* (pp. 178–180). Washington, DC: The National Association for the Education of Young Children.

———. (1982). Stress absorbing systems in black families. *Family Relations, 31* (3), 479–488.

———. (1983). Societal stress; The black family. In H. I. McCubbin & C. R. Figley (Eds.), *Stress and the family. Vol. I: Coping with normative transitions* (pp. 178–187). New York: Brunner/Mazel.

———. (Ed.). (1988). *Black families* (2nd ed.). Newbury Park, CA: Sage.

———. (1993). Ethnic families: Strengths that are found in diversity. In H. P. McAdoo (Ed.), *Family ethnicity: Strength in diversity* (pp. 3–14). Newbury Park, CA: Sage.

McAdoo, J. L. (1988a). Changing perspectives on the role of the black father. In P. Bronstein & C. P. Cowan (Eds.), *Fatherhood today. Men's changing role in the family* (pp. 79–92). New York: Wiley.

———. (1988b). The roles of black fathers in the socialization of black children. In H. P. McAdoo (Ed.), *Black families* (2nd ed.) (pp. 258–268). Newbury Park, CA: Sage.

———. (1997). The roles of African American fathers in the socialization of their children. In H. P. McAdoo (Ed.), *Black families* (3rd ed.) (pp. 183–195). Thousand Oaks, CA: Sage.

McBridge, V. M. (1995). *Strengths and Resiliency of Black Families: Implications for Practitioners.* Paper presented at the National Council for Family Relations Conference, Nov. 16, Portland, Oregon.

McCall, T. (1996, July/Aug.). The best of both worlds. *American Health, 53.*

McChesney, K. L. (1987). *Women without: Homeless mothers and their children.* Unpublished doctoral dissertation, University of Southern California, Los Angeles.

McClelland, D., Constantine, C. A., Regaldo, D., & Stone, C. (1978, June). Making it to maturity. *Psychology Today,* 45–47.

McCloskey, J. C., & Bulechek, G. M. (1996). *Iowa intervention project: Nursing intervention classification (NIC)* (2nd ed.). St. Louis: Mosby.

McClowry, S., Gilliss, C. L., & Martinson, I. M. (1989). The process of grief in the bereaved family. In C. L. Gilliss, B. L. Highley, B. M. Roberts, & I. M. Martinson (Eds.), *Toward a science of family nursing* (pp. 216–225). Reading, MA: Addison-Wesley.

McCown, D., & Davies, B. (1995). Patterns of grief in young siblings. *Journal of Death Studies, 19,* 41–53.

McCown, D., & Pratt, C. (1985). Impact of sibling death on children's behavior. *Journal of Death Studies, 9,* 323–335.

McCown, D. E. (1996). Family recreation and exercise. In P. J. Bomar (Ed.), *Nurses and family health promotion* (2nd ed.) (pp. 264–283). Philadelphia: Saunders.

McCown, D. E., Delamarter, D., Schroeder, B., & Liegler, R. (1989). Family recreation and exercise. In P. J. Bomar (Ed.), *Nurses and family health promotion* (pp. 216–236). Baltimore: Williams & Wilkins.

McCreery, A. (1981). Scapegoating. A survival phenomenon. In C. Getty & W. Humphreys (Eds.), *Understanding the family* (pp. 479–487). New York: Appleton-Century-Crofts.

McCubbin, H., & Figley, D. (Eds.) (1983). *Stress and the family: Vol. 1. Coping with normative transitions.* New York: Wiley.

McCubbin, H. I. (1979). Integrating coping behavior in family stress theory. *Journal of Marriage and the Family, 41,* 237–244.

McCubbin, H. I., & Dahl, B. B. (1985). *Marriage and family: Individuals and life cycles.* New York: Wiley.

McCubbin, H. I., & McCubbin, M. A. (1988). Typologies of resilient families: Emerging roles of social class and ethnicity. *Family Relations, 37* (July), 247–254.

McCubbin, H. I., McCubbin, M., Nevin, R. S., & Cauble, E. (1981). Coping health inventory for parents (CHIP). In H. I. McCubbin & J. M. Patterson (Eds.), *Systematic assessment of family stress resources and coping.* St. Paul, MN: Family Social Sciences Department, University of Minnesota.

McCubbin, H.I., Olson, D., & Larsen, A. (1991). F-COPES: Family crisis oriented personal evaluation scales. In H. I. McCubbin & A. Thompson (Eds.), *Family assessment inventories for research and practice* (pp. 203–216). Madison, WI: University of Wisconsin-Madison.

McCubbin, H. I., & Patterson, J. M. (1982). Family adaptation to crisis. In H. McCubbin, A. Cauble, & J. Patterson (Eds.), *Family stress, coping and social support* (pp. 26–47). Springfield, IL: Charles C. Thomas.

_____. (1983a). The family stress process: The double ABCX model of adjustment and adaptation. In H. I. McCubbin, M. B. Sussman, & J. M. Patterson (Eds.), *Social stress and the family.* (Special Issue). *Marriage and Family Review, 6* (1/2), 7–27.

_____. (1983b). Family transitions: Adaptation to stress. In H. I. McCubbin & C. R. Figley (Eds.), *Stress and the family: Coping with normative transitions* (pp. 5–25). New York: Brunner/Mazel.

_____. (1991). FILE: Family inventory of life events and changes. In H. I. McCubbin & A. Thompson (Eds.), *Family assessment inventories for research and practice* (pp. 81–110). Madison, WI: University of Wisconsin-Madison.

McCubbin, H. I., Patterson, J. M., & Wilson, L. (1983). *FILE: Family inventory of life events.* Madison, WI: University of Wisconsin-Madison.

McCubbin, H. I., Thompson, A., Pirner, P., & McCubbin, M. A. (1988). *Family types and strengths: A life cycle and ecological perspective.* Minneapolis, MN: Burgess.

McCubbin, H. I., Wilson, L., & Patterson, J. M. (1981). Family inventory of life events and changes (FILE). In H. I. McCubbin & J. M. Patterson (Eds.), *Systematic assessment of family stress, resources, and coping.* St. Paul, MN: Family Social Sciences Department, University of Minnesota.

McCubbin, M. A., & McCubbin, H. I. (1987). Family stress theory and assessment: The T-double ABCX model of family adjustment and adaptation. In H. I. McCubbin & A. Thompson (Eds.), *Family assessment inventories for research and practice* (pp. 3–35). Madison, WI: University of Wisconsin-Madison.

_____. (1989). Theoretical orientations to family stress and coping. In C. R. Figley (Ed.), *Treating stress in families* (pp. 3–43). New York: Brunner/Mazel.

_____. (1991). Family stress theory and assessment: The resiliency model of family stress, adjustment, and adaptation. In H. I. McCubbin & A. Thompson (Eds.), *Family assessment inventories for research and practice* (pp. 3–32). Madison, WI: University of Wisconsin-Madison.

_____. (1993). Families coping with illness: The resiliency model of family stress, adjustment and adaptation. In C. Danielson, B. Hamel-Bissell, & P. Winstead-Fry (Eds.), *Families, health, and illness: Perspectives on coping and intervention* (pp. 21–63). St. Louis: Mosby.

McCullough, P. G., & Rutenberg, S. K. (1988). Launching children and moving on. In B. Carter & M. McGoldrick (Eds.), *The changing family life cycle* (pp. 285–308). New York: Gardner Press.

McDonald, G. W. (1977). Family power, reflection and direction. *Pacific Sociological Review, 20,* 609–614.

_____. (1980, Nov.). Family power: The assessment of a decade of theory and research, 1970–1979. *Journal of Marriage and the Family, 42* (4), 841–854.

McFarland, G. K., & McFarlane, E. A. (1989). *Nursing diagnosis and intervention.* St. Louis: Mosby.

_____. (1993). *Nursing diagnosis and intervention* (2nd ed.). St. Louis: Mosby.

McFarlane, J. M. (1986). *The clinical handbook of family nursing.* New York: Wiley.

McGoldrick, M. (1988). The joining of families through marriage: The new couple. In B. Carter & M. McGoldrick (Eds.), *The changing family life cycle* (pp. 209–233). New York: Gardner Press.

_____. (1989). Women and the family life cycle. In B. Carter & M. McGoldrick (Eds.), *The changing family life cycle* (2nd ed.) (pp. 29–68). Boston: Allyn & Bacon.

_____. (1993). Ethnicity, cultural diversity and normality. In F. Walsh (Ed.), *Normal family processes* (2nd ed.) (pp. 331–360). New York: Guilford Press.

_____. (1996). Irish families. In M. McGoldrick, J. Giordano, & J. K. Pierce (Eds.), *Ethnicity and family therapy* (2nd ed.) (pp. 544–566). New York: Guilford Press.

McGoldrick, M., & Gerson, R. (1985). *Genograms in family assessment.* New York: W. W. Norton.

McGoldrick, M., & Giordano, J. (1996). Overview: Ethnicity and family therapy. In M. McGoldrick, J. Giordano, & J. K. Pearce (Eds.), *Ethnicity and family therapy* (pp. 1–30). New York: Guilford Press.

McGoldrick, M., Heiman, M., & Carter, B. (1993). The changing family life cycle, A perspective of normalcy. In F. Walsh (Ed.), *Normal family processes* (pp. 405–443). New York: Guilford Press.

McHale, S. M., & Crouter, A. C. (1992). You can't always get what you want: Incongruence between sex-role attitudes and family work roles and its implication for marriage. *Journal of Marriage and the Family, 46,* 357–364.

McKinley, D. (1964). *Social class and family life.* Glencoe, IL: Free Press.

McLachlan, J. M. (1958). Cultural factors in health and disease. In E. G. Jaco (Ed.), *Patients, physicians, and illness.* New York: Free Press.

McLanahan, S., & Booth, K. (1989). Mother-only families: Problems, prospects and politics. *Journal of Marriage and the Family, 51* (3), 557–580.

McLemore, S. D., & Romo, R. (1985). The origins and development of the Mexican-American people. In R. D. De La Garza, et al. (Eds.), *The Mexican-American experience: An interdisciplinary anthology.* Austin, TX: University of Texas Press.

McLeod, H., & Cooper, J. (1996, July 28). Generation X is active locally. How about nationally? *Los Angeles Times,* pp. M2, M6.

McRae, M. E. (1991). Holding death at bay: The experience of the spouses of patients undergoing cardiovascular surgery. *Canadian Journal of Cardiovascular Nursing, 2* (2), 14–20.

Mead, G. (1934). *Mind, self and society.* Chicago: University of Chicago Press.

Mechanic, D. (1964). Influences of mothers on their children's health attitudes and behavior. *Pediatrics, 33,* 445.

Mederer, H., & Hill, R. (1983). Critical transitions over the family life span. Theory and research. *Marriage and Family Review, 6* (1/2), 39–60.

Mehren, E. (1993, Oct. 21). Number of children living in poverty continues to rise. *Los Angeles Times,* p. E5.

_____. (1996, Oct. 11). Parents want safety, not family values. *Los Angeles Times,* pp. E1, E8.

Meisenhelder, J.B. (1982). Boundaries of personal space. *Image, 14* (1), 16–19.

Meisler, S., & Fulwood, S. (1989, July 17). Number of inner-city single parents on rise. *Los Angeles Times,* p. A14.

Meleis, A. I. (1975). Role insufficiency and role supplementation. *Nursing Research, 24* (2), 264.

Meleis, A. I. (1992). Directions for nursing theory development in the 21st century. *Nursing Science Quarterly, 5,* 112–117.

Meleis, A. I., & Swendsen, L. A. (1978). Role supplementation—an empirical test of a nursing intervention. *Nursing Research, 27* (1), 11.

Melson, G. F. (1983). Family adaptation to environmental demands. In H. I. McCubbin & C. R. Figley (Eds.), *Stress and the family. Vol I: Coping with normative transitions* (pp. 149–162). New York: Brunner/Mazel.

Menaghan, E. G. (1983). Individual coping efforts and family studies. Conceptual and methodological issues. In H. I. McCubbin, M. B. Sussman, & J. M. Patterson (Eds.), *Social stress and the family* (Special Issue). *Marriage and Family Review, 6* (1/2), 113–135.

Mendes, H. A. (1988). Single-parent families: A typology of life-styles. In J. G. Wells, (Ed.), *Current issues in marriage and the family* (4th ed.) (pp. 247–259). New York: Macmillan.

Mercer, R. T. (1989). Theoretical perspectives on the family. In C. L. Gilliss, B. L. Highley, B. M. Roberts, & I. M. Martinson (Eds.), *Toward a science of family nursing* (pp. 9–36). Menlo Park, CA: Addison-Wesley.

Meredith, W. H., & Abbott, D. A. (1995). Chinese families in later life. In B. B. Ingoldsby & S. Smith (Eds.), *Families in multicultural perspective* (pp. 213–230). New York: Guilford Press.

Merton, R. K. (1957). *Social theory and social structure.* New York: Free Press.

Messer, A. (1970). *The individual in his family: An adaptational study.* Springfield, IL: Charles C. Thomas.

Mikhail, B. I. (1994). Hispanic mother's beliefs and practices regarding selected children's health problems. *Western Journal of Nursing, 16* (6), 623–638.

Milardo, R. M. (1988). *Families and social networks.* Newbury Park, CA: Sage.

Miller, B. G., & Myers-Walls, J. A. (1983). Parenthood: Stresses and coping strategies. In H. I. McCubbin & C. R. Figley (Eds.), *Stress and the family. Vol I. Coping with normative transitions* (pp. 54–73). New York: Brunner/Mazel.

Miller, B. G., & Sollie, D. L. (1980). Normal stresses during the transition to parenthood. *Family Relations, 29* (4), 459–465.

Miller, D. (1989). Family violence and the helping system. In L. Combrinck-Graham (Ed.), *Children in family contexts* (pp. 413–434). New York: Guilford Press.

Miller, F. (1986). The people. In B. Coyne & B. Holland (Eds.), *Encyclopedia Americana* (pp. 819–830). Danbury, CT: Grolier.

Miller, J. G. (1969). Living systems. Basic concepts. In W. Gray, F. Duhl, & N. Rizzo (Eds.), *General systems theory and psychiatry.* Boston: Little, Brown.

Miller, S., & Katz, G. (1992). The educational needs of mental health self-help groups. *Psychosocial Rehabilitation Journal, 16,* 160–163.

Miller, S. R., & Winstead-Fry, P. (1982). *Family systems theory in nursing practice.* Reston, VA: Reston Publishing.

Millington, M. J., & Zieball, C. W. (1986). Financial strategies. In S. H. Johnson (Ed.), *Nursing assessment and strategies for the family at risk. High risk parenting* (2nd ed.) (pp. 473–487). Philadelphia: Lippincott.

Milner, J., & Murphy, W. (1995). Assessment of child physical and sexual abuse offenders. *Family Relations, 44,* 478–488.

Min, P. G. (1988). The Korean American family. In C. H. Mindel, R. W. Habenstein, & R. Wright, Jr. (Eds.), *Ethnic families in America* (pp. 199–229). New York: Elsevier.

_____. (1995a). An overview of Asian Americans. In P. G. Min (Ed.), *Asian Americans: Contemporary trends and issues* (pp. 10–37). Thousand Oaks, CA: Sage.

_____. (Ed.). (1995b). *Asian Americans: Contemporary trends and issues.* Thousand Oaks, CA: Sage.

_____. (1995c). Korean Americans. In P. G. Min (Ed.), *Asian Americans: Contemporary trends and issues* (pp. 199–231). Thousand Oaks, CA: Sage.

Minkler, M., & Roe, K. (1995, Spring). Grandparents as surrogate parents. *Generations, XX* (1), 34–38.

Minkler, M., & Stone, R. (1985). The faminization of poverty and older women. *The Gerontologist, 25,* 351–357.

Minuchin, S. (1974). *Families and family therapy.* Cambridge, MA: Harvard University Press.

Minuchin, S., & Fishman, H. G. (1981). *Family therapy techniques.* Cambridge, MA: Harvard University Press.

Minuchin, S., Rosman, B. L., & Baker, L. (1978). *Psychosomatic families. Anorexia nervosa in context.* Cambridge, MA: Harvard University Press.

Mirandé, A. (1977). The Chicano family: A re-analysis of conflicting views. *Journal of Marriage and the Family, 6* (1), 751–755.

_____. (1979, Oct.). A reinterpretation of male dominance in the Chicano family. *The Family Coordinator,* 473–479.

_____. (1985). *The Chicano experience: An alternative perspective.* Notre Dame, IN: The University of Notre Dame Press.

_____. (1991). Ethnicity and fatherhood. In F. W. Bozett & S. M. H. Hanson (Eds.), *Fatherhood and families in cultural context* (pp. 53–82). New York: Springer.

Mirowsky, J., & Ross, C. E. (1984). Mexican culture and its emotional contradictions. *Journal of Health and Social Behavior, 25* (1), 2–13.

Mishel, M. H. (1974). *Patient problems in self-esteem and nursing intervention.* Los Angeles: California State University, Los Angeles, Trident Shop.

Mishel, M. H., & Murdaugh, C. L. (1987). Family adjustment to heart transplantation: Redesigning the dream. *Nursing Research, 36* (6), 332–338.

Mitchell, A. L. (1982). Barriers to therapeutic communication with Black clients. In B. W. Spradley (Ed.), *Readings in community health nursing* (2nd ed.). Boston: Little, Brown.

Mitchell, B. A., Wister, A. V., & Burch, T. K. (1989). The family environment and leaving the parental home. *Journal of Marriage and the Family, 51* (3), 605–613.

Monroe, L. D. (1989, Aug. 19). Culture shock hits health care. *Los Angeles Times,* Part I, pp. 1, 30.

_____. (1990, Nov. 22). Programs tailor tips on health to Latinos. *Los Angeles Times,* pp. E1, E6.

Montgomery, R. (1989). Investigating caregiver burden. In K. S. Markides & C. C. Cooper (Eds.), *Aging, stress and health.* New York: Wiley.

Montgomery, R., & Kosloski, K. (1994). Outcomes of family caregiving: Lessons from the past and challenges for the future. In M. H. Cantor (Ed.), *Family caregiving, agenda for the future* (pp. 123–136). Chicago: American Society on Aging.

Moore, D. (1983, Jan. 30). America's neglected elderly. *New York Times Magazine,* pp. 30–37.

Moore, J. W. (1970). *Mexican Americans.* Englewood Cliffs, NJ: Prentice-Hall.

Moorek, K., Spain, D., & Bianchi, S. (1984). Working wives and mothers. *Marriage and Family Review, 7* (3/4), 77–98.

Morehead, S. A. (1985). Role supplementation. In G. M. Bulechek, J. C. McCloskey, & M. K. Aydelotte (Eds.), *Nursing interventions: Treatments for nursing diagnoses* (pp. 152–159). Philadelphia: Saunders.

Morehead, S. A., McCloskey, J. C., & Bulechek, G. M. (1985). Nursing interventions classification: A comparison with the Omaha system and the home health care classification. *JONA, 23* (10), 23–29.

Morrow, R. (1987). Cultural differences—Be aware. *Academic therapy, 23* (2), 143–149.

Moynihan, D. P. (1965). *The Negro family: A case for national action.* Washington, DC: U.S. Government Printing Office.

Mueller, D. P., & Cooper, P. W. (1986). Children of single parent families: How they fare as young adults. *Family Relations, 35* (1), 169–176.

Mullins, L. C., & Mushel, M. (1992). The existence and emotional closeness of relationships with children, friends and spouses. *Research on Aging, 14,* 448–470.

Mumford, E., Schlesinger, H. J., & Glass, G. V. (1982). The effects of psychological intervention in recovery from surgery and heart attacks: An analysis of the literature. *American Journal of Public Health, 72,* 141–151.

Murata, J. E. (1995). Family stress, mothers' social support, depression, and sons' behavior problems: Modeling nursing interventions for low-income inner city families. *Journal of Family Nursing, 1* (1), 41–62.

Murillo, N. (1976). The Mexican-American family. In C. A. Hernandez, M. J. Haug, & N. N. Wagner (Eds.), *Chicanos: Social and psychological perspectives* (2nd ed.) (pp. 15–25). St. Louis: Mosby.

Murray, C. I., & Leigh, G. K. (1995). Families and sexuality. In R. D. Day, K. R. Gilbert, B. H. Settles, & W. R. Burr (Eds.), *Research and theory in family science* (pp. 186–204). Pacific Grove, CA: Brooks/Cole.

Murray, R., & Zentner, J. (1985). *Nursing concepts for health promotion* (3rd ed.). Englewood Cliffs, NJ: Prentice-Hall.

_____. (1993). *Nursing concepts for health promotion* (4th ed.). Englewood Cliffs, NJ: Prentice-Hall.

Naisbitt, J. (1984). *Megatrends.* New York: Warner Communications.

Nall, F. C., & J. S. Speilberg. (1978). New York social and cultural factors in the responses of Mexican Americans to medical treatment. In R. A. Martinez (Ed.), *Hispanic culture and health care.* St. Louis: Mosby.

Napier, A. Y. (1988). *The fragile bond.* New York: Harper & Row.

National Center for Health Statistics. (1986). *Advance report on final natality statistics, 1984,* Vol. 35, No. 4, Supplement, July 18.

_____. (1989, Sept. 26). *Monthly vital statistics report.* Washington, DC: U.S. Government Printing Office.

_____. (1991). Premarital sexual experience among adolescent women: U.S. 1970–1988. *Morbidity and Mortality Weekly Report, 39,* 932.

_____. (1992). Annual summary of births, marriages, divorces, and deaths: United States, 1991. *Monthly Vital Statistics Report, 40,* 13.

National Committee to Prevent Child Abuse (1996, April). *Current trends in child abuse reporting and fatalities: The results of the 1995 fifty state survey.* Chicago: National Committee to Prevent Child Abuse.

National Council for Family Relations. (1993). *Vision 2010: Families and health care.* Minneapolis, MN: National Council for Family Relations.

_____. (1989, June). Facts shared on rural poverty. *NCFR report* (p. 13). Minneapolis, MN: National Council for Family Relations.

National Institute on Drug Abuse. (1996). *National pregnancy and health survey: Drug use among women delivering livebirths: 1992.* (NIH Publication No. 96-3819). Washington, DC: U.S. Government Printing Office.

National Research Council. (1989). *Executive summary, diet and health: Implications for reducing chronic disease risk.* Washington, DC: National Academy Press.

Neal, M. B., Chapman, N. J., Ingersoll-Dayton, B., & Emlen, A. C. (1993). *Balancing work and caregiving for children, adults, and elders.* Thousand Oaks, CA: Sage.

Neff, J. A., & Hoppe, S. K. (1993). Race/ethnicity, acculturation, and psychological distress: Fatalism and religiosity as cultural resources. *Journal of Community Psychology, 21,* 3–20.

Neimeyer, R. A. (1988). Death anxiety. In H. Wass, F. M. Berardo, & R. A. Neimeyer (Eds.), *Dying: Facing the facts* (2nd ed.) (pp. 97–136). Washington, DC: Hemisphere.

Nelson, H., & Roark, A. (1985, April 7). Health care crisis: Less for more. *Los Angeles Times,* Part I, pp. 1, 24, 25, 27, 28.

Nelson, M. A. (1994). Economic impoverishment and health risk: Methodologic and conceptual issues. *Advances in Nursing Science, 16* (3), 1–12.

Neser, W. (1975). Fragmentation of black families and stroke susceptibility. In B. Kaplan & J. Cassel (Eds.), *Family and health: An epidemiological approach.* Chapel Hill, NC: Institute for Research in Social Science.

Neuman, B. (1982). *The Neuman systems model: Application to nursing education and practice.* Norwalk, CT: Appleton-Century-Crofts.

_____. (1983). Family intervention using the Betty Neuman health care systems model. In I. W. Clements & F. B. Roberts (Eds.), *Family health: A Theoretical approach to nursing care.* New York: Wiley.

Neundorfer, M. (1991). Family caregivers of the frail elderly: Impact of caregiving on their health and implications for interventions. *Family and Community Health, 14* (2), 48–58.

Newman, M., Lamb, G., & Michaels, C. (1991). Nurse case management: The coming together of theory and practice. *Nursing and Health Care, 12,* 404–408.

Nickolls, K. (1975). Life crisis and psychosocial assets: Some clinical implications. In B. H. Kaplan & J. C. Cassell (Eds.), *Family and health: An epidemiological approach.* Chapel Hill, NC: Institute for Research in Social Science.

Nightingale, F. (1859). *Notes on nursing: What it is, and what it is not.* London: Harrison. (Reprinted 1946. Philadelphia: Lippincott.)

_____. (1949). Sick nursing and health nursing. In I. Hampton, et al. (Eds.), *Nursing of the sick: 1893.* New York: McGraw-Hill.

_____. (1979). *Cassandra.* Westbury, NY: Feminist Press.

Nishi, S. M. (1995). Japanese Americans. In P. G. Min (Ed.), *Asian Americans: Contemporary trends and issues* (pp. 95–133). Thousand Oaks, CA: Sage.

Nobles, W. (1974). African root and American fruit: The Black family. *Journal of Social and Behavioral Sciences, 20,* 52–64.

Nock, S. L. (1988). The family and hierarchy. *Journal of Marriage and the Family, 50* (4), 957–966.

Norbeck, J. S., & Tilden, V. P. (1983, March). Life stress, social support, and emotional disequilibrium in complications of pregnancy: A prospective, multivariate study. *Journal of Health and Social Behavior, 24* (1), 30–46.

Nortan, A. J., & Glick, P. G. (1986). One-parent families: A social and economic profile. *Family Relations, 35* (1), 177–181.

North American Nursing Diagnosis Association. (1988). NANDA approved nursing diagnostic categories. *Nursing Diagnoses Newsletter, 15* (1), 1–3.

Nyamathi, A. M. (1987a). The coping responses of female spouses of patients with myocardial infarction. *Heart & Lung, 16* (1), 86–92.

———. (1987b). Coping responses of spouses of MI patients and of hemodialysis patients as measured by the Jalowiec Coping Scale. *Journal of Cardiovascular Nursing, 2* (1), 67–74.

Nye, F. I. (1974). Emerging and declining roles. *Journal of Marriage and the Family, 36* (2), 238.

———. (Ed.). (1976). *Role structure and analysis of the family,* Vol 24. Beverly Hills, CA: Sage.

Nye, F. I., & Berardo, F. (Eds.). (1981). *Emerging conceptual frameworks in family analysis.* New York: Praeger.

Nye, F. I. & Gecas, V. (1976). The role concept: Review and delineation. In F.I. Nye (Ed.), *Structure and analysis of the family, 24.* Beverly Hills, CA: Sage.

Okin, S. M. (1989). *Justice, gender and the family.* New York: Basic Books.

Olson, D. (1993). Circumplex model of marital and family systems: Assessing family functioning. In F. Walsh (Ed.), *Normal family processes* (pp. 104–137). New York: Guilford Press.

Olson, D. H., & Cromwell, R. E. (1975). Methodological issues in family power. In R. E. Cromwell & D. H. Olson (Eds.), *Power in families* (pp. 142–145). New York: Sage.

Olson, D. H., Cromwell, R. E., & Klein, D. M. (1975). Beyond family power. In R. E. Cromwell & D. H. Olson (Eds.), *Power in families* (pp. 236–239). New York: Sage.

Olson, D. H., McCubbin, H. I., et al. (1983). *Families: What makes them work.* Newbury Park, CA: Sage.

Oppenheim, M. (1984, Sept.). The "big four" tests you really need. *American Health,* 80–89.

Orem, D. (1971). *Nursing: Concepts and practice.* New York: McGraw-Hill.

———. (1983a). The family coping with a medical illness: Analysis and application of Orem's theory. In I. Clements & F. Roberts (Eds.), *Family health: A theoretical approach to nursing care.* New York: Wiley.

———. (1983b). The family experiencing emotional crisis: Analysis and application of Orem's self-care deficit theory. In I. Clements & F. Roberts (Eds.), *Family health: A theoretical approach to nursing care.* New York: Wiley.

———. (1980). *Nursing: Concepts and practice* (2nd ed.). New York: McGraw-Hill.

———. (1985). *Nursing: Concepts and practice* (3rd ed.). New York: McGraw-Hill.

Orthner, D. (1995). Families in transition: Changing values and norms. In R. D. Day, K. R. Gilbert, B. H. Settles, & W. R. Burr (Eds.), *Research and theory in family science* (pp. 3–19). Pacific Grove, CA: Brooks/Cole.

Orthner, D. K. (1976). Familia ludens: Reinforcing the leisure component in family life. In E. Eldridge & N. Meredith (Eds.), *Environmental issues: Family impact.* Minneapolis, MN: Burgess.

Ortiz, V. (1995). The diversity of Latino families. In R. E. Zambrana (Ed.), *Understanding Latino families. Scholarship, policy and practice* (pp. 18–38). Thousand Oaks, CA: Sage.

Osborne, P. (1995). The parenting experts. In R. D. Day, K. R. Gilbert, B. H. Settles, & W. R. Burr (Eds.), *Research and theory in family science* (pp. 320–333). Pacific Grove, CA: Brooks/Cole.

Osmond, M. W. (1978). Reciprocity: A dynamic model and a method to study family power. *Journal of Marriage and the Family, 40* (1), 51.

Otten, A. L. (1989, Jan. 27). Extended families: As people live longer, houses become homes to several generations. *Wall Street Journal, CXX* (19), 1.

Otto, H. (1973). A framework for assessing family strengths. In A. Reinhardt & M. Quinn (Eds.), *Family-centered community nursing* (pp. 87–93). St. Louis: Mosby.

Padilla, E. R. (1976). The relationship between psychology and Chicanos: Failures and possibilities. In C. A. Hernandez, M. J. Haug, & N. N. Wagner (Eds.), *Chicanos—Social and psychological perspectives* (2nd ed.) (pp. 282–290). St. Louis: Mosby.

Pagelow, M. D. (1984). *Family violence.* New York: Praeger.

Pallett, P. J. (1990). A conceptual framework for studying family caregiver burden in Alzheimer's-type dementias. *Image, 22* (1), 52–58.

Paniagua, F. A. (1994). *Assessing and treating culturally diverse clients.* Thousand Oaks, CA: Sage.

Papernow, P. L. (1984). The stepparent cycle. An experiential model of stepfamily development. *Family Relations, 33* (3), 355–363.

Parachini, A. (1987, June 9). New guidelines for physical exams. *Los Angeles Times,* Part V, pp. 1–2.

Parad, H. J., & Caplan, G. (1965). A framework for studying families in crisis. In H. J. Parad (Ed.), *Crisis intervention: Selected readings* (pp. 55–60). New York: Family Service of America.

Parsons, R., Bales, R. F., & Shils, E. A. (1953). *Working papers on the theory of action.* Glencoe, IL: Free Press.

Parsons, T. (1951). *The social system.* Glencoe, IL: Free Press.

Parsons, T., & Bales, R. F. (1955). *Family socialization and interaction process.* New York: Free Press.

Pasquali, E. A., Arnold, H. M., De Basio, N., & Alesi, E. G. (1985). *Mental health nursing* (2nd ed.). St. Louis: Mosby.

Patterson, J. M. (1988). Chronic illness in children and the impact on families. In C. S. Chilman, E. W. Nunally, & F. M. Cox (Eds.), *Chronic illness and disability* (pp. 69–107). Newbury Park, CA: Sage.

Patterson, J. M., & Zderad, L. (1976). *Humanistic nursing.* New York: Wiley.

Paz, O. (1973). The sons of La Malenche. In L. I. Duran & H. R. Bernard (Eds.), *Introduction to Chicano studies.* New York: Macmillan.

Pearlin, L., & Schooler, C. (1978). The structure of coping. *Journal of Health and Social Behavior, 19,* 19–21.

Pearlin, L., & Turner, H. A. (1987). The family as a context of the stress process. In S. V. Kasl & C. L. Cooper (Eds.), *Stress and health: Issues in research methodology.* New York: Wiley.

Pearson, G. S. (1995). Pervasive developmental disorders. In B. S. Johnson (Ed.), *Child, adolescent, and family psychiatric nursing* (pp. 270–284). Philadelphia: Lippincott.

Pearson, R. E. (1990). *Counseling and social support. Perspectives and practice.* Newbury Park, CA: Sage.

Peck, J. S., & Manocharian, J. R. (1988). Divorce in the changing family life cycle. In B. Carter & M. McGoldrick (Eds.), *The changing family life cycle* (pp. 335–369). New York: Gardner Press.

Pedersen, P. B., Draguns, J. G., Lonner, W. J., & Trimble, J. E. (1996). Introduction. In P. B. Pedersen, J. G. Draguns, W. J. Lonner, and J. E. Trimble (Eds.), *Counseling across cultures* (4th ed.) (pp. vii–xvii). Thousand Oaks, CA: Sage.

Pederson, P. (1976, Aug. 2). Varighed fra sygdoms begyndelse til henvendelse til prakliserende laege. *Ugekr Laeg, 138,* 32.

Pelletier, K. (1979). *Holistic medicine.* New York: Delta/ Seymour Lawrence.

Pender, N. J. (1986). Health promotion: Implementing strategies. In B. B. Logan & C. E. Dawkins (Eds.), *Family-centered nursing in the community* (pp. 296–334). Reading, MA: Addison-Wesley.

———. (1987). *Health promotion in nursing practice.* (2nd ed.). Norwalk, CT: Appleton & Lange.

———. (1996). *Health promotion in nursing practice* (3rd ed.). Stamford, CT: Appleton & Lange.

Penning, M., & Strain, L. (1994). Gender difference in disability, assistance, and subjective well-being in later life. *Journal of Gerontology, 46* (4), S202–208.

Peplau, H. (1952). *Interpersonal relations in nursing.* New York: GP Putnams' Sons.

Perkins, E. J. (1973). Screening for ophthalmic conditions. *Practitioner, 211,* 171–177.

Perkins, H. W., & Harris, L. B. (1990). Familial bereavement and health in adult life course perspective. *Journal of Marriage and the Family, 52* (1), 233–241.

Perry, S. E. (1983). Attachment theory. In I. W. Clements & F. B. Roberts (Eds.), *Family health: A theoretical approach to nursing care* (pp. 109–122). New York: Wiley.

Perry-Jenkins, M., & Crouter, A. C. (1990). Men's provider role attitudes: Implications for household work and marital satisfaction. *Journal of Family Issues, 11,* 136–156.

Perry-Jenkins, M., & Folk, K. (1994). Class, couples, and conflicts. Effects of the division of labor on assessments of marriage in dual-earner families. *Journal of Marriage and the Family, 56,* 165–180.

Peters, L. R. (1974). Family team or myth. In J. E. Hall & B. R. Weaver (Eds.), *Nursing of families in crisis* (pp. 226–237). Philadelphia: Lippincott.

Peters, M. F. (1981). "Making it" Black family style: Building on the strengths of Black families. In N. Stinnett, J. De Frain, K. King, et al. (Eds.), *Family strengths: Roots of well-being* (pp. 73–91). Lincoln, NE: University of Nebraska Press.

———. (1997). Historical note: Parenting of young children in black families. In H. P. McAdoo (Ed.), *Black families* (3rd ed.) (pp. 167–181). Thousand Oaks, CA: Sage.

Peters, M. F., & Massey, G. (1983). Mundane extreme environmental stress in family stress theories: The case of Black families in White America. In H. I. McCubbin, M. B. Sussman, & J. M. Patterson (Eds.), *Social stress and the family* (Special Issue). *Marriage and Family Review, 6* (1/2), 193–218.

Peterson, G. W. (1995). Autonomy and connectedness in families. In R. Day, K. Gilbert, B. Settles, & W. Burr (Eds.), *Research and theory in family social science* (pp. 20–41). Pacific Grove, CA: Brooks/Cole.

Peterson, G. W., & Rollins, B. C. (1987). Parent–child socialization. In M. B. Sussman & S. K. Steinmetz (Eds.), *Handbook of marriage and the family* (pp. 471–507). New York: Plenum Press.

Peterson, L. R., & Maynard, J. L. (1981, Jan.). Bringing home the bacon doesn't mean I have to cook it too. *Pacific Sociological Review, 24* (1), 87–106.

Petrie, K., & Azariah, R. (1990). Health-promoting variables as predictors of response to a brief pain management program. *Clinical Journal of Pain, 6,* 43–46.

Pew Health Professions Commission. (1991). *Healthy America: Practitioners for 2005.* San Francisco, CA: Pew Health Professions Commission.

Phillips, S., & Lobar, S. (1990). Literature summary of some Navajo child health beliefs and rearing practices within a transcultural nursing framework. *Journal of Transcultural Nursing, 1* (2), 13–20.

Piaget, J. (1971). *Science of education and the psychology of the child.* New York: Viking Press.

Picker, L. (1996, May). Herbal medicine goes mainstream. *American Health,* 68–75.

Pifer, A., & Bronte, L. (1986). Introduction: Squaring the pyramid. In A. Pifer & L. Bronte (Eds.), *Our aging society.* New York: Norton.

Pilisuk, M., & Parks, S. H. (1983). Social support and family stress. In H. I. McCubbin, M. B. Sussman, & J. M. Patterson (Eds.), *Social stress and the family* (Special Issue). *Marriage and Family Review, 6* (1/2), 137–156.

Pillari, V. (1992). Family myths among female adolescents in a residential setting. *Child and Adolescent Social Work Journal, 9,* 77–88.

Piotrkowski, C. S., & Hughes, D. (1993). Dual-earner families in context. In F. Walsh (Ed.), *Normal family processes* (2nd ed.) (pp. 185–208). New York: Guilford Press.

Pipes, W. H. (1988). Old-time religion. Benches can't say amen. In H. P. McAdoo (Ed.), *Black families* (2nd ed.) (pp. 54–76). Newbury Park, CA: Sage.

_____. (1997). Old-time religion: Benches can't say "Amen." In H. P. McAdoo (Ed.). *Black families* (3rd ed.) (pp. 41–66). Thousand Oaks, CA: Sage.

Pleck, J. H. (1985). *Working wives/working husbands.* Beverly Hills, CA: Sage.

Pollack, D. (1981, April 5). The stepparent. How to put your best foot forward. *Fresno Bee,* Part B1, B4.

Popenoe, D. (1995). The American family crisis. *National Forum, 75* (3), 15–19.

Power, P. W., & Dell Orto, A. E. (1988). Approaches to family intervention. In P. W. Power, A. E. Dell Orto, & M. Gibbons (Eds.), *Role of the family in the rehabilitation of the physically disabled* (pp. 321–330). Baltimore: University Park Press.

Prater, L. P. (1995). Never married/biological teen mother headed household. In S. Hanson, M. Heims, D. Julian, & M. Sussman (Eds.), *Single parent families: Diversity, myths and realities* (pp. 305–323). New York: Haworth Press.

Pratt, L. (1976). *Family structure and effective health behavior. The energized family.* Boston: Houghton-Miffin.

_____. (1977). Changes in health care ideology in relation to self-care by families. *Health Education Monograph, 5* (2), 121–122.

_____. (1982). Family structure and health work: Coping in the context of social change. In H. I. McCubbin, A. E. Cauble, & J. M. Patterson (Eds.), *Family stress, coping, and social support* (pp. 73–89). Springfield, IL: Charles C. Thomas.

Prattes, O. (1973). Beliefs of the Mexican American family. In D. Hymovich & M. V. Barnard (Eds.), *Family health care* (pp. 131–137). New York: McGraw-Hill.

Pravikoff, D. (1985). *Family coping and perception of the situation in families with an actual or suspected myocardial infarction.* Unpublished master's thesis, California State University, Los Angeles.

Preto, N. G. (1988). Transformation of the family system in adolescence. In B. Carter & M. McGoldrick (Eds.), *The changing family life cycle* (2nd ed.) (pp. 255–283). New York: Gardner Press.

Price, J. A. (1976). North American Indian families. In C. H. Mindel & R. Haberstein (Eds.), *Families in America: Patterns and variations.* New York: Elsevier.

Price, R. (1990). Borderline disorders of the self: Toward a reconceptualization. *Transactional Analysis Journal, 20,* 128–134.

Prohaska, T. R., Leventhal, E. A., Leventhal, H., et al. (1985). Health practices and illness cognition in young, middle aged and elderly adults. *Journal of Gerontology, 40* (5), 569–578.

Pruchno, R. A., & Resch, N. L. (1989). Husbands and wives as caregivers: Antecedents of depression and burden. *The Gerontologist, 29,* 159–165.

Queen, S. A., & Haberstein, R. W. (1974). *The family in various cultures.* Philadelphia: Lippincott.

Quinn, P. (1995). Gender interactions in families. In R. D. Day, K.R. Gilbert, B. H. Settles, & W. R. Burr (Eds.), *Research and theory in family science* (pp. 42–53). Pacific Grove, CA: Brooks/Cole.

Quinn, W. H. (1993). Personal and family adjustment in later life. *Journal of Marriage and the Family, 51,* 581–591.

Rafael, A. R. (1995). Advocacy and empowerment: Dichotomous or synchronous concepts? *Advances in Nursing Science, 18* (2), 25–32.

Rainwater, L. (1971). Crucible of identity: The Negro lower-class family. In J. H. Bracey, A. Meier, & E. Rudwick (Eds.), *Black matriarchy: Myth or reality?* (pp. 76–109). Belmont, CA: Wadsworth.

_____. (1972). Fear and house as haven in the lower class. In R. Gutman (Ed.), *People and buildings.* New York: Basic Books.

Ramirez, O., & Arce, C. (1981). The contemporary Chicano family: An empirically-based review. In A. Baron (Ed.), *Explorations in Chicano psychology.* New York: Praeger.

Rando, T. (Ed.). (1986). *Loss and anticipatory grief.* Lexington, MA: Lexington Books.

Rankin, S. H., & Stallings, K. D. (1996). *Patient education: Issues, principles and practices* (3rd ed.). Philadelphia: Lippincott.

Rapoport, R., Rapoport, R., & Thiessen, V. (1974). Couple symmetry and enjoyment. *Journal of Marriage and the Family, 36* (3), 588–591.

Raths, L. E., Harmin, M., & Simon, S. B. (1978). *Values and teaching: Working with values in the classroom* (2nd ed.). Columbus, OH: Charles E. Merrill.

Rauckhorst, L. M., Stokes, S. A., & Mezey, M. D. (1982). Community and home assessment. In B. W. Spradley (Ed.), *Readings in community health nursing* (2nd ed.) (pp. 154–165). Boston: Little, Brown.

Raush, H., Goodrich, W., & Campbell, J. D. (1969). Adaptation to the first years of marriage. *Psychiatry, 26,* 368–371.

Raven, B. H., Center, R., & Rodrigues, A. (1975). The bases of conjugal power. In R. E. Cromwell & D. H. Olson (Eds.), *Power in families* (pp. 217–232). New York: Sage.

Rayner, J. F. (1970). Socioeconomic status and factors influencing the dental health practices of mothers. *American Journal of Public Health, 60,* 1250.

Rebelsky, F. G. (1967). Infancy in two cultures. *Psychologie Ned Tydschr Psychol Grensgebieden, 22,* 379.

Reinhard, S. C., & Horwitz, A. V. (1995). Caregiver burden: Differentiating the content and consequences of family caregiving. *Journal of Marriage and the Family, 57,* 741–750.

Reinhardt, A., & Quinn, M. (Eds.). (1973). *Current practices in family-centered community nursing.* St. Louis: Mosby.

Reiss, D. (1981). *The family's construction of reality.* Cambridge, MA: Harvard University Press.

Reiss, D., Gonzalez, S., & Kramer, N. (1986). Family process, chronic illness, and death: On the weakness of strong bonds. *Archives of General Psychiatry, 43,* 975.

Reiss, D., & Oliveri, M. E. (1983, Spring/Summer). Family stress as community frame. *Marriage and Family Review, 6* (1/2), 61–83.

Reiss, D., Steinglass, P., & Howe, G. (1993). The family's organization around the illness. In R. Cole & D. Reiss (Eds.), *How do families cope with chronic illness?* (pp. 173–213). Hillsdale, NJ: Erlbaum.

Reiss, I. L. (1965). The universality of the family: A conceptual analysis. *Journal of Marriage and the Family, 27,* 443.

———. (1976). *Family systems in America* (2nd ed.). Hinsdale, IL: Dryden Press.

Richards, B. S. (1996). Gerontological family nursing. In S. M. H. Hanson & S. T. Boyd (Eds.), *Family health care nursing: Theory, practice, and research.* Philadelphia: Davis.

Richards, E., & Lansberry, C. R. (1995). A national survey of graduate family nursing educators. *Journal of Family Nursing, 1* (4), 382–396.

Richardson, W. (1970). Measuring the urban poor's use of physicians' services in response to illness episodes. *Medical Care, 8,* 132.

Riche, M. F. (1991, March). The future of the family. *American Demographics,* 43–46.

Ridley, C. R., & Lingle, D. W. (1996). Cultural empathy in multicultural counseling. In P. B. Pedersen, J. G. Draguns, W. J. Lonner, & J. E. Trimble (Eds.), *Counseling across cultures* (4th ed.) (pp. 21–46). Thousand Oaks, CA: Sage.

Riesch, S. K., et al. (1993). Effects of communication training on parents and young adolescents. *Nursing Research, 42* (1), 10–16.

Rippe, J. M. (1989, Feb. 13). For a life long healthy heart: Choose exercise. *Newsweek,* S-8, S-10.

Roack, A. C. (1988, July 24). Parenting: Fads, theories change with the years. *Los Angeles Times,* pp. A1, A24.

Roan, S. (1995, July 9). Who's to blame for teenage pregnancy? *Los Angeles Times,* p. E3.

Robbins, L. C. & Hall, J. H. (1970). *How to practice medicine.* Indianapolis, IN: Methodist Hospital.

Roberto, K. A. (1993). Family caregivers of aging adults with disabilities: A review of the caregiving literature. In K. A. Roberto (Ed.), *The elderly caregiver: Caring for adults with developmental disabilities.* Newbury Park, CA: Sage.

Roberts, R. H. (1975). Perceptual views of family members of the identified patient. In S. Smoyak (Ed.). *The psychiatric nurse as a family therapist* (pp. 156–163). New York: Wiley.

Roberts, S. (1995). *Who we are: A portrait of America based on the latest U.S. Census.* New York: Times Books.

Robinson, C. A. (1994). Nursing interventions with families: A demand or an invitation to change? *Journal of Advanced Nursing, 19,* 897–904.

———. (1995). Unifying distinctions for nursing research with persons and families. *Journal of Family Nursing, 1* (1), 8–29.

———. (1996). Health care relationships revisited. *Journal of Family Nursing, 2* (2), 152–173.

Robinson, C. A., & Wright, L. M. (1995). Family nursing interventions: What families say makes a difference. *Journal of Family Nursing, 1* (3), 327–345.

Robiscon, R., & Smith, J. A. (1973). Family assessment. In A. M. Reinhardt & M. D. Quinn (Eds.), *Current practice in family-centered community nursing,* Vol I. St. Louis: Mosby.

Rodgers, H. R., Jr. (1990). *Poor women, poor families and the economic plight of America's female-headed households* (rev. ed.). Armonk, NY: M. E. Sharpe.

Rodgers, J. (1993, June). Higher education: Preparing the post-reform nurse. *The American Nurse,* p. 6.

Rodgers, R. H. (1973). *Family interaction and transaction: The developmental approach.* Englewood Cliffs, NJ: Prentice-Hall.

Rodman, H. (1965). *Marriage, family and society.* New York: Random House.

Rodman, H., & Sidden, J. (1992). A critique of pessimistic views about U.S. families. *Family Relations, 41,* 436–439.

Rodwell, C. M. (1996). An analysis of the concept of empowerment. *Journal of Advanced Nursing, 23,* 305–313.

Roessler, R., & Bolton, B. (1978). Coordination of human services. In R. Roessler & B. Bolton (Eds.), *Psychological adjustment to disability* (pp. 145–161). Baltimore: University Park Press.

Rogers, C. (1951). *Client-centered therapy: Implications and theory.* Boston: Houghton Mifflin.

Rogers, M. (1970). *Introduction to the theoretical basis of nursing.* Philadelphia: Davis.

———. (1986). Science of unitary human beings. In V. Malinski (Ed.), *Explorations on Martha Rogers' science of unitary human beings* (pp. 3–8). Norwalk, CT: Appleton-Century-Crofts.

————. (1990). Nursing: Science of unitary, irreducible, human beings: Update, 1900. In E. Barret (Ed.), *Visions of Rogers' science-based nursing* (pp. 5–11). New York: National League for Nursing.

Rokeach, M. (1973). *The nature of human values.* New York: Free Press.

Rolland, J. (1988). Model of chronic and life-threatening illness. In C. S. Chilman, E. W. Nunnally, & F. M. Cox (Eds.), *Chronic illness and disability* (pp. 17–68). Newbury Park, CA: Sage.

————. (1993). Serious illness and disability. In F. Walsh (Ed.), *Normal family processes* (2nd ed.) (pp. 444–473). New York: Guilford Press.

Rolland, J. S. (1994). *Families, illness, & disability: An integrative treatment model.* New York: Basic Books.

Rollins, B. C., & Feldman, H. (1970). Marital satisfaction over the family life cycle. *Journal of Marriage and the Family, 32* (1), 20–25.

Rollins, B. C., & Thomas, D. L. (1979). Parental support, power and control techniques in the socialization of children. In W. R. Burr, R. Hill, F. I. Nye, & I. L. Reiss (Eds.), *Contemporary theories about the family,* Vol. I. New York: Free Press.

Roney, R. G., & Nall, M. L. (1966). *Medication practices in a community: An exploratory study.* Menlo Park, CA: Stanford Research Institute.

Ropers, R. H. (1991). *Persistent poverty.* New York: Plenum Press.

Rose, A. M. (1962). *Human behavior and social processes.* Boston: Houghton Mifflin.

Rosenblatt, R. A. (1996, March 4). Latinos, Asians to lead rise in U.S. population. *Los Angeles Times,* pp. A1, A4.

Rosenbloom, C. A., & Whittington, F. J. (1993). The effects of bereavement on eating behavior and nutrient intake in elderly widowed persons. *Journal of Gerontology; Social Sciences, 48* (4), 223–229.

Rosenstock, I. M. (1974). Historical origins of the health belief model. In M. Becker (Ed.), *The health belief model and personal health behavior* (pp. 1–8). Thorofare, NJ: Charles Slack.

Ross, B., & Cobb, K. H. (1990). *Family nursing: A nursing process approach.* Redwood City, CA: Addison-Wesley.

Ross, C. E., Mirowsky, J., & Goldstein, K. (1990). The impact of the family on health: The decade in review. *Journal of Marriage and the Family, 52* (4), 1059–1078.

————. (1991). The impact of the family on health. The decade in review. In A. Booth (Ed.), *Contemporary families: Looking forward, looking back* (pp. 341–360). Minneapolis, MN: National Council for Family Relations.

Rossi, A. S. (1986). Sex and gender in the aging society. In A. Pifer & L. Bronte (Eds.), *Our aging society* (pp. 111–139). New York: Norton.

Roth, P. (1989). Family social support. In P. J. Bomar (Ed.), *Nurses and family health promotion* (pp. 90–102). Baltimore, MD: Williams & Wilkins.

————. (1996a). Family health promotion during transitions. In P. J. Bomar (Ed.), *Nurses and family health promotion* (2nd ed.) (pp. 365–394). Philadelphia: Saunders.

————. (1996b). Family social support. In P. J. Bomar (Ed.), *Nurses and family health promotion* (2nd ed.) (pp. 107–120). Philadelphia: Saunders.

Roy, C. (1976). *Introduction to nursing: An adaptation model.* Englewood Cliffs, NJ: Prentice-Hall.

Roy, C., & Roberts, S. (1981). *Theory construction in nursing: An adaptation model.* Englewood Cliffs, NJ: Prentice-Hall.

Rubin, L. (1976). *Worlds of pain: Life in the working class family.* New York: Basic Books.

Rubin, L. B. (1994). *Families on the fault line: America's working class speaks about the family. The economy, race and ethnicity.* New York: HarperCollins.

Rubin, R. (1967). Attainment of the maternal role. 1. Processes. *Nursing Research, 16,* 237.

————. (1967). Attainment of maternal role. 2. Models and referrants. *Nursing Research, 16,* 342.

Rubin, R., & Neiswiadomy, M. (1995, Dec.). Economic adjustments of households on entry into retirement. *Journal of Applied Gerontology, 14* (4), 467–482.

Ruesch, H., Barry, W., Hertel, R., & Swain, M. (1974). *Communication conflict and marriage.* San Francisco: Jossey-Bass.

Rumbaut, R. G. (1995). Vietnamese, Laotian, and Cambodian Americans. In P. G. Min (Ed.), *Asian Americans: Contemporary trends and issues* (pp. 232–270). Thousand Oaks, CA: Sage.

Rushing, W. (1968). Individual behavior and suicides. In J. P. Gibbs (Ed.), *Suicide* (pp. 96–121). New York: Harper & Row.

Russell, G. (1977, Aug. 29). The American underclass. *Time,* 16–19.

Russell, G., & Satterwhite, B. (1978, Oct. 16). It's your turn in the sun. *Time,* 48.

Ryan, K. O. (1996, April 24). The road to wellville. *Los Angeles Times,* p. E3.

Ryan, M. C., & Austin, A. L. (1989). Social supports and social networks in the aged. *Image, 21* (3), 176–179.

Ryland, E. K., & Greenfeld, S. (1990). An investigation of gender differences in occupational stress and general well-being. *Journal of Applied Business Research, 6,* 35–43.

Safilios-Rothschild, C. (1976a). A macro and micro-examination of family power and love: An exchange model. *Journal of Marriage and the Family, 38* (2), 355–362.

————. (1976b). The dimensions of power distribution in the family. In H. Grunebaum & J. Christ (Eds.), *Contemporary marriage: Structure, dynamics and therapy.* Boston: Little, Brown.

Saluter, A. F. (1993). Marital status and living arrangements: March, 1992. *Current Population Reports* (Series P. 20, No. 468). Washington, DC: U.S. Government Printing Office.

———. (1994). Marital status and living arrangements: March, 1993. *Current population reports* (Series P. 20, No. 478). Washington, DC: U.S. Government Printing Office.

Samuelson, R. J. (1986, Oct. 20). The discovery of money. *Newsweek*, 58.

Santi, L. L. (1987, Nov.). Changes in the structure and size of American households: 1970 to 1985. *Journal of Marriage and the Family, 49* (4) 833–837.

Santiago, A. M., & Muschkin, C. G. (1996). Disentangling the effects of disability status and gender on the labor supply of Anglo, Black, and Latino older workers. *The Gerontologist, 36* (3), 299–310.

Satir, V. (1967). *Conjoint family therapy* (2nd ed.). Palo Alto, CA: Science and Behavior Books.

———. (1972). *Peoplemaking*. Palo Alto, CA: Science and Behavior Books.

———. (1975). Intervention for congruence. In V. Satir, J. S. Stachowiak, & H. A. Taschman (Eds.), *Helping families to change* (pp. 79–104). New York: Aronson.

———. (1982). The therapist and family therapy: Process model. In A. M. Horne & M. M. Ohlsen (Eds.), *Family counseling and therapy* (pp. 12–42). Itasca, IL: Peacock.

———. (1983). *Conjoint family therapy* (3rd ed.). Palo Alto, CA: Science and Behavior Books.

Satir, V., Banmen, J., Gerber, J., & Gomori, M. (1991). *The Satir model: Family therapy and beyond*. Palo Alto, CA: Science and Behavior Books.

Saunders, L. (1954). *Cultural differences & medical care: The case of the Spanish-speaking people of the Southwest*. New York: Sage Foundation.

Savage, D. G. (1990, Feb. 27). One in four young black males in jail or in court control, study says. *Los Angeles Times*, pp. A1, A16.

———. (1996, Sept. 18). Clinton not to blame for rise in teen drug use, experts say. *Los Angeles Times*, p. A5.

Scanzoni, J. (1971). *The Black family in modern society*. Boston: Allyn & Bacon.

———. (1987). Families in the 1990's. *Journal of Family Issues, 8* (4), 394–421.

Scanzoni, J., & Marsiglio, W. (1993). New action theory and contemporary families. *Journal of Family Issues, 14* (1), 105–132.

Scanzoni, J., & Szinovacz, M. (1980). *Family decision-making. A developmental sex role model*. Newbury Park, CA: Sage.

Scarr, S. (1995). The two worlds of child care. *National Forum, 75* (3), 39–41.

Schmall, V. L. (1994). A training and education perspective on family caregiving. In Schmall, V. L. (Ed.), *Family caregiving: Agenda for the future*. Chicago: American Society on Aging.

Schnittger, M., & Bird, G. (1990). Coping among dual-career men and women across the family life cycle. *Family Relations, 39*, 199–205.

Schonfield, D. (1982). Who is stereotyping whom and why? *The Gerontologist, 22*, 267–272.

Schor, E. L. (Ed.). (1995). *Caring for your school-age child* (American Academy of Pediatrics Publication). New York: Bantam Books.

Schorr, A. L. (1970). Housing and its effects. In H. M. Proshansky, et al. (Eds.), *Environmental psychology*. New York: Holt, Rinehart, & Winston.

Schraneveldt, J. D. (1973). The interactionist framework in the study of the family. In A. Reinhardt & M. Quinn (Eds.), *Family-centered community nursing*. St. Louis: Mosby.

Schraneveldt, J. D., & Young, M. H. (1992). Strengthening families: New horizons in family life education. *Family Relations, 41*, 385–389.

Schreiber, K. (1992). The adolescent crack dealer: A failure in the development of empathy. *Journal of the American Academy of Psychoanalysis, 20*, 241–249.

Schulte, B. (1995, Feb. 23). Black families' income unchanged since 1969. *Daily News*, p. 13.

Schultz, D. A. (1972). *The changing family*. Englewood Cliffs, NJ: Prentice-Hall.

Schwab, J. (Ed.). (1990). *Resource handbook for Satir concepts*. Palo Alto, CA: Science and Behavior Books.

Schwartz, G., & Merton, D. (1967). The language of adolescents: An anthropological approach to the youth culture. *American Journal of Sociology, 72*, 459.

Schwartz, P. (1987). The family as a changed institution. *Journal of Family Issues, 8* (4), 455–459.

Schwartz, S. H. (1990). Individualism–collectivism: Critique and proposed refinements. *Journal of Cross-Cultural Psychology, 21*, 139–157.

Scotch, N., & Greiger, J. (1962). The epidemiology of rheumatoid arthritis—A review with special attention to social factors. *Journal of Chronic Diseases, 15*, 1037.

Sears, R., Maccoby, E., & Levin, H. (1957). *Patterns of child rearing*. New York: Harper & Row.

Sells, J. W. (1973). *Seven steps to effective communication*. Atlanta: Forum House.

Seltzer, M. M., Litchfield, L. C., Lowy, L., & Levin, R. J. (1989). Families as case managers: A longitudinal study. *Family Relations, 38* (3), 332–336.

Selye, H. (1974). *Stress without distress*. New York: Lippincott.

Seuntjens, A. D. (1995). Case management/care management. In M. Snyder & M. P. Mirr (Eds.), *Advanced practice nursing* (pp. 135–152). New York: Springer.

Shanas, E. (1980, Feb.). Older people and their families. The new pioneers. *Journal of Marriage and the Family, 42* (1), 9–15.

Shanas, E., et al. (1968). *Old people in three industrial societies*. New York: Atherton.

Shapiro, E. (1994). *Grief as a family process.* New York: Guilford Press.

Shapiro, J. (1989). Stress, depression and support group participation in mothers of developmentally delayed children. *Family Relations, 38* (2), 169–173.

Shapiro, V. (1983). Growing hand in hand: Infants and parents at risk. In V. J. Sasserath & R. A. Hoekelman (Eds.), *Minimizing high-risk parenting.* Skillman, NJ: Johnson & Johnson.

Shaw, S. M. (1988). Gender differences in the definition and perception of household labor. *Family Relations, 37* (3), 333–337.

Shelov, S. P. (Ed.). (1991). *Caring for your baby and young child* (American Academy of Pediatrics Publication). New York: Bantam Books.

Shepard, M. P., & Mahon, M. M. (1996). Chronic conditions in the family. In P. L. Jackson & J. A. Vessey (Eds.), *Primary care of the child with a chronic condition* (2nd ed.) (pp. 41–46). St. Louis: Mosby.

Sheppard, H. (1990, Feb. 5). How Hispanic cultural patterns affect caregivers. *The Nurse's Newspaper,* pp. 15–16.

Shon, S., & Ja, D. (1982). Asian families. In M. McGoldrick, J. Pierce, & J. Giordano (Eds.), *Ethnicity and family therapy* (pp. 208–229). New York: Guilford Press.

Shrestha, L. B., & Rosenwaike, I. (1996). Can data from the decennial census measure trends in mobility limitation among the aged? *The Gerontologist, 36* (1), 106–109.

Sillars, A. L. (1995). Communication and family culture. In M. A. Fitzpatrick & A. L. Vangelisti (Eds.), *Explaining family interactions* (pp. 375–399). Thousand Oaks, CA: Sage.

Silver, J. (1975). Solidarity versus pseudomutuality. In S. Smoyak (Ed.), *The psychiatric nurse as a family therapist* (pp. 106–113). New York: Wiley.

Silverstein, S. (1996, March 20). Study finds gap growing between rich and poor in U.S. *Los Angeles Times,* pp. A1, A16.

Simmel, G. (1955). *Conflict and the web of group affiliations.* Englewood Cliffs, NJ: Prentice-Hall.

Sistler, A. (1989). Adaptive coping of older caregiving spouses. *Social Work, 34* (5), 415–420.

Skinner, D. (1984). Dual-career families: Strains of sharing. In H. I. McCubbin & C. R. Figley (Eds.), *Stress and the family. Vol I: Coping with normative transitions.* New York: Brunner/Mazel.

Slater, P. (1970, July). Culture in collision. *Psychology Today,* 31–33, 66–68.

Slater, S. (1995). *The lesbian family life cycle.* New York: Free Press.

Sloan, M., & Schommer, B. (1975). The process of contracting in community nursing. In B. Spradley (Ed.), *Contemporary community nursing* (pp. 221–229). Boston: Little, Brown.

Smelzer, N. J., & Halpern, S. (1978). The historical triangulations of family, economy and education. In J. Demos & S. S. Boocock (Eds.), *Turning points: Historical and sociological essays on the family.* Chicago: The University of Chicago Press.

Smerglia, V. L., Deimling, G. T., and Baresi, C. M. (1988). Black/white family comparisons in helping and decision making networks of impaired elderly. *Family Relations, 37,* 305–309.

Smith, G. (1993). *Hospital-based case management: Reforming health care for the 21st century.* Sacramento, CA: CME Resources.

Smith, G.R. (1988, June 13). *Exploiting the Public Agenda. Advancing New Opportunities for Public Health Nursing.* Paper presented at American Nurses Foundation, Louisville, KY.

Smith, G. R., & Wesley, R. L. (1993). Health promotion: Public policy goals. In R. N. Knollmueller (Ed.), *Prevention across the life span.* Kansas City, MO: American Nurses Association Council of Community Health.

Smith, H. (1985). What research is telling us about family recreation. *Perspectives on family recreation and leisure.* Centennial National Conference American Alliance for Health, Physical Education and Dance (ERIC Document Reproduction Service, No. ED 263–1061).

Smith, L. (1995, Jan. 18). Can we really legislate good parenting? *Los Angeles Times,* pp. E1, E8.

Smith, S. (1995). Family theory and multicultural family studies. In B. B. Ingoldsby & S. Smith (Eds.), *Families in multicultural perspective,* (pp. 5–35). New York: Guilford Press.

Smith, T. E., & Graham, P. B. (1995). Socioeconomic stratification in family research. *Journal of Marriage and the Family, 57* (Nov.), 930–940.

Smoyak, S. (1969). Threat: A recurring family dynamic. *Perspectives in Psychiatric Care, 7,* 267–268.

————. (1975). Introducing families to family therapy. In S. Smoyak (Ed.), *The psychiatric nurse as a family therapist.* New York: Wiley.

Snarey, J. (1993). *How fathers care for the next generation: A four decade study.* Cambridge, MA: Harvard University Press.

Sobel, E. G., & Robischon, P. (1975). *Family nursing: A study guide.* St. Louis, Mosby.

Sorofman, B. (1986). Research in cultural diversity. Defining diversity. *Western Journal of Nursing Research, 8,* 121–123.

Sotomayor, M. (1991). Introduction. In M. Sotomayor (Ed.), *Empowering Hispanic families: A critical issue for the 90's* (pp. xi–xxiii). Milwaukee, WI: Family Service America.

Sparks, R. K. (1995). Client education. In M. Snyder & M. P. Mirr (Eds.), *Advanced practice nursing* (pp. 117–133). New York: Springer.

Speck, R. V., & Attneave, C. (1973). *Family networks.* New York: Random House.

Spector, R. E. (1991). *Cultural diversity in health and illness* (3rd ed.). Norwalk, CT: Appleton & Lange.

Spence, W. R. (1989). *Weight control.* Waco, TX: Health EDCO.

Spiegel, J. (1957). The resolution of role conflict within the family. *Psychiatry, 25,* 1.

Spinetta, J. J., & Deasy-Spinetta, P. (1981). *Living with childhood cancer.* St. Louis: Mosby.

Spitze, G. (1988). Women's employment and family relations: A review. *Journal of Marriage and the Family, 50* (3), 595–618.

Spitzer, W., & Brown, B. (1975). Unanswered questions about the periodic health examination. *Annals of Internal Medicine, 83,* 257.

Sprey, J. (1969). The family as a system in conflict. *Journal of Marriage and the Family, 31* (4), 699–706.

————. (1972). Family power structure: A critical comment. *Journal of Marriage and the Family, 34* (2), 235.

————. (1979). Conflict theory and the study of marriage and the family. In W. R. Burr, R. Hill, F. I. Nye, & I. L. Reiss (Eds.), *Contemporary theories about the family, Vol. II* (pp. 130–159). New York: Free Press.

Sprey, J., & Matthews, S. (1982). Contemporary grandparenthood. A systematic transition. *Annals of the American Academy of Political and Social Science, 464,* 91–103.

Stachowiak, J. (1975). Family structure and intervention strategies. In V. Satir, J. Stachowiak, & H. A. Taschman (Eds.), *Helping families to change* (pp. 105–131). New York: Aronson.

Staight, P. R., & Harvey, S. M. (1990). Caregiver burden: A comparison between elderly women as primary and secondary caregiver to their spouses. *Journal of Gerontological Social Work, 15* (1/2), 89–104.

Stanley, M. J. B., & Frantz, R. A. (1988). Adjustment problems of spouses of patients undergoing coronary artery bypass graft surgery during early convalescence. *Heart & Lung, 17* (6), 677–682.

Staples, R. (1976). The Black American family. In C. H. Mindel & R. W. Habersteiॱ (Eds.), *Ethnic families in America.* New York: Elsevier.

————. (1985). Changes in black family structure: The conflict between family ideology and structural conditions. *Journal of Marriage and the Family, 47* (4), 1005–1013.

————. (1989). Family life in the 21st century. In C. L. Gilliss, B. L. Highley, B. M. Roberts, & I. M. Martinson (Eds.), *Toward a science of family nursing* (pp. 156–170). Menlo Park, CA: Addison-Wesley.

Starr, B. D. (1985). Sexuality and aging. In C. Eisdorfer (Ed.), *Annual review of gerontology and geriatrics, Vol. 5.* New York: Springer.

Starrels, M. E., Bould, S., & Nicholas, L. J. (1994). The feminization of poverty in the United States. *Journal of Family Issues, 15* (4), 590–607.

Stauffer, R. Y. (1995). Vietnamese Americans. In J. N. Giger & R. E. Davidhizar (Eds.), *Transcultural nursing: Assessment and intervention* (pp. 441–472). St. Louis: Mosby.

Stea, D. (1965, Autumn). Space, territory, and human movement. *Landscape,* 14.

Steen, S., & Schwartz, P. (1995). Communication and gender. In M. A. Fitzpatrick & A. L. Vangelisti (Eds.), *Explaining family interactions* (pp. 310–343). Thousand Oaks, CA: Sage.

Steiger, N. J., & Lipson, J. G. (1985). *Self-care nursing: Theory and practice.* Bowie, MD: Brady.

————. (1970). Space, territory, and human movements. In Proshansky, H. M., et al. (Eds.), *Environmental psychology* (pp. 37–44). New York: Holt, Rinehart, & Winston.

Steinberg, R. M., & Carter, G. W. (1983). *Case management and the elderly.* Lexington, MA: Lexington Books.

Steinglass, P. (1978). The conceptualization of marriage from a systems theory perspective. In T. J. Paolino & B. S. McCrady (Eds.), *Marriage and marital therapy: Psychoanalytic, behavioral, and systems theory perspectives.* New York: Brunner/Mazel.

Steinglass, P., Bennett, L. A., Wolin, S. J., & Reiss, D. (1987). *The alcoholic family.* New York: Basic Books.

Steinmetz, S. (1995). Violence in families. In R. D. Day, K. R. Gilbert, B. H. Settles, & W. R. Burr (Eds.), *Research and theory in family science* (pp. 255–267). Pacific Grove, CA: Brooks/Cole.

Steinmetz, S. K. (1987). Family violence. Past, present and future. In M. B. Sussman & S. K. Steinmetz (Eds.), *Handbook of marriage and the family* (pp. 725–765). New York: Plenum Press.

Stetz, K., Lewis, J., & Primomo, J. (1986). Family coping strategies and chronic illness in the mother. *Family Relations, 35,* 515–522.

Stewart, E. C., & Bennett, M. J. (1991). *American cultural patterns.* Yarmouth, ME: Intercultural Press.

Stewart, M. J. (1993). *Integrating social support in nursing.* Newbury Park, CA: Sage.

Stinnett, N. (1979). In search of strong families. In N. Stinnett, B. Chesser, & J. De Frain (Eds.), *Building family strengths—Blueprints for action.* Lincoln, NE: University of Nebraska Press.

Stokes, L. G. (1974). Delivering health services in a Black community. In A. Reinhardt & M. Quinn (Eds.), *Family-centered community nursing.* St. Louis: Mosby.

Stolberg, S. (1996a, June 16). Fathers try to learn what it takes. *Los Angeles Times,* pp. A1, A16.

————. (1996b, June 16). No longer missing in action. *Los Angeles Times,* pp. A1, A5.

Stone, R., Cafferata, G. L., & Sangle, J. (1987). Caregivers of the frail elderly: A national profile. *The Gerontologist, 27,* 616–626.

Straus, M. A. (1968). Communication, creativity, and problem-solving ability of middle and working class families in three societies. *American Journal of Sociology, 73,* 417–430.

———. (1991). Discipline and deviance: Physical punishment of children and violence and other crime in adulthood. *Social Problems, 38,* 101–123.

Straus, M. A., & Gelles, R. (1990). *Physical violence in American families: Risk factors and adaptations to violence in 8,145 families.* New Brunswick, NJ: Transaction.

Straus, M. A., Gelles, R. J., & Steinmetz, S. K. (1980). *Behind closed doors: Violence in the American family.* New York: Anchor Press.

Strayhorn, J. M., Jr. (1977). *Talking it out: Guide to effective communication.* Champagne, IL: Research Press.

Strodtbeck, F. L. (1978). Family interaction, values, and achievement. In D. C. McClelland, et al. (Eds.), *Talent and society* (pp. 135–194). New York: Van Nostrand.

Suchman, E. A. (1965, Fall). Stages of illness and medical care. *Journal of Health and Human Behavior, 6,* 114–128.

Sung, S. L. (1967). *The story of the Chinese in America.* New York: Collier.

Sussman, M. B. (1974). Family systems in the 1970s: Analysis, policies, and programs. In A. Skolnick, & J. H. Skolnick (Eds.), *Intimacy, family and society* (pp. 579–598). Boston: Little, Brown.

Sussman, M. B., & Slater, S. B. (1963, Aug. 28). *Reappraisal of Urban Kin Networks—Empirical Evidence.* Paper presented at the Annual Meeting of the American Sociological Association, Los Angeles, CA.

Suzuki, B. H. (1985). Asian American families. In J. H. Henslin (Ed.), *Marriage and family in a changing society* (pp. 104–119). New York: Macmillan.

Svavarsdottir, E., & McCubbin, M. (1996). Parenthood transition for parents of an infant diagnosed with a congenital heart condition. *Journal of Pediatric Nursing, 11* (4), 207–216.

Swendsen, L. A., & Meleis, A. I. (1978, March/April). Role supplementation for new parents—a role mastery plan. *American Journal of Maternal-Child Nursing, X* (2), 84.

Syme, S., Hyman, M., & Enterline, P. (1964). Some social and cultural factors associated with the occurrence of coronary heart disease. *Journal of Chronic Disease, 17,* 277.

Synder, W. K. (1988). *Sudden infant death syndrome. Self-help support groups. An annotated bibliography* (Fall, 1988). McLean, VA: National Sudden Infant Death Syndrome Clearinghouse.

Szafran, K. K. (1996). Family health protective behaviors. In P. J. Bomar (Ed.), *Nurses and family health promotion* (2nd ed.) (pp. 306–338). Philadelphia: Saunders.

Szinovacz, M., & Egley, L. (1995). Comparing one-partner and couple data on sensitive marital behaviors: The case of marital violence. *Journal of Marriage and the Family, 57,* 995–1010.

Szinovacz, M. E. (1987). Family power. In M. B. Sussman & S. K. Steinmetz (Eds.), *Handbook of marriage and the family* (pp. 651–693). New York: Plenum Press.

Tadych, R. (1985). Nursing in multiperson units: The family. In Riehl-Sisca, J (Ed.). *The science and art of self-care* (pp. 49–55), Norwalk, CT: Appleton & Lange.

Taeuber, C. M. (1993). Sixty-five in America. *U.S. Bureau of the Census, Current population reports, special studies,* No. 23-178. Washington, DC: U.S. Government Printing Office.

Tannen, D. (1990). *You just don't understand: Women and men in conversation.* New York: Ballantine.

Tapp, D. (1995). Impact of ischemic heart disease: Family nursing research, 1984–1993. *Journal of Family Nursing, 1* (1), 79–104.

Taylor, C. (1970). In horizontal orbit. New York: Holt, Rinehart & Winston.

Taylor, C. W. (1995). Homeless families. In B. S. Johnson (Ed.), *Child, adolescent and family psychiatric nursing* (pp. 180–198). Philadelphia: Lippincott.

Taylor, R. J. (1990). Need for support and family involvement among Black Americans. *Journal of Marriage and the Family, 52* (3), 584–590.

Taylor, R. J., Chatters, C. M., & Mays, V. M. (1988). Parents, children, siblings, in-laws, and non-kin as sources of emergency assistance to Black Americans. *Family Relations, 37* (3), 298–304.

Taylor, R. J., Chatters, C. M. Tucker, M. B., & Lewis, E. (1990). Developments in research on black families: A decade review. *Journal of Marriage and the Family, 52* (4), 993–1014.

Teachman, J. D., Polonko, K. A., & Scanzoni, J. (1987). Demography of the family. In M. B. Sussman, & S. Steinmetz (Eds.), *Handbook of marriage and the family* (pp. 3–36). New York: Plenum Press.

Thoits, P. A. (1982). Conceptual, methodological and theoretical problems in studying social support as a buffer against life stress. *Journal of Health and Social Behavior, 23* (June), 145–159.

Thomas, R. B., Barnard, K. E., & Sumner, G. A. (1993). Family nursing diagnosis as a framework for family assessment. In S. L. Feetham, S. B. Meister, J. M. Bell, & C. L. Gilliss (Eds.), *The nursing of families: Theory, research, education, practice.* Newbury Park, CA: Sage.

Thomas, W. I. (1923). *The unadjusted girl.* New York: The Social Science Research Council (Later publication in 1967 by New York: Harper & Row).

Thompson, L., & Walker, A. J. (1991). Gender in families: Women and men in marriage, work, and parenthood. In A. Booth (Ed.), *Contemporary families: Looking forward, looking back* (pp. 76–102). Minneapolis, MN: National Council on Family Relations.

Thorne, S. E., & Robinson, C. A. (1989). Guarded alliance: Health care relationships in chronic illness. *Image, 21*, 153–157.

Tiesel, J. W., & Olson, D. H. (1992). Preventing family problems: Troubling trends and promising opportunities. *Family Relations, 41*, 398–403.

Tiller, C. M. (1995). Fathers parenting attitudes during a child's first year. *Journal of Obstetric, Gynecologic, and Neonatal Nursing, 24* (6), 508–514.

Tinkham, G., & Voorhies, E. (1977). *Community health nursing—Evolution and process.* New York: Appleton-Century-Crofts.

———. (1984). *Community health nursing—Evolution and process* (2nd ed.). New York: Appleton-Century-Crofts.

Toffler, A. (1970). *Future shock.* New York: Warner Communications.

———. (1990, Oct. 15). Power shift. Knowledge, wealth, and violence at the edge of the 21st century. *Newsweek*, 85–92.

Toman, W. (1961). *Family constellation: Its effects on personality and social behavior.* New York: Springer.

Tomlinson, P., & Anderson, K. (1995). Family health and the Neuman systems model. In B. Neuman (Ed.), *The Neuman systems model* (3rd ed.). Stamford, CT: Appleton & Lange.

Toynbee, A. J. (1955, March). We must pay for freedom. *Women's Home Companion*, 52–53.

Trainor, M. G. (1983). Self-help groups as a resource for individual clients and families. In I. W. Clements & F. B. Roberts (Eds.), *Family health: A theoretical approach to nursing care* (pp. 45–56). New York: Wiley.

Tran, T. V. (1988). The Vietnamese American family. In C. H. Mindel, R. W. Habenstein, & R. Wright, Jr. (Eds.), *Ethnic families in America* (pp. 276–299). New York: Elsevier.

Travelbee, J. (1969). *Intervention in psychiatric nursing.* Philadelphia: Davis.

Travis, J. (1976). *Wellness workbook.* Mill Valley, CA: Wellness Resource Center.

Tripp, S. L., & Stachowiak, B. (1992). Health maintenance, health promotion. Is there a difference? *Public Health Nursing, 9* (3), 155–161.

Tripp-Reimer, T., Brink, P. J., & Saunders, J. M. (1984, March/April). Cultural assessment: Content and process. *Nursing Outlook, 32* (2), 78–82.

Tripp-Reimer, T., & Lauer, G. M. (1987). Ethnicity and families with chronic illness. In L. M. Wright & M. Leahey (Eds.), *Families and chronic illness* (pp. 77–100). Springhouse, PA: Springhouse Corporation.

Tripp-Reimer, T., & Lively, S. (1988). Cultural considerations in therapy. In C. K. Beck, R. P. Rawlins, & S.

Williams (Eds.), *Mental health and psychiatric nursing* (pp. 185–199). St. Louis: Mosby.

Troll, L. (1971). The family of later life: A decade review. *Journal of Marriage and the Family, 33*, 263–275.

Truax, C., & Carkhuff, R. (1967). *Toward effective counseling and psychotherapy.* Chicago: Aldine.

Turner, R. H. (1962). Role taking: Process vs. conformity. In A. M. Rose (Ed.). *Human behavior and social processes* (pp. 20–40). Boston: Houghton-Mifflin.

———. (1970). *Family interaction.* New York: Wiley.

Turner, V. (1990, Winter). A look at methamphetamine. *People reaching out newsletter.* New York: Youth and Family Center for Substance Abuse Counseling and Information.

Uba, L. (1994). *Asian Americans: Personality patterns, identity, and mental health.* New York: Guilford Press.

United Press International. (1990, Feb. 6). Tax report says rich gained, poor lost during the 80's. *Los Angeles Times*, p. A4.

U.S. Bureau of the Census. (1980). *Statistical abstracts of the U.S.* (101st ed.). Washington, DC: U.S. Government Printing Office.

———. (1981). *Statistical abstracts of the U.S.* (102nd ed.). Washington, DC: U.S. Government Printing Office.

———. (1982). *Statistical abstracts of the U.S.* (103rd ed.). Washington, DC: U.S. Government Printing Office.

———. (1983a). *1980 census of population, general population characteristics, United States summary* (PC80-1-D1). Washington, DC: U.S. Government Printing Office.

———. (1983b). *Statistical abstracts of the U.S.* (104th ed.). Washington, DC: U.S. Government Printing Office.

———. (1984). Projections of the population of the United States, by age, sex, and race: 1983–2080. *Current populations reports,* Series No. 952, p. 25. Washington, DC: U.S. Government Printing Office.

———. (1985, March). Households, families, marital status and living arrangements. *Current population reports,* Series P-20, No. 402. Washington, DC: U.S. Government Printing Office.

———. (1986). Marital status and living arrangements: March 1985. *Current population reports,* Series P-20, No. 410. Washington, DC: U.S. Government Printing Office.

———. (1988). *Statistical abstracts of the U.S., 1988.* (108th ed.). Washington, DC: U.S. Government Printing Office.

———. (1989). *Statistical abstracts of the U.S.* (109th ed.). Washington, DC: U.S. Government Printing Office.

———. (1990, Jan.). How we're changing. *Current population reports,* Series No. 164, p. 23. Washington, DC: U.S. Government Printing Office.

———. (1991a). *Census & you, 26* (2) & (4). Washington, DC: U.S. Government Printing Office.

———. (1991b, Aug.). Poverty in the United States: 1990. *Current population reports,* P-60, No. 175. Washington, DC: U.S. Government Printing Office.

———. (1992). Household and family characteristics—March, 1991. *Current population reports,* Series P-20, No. 458. Washington, DC: U.S. Government Printing Office.

———. (1993a). *1990 census of population, Asian and Pacific Islanders in the United States* (CP-3-5). Washington, DC: U.S. Government Printing Office.

———. (1993b). *1990 census of population, general population characteristics, the United States* (CP-1-1). Washington, DC: U.S. Government Printing Office.

———. (1994). *1990 census of population, general social and economic characteristics, the United States* (CP-2-1). Washington, DC: U.S. Government Printing Office.

U.S. Department of Agriculture. (1985). *Dietary guidelines for Americans* (2nd ed.). Washington, DC: USDA, Dept. of Health and Human Services.

U.S. Department of Health, Education and Welfare. (1972, June). *Periodontal disease and oral hygiene among children.* U.S. Public Health Services, Series 11, No. 117.

———. (1983, May 30). *Monthly Vital Statistics Report, 23,* 13.

U.S. Department of Health and Human Services. (1988). *Health care financing review, 1988 supplement, national sample of registered nurses.* Washington, DC: U.S. Government Printing Office.

———. (1989a). *A profile of uninsured Americans.* National Center for Health Services Research and Health Care Technology Assessment (DHHS Publication No. [PHS] 89-3443). Washington, DC: U.S. Government Printing Office.

———. (1989b). *Child health USA '89.* Office of Maternal and Child Health. HRS-M-CH 8915, October, 1989.

———. (1990). *The seventh special report to the U.S. Congress on: Alcohol and health.* Alcohol, Drug Abuse, and Mental Health Administration. Washington, DC: U.S. Government Printing Office.

———. (1991). *Healthy people 2000: National health promotion and disease prevention objectives* (DHHS Publication No. [PHS] 91-50213). Washington, DC: U.S. Government Printing Office.

———. (1993). *Toward equality of well-being: Strategies for improving minority health. Strategic planning and coordination process* (PHS Publication No. 93-50217). Washington, DC: U.S. Government Printing Office.

———. (1995). *Nutrition and your health: Dietary guidelines for Americans* (4th ed.). U.S. Department of Agriculture. Home & Garden Bulletin No. 232.

———. (1996). *Preliminary estimates from the 1995 national household survey on drug abuse.* Substance Abuse and Mental Health Services Administration, Office of Applied Studies. Advanced Report No. 18. (DHHS Publication No. [SMA] 96-3107). Washington, DC: U.S. Government Printing Office.

U.S. Department of Health and Human Services, Center for Disease Control. (1985). *Diphtheria, tetanus, and per-tussis: Guidelines for vaccine prophylaxis and other preventive measures.* Atlanta, MMWR July 12, pp. 405–426.

———. (1987). *The 21st immunization conference proceedings.* CDC, Atlanta, June 8–11.

U.S. Environmental Protection Agency. (1988). *The inside story: A guide to indoor pollution quality.* United States Consumer Product Safety Commission. EPA 400/1-88/004. Washington, DC: U.S. Government Printing Office.

U.S. Public Health Service. (1979). *Healthy people: The surgeon general's report on health promotion and disease prevention.* (DHEW [PHS] No. 79-55071). Washington, DC: U.S. Government Printing Office.

———. (1980). *Promoting health/preventing disease: Objectives for the nation.* USDHEW (PHS). Washington, DC: U.S. Government Printing Office.

———. (1990). *Healthy people 2000: National health promotion and disease prevention objectives.* Washington, DC: U.S. Government Printing Office.

———. (1991). *Healthy people 2000: National health promotion and disease prevention objectives* (DHHS Publication No. [PHS] 91-50213). Washington, DC: U.S. Government Printing Office.

U.S. Senate Special Committee on Aging (in conjunction with the American Association of Retired Persons, the Federal Council on Aging and the U.S. Administration on Aging). (1987–1988). *Aging America: Trends and projections.* Washington, DC: U.S. Government Printing Office.

Valdez, R. (1991). Latino access to health care. *Health, 10* (1), 3.

Vannoy-Hiller, D., & Philliber, W. W. (1992). Wife's employment and quality of marriage. *Journal of Marriage and the Family, 54,* 387–398.

Vaux, A. (1990). An ecological approach to understanding and facilitating support. *Journal of Social and Personal Relationships, 7* (4), 507–518.

Vega, W. A. (1990). Hispanic families in the 1980s: A decade of research. *Journal of Marriage and the Family, 52* (Nov.), 1015–1024.

———. (1995). The study of Latino families. In R. E. Zambrana (Ed.), *Understanding Latino families: Scholarship, policy and practice* (pp. 3–17). Thousand Oaks, CA: Sage.

Vega, W. A., & Amaro, H. (1994). Latino outlook: Good health, uncertain prognosis. *Annual Review of Public Health, 15,* 39–67.

Vega, W. A., Hough, R. L., & Romero, A. (1983). Family life patterns of Mexican Americans. In A. J. Powell (Ed.), *The psychological development of minority children* (pp. 194–215). New York: Brunner/Mazel.

Vega, W. A., et al. (1986). Cohesion and adaptability in Mexican-American and Anglo families. *Journal of Marriage and the Family, 48*(4), 857–867.

Venegoni, S. L. (1995). Primary care: Improving health promotion and disease prevention. In J. V. Hickey, R. M. Ouimette, & S. L. Venegoni (Eds.), *Advanced practice nursing. Changing roles and clinical applications* (pp. 255–256). Philadelphia: Lippincott.

Venters, M. H. (1981). Familial coping with chronic and severe childhood illness: The case of cystic fibrosis. *Social Science and Medicine, 19A,* 189–197.

Ventura, J. N. (1987). The stresses of parenthood reexamined. *Family Relations, 36* (1), 26–29.

———. (1989). First births to older mothers, 1970–1986. *American Journal of Public Health, 79* (12), 1675–1677.

Vernez, G., Burnam, M. A., McGlynn, E. A., Trude, S., & Mittman, B. S. (1988, Feb.). *Review of California's program for the homeless mentally disabled.* Santa Monica, CA: Rand Corporation.

Vickers, G. (1971). Institutional and personal roles. *Human Relations, 24* (5), 433.

Vincent, C. E. (1970). Mental health and the family. In P. H. Glasser & L. N. Glasser (Eds.), *Families in crisis.* New York: Harper & Row.

Vincent, J., & Ransford, H. E. (1980). *Social stratification.* Boston: Allyn & Bacon.

Visher, E. B., & Visher, J. S. (1979). *Stepparent families: Myths and realities.* Secaucus, NJ: Citadel.

———. (1990). Dynamics of successful stepfamilies. *Journal of Divorce and Remarriage, 14,* 3–11.

———. (1993). Remarriage families and stepparenting. In F. Walsh (Ed.), *Normal family processes* (pp. 235–253). New York: Guilford Press.

Visiting Nurse Association of Omaha. (1986). *Client management information system for community health nursing agencies. An implementation manual.* Bethesda, MD: USDHHS, Division of Nursing. Pub. No. NTIS HRP-0907023. For sale by the National Technical Information Service, 5285 Port Royal Rd., Springfield, VA 22161.

Vogel, E., & Bell, N. (1960). The emotionally disturbed child as a family scapegoat. In N. Bell & E. Vogel (Eds.), *A modern introduction to the family.* New York: Free Press.

von Bertalanffy, L. (1950). The theory of open systems in physics and biology. *Science, 111,* 23–29.

———. (1966). General system theory and psychiatry. In S. Arieti (Ed.), *American handbook of psychiatry,* Vol. 3 (pp. 705–721). New York: Basic Books.

———. (1968a). *General systems theory.* New York: George Braziller.

———. (1968b). General system theory: A critical review. In W. Buckley (Ed.), *Modern systems research for the behavioral scientist.* Chicago: Aldine.

Vosburgh, D., & Simpson, P. (1993). Linking family theory and practice: A family nursing program. *Image, 25* (3), 231–234.

Voydanoff, P. (1991). Economic distress and family relations: A review in the eighties. In Booth, A. (Ed.), *Contemporary families. Looking forward, looking back.* Minneapolis, MN: National Council for Family Relations.

Voydanoff, P., & Donnelly, B. W. (1988). Economic distress, family coping and quality of family life. In P. Voydanoff & L. C. LeMajka (Eds.), *Families and economic distress* (pp. 97–115). Newbury Park, CA: Sage.

Vuchinich, S. (1987). Starting and stopping spontaneous family conflicts. *Journal of Marriage and the Family, 49* (3), 591–601.

Wade, C., Howell, F., & Wells, J. G. (1994). Turning to family, friends, or others: A model of social network usage during stressful events. *Sociological Spectrum, 14,* 385–407.

Wahlstedt, P., & Blaser, W. (1986). Nurse case management for the frail elderly: A curriculum to prepare nurses for that role. *Home Healthcare Nurse, 4* (2), 30–35.

Walker, A. J. (1990). Gender and families. In National Council on Family Relations. *2001: Preparing families for the future* (pp. 16–17). Minneapolis, MN: National Council on Family Relations.

Walker, A. J., Pratt, C. C., & Oppy, N. C. (1992). Perceived reciprocity in family caregiving. *Family Relations, 41,* 82–85.

Wallace, H. (1996). *Family violence: Legal, medical and social perspectives.* Boston: Allyn & Bacon.

Waller, W. (1938). *The family: A dynamic interpretation.* New York: Dryden Press.

Wallerstein, J., & Kelly, J. B. (1980). *Surviving the break-up: How children and parents cope with divorce.* New York: Basic Books.

Walsh, F. (1989). The family in later life. In B. Carter & M. McGoldrick (Eds.), *The changing family life cycle: A framework for family therapy* (2nd ed.). Boston: Allyn & Bacon.

Walters, D. H. (1995, May 11). Working women play key role at home, study finds. *Los Angeles Times,* pp. A1, A22.

Walters, J. (Ed.). (1976). Fatherhood (Special Issue). *Family Coordinator, 25.*

Warner, W. L. (1953). *American life.* Chicago: University of Chicago Press.

Watson, J. (1985). *Nursing. The philosophy and science of caring.* Denver, CO: Colorado Associated University Press.

Watson, W. L. (1992). Family therapy. In G. M. Bulechek & J. C. McCloskey (Eds.), *Nursing interventions: Essential nursing treatments* (2nd ed.) (pp. 379–391). Philadelphia: Saunders.

Watzlawick, P., Beavin, J. H., & Jackson, D. D. (1967). *Pragmatics of human communication.* New York: Norton.

Watzlawick, P., Weakland, J., & Fisch, R. (1974). *Change: Principles of problem formulation and problem resolution.* New York: Norton.

Weaver, G. R. (1976). American identity movements: A cross-cultural confrontation. In E. Eldridge & N. Meredith (Eds.), *Environmental issues: Family impact.* Minneapolis, MN: Burgess.

Weed, J. A. (1990). National estimates of marriage dissolution and survivorship (DHHS Publication No. 581-1403, Series 3). Washington, DC: National Center for Health Statistics.

Weeks, G., & Jackson, J. (1982). The power of powerlessness. *American Journal of Family Therapy, 44–47.*

Weil, M., Karl, J. M., et al. (1985). *Case management in human services practice.* San Francisco: Jossey-Bass.

Weiner, N. (1948). *Cybernetics.* New York: Wiley.

Weinert, C., & Long, K. A. (1987). Understanding the health care needs of rural families. *Family Relations, 36* (4), 450–455.

Weiss, R. S. (1988). On the current state of the American family. *Journal of Family Issues, 8* (4), 468–470.

———. (1994). A different kind of parenting. In G. Handel & G. G. Whitchurch (Eds.), *The psychosocial interior of the family* (4th ed.) (pp. 609–639). New York: Aldine de Gruyter.

Wenk, D., Hardesty, C., Morgan, C., & Blair, S. (1994). The influence of parental involvement on well-being of sons and daughters. *Journal of Marriage and the Family, 56,* 229–234.

Wessell, M. L. (1975). Use of humor by an immobilized adolescent girl during hospitalization. *Maternal Child Nursing Journal, 4* (1), 35–48.

West, P., & Merriam, L. E. (1969). Camping and cohesiveness: A sociological study of the effect of outdoor recreation on family solidarity. *Minnesota Forestry Research Notes,* 201.

———. (1970). Outdoor recreation and family cohesivensss: A research approach. *Journal of Leisure Research, 2,* 251–259.

Whall, A. L. (1983). Family system theory. Relationship to nursing conceptual models. In J. Fitzpatrick & A. Whall (Eds.), *Conceptual models of nursing: Analysis and application* (pp. 69–93). Bowie, MD: Brady.

———. (1986a). The family as the unit of care in nursing: A historical review. *Public Health Nursing, 3* (4), 240–249.

———. (1986b). *Family therapy theory for nursing.* Norwalk, CT: Appleton & Lange.

Whall, A. L., & Fawcett, J. (1991a). *Family therapy development in nursing: State of the science and art.* Philadelphia: Davis.

———. (1991b). Introduction. In A. L. Whall & J. Fawcett (Eds.), *Family theory development in nursing: State of the science and art* (pp. 3–6). Philadelphia: Davis.

Whitaker, C. A., & Keith, D. V. (1981). Symbolic–experiential family therapy. In A. S. Gurman & D. P. Kriskern (Eds.), *Handbook of family therapy.* New York: Brunner/Mazel.

Whitchurch, G., & Constantine, L. (1993). Systems theory. In P. Boss, W. Boherty, R. LaRossa, W. Schumm, & S. Steinmetz (Eds.), *Sourcebook of family theories and methods. A contextual approach* (pp. 325–352). New York: Plenum Press.

White, B. B. (1989). Gender differences in marital communication patterns. *Family Relations, 28* (2), 89–105.

White, J. (1972). Towards a black psychology. In R. Jones (Ed.), *Black psychology* (pp. 43–50). New York: Harper & Row.

White, L. (1988). Freedom versus constraint. *Journal of Family Issues, 8* (4), 468–470.

White, M. (1986). Case management. In M. Maddox (Ed.), *The encyclopedia of aging.* New York: Springer.

White, M., & Epston, D. (1990). *Narrative means to therapeutic ends.* New York: Norton.

White, R. W. (1974). Strategies of adaptation: An attempt at systematic description. In G. V. Coehlo, D. A. Hamburg, & J. E. Adams (Eds.), *Coping and adaptation.* New York: Basic Books.

Whiting, B. (1974). Folk wisdom and child rearing. *Merrill-Palmer Quarterly, 20* (1), 9.

Wilberding, J. Z. (1985). Values clarification. In G. M. Bulechek & J. C. McCloskey (Eds.), *Nursing interventions: Treatments for nursing diagnosis* (pp. 173–184). Philadelphia: Saunders.

Wiley, D. J. D. (1989). Family environmental health. In P. J. Bomar (Ed.), *Nurses and family health promotion* (pp. 293–319). Baltimore: Williams & Wilkins.

———. (1996). Family environmental health. In P. J. Bomar (Ed.), *Nurses and family health promotion* (2nd ed.) (pp. 339–364). Philadelphia: Saunders.

Wilkinson, D. (1987). Ethnicity. In M. B. Sussman & S. K. Steinmetz (Eds.), *Handbook of marriage and the family* (pp. 183–210). New York: Plenum Press.

Williams, C. A. (1996). Community-based, population-focused practice: The foundation of specialization on public health nursing. In M. Stanhope & J. Lancaster (Eds.), *Community health nursing: Promoting health of aggregates, families and individuals* (4th ed.) (pp. 21–34). St. Louis: Mosby.

Williams, D. A., & Lord, M. (1978, May 15). Blacks: Fresh trials. *Newsweek,* 77–78.

Williams, J. I., & Leaman, T. (1973). Family structure and function. In H. Conn & R. Rakel (Eds.), *Family practice.* Philadelphia: Saunders.

Williams, L. R., & Cooper, M. K. (1993). Nurse-managed postpartum home care. *Journal of Obstetric, Gynecologic, and Neonatal Nursing, 22* (1), 25–31.

Williams, R. M. (1960). *American society: A sociological interpretation* (3rd ed.). New York: Knopf.

Willie, C. V. (1976). *A new look at black families.* Bayside, NY: General Hall, Inc.

Willie, C. V., & Greenblatt, S. (1978). Four classic studies of power relationships in Black families: A review and look to the future. *Journal of Marriage and the Family, 40,* 691–694.

Wills, T. A. (1985). Supportive functions of interpersonal relationships. In S. Cohen & S. L. Syme (Eds.), *Social support and health* (pp. 61–82). Orlando, FL: Academic Press.

Wilson, M., Lewis, J., Hinton, I., Kohn, and associates (1995). Promotion of African American family life: Families, poverty and social programs. *New Directions for Child Development, 68,* 85–99.

Wilson, M. T. (1988). The family with a school-age child and the family with an adolescent. In B. J. Bradshaw (Ed.), *Nursing of the family in health and illness* (pp. 176–213, 214–255). Norwalk, CT: Appleton & Lange.

Wilson, W. J. (1987). *The truly underclass.* Chicago: University of Chicago Press.

Winder, P. G. (1988, July). Case management by nurses at a county facility. *Quality Review Bulletin,* 215–219.

Winnick, A. J. (1988). The changing distribution of income and wealth in the United States, 1960–1985: An examination of the movement toward two societies, "separate and unequal." In P. Voydanoff & L. C. Majka (Eds.), *Families and economic distress* (pp. 232–260). Newbury Park, CA: Sage.

Winton, C. A. (1995). *Frameworks for studying families.* Guilford, CT: Dushkin.

Wong, D. (1995). Health promotion of the infant and family. In L. Whaley & D. Wong (Eds.), *Nursing care of infants and children* (5th ed.) (pp. 548–561). St. Louis: Mosby.

Wong, M. G. (1988). The Chinese American family. In C. H. Mindel, R. W. Habenstein, & R. Wright, Jr. (Eds.), *Ethnic families in America* (pp. 230–257). New York: Elsevier.

_____. (1995). Chinese Americans. In P. G. Min (Ed.), *Asian Americans: Contemporary trends and issues* (pp. 58–94). Thousand Oaks, CA: Sage.

Woo, E., & Lee, P. (1996, July 3). Latino immigrants' wages, education lag, studies find. *Los Angeles Times,* pp. A1, A19.

Woods, N. (1996). Personal communication. University of Washington School of Nursing.

Woods, N., Laffrey, S., Duffy, M., Lentz, M., Mitchell, E., Taylor, D., & Cowan, K. (1988). Being healthy: Women's images. *Advances in Nursing Science, 11* (1), 36–46.

Woods, N. J., Yates, B. L., & Primomo, J. (1988). Supporting families during chronic illness. *Image, 21* (1), 1989, 46–50.

Woodward, K. L. (1990, Winter/Spring). Young beyond their years. *Newsweek* (Special Issue), 54–60.

Woodward, K. L., Lord, M., Maier, F., Foote, D. M., & Malamud, P. (1978, May 15). Saving the family. *Newsweek,* 67–71.

Woodward, S. (1994, Feb. 13). The anguish of the Black middle class. *The Oregonian,* p. L1.

Woolf, S., & Lawrence, R. (1996). The physical examination: Where to look for preclinical disease. In S. Woolf,

S. Jonas, & R. Lawrence (Eds.), *Health promotion and disease prevention in clinical practice* (pp. 49–84). Baltimore: Williams & Wilkins.

Wooten, P. (1996). Humor: An antidote for stress. *Holistic Nursing Practice, 10* (2), 49–56.

Worden, J. W., Davies, B., & McCown, D. (1996). *Comparing childhood parent loss with sibling loss.* Unpublished manuscript.

World Health Organization. (1974). *Community health nursing report of the WHO expert committee.* Technical Report Series No. 558. Geneva: WHO.

Wright, L. M., & Bell, J. M. (1994). The future of family nursing research: Interventions, interventions, interventions. *Japanese Journal of Nursing Research, 27* (2–3), 4–15.

Wright, L. M., & Leahey, M. (1984). *Nurses and families, A guide to family assessment and intervention.* Philadelphia: Davis.

_____. (1987). Families and life-threatening illness: Assumptions, assessment, and intervention. In M. Leahey & L. M. Wright (Eds.), *Families and life-threatening illness* (pp. 45–58). Springhouse, PA: Springhouse Corporation.

_____. (1988). Family nursing trends in academic and clinical settings. *Proceedings of the international family nursing conference.* May, 1988. Calgary, Alberta, Canada.

_____. (1988). Nursing and family therapy training. In H. A. Liddle, D. C. Breunlin, and R. C. Schwartz (Eds.), *Handbook of family therapy and supervision* (pp. 278–289). New York: Guilford Press.

_____. (1990). Trends in nursing of families. *Journal of Advanced Nursing, 15,* 148–154.

_____. (1994). *Nurses and families: A guide to family assessment and intervention* (2nd ed.). Philadelphia: Davis.

Wright, L. M., & Watson, W. L. (1988). Systemic family therapy and family development. In C. J. Falicox (Ed.), *Family transitions: Continuity and change over the life cycle* (pp. 407–430). New York: Guilford Press.

Wright, L. M., Watson, W. L., & Bell, J. M. (1997). *Beliefs: The heart of healing in families and illness.* New York: Basic Books.

Wright, L. M., Watson, W. L., & Tapp, D. M. (1995). The influence on the beliefs of nurses: A clinical example of a post-myocardial-infarction couple. *Journal of Family Nursing, 1* (3), 238–256.

Wright, L. M., & Levac, A. M. (1993). The nonexistence of noncompliant families: The influence of Humberto Maturana. In S. L. Feetham, S. B. Meister, J. M. Bell, & C. L. Gilliss (Eds.), *The nursing of families: Theory, research, education, practice.* Newbury Park, CA: Sage.

Wright, R. (1996, June 12). U.S. child poverty worst among richest nations. *Los Angeles Times,* p. 22.

Wynne, L. G., et al. (1958). Pseudomutuality in the family relationships of schizophrenics. *Psychiatry, 21,* 205.

Yankelovich, D., & Gurin, J. (1989, March). The new American dream. *American Health,* 63–67.

————. (1979). *Family health in an era of stress. General Mills family report: Report 1978–1979.* Minneapolis: General Mills.

Ybarra, L. (1982, Feb.). When wives work: The impact on the Chicano family. *Journal of Marriage and the Family, 44,* 169–180.

Young, C. (1982). Family systems model. In I. W. Clements & D. M. Buchanan. *Family therapy, A nursing perspective* (pp. 101–109). New York: Wiley.

Yu, K., & Kim, L. (1983). The growth and development of Korean-American children. In G. Powell (Ed.), *The psychosocial development of minority group children* (pp. 147–158). New York: Brunner/Mazel.

Yura, H., & Walsh, M. (1988). *The nursing process* (5th ed.). Norwalk, CT: Appleton & Lange.

Zambrana, R. E., Dorrington, D., & Hayes-Bautista, D. (1995). Family and child health: A neglected vision. In R. E. Zambrana (Ed.), *Understanding Latino families: Scholarship, policy and practice* (pp. 157–176). Thousand Oaks, CA: Sage.

Zander, K. (1988). Nursing case management: Strategic management of cost and quality outcomes. *Journal of Nursing Administration, 18* (5), 23–30.

————. (1995). Case management series. Part III: Case manager role dimensions. *The New Definition* (Center for Case Management), *10* (1), 1–4.

Zerwekh, J. V. (1992). Laying the groundwork for family self-help. Locating families, building trust, and building strength. *Public Health Nursing, 9* (1), 15–21.

Zisook, S., & Shuchter, S. R. (1993, Fall). Major depression associated with widowhood. *American Journal Geriatric Psychiatry, 1* (4), 316–326.

Zuk, G. H. (1966). The go-between process in family therapy. *Family Process, 5,* 162.

Index